ZOONOSES AND COMMUNICABLE DISEASES COMMON TO MAN AND ANIMALS

Third Edition

Volume I

Bacterioses and Mycoses

Scientific and Technical Publication No. 580

PAN AMERICAN HEALTH ORGANIZATION
Pan American Sanitary Bureau, Regional Office of the
WORLD HEALTH ORGANIZATION
525 Twenty-third Street, N.W.
Washington, D.C. 20037 U.S.A.

2001

Also published in Spanish (2001) with the title:
Zoonosis y enfermedades transmisibles comunes al hombre a los animales
ISBN 92 75 31580 9

PAHO Cataloguing-in-Publication
Pan American Health Organization
  Zoonoses and communicable diseases common to man and animals
3rd ed. Washington, D.C.: PAHO, © 2001.
3 vol.—(Scientific and Technical Publication No. 580)

ISBN 92 75 11580 X
I. Title II. Series
1. ZOONOSES
2. BACTERIAL INFECTIONS AND MYCOSES
3. COMMUNICABLE DISEASE CONTROL
4. FOOD CONTAMINATION
5. PUBLIC HEALTH VETERINARY
6. DISEASE RESERVOIRS

NLM WC950.P187 2001 En

CONTENTS

PART I: BACTERIOSES

PART II: MYCOSES

LIST OF TABLES AND ILLUSTRATIONS

Bacterioses

Tables

Figures

PROLOGUE

Zoonoses and communicable diseases common to man and animals continue to have high incidence rates and to cause significant morbidity and mortality. Infections and parasitoses of cattle can reduce meat or milk production and can lead to the death or destruction of the animals, all of which diminishes the supply of available food for man. These diseases are also an obstacle for international trade, as well as a serious financial drain for cattle farmers and, more broadly, for a community's or a country's economy, which can have wide repercussions for a society's health.

With the aim of helping to solve these problems, the Pan American Health Organization (PAHO)—an international public health organization that has devoted itself to improving the health and living conditions of the people of the Americas for nearly one hundred years—established the Veterinary Public Health Program. The Program's overall objective is to collaborate with PAHO's Member Countries in the development, implementation, and evaluation of policies and programs that lead to food safety and protection and to the prevention, control, or eradication of zoonoses, among them foot-and-mouth disease.

To this end, PAHO's Veterinary Public Health Program has two specialized regional centers: the Pan American Foot-and-Mouth Disease Center (PANAFTOSA), created in 1951 in Rio de Janeiro, Brazil, and the Pan American Institute for Food Protection and Zoonoses (INPPAZ), established on November 15, 1991 in Buenos Aires, Argentina. INPPAZ's precursor was the Pan American Zoonoses Center (CEPANZO), which was created through an agreement with the Government of Argentina to help the countries of the Americas combat zoonoses, and which operated from 1956 until 1990.

Since its creation in 1902, PAHO has participated in various technical cooperation activities with the countries, among them those related to the surveillance, prevention, and control of zoonoses and communicable diseases common to man and animals, which cause high morbidity, disability, and mortality in vulnerable human populations. PAHO has also collaborated in the strengthening of preventive medicine and public health through the promotion of veterinary health education in learning, research, and health care centers. An example of this work is the preparation of several publications, among which the two previous Spanish and English editions of *Zoonoses and Communicable Diseases Common to Man and Animals* stand out.

Scientific knowledge has progressed since the last edition. Also, the countries of the Americas have modified their livestock production strategies in recent years, which has affected the transmission of zoonotic infections and their distribution. The publication of this third edition is an attempt to address these changes. The third edition is presented in three volumes: the first contains bacterioses and mycoses; the second, chlamydioses, rickettsioses, and viroses; and the third, parasitoses.

We believe that this new edition will continue to be useful for professors and students of public health, medicine, and veterinary medicine; workers in public health and animal health institutions; and veterinarians, researchers, and others interested in the subject. We also hope that this publication is a useful tool in the elaboration of national zoonosis control or eradication policies and programs, as well as in risk evaluation and in the design of epidemiological surveillance systems for the prevention and timely control of emerging and reemerging zoonoses. In summary, we are confident that this book will contribute to the application of the knowledge and resources of the veterinary sciences for the protection and improvement of public health.

GEORGE A.O. ALLEYNE
DIRECTOR

PREFACE TO THE FIRST EDITION

This book considers two groups of communicable diseases: those transmitted from vertebrate animals to man, which are—strictly speaking—zoonoses; and those common to man and animals. In the first group, animals play an essential role in maintaining the infection in nature, and man is only an accidental host. In the second group, both animals and man generally contract the infection from the same sources, such as soil, water, invertebrate animals, and plants; as a rule, however, animals do not play an essential role in the life cycle of the etiologic agent, but may contribute in varying degrees to the distribution and actual transmission of infections.

No attempt has been made to include all infections and diseases comprised in these two groups. A selection has been made of some 150 that are of principal interest, for various reasons, in the field of public health. The number of listed zoonoses is increasing as new biomedical knowledge is acquired. Moreover, as human activity extends into unexplored territories containing natural foci of infection, new zoonotic diseases are continually being recognized. In addition, improved health services and better differential diagnostic methods have distinguished zoonoses previously confused with other, more common diseases. A number of diseases described in this book have only recently been recognized, examples of which include the Argentine and Bolivian hemorrhagic fevers, angiostrongyliasis, rotaviral enteritis, Lassa fever, Marburg disease, and babesiosis.

The principal objective in writing this book was to provide the medical professions a source of information on the zoonoses and communicable diseases common to man and animals. Toward that end, both medical and veterinary aspects, which have traditionally been dealt with separately in different texts, have been combined in a single, comprehensive volume. As a result, physicians, veterinarians, epidemiologists, and biologists can all gain an overview of these diseases from one source.

This book, like most scientific works, is the product of many books, texts, monographs, and journal articles. Many sources of literature in medicine, veterinary medicine, virology, bacteriology, mycology, and parasitology were consulted, as were a large number of reports from different biomedical disciplines, in order to provide up-to-date and concise information on each disease. It is expected that any errors or omissions that may have been committed can, with the collaboration of the readers, be corrected in a future edition.

Where possible, explanations were attempted with special emphasis on the Americas, particularly Latin America. An effort was made, one which was not always successful, to collect available information on diseases in this Region. Data on the incidence of many zoonoses are fragmentary and frequently not reliable. It is hoped that the establishment of control programs in various countries will lead to improved epidemiologic surveillance and disease reporting.

More space has been devoted to those zoonoses having greatest impact on public health and on the economy of the countries of the Americas, but information is also included on those regionally less important or exotic diseases.

The movement of persons and animals over great distances adds to the risk of introducing exotic diseases that may become established on the American continent given the appropriate ecologic factors for existence of the etiologic agents. Today, public health and animal health administrators, physicians, and veterinarians must be familiar with the geographic distribution and pathologic manifestations of the various infectious agents so that they can recognize and prevent the introduction of exotic diseases.

We, the authors, would like to give special recognition to Dr. Joe R. Held, Assistant Surgeon-General of the United States Public Health Service and Director of the Division of Research Services of the U.S. National Institutes of Health, who gave impetus to the English translation and reviewed the bacterioses sections.

We would also like to express our utmost appreciation to the experts who reviewed various portions of this book and offered their suggestions for improving the text. These include: Dr. Jeffrey F. Williams, Professor in the Department of Microbiology and Public Health, Michigan State University, who reviewed the chapters dealing with parasitic zoonoses; Dr. James Bond, PAHO/WHO Regional Adviser in Viral Diseases, who read the viroses; Dr. Antonio Pío, formerly PAHO/WHO Regional Adviser in Tuberculosis and presently with WHO in Geneva, and Dr. James H. Rust, PAHO/WHO Regional Adviser in Enteric Diseases, both of whom reviewed the bacterioses; and Dr. F. J. López Antuñano, PAHO/WHO Regional Adviser in Parasitic Diseases, who read the metazooses.

We would like to thank Dr. James Cocozza, PAHO/WHO Veterinary Adviser, for his review of the translation and Dr. Judith Navarro, Editor in the Office of Publications of PAHO, for her valuable collaboration in the editorial revision and composition of the book.

PEDRO N. ACHA
BORIS SZYFRES

PREFACE TO THE SECOND EDITION

The fine reception accorded the Spanish, English, and French versions of this book has motivated us to revise it in order that it still may serve the purpose for which it was written: to provide an up-to-date source of information to the medical profession and allied fields. This book has undoubtedly filled a void, judging by its wide use in schools of public health, medicine, and veterinary medicine, as well as by bureaus of public and animal health.

The present edition has been considerably enlarged. In the seven years since the first edition was published, our knowledge of zoonoses has increased broadly and rapidly, and new zoonotic diseases have emerged. Consequently, most of the discussions have been largely rewritten, and 28 new diseases have been added to the original 148. Some of these new diseases are emerging zoonoses; others are pathologic entities that have been known for a long time, but for which the epidemiologic connection between man and animal has been unclear until recently.

The use this book has had outside the Western Hemisphere has caused us to abandon the previous emphasis on the Americas in favor of a wider scope and geomedical view. Moreover, wars and other conflicts have given rise to the migration of populations from one country or continent to another. A patient with a disease heretofore known only in Asia may now turn up in Amsterdam, London, or New York. The physician must be aware of these diseases in order to diagnose and treat them. "Exotic" animal diseases have been introduced from Africa to Europe, the Caribbean, and South America, causing great damage. The veterinary physician must learn to recognize them to be able to prevent and eradicate them before they become entrenched. It must be remembered that parasites, viruses, bacteria, and other agents of zoonotic infection can take up residence in any territory where they find suitable ecologic conditions. Ignorance, economic or personal interests, and human customs and needs also favor the spread of these diseases.

Research in recent years has demonstrated that some diseases previously considered to be exclusively human have their counterparts in wild animals, which in certain circumstances serve as sources of human infection. On the other hand, these animals may also play a positive role by providing models for research, such as in the case of natural leprosy in nine-banded armadillos or in nonhuman primates in Africa. Of no less interest is the discovery of *Rickettsia prowazekii* in eastern flying squirrels and in their ectoparasites in the United States, and the transmission of the infection to man in a country where epidemic typhus has not been seen since 1922. A possible wild cycle of dengue fever is also discussed in the book. Is Creutzfeldt-Jakob disease a zoonosis? No one can say with certainty, but some researchers believe it may have originated as such. In any case, interest is aroused by the surprising similarity of this disease and of kuru to animal subacute spongiform encephalopathies, especially scrapie, the first known and best studied of this group. Discussion of human and animal slow viruses and encephalopathies is included in the spirit of openness to possibilities and the desire to bring the experience of one field of medicine to another. In view of worldwide concern over acquired immunodeficiency syndrome (AIDS), a brief section on retroviruses has also been added, in which the relationship between the human disease and feline and simian AIDS is noted. Another topic deeply interesting to researchers is the mystery of the radical antigenic changes of type A influenza virus, a cause of explosive pandemics that affect millions of persons around the world. Evidence is mounting that these changes result from recombination with a virus of animal origin (see Influenza). That this should occur is not surprising, given the constant interaction between man and animals. As a rule, zoonoses are transmitted from animal to man, but the reverse may also occur, as is pointed out in the chapters on hepatitis, herpes simplex, and measles. The victims in these cases are nonhuman primates, which may in turn retransmit the infection to man under certain circumstances.

Among emerging zoonoses we cite Lyme disease, which was defined as a clinical entity in 1977; the etiologic agent was found to be a spirochete (isolated in 1982), for which the name *Borrelia burgdorferi* was recently proposed. Emerging viral zoonoses of note in Latin America are Rocio encephalitis and Oropouche fever; the latter has caused multiple epidemics with thousands of victims in northeast Brazil. Outstanding among new viral disease problems in Africa are the emergence of Ebola disease and the spread of Rift Valley fever virus, which has caused tens of thousands of human cases along with great havoc in the cattle industry of Egypt and has evoked alarm around the world. Similarly, the protozoan *Cryptosporidium* is emerging as one of the numerous agents of diarrheal diseases among man and animals, and probably has a worldwide distribution.

As the English edition was being prepared, reports came to light of two animal diseases not previously confirmed in humans. Three cases of human pseudorabies virus infection were recognized between 1983 and 1986 in two men and one woman who had all had close contact with cats and other domestic animals. In 1986, serologic testing confirmed infection by *Ehrlichia canis* in a 51-year-old man who had been suspected of having Rocky Mountain spotted fever. This is the first known occurrence of *E. canis* infection in a human. These two diseases bear watching as possible emerging zoonoses.

The space given to each zoonosis is in proportion to its importance. Some diseases that deserve their own monographs were given more detailed treatment, but no attempt was made to cover the topic exhaustively.

We, the authors, would like to give special recognition to Dr. Donald C. Blenden, Professor in the Department of Medicine and Infectious Diseases, School of Medicine, and Head of the Department of Veterinary Microbiology, College of Veterinary Medicine, University of Missouri; and to Dr. Manuel J. Torres, Professor of Epidemiology and Public Health, Department of Veterinary Microbiology, College of Veterinary Medicine, University of Missouri, for their thorough review of and valuable contributions to the English translation of this book.

We would also like to recognize the support received from the Pan American Health Organization (PAHO/WHO), the Pan American Health and Education Foundation (PAHEF), and the Pan American Zoonoses Center in Buenos Aires, Argentina, which enabled us to update this book.

We are most grateful to Dr. F. L. Bryan for his generous permission to adapt his monograph "Diseases Transmitted by Foods" as an Appendix to this book.

Mr. Carlos Larranaga, Chief of the Audiovisual Unit at the Pan American Zoonosis Center, deserves our special thanks for the book's artwork, as do Ms. Iris Elliot and Mr. William A. Stapp for providing the translation into English. We would like to express our most sincere gratitude and recognition to Ms. Donna J. Reynolds, editor in the PAHO Editorial Service, for her valuable collaboration in the scientific editorial revision of the book.

PEDRO N. ACHA
BORIS SZYFRES

INTRODUCTION

This new edition of *Zoonoses and Communicable Diseases Common to Man and Animals* is published in three volumes: I. Bacterioses and mycoses; II. Chlamydioses and rickettsioses, and viroses; and III. Parasitoses. Each of the five parts corresponds to the location of the etiologic agents in the biological classification; for practical purposes, chlamydias and rickettsias are grouped together.

In each part, the diseases are listed in alphabetical order to facilitate reader searches. There is also an alphabetical index, which includes synonyms of the diseases and the etiologic agents' names.

In this edition, the numbers and names of the diseases according to the *International Statistical Classification of Diseases and Related Health Problems*, Tenth Revision (ICD-10), are listed below the disease title. However, some zoonoses are not included in ICD-10 and are difficult to classify within the current scheme.

In addition, for each disease or infection, elements such as synonyms; etiology; geographical distribution; occurrence in man and animals; the disease in man and animals; source of infection and mode of transmission; role of animals in the epidemiology; diagnosis; and control are addressed. Patient treatment (for man or other species) is beyond the scope of this work; however, recommended medicines are indicated for many diseases, especially where they are applicable to prophylaxis. Special attention is paid to the epidemiological and ecological aspects so that the reader can begin to understand the determining factors of the infection or disease. Some topics include simple illustrations of the etiologic agent's mode of transmission, showing the animals that maintain the cycle of infection in nature. Similarly, other graphics and tables are included to provide additional information on the geographical distribution or prevalence of certain zoonoses.

The data on the occurrence of the infection in man and animals, along with data on the geographical distribution, may help the reader judge the relative impact that each disease has on public health and the livestock economy in the different regions of the world, given that the importance of different zoonoses varies greatly. For example, foot-and-mouth disease is extremely important from an economic standpoint, but of little importance in terms of public health, if animal protein losses are not considered. In contrast, Argentine and Bolivian hemorrhagic fevers are important human diseases, but their economic impact is minimal, if treatment costs and loss of man-hours are not taken into account. Many other diseases, such as brucellosis, leptospirosis, salmonellosis, and equine encephalitis, are important from both a public health and an economic standpoint.

Finally, each disease entry includes an alphabetical bibliography, which includes both the works cited and other relevant works that the reader may consult for more information about the disease.

Part I

BACTERIOSES

ACTINOMYCOSIS

ICD-10 A42.9

Synonyms: Actinostreptotrichosis, mandibular cancer, ray fungus disease.

Etiology: *Actinomyces israelii* is the principal etiologic agent in man, and *A. bovis* the main one in animals. *A. naeslundi*, *A. viscosus*, *A. odontolytical*, *A. meyeri* and *Arachnia propionica* (*A. propionicus*) are isolated less often, although *A. viscosus* plays an important role in canine actinomycosis. Some reports indicate isolation of *A. israelii* from animals (Georg, 1974) and *A. bovis* from man (Brunner *et al.*, 1973). Actinomyces are higher bacteria with many characteristics of fungi. They are gram-positive, do not produce spores, are non–acid-fast, range from anaerobic to microaerophilic, and are part of the normal flora of the mouth and of women's genital tract (Burden, 1989).

Geographic Distribution: Worldwide.

Occurrence in Man: Infrequent; however, data are very limited. Fewer than 100 cases of the disease are recorded each year by the Public Health Laboratory Service's Communicable Disease Surveillance Centre in Great Britain (Burden, 1989). According to older data, 368 cases were recorded in Wales and England over 12 years (1957–1968), with an incidence of 0.665 per million inhabitants, with a higher incidence among industrial workers (Wilson, 1984). In Scotland, the annual incidence was three per million and the rate of attack was 10 times higher in agricultural workers than among others.

The historical ratio of two cases in men to one in women is probably no longer valid because of the number of cases of genital actinomycosis in women using intrauterine contraceptive devices (IUDs).

Occurrence in Animals: The frequency of the disease varies widely among regions and is also influenced by different livestock management practices. The disease usually appears as sporadic cases. Small outbreaks have occurred in some marshy areas of the United States and the former Soviet Union.

The Disease in Man: *A. israelii*, the main causal agent in man, is a normal component of the flora of the mouth. As a result of wounds or surgery, it can enter the soft tissues and bones, where it causes a suppurative granulomatous process that opens to the surface through fistulas. Several clinical forms have been identified according to their location: cervicofacial, thoracic, abdominal, and generalized. Cervicofacial, which is the most common (from 50% to more than 70% of cases), is usually caused by a tooth extraction or a jaw injury; it begins with a hard swelling under the mucous membrane of the mouth, beneath the periosteum of the mandible, or in the skin of the neck. At a later stage, softened areas, depressions, and openings to the exterior with a purulent discharge are evident. These secretions usually contain the characteristic "sulphur granules," which are actinomyces colonies. The thoracic form is generally caused by breathing the etiologic agent into the bronchial tubes where it establishes a chronic bronchopneumonia that affects the lower portions of the right lung (Burden, 1989), with symptoms similar to pulmonary tuberculosis. As the disease progresses, invasion of the thoracic wall and its perforation

3

by fistulous tracks may occur. The abdominal form usually occurs after surgery and appears as an encapsulated lesion that often becomes localized in the cecum and the appendix, where it produces hard tumors that adhere to the abdominal wall.

The generalized form is infrequent and results from the erosive invasion of blood vessels and lymphatic system, resulting in liver and brain disease.

In recent years, reports of actinomycosis in the genital tract of women using intrauterine contraceptive devices have multiplied, with the rate of infection increasing in proportion to the duration of IUD use. In one study (Valicenti et al., 1982), the infection was found in 1.6% of women in the general population of IUD users and in 5.3% of those attending the clinics. Another study of 478 IUD users found a rate of infection of 12.6% based on Papanicolaou (Pap) smears (Koebler et al., 1983). Attempts to isolate the bacteria in Pap smears rarely yield positive results. However, A. israelii is also isolated from the genital tract of women who do not use IUDs, indicating that actinomyces are part of the normal flora (Burden, 1989). In the vast majority of cases, colonization by actinomyces produces only a superficial or asymptomatic infection.

Treatment consists of prolonged high doses of penicillin (weeks or months). Erythromycin, clindamycin, and tetracycline may also be used. Surgical drainage of abscesses is important. In women with an endometrium colonized by actinomyces, removing the IUD is sometimes enough for the endometrium to return to normal.

The Disease in Animals: A. bovis is the principal agent of actinomycosis in bovines and, occasionally, in other animal species. In bovines, it centers chiefly in the maxillae where it forms a granulomatous mass with necrotic areas that develop into abscesses. These open via fistulous passages and discharge a viscous, odorless, yellow pus. The pus contains small, yellow, sulphur granules, which are rosette-shaped when viewed under a microscope. In some cases chewing becomes very difficult, and the animal stops eating and loses weight.

The cost-benefit ratio must be measured when treating bovine and equine actinomycosis. Long-standing chronic lesions do not respond readily to treatment. If the lesions are small and circumscribed, they may be removed surgically. In other cases, curettage can be performed on the abscesses and fistulas, which are then packed with gauze saturated with iodine tincture. Medical treatment is the same as for human actinomycosis, preferably using penicillin.

In swine the etiologic agent localizes principally in the sow's udder, where it gives rise to abscesses and fistulas. Its pathway of penetration is the lesion caused by the teeth of suckling pigs. This infection is attributed to *Actinomyces suis*, whose taxonomy is still uncertain.

In dogs, the disease produces cervicofacial abscesses, empyemas accompanied by pleurisy and osteomyelitis, and, more rarely, abdominal abscesses and cutaneous granulomas. The most common agent encountered prior to 1982 was A. viscosus (Hardie and Barsanti, 1982).

Source of Infection and Mode of Transmission: The infection is endogenous. Actinomyces develop as saprophytes within and around carious teeth, in the mucin on dental enamel and in the tonsillar crypts. In studies carried out in several countries, actinomyces have been found in 40% of excised tonsils and have been isolated in 30% to 48% of saliva samples or material from decayed teeth, as well as from the vaginal secretions of 10% of women using IUDs (Benenson, 1992).

Infections and pathological developments are the product of tissue trauma, lesions, or prolonged irritation. It has not been possible to isolate the agent of actinomycosis from the environment. It is believed that the causal agent penetrates the tissues of the mouth through lesions caused by foods or foreign objects, or by way of dental defects. From the oral cavity, the bacteria can be swallowed or breathed into the bronchial tubes.

Role of Animals in the Epidemiology of the Disease: The species of *Actinomyces* that attack man are different from those that affect animals. Rarely is *A. israelii* found in animals or *A. bovis* found in man. The designation of species prior to 1960 is doubtful (Lerner, 1991) and thus, distinguishing one species from another presents great problems. The infection in animals is not transmitted to man, nor is it transmitted from person to person or animal to animal.

Diagnosis: The clinical picture may be confused with other infections, such as actinobacillosis, nocardiosis, and staphylococcosis, as well as neoplasia and tuberculosis. The first step in confirming the diagnosis is to obtain pus, sputum, or tissue samples for microscopic examination and culture, and to inspect them for granules. Filament masses are visible by direct observation. In smears of crushed granules or pus stained by the Gram and Kinyoun methods, gram-positive and non–acid-fast filaments or pleomorphic forms, occasionally with bacillary-sized branching, may be seen (Cottral, 1978). It is possible to identify the species of actinomyces causing the disease only by culturing and typing the isolated microorganism. In testing women who use IUDs, direct immunofluorescence has yielded good results (Valicenti *et al.*, 1982).

Control: Prevention in man consists of proper oral hygiene and care after dental extractions or other surgery in the oral cavity. No practical means have been established yet to prevent actinomycosis in animals.

Bibliography

Ajello, L., L.K. Georg, W. Kaplan, L. Kaufman. *Laboratory Manual for Medical Mycology*. Washington, D.C.: U.S. Government Printing Office; 1963. (Public Health Service Publication 994).

Benenson, A.S., ed. *Control of Communicable Diseases in Man*. 15th ed. An official report of the American Public Health Association. Washington, D.C.: American Public Health Association; 1990.

Brunner, D.W., J.H. Gillespie. *Hagan's Infectious Diseases of Domestic Animals*. 6th ed. Ithaca: Comstock; 1973.

Burden P. Actinomycosis [editorial]. *J Infect* 19:95–99, 1989.

Cottral, G.E., ed. *Manual of Standardized Methods for Veterinary Microbiology*. Ithaca: Comstock; 1978.

Dalling, T., A. Robertson, eds. *International Encyclopaedia of Veterinary Medicine*. Edinburgh: Green; 1966.

Georg, L.K. The agents of human actinomycosis. Cited in: Lerner, P.L. *Actinomyces* and *Arachnia* species. *In*: Mandell, G.L., R.G. Douglas, Jr., J.E. Bennett, eds. *Principles and Practice of Infectious Diseases*. 3rd ed. New York: Churchill Livingstone, Inc.; 1990.

Hardie, E.M., J.A. Barsanti. Treatment of canine actinomycosis. *J Am Vet Assoc* 180:537–541, 1982.

Koebler, C., A. Chatwani, R. Schwartz. Actinomycosis infection associated with intrauterine contraceptive devices. *Am J Obstet Gynecol* 145:596–599, 1983.

Lerner, P.L. *Actinomyces* and *Arachnia* species. *In*: Mandell, G.L., R.G. Douglas, Jr., J.E. Bennett, eds. *Principles and Practice of Infectious Diseases*. 3rd ed. New York: Churchill Livingstone, Inc.; 1990.

Pier, A.C. The actinomycetes. *In*: Hubbert, W.T., W.F. McCulloch, P.R. Schnurrenberger, eds. *Diseases Transmitted from Animals to Man*. 6th ed. Springfield: Thomas; 1975.

Valicenti, J.F., Jr., A.A. Pappas, C.D. Graber, H.O. Williamson, N.F. Willis. Detection and prevalence of IUD-associated *Actinomyces* colonization and related morbidity. A prospective study of 69,925 cervical smears. *JAMA* 247:1149–1152, 1982.

Wilson, G. Actinomycosis, actinobacillosis, and related diseases. *In*: Smith, G.R., ed. Vol 3: *Topley and Wilson's Principles of Bacteriology, Virology and Immunity*. Baltimore: Williams & Wilkins; 1984.

AEROMONIASIS

ICD-10 AO5.8 other specified bacterial foodborne intoxications

Etiology: The genus *Aeromonas* is classified within the family *Vibrionaceae* and shares some characteristics with members of other genera of this family. However, genetic hybridization studies indicate that the genus *Aeromonas* is sufficiently different to place it in a new family, with the suggested name of *Aeromonadaceae*. Two groups can be distinguished in the genus *Aeromonas*. The first group is psychrophilic and nonmotile and is represented by *Aeromonas salmonicida*, an important pathogen for fish (the agent of furunculosis). It does not affect man because it cannot reproduce at a temperature of 37°C. The second group is mesophilic and motile, and it is this group that causes aeromoniasis, a disease common to man and animals. These aeromonas are gram-negative, straight bacilli ranging from 1 to 3 microns in length. They have a polar flagellum and are oxidase positive and facultatively anaerobic. They essentially include the species *A. hydrophila*, *A. sobria*, and *A. caviae* (Janda and Duffey, 1988), to which *A. veronii* and *A. schuberti* were added later, as well as the genospecies *A. jandae* and *A. trota*. However, only *A. hydrophila* and *A. sobria* are of clinical interest.

More recent hybridization studies show that the *A. hydrophila* complex is genetically very variable. Thirteen different genospecies have been established, but from a practical standpoint the three principal phenospecies are retained. It is possible to identify 95% of isolates on the basis of their biochemical properties (Janda, 1991).

A system of 40 serogroups was established based on the somatic antigens (O) of *A. hydrophila* and *A. caviae*. All the O antisera contain antibodies to the rugose form (R) of the bacillus, and thus the antisera must be absorbed by culturing the R form before being used (Sakazaki and Shimada, 1984). Typing is done by gel protein electrophoresis, isoenzyme analysis, and genetic analysis. Isoenzyme analysis made it possible to identify genospecies through four enzymes. All these methods have shown that the clinical strains are very diverse and that no single clone is responsible for most of the infections (Von Graevenitz and Altwegg, 1991).

Over the last decade, researchers have tried to define the virulence factors of this genus, both in terms of structural characteristics and the extracellular products they secrete. Considered important among the structural characteristics is a type of pilus, the "flexible" or curvilinear pilus. It is expressed when stimulated by certain environmental conditions that give the bacteria the ability to colonize. Another structural characteristic that was first discovered in autoagglutinating strains of *A. salmonicida* is the S layer, which is outside the cell wall. The loss of this layer—which can be seen with an electron microscope—decreases pathogenicity for fish 1,000 to 10,000 times. A similar layer was later discovered in certain strains of *A. hydrophila* and *A. sobria* in infected fish and mammals, but their functional role seems to differ substantially from the same S layer in *A. salmonicida* (it does not make the surface of the bacteria hydrophobic).

The substances externally secreted by aeromonas include beta-hemolysin that is produced by certain strains of *A. hydrophila* and *A. sobria*. It has been determined that this hemolysin has enterotoxigenic effects on lactating mice and ligated ileal loops of rabbits. Purified beta-hemolysin inoculated intravenously into mice is lethal at a dose of 0.06 µg. The cytotonic enterotoxin that causes an accumulation of fluid in the ligated ileal loop of the rabbit, as well as other effects, has also been described. Between 5% and 20% of the strains produce a toxin that cross reacts with the cholera toxin in the ELISA test (Janda, 1991).

Based on tests conducted in mice and fish (the latter are much more susceptible), it can be concluded that *A. hydrophila* and *A. sobria* are more virulent than *A. caviae*. In addition, there is a great difference in the virulence of the strains within each species (Janda, 1991). These variations cannot be attributed to a single virulence factor. In addition, it was not possible to detect a common mechanism in the pathogenic capacity of *Aeromonas* spp. in humans or in animals.

An enzyme (acetylcholinesterase) isolated from fish infected by *A. hydrophila* proved to be highly active against the central nervous system. The toxin was lethal for fish at a dose of 0.05 µg/g of bodyweight; no lesions were observed in the tissues. The same toxin was obtained from six different strains (Nieto *et al.*, 1991).

A comparison was made of 11 environmental strains and 9 human strains. All the environmental strains and four of the human strains proved to be pathogenic for trout, at a dose of 3 x 10^7 colony forming units (CFU). Only the human strains caused death or lesions through intramuscular inoculation of mice. The virulent strains produced more hemolysis and cytotoxins in cultures at 37°C than at 28°C (Mateos *et al.*, 1993).

Geographic Distribution: The motile aeromonas appear worldwide. Their principal reservoir is in river and estuary waters, as well as in salt water where it meets fresh water. Population density is lower in highly saline waters and waters with limited dissolved oxygen. It has sometimes been possible to isolate *Aeromonas* from chlorinated water, including muncipal water supplies. These bacteria are more prolific in summer than in winter (Stelma, 1989).

Occurrence in Man: Aeromoniasis generally occurs sporadically. There is no evidence that water or foods contaminated by *Aeromonas* spp. have been the source of outbreaks (as happens with other agents, such as enterobacteria). The only cases that suggest the possibility of outbreaks are those described in 1982 and 1983. In late 1982, some 472 cases of gastroenteritis associated with the consumption of raw oysters occurred in Louisiana (USA). One year later, another outbreak affected seven people in Florida. This was also attributed to raw oysters that came from Louisiana. Pathogenicity tests were performed on 23 of the 28 strains identified as *A. hydrophila*; 70% tested positive in at least one of the virulence tests (Abeyta *et al.*, 1986). There may have been other outbreaks that were not recognized because food and patient stools were not examined for detection and identification of *A. hydrophila* (Stelma, 1989).

Occurrence in Animals: *A. hydrophila* is a recognized pathogen in fish, amphibians, and reptiles. The disease may occur individually or epidemically, particularly in fish-farming pools. The agent affects many fish species, particularly fresh water species. Its economic impact varies, but can be severe (Stoskopf, 1993). Aeromoniasis due to *A. hydrophila* also causes significant illness in colonies of amphibians and reptiles bred for experimental purposes.

The Disease in Man: For some time the aeromonas were considered opportunistic bacteria. Clinical and epidemiological information amassed in recent years seems to confirm that *A. hydrophila* and *A. sobria* are the primary human pathogens, particularly as agents of enteritis in children.

The disease appears in two forms: enteric and extraenteric. Studies on the pathogenic role of *Aeromonas* spp. in gastroenteritis have been conducted in Australia, the United States, England, Thailand, and, more recently, in Rosario, Argentina (Notario *et al.*, 1993). Patients with and without diarrhea have been compared, with the latter group consisting of patients suffering from other diseases or healthy individuals. In Argentina, 8 strains (2%) were isolated from 400 fecal samples and from a colon biopsy in children with diarrhea, and no strains were isolated from 230 children without diarrhea. In the United States, the agent was found in 1.1% of the cases and in none of the controls (Agger *et al.*, 1985). The tests in the other countries also isolated *A. hydrophila* and *A. sobria* with greater frequency and in greater numbers from diarrheal feces than from nondiarrheal feces.

Enteritis due to *Aeromonas* spp. occurs more frequently in summer and predominantly in children from 6 months to 5 years of age. The clinical symptoms include profuse diarrhea, slight fever, and abdominal pains; vomiting is occasionally seen in patients under 2 years of age. Cases of gastroenteritis with blood and mucus in the feces have also been described. The disease is generally benign in children and lasts only a few days. Gastroenteritis is much less frequent in adults, but can occur with diarrhea of longer duration (from 10 days to several weeks or months), weight loss, and dehydration. The predominant species are *A. hydrophila* and *A. sobria*, but *A. caviae* has also been implicated in some cases (Janda and Duffey, 1988).

The extra-intestinal clinical form can affect different organs and tissues. One very common form of contamination is through wounds and various traumas. The wound generally becomes infected through contact with river water, ponds, or other water reservoirs. The most common clinical expression is cellulitis. The patient recovers completely in such cases.

Some 20 cases have been described of infection caused by medicinal leeches (*Hirudo medicinalis*) used to treat postoperative venous congestion after grafts or replantations. The leeches inject a very powerful anticoagulant, causing the congested area to bleed for one to two hours (or longer) and preventing loss of the graft. Leeches may harbor *A. hydrophila* in their digestive tract and suckers and transmit the bacteria to the patient. These infections are usually limited to contamination of the wound, but can cause extensive tissue loss and septicemia (Lineaweaver *et al.*, 1992).

Untreated cellulitis can become complicated by myonecrosis and require amputation of a limb. If there is bacteremia, the infection may ultimately be fatal. Septicemia occurs primarily in immunodeficient patients and rarely in immunocompetent patients. The clinical manifestations are similar to septicemia caused by other gram-negative bacteria and consist of fever and hypotension. Mortality is high in these cases (Janda and Duffey, 1988). Other clinical forms are rare.

Gastroenteritis in children is a self-limiting disease and does not require treatment, except in prolonged cases. All other forms should be treated with antibiotics, such as gentamicin, amikacin, chloramphenicol, and cyprofloxacin. All strains of *A. hydrophila* and *A. sobria* are resistant to ampicillin (Gutierrez *et al.*, 1993), *A. trota* is not.

The Disease in Animals: Aeromoniasis is primarily a disease that affects fish, amphibians, and reptiles. The disease is rare in wild or domestic mammals and birds.

FISH: *A. hydrophila* is the agent of bacterial hemorrhagic septicemia in fish. All species of fresh water fish are considered susceptible to this disease. The clinical picture is very varied and sometimes other pathogens are isolated that can confuse the diagnosis and signs of the disease. In the very acute form of the disease, death may occur without warning signs. In other cases, scales are lost and localizaed hemorrhages appear in the gills, mouth, and base of the fins. Ulcers in the skin, exophthalmia, and abdomen-distending ascites may also be found. Renal and hepatic lesions are seen in very prolonged cases (Stoskopf, 1993). The disease occurs sporadically or in outbreaks. Mortality is variable but can be high.

Intensive fish farming can create conditions that favor infection, such as overpopulation and adverse environmental factors (increase in organic material and decrease in dissolved oxygen). These factors reduce the resistance of the fish and favor the pathogenic action of *A. hydrophila* and other bacteria. *Pseudomonas* spp. often accompanies *A. hydrophila* in ulcerous lesions in the skin of fish (erythrodermatitis, fin disease). In northern Greece, where great losses of carp (*Cyprinus carpio*) occurred in ponds due to a disease characterized primarily by cutaneous ulcers, both *A. hydrophila* and various species of *Pseudomonas* were isolated. It was possible to reproduce the disease experimentally through subcutaneous inoculation of *A. hydrophila* without the simultaneous presence of other bacteria (Sioutas *et al.*, 1991). Previously, there was an outbreak in Argentina of fin disease in young black catfish (*Rhamdia sapo*). Both *A. hydrophila* and *Pseudomonas aeruginosa* were isolated from fin lesions. When the disease was reproduced experimentally, there was not much difference between the fish inoculated with *A. hydrophila* alone and those inoculated with both bacteria (Angelini and Seigneur, 1988).

Infection of striped (grey) mullet (*Mugil cephalus*) by *A. hydrophila* results in an acute septicemic disease. The agent can be isolated from the blood of mullet with the experimentally reproduced disease one or two days after inoculation. The disease is characterized by inflammatory and proliferative changes and later by necrotic lesions. Enteritis and hepatic necrosis are constant lesions (Soliman *et al.*, 1989).

Aeromoniasis in fish can be treated with antibiotics.

AMPHIBIANS: Frogs used for experimental purposes—whether in laboratory colonies or under natural conditions—die from a disease called "red leg" that causes cutaneous ulceration and septicemia. The Louisiana frog (*Rana catesbeiana*) suffered various epizootics in 1971 and 1972. Of 4,000 tadpoles separated from their natural habitat and kept under laboratory conditions, 70% died during metamorphosis and 20% died after completing it.

Of the wild frogs brought to the laboratory, 10% became ill and died during the first year. The tadpoles born in the laboratory that became ill during metamorphosis demonstrated lassitude, edema, and hemorrhage in the tail; accumulation of bloody lymph around the leg muscles; and small ulcers on the operculum and the skin of the abdomen. Death occurred 24 hours after onset of the disease. The disease progressed slowly in adults; it sometimes lasted up to six months and ended in death. Sick frogs had petechial or diffuse hemorrhages on the skin of their entire bodies. The lymphatic sacks were full of a bloody serous fluid and intramuscular hemorrhages were found on the hind legs and on the periosteum (Glorioso *et al.*, 1974).

"Red leg" disease in *Xenopus leavis* (a frog of African origin of the family *Pipidae*) was described in Cuba, the United States, Great Britain, and South Africa. In Cuba, the outbreak of the disease occurred three weeks after the frogs were transferred from the laboratory (where they were kept at 22°C) to ambient temperature in order to acclimate them. The disease lasted for about 48 days and the principal symptoms were lethargy, anorexia, petechiae, and edema. Autopsy revealed subcutaneous edemas, hemorrhages, and ascites. *Aeromonas hydrophila* was isolated from 14 of the 50 frogs (Bravo Fariñas *et al.*, 1989). According to the authors, the disease was unleashed by environmental changes, infrequent changes of water, and traumas, as well as other factors.

In Johor, Malaysia, where there is a small frog-breeding industry, an outbreak occurred that affected 80% of the animals in a population of 10,000. The disease was characterized by ulcers and petechial hemorrhages on the skin and opaque corneas, but no visceral lesions. In a second outbreak, the disease followed a more chronic course, with symptoms such as ascites, visceral tumefaction, and nervous disorders (Rafidah *et al.*, 1990).

The indicated treatment is antibiotics to which *A. hydrophila* is susceptible.

REPTILES: In a variety of lizards and snakes, infection due to *Aeromonas* is associated with ulcerous stomatitis. The lesions may result in septicemia, with hemorrhages and areas with ecchymoses on the integument. The animals are anorexic and suffer deterioration in their general health. One complication is pneumonia. At autopsy, exudates are found in the lungs and secondary air passages. The viscera and gastrointestinal tract show pronounced congestion with hemorrhagic areas. Treatment consists of removing the necrotic tissue from the mouth, followed by irrigation with 10% hydrogen peroxide. The use of such antibiotics as chloramphenicol and gentamicin is indicated (Jacobson, 1984).

OTHER ANIMALS: A case was described in Nigeria of aeromoniasis in a caracal lynx (*Felis caracal*) at a zoo. The animal was found with profuse diarrhea, anorexia, and depression. Despite antidiarrheal treatment, it died in a month. The lesions suggested that the cause of death was acute septicemia. *A. hydrophila* was isolated from the animal's internal organs (Ocholi and Spencer, 1989). Similar cases had appeared in young ferrets at a research institute in Japan. The agent isolated was identified as *A. sobria* (Hiruma *et al.*, 1986). A case of polyarthritis in a 3-day-old calf was described in Australia. *A. hydrophila* was isolated from the synovial fluid (Love and Love, 1984). In Germany, a septicemic condition attributed to *A. hydrophila* has been described in turkeys at 3 to 16 weeks of life, with morbidity of 10% and mortality of 1%. Cases have also been recorded in canaries and in a toucan suffering from enteritis; *A. hydrophila* was isolated from the viscera. *A. hydrophila* was isolated in a routine postmortem examination of 15 wild, farm, and pet birds. The isolates were taken primarily in the cold months (Shane *et al.*, 1984). A pure culture of *A. hydrophila* was isolated from a parrot (*Amazona versicolor*) with bilateral conjunctivitis (García *et al.*, 1992). In all cases, the stressful conditions that contributed to the development of the disease were emphasized.

Source of Infection and Mode of Transmission: The primary reservoir of *A. hydrophila* and *A. sobria* is fresh water in rivers, ponds, and lakes. It is also found in estuaries and in low-salinity salt water. Even treated municipal water supplies can contain *Aeromonas*. In a French hospital, intestinal and extraintestinal aeromoniasis in 12 patients was attributed to the drinking water (Picard and Goullet, 1987).

Due to the increased numbers of motile *Aeromonas* in the water supply in The Netherlands, health authorities established maximum indicative values for the density of these bacteria in drinking water. These values are 20 CFU/100 ml for the drinking water in water treatment plants and 200 CFU/100 ml for water being distributed (Van der Kooij, 1988).

Motile *Aeromonas* have not caused outbreaks with multiple cases (Altwegg *et al.*, 1991). It is difficult to understand why, since the bacteria are widely distributed in nature, water, animal feces, and foods of animal origin, and since they also multiply at refrigeration temperatures.

The distribution of the agents in water reaches its highest level during the warm months, as does the disease. The situation seems to be different in tropical countries. In India, the most frequent isolates from river water occur in late winter, declining in summer and the monsoon season (Pathak *et al.*, 1988). These authors believe that fish are an independent or additional reservoir, since *Aeromonas* can be isolated from them independent of the bacteria's density in river water.

Water contaminated by virulent strains of *A. hydrophila* or *A. sobria* is the source of infection for man and other animals. Domestic animals, especially cattle and pigs, eliminate in their feces a large amount of *Aeromonas* that are probably of aquatic origin. There are indications that, in addition to water, other contaminated foods, such as oysters and shrimp, may be a source of infection for man. A case of enteritis caused by eating a shrimp cocktail occurred in Switzerland in a healthy 38-year-old. Only *A. hydrophila* and no other pathogen was isolated from the patient's stool. The strain isolated from the shrimp was biochemically identical and had the same ribosomal DNA sequence (Altwegg *et al.*, 1991).

Enteric disease occurs in normal children and the route of infection is through the mouth. In contrast, both enteric and extraintestinal aeromoniasis in individuals older than 5 years of age occurs in combination with other conditions, such as an underlying disease, trauma, or other stress factors. Wounds become infected upon contact with water. Medicinal leeches can infect the wound they produce with the aeromonas they harbor in their digestive tract and suckers. The most serious form of the disease, septicemia and its various organic complications, occurs in immunodeficient individuals and the route of infection is usually extraintestinal.

Fish, amphibians, and reptiles—especially in intensive breeding programs—are infected through the mouth. The factors that contribute to infection are stress from overpopulation, temperature changes, lack of hygiene, and inadequate feeding.

Role of Animals in the Epidemiology of the Disease: Aeromoniasis is primarily a disease common to man and animals. Fish may act as a reservoir in addition to water. Other animals contribute to contamination of the environment with their feces.

Diagnosis: Diagnosis can be obtained by isolating and identifying the species of the etiologic agent. As a selective medium, Rimler-Shotts agar can be used; it contains citrate, novobiocin, and sodium deoxycholate as selective agents, and lysine, ornithine, and maltose as differential agents. Another commonly used medium is agar with ampicillin and sodium deoxycholate as selective agents and trehalose as a differential agent (García-López *et al.*, 1993).

Control: Until more is known about the disease's epidemiology and the factors that determine its virulence, the consumption of raw foods of animal origin should be avoided.

Aeromonas are sensitive to heat, and pasteurization is an effective means for destroying them in milk.

The measure introduced by health authorities in The Netherlands of setting a maximum indicative value for the density of aeromonas in the water in water treatment plants and in the water distribution network should be considered by other countries when warranted by the number of human cases.

Wounds should be cleaned and disinfected to prevent contamination.

In cases of replantation surgery that require the application of medical leeches, it is recommended that the patient be given antibiotics to which *A. hydrophila* and *A. sobria* are sensitive a few days prior to surgery, so as to eliminate them from the digestive tract of the leeches.

Preventing aeromoniasis in aquatic and semi-aquatic animals in intensive breeding programs requires avoiding overpopulation, changing the water, and maintaining proper temperature and feeding regimes. Work is being done to develop vaccines for fish. Tests indicate that they can provide good protection (Plumb, 1984; Lamers *et al.*, 1985; Ruangpan *et al.*, 1986).

Bibliography

Abeyta, C., C.A. Kaysner, M.A. Wekell, *et al.* Recovery of *Aeromonas hydrophila* from oysters implicated in an outbreak of foodborne illness. *J Food Protect* 49:643–644, 1986.

Agger, W.A., J.D. McCormick, M.J. Gurwith. Clinical and microbiological features of *Aeromonas hydrophila* associated diarrhea. *J Clin Microbiol* 21:909–913, 1985.

Altwegg, M., G. Martinetti Lucchini, J. Lüthy-Hottenstein, M. Rohr-Bach. *Aeromonas*-associated gastroenteritis after consumption of contaminated shrimp. *Europ J Clin Microbiol Infect Dis* 10:44–45, 1991.

Angelini, N.M., G.N. Seigneur. Enfermedad de las aletas de *Rhamdia sapo*. Aislamiento de los agentes etiológicos e infección experimental. *Rev Argent Microbiol* 20:37–48, 1988.

Bravo Fariñas, L., R.J. Monté Boada, R. Cuellar Pérez, S.C. Dumas Valdiviezo. *Aeromonas hydrophila*, infección en *Xenopus leavis*. *Rev Cubana Med Trop* 41:208–213, 1989.

García, M.E., A. Domenech, L. Dominguez, *et al. Aeromonas hydrophila* in a pet parrot (*Amazona versicolor*). *Avian Dis* 36:1110–1111, 1992.

García-López, M.L., A. Otero, M.C. García-Fernández, J.A. Santos. Incidencia, comportamiento y control de *Aeromonas hydrophila* en productos cárnicos y lácteos. *Microbiología* 9:49–56, 1993.

Glorioso, J.C., R.L. Amborski, G.F. Amborski, D.D. Culley. Microbiological studies on septicemic bullfrogs (*Rana catesbeiana*). *Am J Vet Res* 35:1241–1245, 1974.

Gutiérrez, J., M.C. Nogales, M.C. Aretio, E. Martín. Patrón de sensibilidad de las *Aeromonas* spp. productoras de infecciones extraintestinales. *An Med Interna* 10:65–67, 1993.

Hiruma, M., K. Ike, T. Kume. Focal hepatic necrosis in young ferrets infected with *Aeromonas* spp. *Jpn J Vet Sci* 48:159–162, 1986.

Jacobson, E.R. Biology and diseases of reptiles. *In:* Fox, J.G., B.J. Cohen, F.M. Loew, eds. *Laboratory Animal Medicine*. Orlando: Academic Press; 1984.

Janda, J.M. Recent advances in the study of taxonomy, pathogenicity, and infectious syndromes associated with the genus *Aeromonas*. *Clin Microbiol Rev* 4:397–410, 1991.

Janda, J.M., P.S. Duffey. Mesophilic aeromonads in human disease: Current taxonomy, laboratory identification, and infectious disease spectrum. *Rev Infect Dis* 10:980–997, 1988.

Lamers, C.H., M.J. De Haas, W.B. Muiswinkel. Humoral response and memory formation in carp after infection of *Aeromonas hydrophila* bacterin. *Dev Comp Immunol* 9:65–75, 1985.

Lineaweaver, W.C., M.K. Hill, G.M. Buncke, *et al. Aeromonas hydrophila* infections following use of medicinal leeches in replantation and flap surgery. *Ann Plast Surg* 29:238–244, 1992.

Love, R.J., D.N. Love. *Aeromonas hydrophila* isolated from polyarthritis in a calf. *Aust Vet J* 61:65, 1984.

Mateos, O., J. Anguita, G. Navarro, C. Paniagua. Influence of growth temperature on the production of extracellular virulence factors and pathogenicity of environmental and human strains of *Aeromonas hydrophila*. *J Appl Bacteriol* 74:111–118, 1993.

Nieto, T.P., Y. Santos, L.A. Rodríguez, A.E. Ellis. An extracellular acetylcholinesterase produced by *Aeromonas hydrophila* is a major toxin for fish. *Microbiol Pathogenesis* 11:101–110, 1991.

Notario, R., E. Careno, N. Borda, *et al. Aeromonas* spp. en niños con síndrome diarreico agudo. *Infect Microbiol Clin* 5:85–89, 1993.

Ocholi, R.A., T.H. Spencer. Isolation of *Aeromonas hydrophila* from a captive caracal lynx (*Felis caracal*). *J Wildl Dis* 25:122–123, 1989.

Pathak, S.P., J.W. Bhattache, N. Kalra, S. Chandra. Seasonal distribution of *Aeromonas hydrophila* in river water and isolation from river fish. *J Appl Bacteriol* 65:347–352, 1988.

Picard, B., Goullet P. Epidemiological complexity of hospital aeromonas infections revealed by electrophoretic typing of esterases. *Epidemiol Infect* 98:5–14, 1987.

Plumb, J.A. Immunisation des poissons d'eau chaude contre cinq agents pathogenes impartants. Symposium sur la vaccination des poissons. Paris, Office Internationale des Epizooties (OIE), 20–22 février 1984.

Rafidah, J., B.L. Ong, S. Saroja. Outbreak of "red leg"—An *Aeromonas hydrophila* infection in frogs. *J Vet Malaysia* 2:139–142, 1990.

Ruangpan, L., I. Kitao, I. Yoshida. Protective efficacy of *Aeromonas hydrophila* vaccines in nile tilapia. *Vet Immunol Immunopathol* 12:345–350, 1986.

Sakazaki, R., T. Shimada. O-serogrouping scheme for mesophilic *Aeromonas* strains. *Jpn J Med Sci Biol* 37:247–255, 1984.

Shane, S.M., K.S. Harrington, M.S. Montrose, R.G. Roebuck. The occurrence of *Aeromonas hydrophila* in avian diagnostic submissions. *Avian Dis* 28:804–807, 1984.

Sioutas, S., R.W. Hoffmann, C. Pfeil-Putzien, T. Scherl. Carp erythrodermatitis (CE) due to an *Aeromonas hydrophila* infection. *J Vet Med B* 38:186–194, 1991.

Soliman, M.K., M. el S. Easa, M. Faisal, *et al.* Motile *Aeromonas* infection of striped (grey) mullet, *Mugil cephalus. Antonie Van Leeuwenhoek* 56:323–335, 1989.

Stelma, G.N. *Aeromonas hydrophila. In*: Doyle, M.T., ed. *Foodborne Bacterial Pathogens.* New York: Marcel Dekker; 1989.

Stoskopf, M.K. Bacterial diseases of goldfish, koi and carp. *In*: Stoskopf, M.K., ed. *Fish Medicine*. Philadelphia: W.B. Saunders; 1993.

Van der Kooij, D. Properties of aeromonads and their occurrence and hygienic significance in drinking water. *Zbl Bakteriol Mikrobiol Hyg* 187B:1–17, 1988.

Von Graevenitz, A., M. Altwegg. *Aeromonas* and *Plesiomonas. In*: Balows, A., K.L. Herrmann, H.D. Isenberg, H.J. Shadomy, eds. *Manual of Clinical Microbiology.* 5th ed. Washington, D.C.: American Society for Microbiology; 1991.

ANIMAL ERYSIPELAS AND HUMAN ERYSIPELOID

ICD-10 A26.0 cutaneous erysipeloid

Synonyms: Rosenbach's erysipeloid, erythema migrans, erysipelotrichosis, rose disease (in swine).

Etiology: The etiologic agent is *Erysipelothrix rhusiopathiae* (*E. insidiosa*), a gram-positive (with uneven coloration), facultatively aerobic or anaerobic, non-motile bacillus 0.6 to 2.5 microns long that does not produce spores. When found in the rugose phase it tends to form filaments. It is resistant to environmental factors, and survives 5 days in water and 15 days in mud (Jones, 1986). The number of serotypes is increasing: in 1987, 23 (from 1 to 23) had been recognized, with sub-serotypes 1a, 1b and 2a, 2b (Norrung *et al.*, 1987), and by 1991, there were already 26 serotypes (Norrung and Molin, 1991). Serotyping is important in epidemiology and immunization.

A second species, *E. tonsillarum*, was isolated from the tonsils of apparently healthy swine (Takahashi *et al.*, 1987).

The classification and nomenclature of the genus *Erysipelothrix* is still under investigation. DNA:DNA hybridization studies have shown that one group of *E. rhusiopathiae* serotypes is genetically more related to this species, while another is genetically more related to *E. tonsillarum*. Two serotypes, 13 and 18, possibly belong to a new species, given their low level of hybridization with both species (Takahashi *et al.*, 1992).

Geographic Distribution: The etiologic agent is distributed on all continents among many species of domestic and wild mammals and birds. It has also been isolated from aquatic animals, such as dolphins, American alligators and crocodiles, and sea lions.

Occurrence in Man: Human erysipeloid is for the most part an occupational disease affecting workers in slaughterhouses and commercial fowl-processing plants, fishermen and fish-industry workers, and those who handle meat (particularly pork) and seafood products. It is not a notifiable disease and little is known of its incidence. In the former Soviet Union, nearly 3,000 cases were reported between 1956 and 1958 in 13 slaughterhouses in the Ukraine, and 154 cases were reported in the Tula region in 1959. From 1961 to 1970, the U.S. Centers for Disease Control and Prevention confirmed the diagnosis of 15 cases in the US. A few isolated cases have occurred in Latin America. Some epidemic outbreaks have occurred in the former Soviet Union, in the United States, and on the southern Baltic coast (see section on source of infection and mode of transmission).

Occurrence in Animals: The disease in swine (rose disease, swine erysipelas) is important in Asia, Canada, Europe, Mexico, and the United States. It has also been seen in Brazil, Chile, Guatemala, Guyana, Jamaica, Peru, and Suriname, but the incidence is low in these countries. However, the disease seems to be increasing in importance in Chile (Skoknic *et al.*, 1981). Polyarthritis in sheep due to *E. rhusiopathiae* has been described in many sheep-breeding areas of the world.

The Disease in Man: The cutaneous form is known by the name erysipeloid to distinguish it from erysipelas caused by a hemolytic streptococcus. The incubation period ranges from one to seven days. Erysipeloid localizes primarily in the hands and fingers and consists of an erythematous, edematous skin lesion with violet coloration around a wound (the inoculation point) that may be a simple abrasion. Arthritis in the finger joints occurs with some frequency. The patient experiences a burning sensation, a pulsating pain, and at times an intense pruritus.

The course of the disease is usually benign and the patient recovers in two to four weeks. If the infection becomes generalized, septicemia and endocarditis may cause death. In the US, most cases reported in recent years have been the septicemic form generally associated with endocarditis (McClain, 1991). An analysis of 49 cases of systemic infection occurring over a 15-year period (Gorby and Peacock, 1988) found that *E. rhusiopathiae* has a peculiar tropism toward the aortic valve. In 40% of the cases, there was a concomitant cutaneous erysipeloid lesion and fatality was 38%. In slightly more than 40%, there was a history of prior valvular disease. Only 17% had a history that could be characterized as involving a compromised immune system. The principal symptoms were fever (92%), splenomegaly (36%), and hematuria (24%).

Nelson (1955) did not record any cases of endocarditis among 500 cases of erysipeloid in the US, which would indicate that the systemic disease is rather rare. The first case of endocarditis in Brazil was described by Rocha *et al.* (1989). The disease began with an erysipeloid and progressed to septicemia and endocarditis. The patient was an alcoholic with a prior history of aortic insufficiency, who had pricked himself with a fishbone.

The preferred treatment is penicillin, to which *E. rhusiopathiae* is very sensitive. Treatment with cephalosporins can be substituted for patients who are allergic to penicillin (McClain, 1991).

The Disease in Animals: Many species of domestic and wild mammals and birds are hosts to the etiologic agent. In several animal species, *E. rhusiopathiae* produces pathologic processes. Swine are the most affected species.

SWINE: Swine erysipelas is an economically important disease in many countries. In several central European countries, swine can only be raised profitably where systematic vaccination is practiced. Morbidity and mortality vary a great deal from one region to another, perhaps due to differences in the virulence of the etiologic agent. At present, acute forms are infrequent in western Europe and in North America.

The incubation period lasts from one to seven days. There are three main clinical forms: acute (septicemia), subacute (urticaria), and chronic (arthritis, lymphadenitis, and endocarditis). These forms may coexist in a herd or appear separately. The acute form begins suddenly with a high fever. Some animals suffer from prostration, anorexia, and vomiting, while others continue to feed despite the high fever. In some animals, reddish purple spots appear on the skin, particularly in the ears. There is splenomegaly and swelling of the lymph nodes. In the final phase of septicemic erysipelas, dyspnea and diarrhea are the most obvious symptoms. The disease has a rapid course and mortality is usually very high (Timoney *et al.*, 1988). The subacute form is characterized by urticaria, which initially appears as reddish or purple rhomboid-shaped spots on the skin. These spots are found particularly on the abdomen, the inside of the thighs, the neck, and the ears. The plaques later become necrotic, dry up, and fall off.

The chronic form is characterized by arthritis. At first, the joints swell and movement is painful; later, the lesion may develop into ankylosis. Losses from arthritis are considerable because the animals' development and weight gain are affected and because they may be confiscated from the abattoirs. The chronic form may also appear as endocarditis, with progressive emaciation or sudden death. Lymphadenitis is another manifestation of the chronic form (Timoney *et al.*, 1988; Blood and Radostits, 1989).

Among the isolates of *E. rhusiopathiae* obtained from swine with clinical erysipelas, serotypes 1 (subtypes 1a and 1b) and 2 predominate. Subtype 1a is usually isolated from the septicemic form, serotype 2 from the urticarial and arthritic form, and serotypes 1 and 2 from endocarditis. A study conducted in Japan typed 300 isolates from swine with erysipelas. Most belonged to serotypes 1a, 1b, or 2. Serotype 1a was also isolated in 9.7% of arthritis and lymphadenitis cases. Only 6.7% belonged to other serotypes: 3, 5, 6, 8, 11, 21, and N (could not be typed), isolated from the chronic form of erysipelas. These latter strains were analyzed experimentally for their pathogenicity in swine and were found to produce the urticarial form.

The strains of serotype 1a isolated from swine with arthritis or lymphadenitis produced various symptoms: generalized urticaria with depression and anorexia in some animals, localized urticaria lesions in other animals, and no symptoms in the remaining animals (Takahashi, 1987).

Acute cases can be treated with simultaneous administration of penicillin and antiserum.

SHEEP AND CATTLE: *E. rhusiopathiae* causes arthritis in lambs, usually after tail docking or sometimes as a result of an umbilical infection. The infection becomes established about two weeks after tail docking or birth, and the main symptoms are difficulty in movement and stunted growth. Recovery is slow.

In Argentina, Brazil, Chile, Great Britain, and New Zealand, a cutaneous infection caused by *E. rhusiopathiae* has been observed on the hooves of sheep a few

Figure 1. Animal erysipelas and human erysipeloid
(*Erysipelothrix rhusiopathiae*). Mode of transmission.

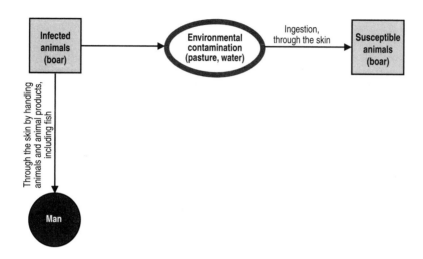

days after they have undergone a benzene hexachloride dip. The lesions consist of laminitis and the animals experience difficulty moving. The disease lasts about two weeks. As with human erysipeloid, the infection gains entry through small skin abrasions. It can be prevented by adding a disinfectant such as a 0.03% solution of cupric sulfate to the dip. Serotype 1b was the most common of the isolates found in Australia, not only in swine but in domestic and wild sheep and fowl as well. Serotypes 1a and 2 were less frequent in sheep (Eamens *et al.*, 1988).

Other forms of erysipelas in sheep are valvular endocarditis, septicemia, and pneumonia (Griffiths *et al.*, 1991).

Arthritis has been observed in calves, and the agent has been isolated from the tonsils of healthy adult cows.

FOWL: A septicemic disease caused by *E. rhusiopathiae* occurs in many species of domestic and wild fowl; turkeys are the most frequently affected. Symptoms include general weakness, diarrhea, cyanosis, and a reddish-purple swollen comb. The disease tends to attack males in particular. Mortality can vary between 2.5% and 25%. The lesions consist of large hemorrhages and petechiae of the pectoral and leg muscles, serous membranes, intestine, and gizzard. The spleen and liver are enlarged. Symptoms and lesions are similar in chickens, ducks, and pheasants.

Source of Infection and Mode of Transmission (Figure 1): Many animal species harbor *E. rhusiopathiae*. The principal reservoir seems to be swine; the etiologic agent has been isolated from the tonsils of up to 30% of apparently healthy swine. In a study carried out in Chile, the agent was isolated from tonsil samples of 53.5% of 400 swine in a slaughterhouse (Skoknic *et al.*, 1981). *E. rhusiopathiae* was isolated from 25.6% of soil samples where pigs live and from their feces (Wood and

Harrington, 1978). Alkaline soil is particularly favorable to the agent's survival. A great variety of serotypes may be isolated from apparently healthy swine. In experimental tests, some serotypes prove to be highly virulent, others moderately pathogenic (producing only localized urticaria), and others avirulent (Takahashi, 1987).

Fish, mollusks, and crustaceans are an important source of infection. The etiologic agent has been isolated from fish skin. In the former Soviet Union, an epidemic of erysipeloid was caused by handling fish brought in by several different boats; on the Baltic coast there was another outbreak of 40 cases. In Argentina, where swine erysipelas has not been confirmed but where cases of human erysipeloid have been described, the agent was isolated from 2 out of 9 water samples from the Atlantic coast, and from 1 out of 40 samples of external integument of fish (de Diego and Lavalle, 1977). Subsequently, these strains were identified as belonging to serotypes 21 and 22.

In meat and poultry processing plants, rodents can be important reservoirs and disseminators of the infection. Fourteen different serotypes of *E. rhusiopathiae* were isolated from 38 samples (33.9%) obtained from pork in 112 shops in Tokyo. Some samples contained more than one serotype (Shiono *et al.*, 1990).

E. rhusiopathiae can survive a long time outside the animal organism, both in the environment and in animal products, which contributes to its perpetuation.

Man is infected through wounds and skin abrasions, but is very resistant to other entry routes. The infection is contracted by handling animals and animal products, including fish. Veterinarians have contracted the infection when they pricked themselves while administering the simultaneous vaccination (virulent culture and serum). This procedure is no longer in use. In Chile, a case of human endocarditis was attributed to the ingestion of smoked fish sold on the street (Gilabert, 1968).

The agent can multiply in an apparently healthy carrier under stress, and can cause disease and contaminate the environment. A pig with the acute form of erysipelas sheds an enormous amount of the bacteria in its feces, urine, saliva, and vomit, thus becoming a source of infection for the other pigs on the farm (Timoney *et al.*, 1988).

The routes of infection are believed to be digestive and cutaneous, through abrasions and wounds. The long survival of the agent in the environment ensures endemism in affected areas. Other animals and fowl may also contribute to maintaining the infection or to causing outbreaks.

Role of Animals in the Epidemiology of the Disease: Man is an accidental host who contracts the infection from sick animals, carriers, animal products, or objects contaminated by animals.

Diagnosis: Clinical diagnosis, based on the patient's occupation and on the characteristics of the cutaneous lesion, can be confirmed by isolation and identification of the etiologic agent. *E. rhusiopathiae* can be isolated from biopsies of the lesion. The sample is cultured in trypticase soy broth and incubated at 35°C for seven days; if there is growth, the culture is repeated in blood agar. The blood of septicemic patients can be cultured directly in blood agar (Bille and Doyle, 1991).

In septicemic cases in animals, the etiologic agent can be isolated from the blood and internal organs. In cases of arthritis or skin infections, cultures are made from localized lesions. Isolations from contaminated materials are accomplished through inoculation of mice, which are very susceptible.

Diagnosis of animal erysipelas makes use of several serologic tests, such as agglutination, growth inhibition, passive hemagglutination, and complement fixation. Given the frequency of subclinical infections and vaccination in animals, serologic tests are often difficult to interpret. A comparative study of the growth inhibition test and the complement fixation test concluded that the latter is more useful for diagnosis, since it eliminates low titers caused by subclinical infection or vaccination (Bercovich *et al.*, 1981). Another serologic method is the indirect enzyme-linked immunosorbent assay (ELISA), which is as sensitive as the growth inhibition test and is easier and less expensive to conduct (Kirchhoff *et al.*, 1985).

Control: In persons exposed as a result of their occupations, prevention of erysipeloid primarily involves hygiene, namely frequent hand washing with disinfectant and proper treatment of wounds. Establishments where foods of animal origin are processed should control rodent populations.

The control of swine erysipelas depends mostly on vaccination. There are two vaccines in use that have given good results: a bacterin adsorbed on aluminum hydroxide and a live avirulent vaccine (EVA=*erysipelas vaccine avirulent*). Vaccination confers immunity for five to eight months. The bacterin is first administered before weaning, followed by another dose two to four weeks later. The avirulent vaccine is administered orally via drinking water. The vaccines are not entirely satisfactory in preventing chronic erysipelas and it is even suspected that vaccination may contribute to arthritic symptoms (Timoney *et al.*, 1988). On the other hand, the great reduction or near elimination of the acute form in western Europe, Japan, and the US is probably due to systematic vaccination. In the case of an outbreak of septicemic erysipelas, it is important to destroy the carcasses immediately, disinfect the premises, and to treat sick animals with penicillin and the rest of the herd with anti-erysipelas serum. Rotation of animals to different pastures and environmental hygiene measures are also of great help in control.

Bacterins are used on turkey-raising establishments, where the infection is endemic. A live vaccine administered orally via drinking water has yielded good results in tests (Bricker and Saif, 1983).

Bibliography

Bercovich, Z., C.D. Weenk van Loon, C.W. Spek. Serological diagnosis of *Erysipelothrix rhusiopathiae*: A comparative study between the growth inhibition test and the complement fixation test. *Vet Quart* 3:19–24, 1981.

Bille, J., M.P. Doyle. *Listeria* and *Erysipelothrix*. *In*: Ballows, A., W.J. Hausler, Jr., K.L. Hermann, *et al. Manual of Clinical Microbiology*. 5th ed. Washington, D.C.: American Society for Microbiology; 1991.

Blood, D.C., O-M. Radostits. *Veterinary Medicine*. 7th ed. London: Baillière Tindall; 1989.

Bricker, J.M., Y.M. Saif. Drinking water vaccination of turkeys, using live *Erysipelothrix rhusiopathiae*. *J Am Vet Med Assoc* 183:361–362, 1983.

de Castro, A.F.P., O. Campedelli Filho, C. Troise. Isolamento de *Erysipelothrix rhusiopathiae* de peixes maritimos. *Rev Inst Med Trop Sao Paulo* 9:169–171, 1967.

de Diego, A.I., S. Lavalle. *Erysipelothrix rhusiopathiae* en aguas y pescados de la costa atlántica de la provincia de Buenos Aires (Argentina). *Gac Vet* 39:672–677, 1977.

Eamens, G.J., M.J. Turner, R.E. Catt. Serotypes of *Erysipelothrix rhusiopathiae* in Australian pigs, small ruminants, poultry, and captive wild birds and animals. *Aust Vet J* 65:249–252, 1988.

Gilabert, B. Endocarditis bacteriana producida por *Erysipelothrix*. Primer caso humano verificado en Chile. *Bol Hosp San Juan de Dios* 15:390–392, 1968. Cited in: Skoknic, A., I. Díaz, S. Urcelay, R. Duarte, O. González. Estudio de la erisipela en Chile. *Arch Med Vet* 13:13–16, 1981.

Gledhill, A.W. Swine erysipelas. *In*: Stableforth, A.W., I.A. Galloway, eds. *Infectious Diseases of Animals*. London: Butterworths; 1959.

Gorby, G.L., J.E. Peacock, Jr. *Erysipelothrix rhusiopathiae* endocarditis: Microbiologic, epidemiologic, and clinical features of an occupational disease. *Rev Infect Dis* 10:317–325, 1988.

Griffiths, I.B., S.H. Done, S. Readman. *Erysipelothrix* pneumonia in sheep. *Vet Rec* 128:382–383, 1991.

Jones, D. Genus *Erysipelothrix*, Rosenbach 1909. *In*: Sneath, P.H., H.S. Mair, M.E. Sharpe, eds. Vol. 2: *Bergey's Manual of Systemic Bacteriology*. Baltimore: Williams & Wilkins; 1986.

Kirchhoff, H., H. Dubenkroop, G. Kerlen, *et al*. Application of the indirect enzyme immunoassay for the detection of antibodies against *Erysipelothrix rhusiopathiae*. *Vet Microbiol* 10:549–559, 1985.

Levine, N.D. Listeriosis, botulism, erysipelas, and goose influenza. *In*: Biester, H.E., L.H. Schwarte, eds. *Diseases of Poultry*. 4th ed. Ames: Iowa State University Press; 1959.

McClain, J.B. *Erysipelothrix rhusiopathiae In*: Mandell, G.L., R.G. Douglas, Jr., J.E. Bennett, eds. *Principles and Practice of Infectious Diseases*. 3rd ed. New York: Churchill Livingstone, Inc.; 1990.

Nelson, E. Five hundred cases of erysipeloid. *Rocky Mt Med J* 52:40–42, 1955. Cited in: Gorby, G.L., J.E. Peacock, Jr. *Erysipelothrix rhusiopathiae* endocarditis: Microbiologic, epidemiologic, and clinical features of an occupational disease. *Rev Infect Dis* 10:317–325, 1988.

Norrung, V., G. Molin. A new serotype of *Erysipelothrix rhusiopathiae* isolated from pig slurry. *Acta Vet Hung* 39:137–138, 1991.

Norrung, V., B. Munch, H.E. Larsen. Occurrence, isolation and serotyping of *Erysipelothrix rhusiopathiae* in cattle and pig slurry. *Acta Vet Scand* 28:9–14, 1987.

Rocha, M.P., P.R.S. Fontoura, S.N.B. Azevedo, A.M.V. Fontoura. *Erysipelothrix* endocarditis with previous cutaneous lesion: Report of a case and review of literature. *Rev Inst Med Trop Sao Paulo* 31:286–289, 1989.

Shiono, H., H. Hayashidani, K-I. Kaneko, *et al*. Occurrence of *Erysipelothrix rhusiopathiae* in retail raw pork. *J Food Protect* 53:856–858, 1990.

Shuman, R.D., R.L. Wood. Swine erysipelas. *In*: Dunne, H.W., ed. *Diseases of Swine*. 3rd ed. Ames: Iowa State University Press; 1970.

Skoknic, A., I. Díaz, S. Urcelay, R. Duarte, O. González. Estudio de la erisipela en Chile. *Arch Med Vet* 13:13–16, 1981.

Takahashi, T. Studies on serotypes, antibiotic resistance, and pathogenic characteristics of *Erysipelothrix rhusiopathiae*. *Bull Nipon Vet Zootechn College* 36:153–156, 1987.

Takahashi, T., T. Fujisawa, T. Benno, *et al*. *Erysipelothrix tonsillarum* sp. nov. isolated from tonsils of apparently healthy pigs. *Int J Syst Bacteriol* 37:166–169, 1987.

Takahashi, T., T. Fujisawa, Y. Tamura, *et al*. DNA relatedness among *Erysipelothrix rhusiopathiae* strains representing all twenty-three serovars and *Erysipelothrix tonsillarum*. *Int J Syst Bacteriol* 42:469–473, 1992.

Timoney, J.F., J.H. Gillespie, F.W. Scott, J.E. Barlough. *Hagan and Bruner's Microbiology and Infectious Diseases of Domestic Animals*. 8th ed. Ithaca: Comstock; 1988.

Wood, R.L. *Erysipelothrix infection*. *In*: Hubbert, W.T., W.F. McCulloch, P.R. Schnurrenberger, eds. *Diseases Transmitted from Animals to Man*. 6th ed. Springfield: Thomas; 1975.

Wood, R.L., R. Harrington. Serotypes of *Erysipelothrix rhusiopathiae* isolated from swine and from soil and manure of swine pens in the United States. *Am J Vet Res* 39:1833–1840, 1978.

Wood, R.L., R. Harrington, D.R. Hubrich. Serotypes of previously unclassified isolates of *Erysipelothrix rhusiopathiae* from swine in the United States and Puerto Rico. *Am J Vet Res* 42:1248–1250, 1981.

ANTHRAX

**ICD-10 A22.0 cutaneous anthrax; A22.1 pulmonary anthrax;
A22.2 gastrointestinal anthrax**

Synonyms: Malignant pustule, malignant carbuncle, charbon, hematic anthrax, bacterial anthrax, splenic fever, woolsorters' disease.

Etiology: *Bacillus anthracis*, an aerobic, nonmotile, gram-positive bacillus 3–5 microns long that forms centrally located spores. It should be differentiated from *B. cereus*, which is quite similar. One of the media used to differentiate them is the gamma phage specific for *B. anthracis*. The etiologic agent is found in a vegetative state in man and animals. When exposed to oxygen in the air, it forms spores that are highly resistant to physical and chemical agents.

In nature, *B. anthracis* occurs in a virulent form—the pathogenic agent of anthrax—and in an avirulent form. Virulence is determined by a capsule that inhibits phagocytosis and an exotoxin, both of which are plasmid mediated. In turn, the toxin consists of three protein factors: the protective antigen, the lethal factor, and the edema factor. None of these factors is toxic by itself. When injected intravenously at the same time, the protective antigen and the lethal factor are lethal in some animal species. The combination of the protective agent and the edema factor produces edema when injected subcutaneously (Little and Knudson, 1986).

Geographic Distribution: Worldwide, with areas of enzootic and sporadic occurrence.

Occurrence in Man: The infection in humans is correlated with the incidence of the disease in domestic animals. In economically advanced countries, where animal anthrax has been controlled, it occurs only occasionally among humans. Some cases stem from the importation of contaminated animal products. Human anthrax is most common in enzootic areas in developing countries, among people who work with livestock, eat undercooked meat from infected animals, or work in establishments where wool, goatskins, and pelts are stored and processed. The incidence of human illness in developing countries is not well known because those sick with the disease do not always see a doctor, nor do doctors always report the cases; in addition, the diagnosis often is based only on the clinical syndrome.

According to data from recent years, epidemic outbreaks continue to occur despite the availability of excellent preventive measures for animal anthrax and, therefore, for the occurrence of the disease in humans. There are some hyperendemic areas, as was shown in Haiti when an American woman contracted the infection after acquiring some goatskin drums. Compilation of data in that country revealed a high incidence of human anthrax in the southern peninsula, Les Cayes, which has a population of approximately 500,000. From 1973 to 1977, 1,587 cases were recorded in the 31 clinics in that region (La Force, 1978).

In Zambia, at least 30 people died from anthrax in 1992. Eastern Nigeria has a very high incidence of human anthrax (Okolo, 1985). On the borders between Thailand, Myanmar (Burma), and Laos that are crossed by animals transported from as far away as India, outbreaks occur frequently. In one Thai village, several of the approximately 200 inhabitants participated in cutting up a buffalo that had supposedly drowned; eight of them became ill and one died with symptoms suspected of being anthrax (Ngampachjana *et al.*, 1989). In a settlement in eastern Algeria, 6 cases of anthrax occurred in an extended family of 59 members. Those who fell ill had participated in slaughtering and butchering a sheep with symptoms that included hemorrhage, black blood, and splenomegaly. Fourteen animals of various ruminant species had died before the appearance of the index case, a child who later died (Abdenour *et al.*, 1987). In the former Soviet Union, at least 15,000 cases of human anthrax occurred prior to 1917 and 178 cases were reported as late as 1985 (Marshall, 1988).

In enzootic areas, the human disease is usually endemosporadic with epidemic outbreaks. The latter are caused primarily by ingestion of meat, often by many people, from animals who were dead or dying from anthrax when slaughtered (Rey *et al.*, 1982; Fragoso and Villicaña, 1984; Sirisanthana *et al.*, 1984). In 1978, in a region in the Republic of Mali, there were 84 cases with 19 deaths. High mortality, possibly due to intestinal anthrax, was also seen in Senegal in 1957, with 237 deaths out of 254 cases (Simaga *et al.*, 1980).

In 1979, an epidemic outbreak in Sverdlovsk, in the former Soviet Union, led to a controversy between that country and the United States. According to the former Soviet Union, fewer than 40 people died from gastric anthrax in this epidemic, while US intelligence sources claimed that several hundred to a thousand people perished from pulmonary anthrax within a few weeks. Later Soviet sources indicated a total of 96 victims, 79 suffering from intestinal infection (64 of whom died), and no pulmonary cases (Marshall, 1988). The controversy centered on whether the epidemic was natural or man-induced, since the US intelligence source suspected that an accident had occurred at a plant presumably engaged in biological warfare projects. If so, this would have indicated a violation of the 1975 treaty against biological weapons (Wade, 1980). Sverdlovsk is located in an enzootic area and, according to Marshall (1988), the source of infection was probably a bone meal food supplement on State-run and private farms. Using preserved tissue, Russian and American researchers were ultimately able to determine that at least 42 people had died from inhaling rather than ingesting the etiological agent. They thus confirmed the suspicion that the source of infection was airborne and probably came from an illegal plant that the Soviet authorities did not allow to be inspected.

Occurrence in Animals: Anthrax is common in enzootic areas where no control programs have been established.

In a hyperenzootic area of eastern Nigeria, animals submitted for emergency slaughter were studied. There is no *ante mortem* inspection of animals in that region, thus increasing the risk of human exposure. Of 150 animals, 34 (22.7%) were positive through culture and inoculation of laboratory animals. Of 35 cows, 42.9% were positive, and of 70 bulls, 14.3% were positive. The milk from 43 cows and 8 sheep was also examined; 15 and 2 of the samples, respectively, were positive (Okolo, 1988).

Some outbreaks and occasional cases of human infection have also been reported in industrialized countries, such as the US (Hunter *et al.*, 1989).

In Africa, wildlife reserves periodically suffer great losses, especially among herbivores. A thesis presented at the University of Nairobi, Kenya, estimated that anthrax accounts for about 11% of the mortality in the animal population each year, excluding calves. At Etosha National Park in Namibia, anthrax caused the death of 1,635 wild animals of 10 species, or 54% of total mortality between January 1966 and June 1974. The source of infection was artificial ponds (Ebedes, 1976). An outbreak occurred on a reserve in Zambia between June and November of 1987, with a total loss of over 4,000 animals. The victims were primarily hippopotamuses (*Hippopotamus amphibius*). Other species, such as the Cape buffalo (*Syncerus caffer*) and the elephant (*Loxodonta africana*), also seem to have been affected (Turnbull *et al.*, 1991).

The Disease in Man: The incubation period is from two to five days. Three clinical forms are recognized: cutaneous, pulmonary or respiratory, and gastrointestinal.

The cutaneous form is the most common and is contracted by contact with infected animals (usually carcasses) or contaminated wool, hides, and fur. The exposed part of the skin begins to itch and a papule appears at the inoculation site. This papule becomes a vesicle and then evolves into a depressed, black eschar. Generally, the cutaneous lesion is not painful or is only slightly so; consequently, some patients do not consult a doctor in time. If left untreated, the infection can lead to septicemia and death. The case fatality rate for untreated anthrax is estimated at between 5% to 20%.

The pulmonary form is contracted by inhalation of *B. anthracis* spores. At the onset of illness, the symptomatology is mild and resembles that of a common upper respiratory tract infection. Thus, many patients do not see a doctor in the early stage of the disease when it would be easily cured. Some three to five days later the symptoms become acute, with fever, shock, and resultant death. The case fatality rate is high.

Gastrointestinal anthrax is contracted by ingesting meat from infected animals and is manifested by violent gastroenteritis with vomiting and bloody stools. Mortality ranges from 25% to 75% (Brachman, 1984).

The recommended treatment for cutaneous anthrax is intramuscular administration of 1 million units of procaine penicillin every 12 to 24 hours for five to seven days. In the case of serious illness, as in pulmonary anthrax, the recommendation is 2 million units of penicillin G per day administered intravenously or 500,000 units administered intravenously through a slow drip every four to six hours until temperature returns to normal. Streptomycin, in 1 g to 2 g doses per day, has a synergistic effect if administered at the same time as penicillin. Some penicillin-resistant strains of *B. anthracis* have been found (Braderic and Punda-Polic, 1992). Penicillin sterilizes the organism in a short time, even in a single day in patients suffering from cutaneous anthrax, but it should be borne in mind that the toxin remains and the patient is still not cured.

The Disease in Animals: It takes three forms: apoplectic or peracute, acute and subacute, and chronic. The apoplectic form is seen mostly in cattle, sheep, and goats, and occurs most frequently at the beginning of an outbreak. The onset is sudden and death ensues rapidly. The animals show signs of cerebral apoplexy and die.

The acute and subacute forms are frequent in cattle, horses, and sheep. The symptomatology consists of fever, a halt to rumination, excitement followed by depression, respiratory difficulty, uncoordinated movements, convulsions, and death. Bloody discharges from natural orifices as well as edemas in different parts of the body are sometimes observed.

Chronic anthrax occurs mainly in less susceptible species, such as pigs, but is also seen in cattle, horses, and dogs. During outbreaks in swine herds, some animals fall victim to the acute form, but most suffer from chronic anthrax. The main symptom of this form is pharyngeal and lingual edema. Frequently, a foamy, sanguinolent discharge from the mouth is observed. The animals die from asphyxiation. Another localized chronic form in pigs is intestinal anthrax.

Anthrax also affects free-roaming wild animals and those in zoos and national parks (see section on occurrence in animals).

Autopsies of acute cases reveal bloody exudate in the natural orifices. Decomposition is rapid and the carcass becomes bloated with gases. Rigor mortis is incomplete. Hemorrhages are found in the internal organs; splenomegaly is almost always present (but may not be in some cases), with the pulp being dark red or blackish and having a soft or semifluid consistency; the liver, kidneys, and lymph nodes are congested and enlarged; and the blood is blackish with little clotting tendency.

Animals treated early with penicillin recover. Treatment consists of intravenous administration of 12,000 to 17,000 units/kg of bodyweight of sodium benzylpenicillin followed by intramuscular administration of amoxicillin.

Source of Infection and Mode of Transmission (Figure 2): Soil is the reservoir for the infectious agent. The process followed by spores in the earth is a subject of controversy. It has been suggested that there is a cycle of germination and subsequent resporulation, but there is no evidence to this effect. The lifecycle of spores under laboratory conditions (in culture media) or in sterile soil is extremely long. However, under natural conditions, it seems that their survival is limited to a few years, due to the activity of saprophytic microbes in the soil. This is probably the case in wild animal reserves in Africa, where attempts to isolate *B. anthracis* from the soil or water one or two years after an epizootic yielded negative results, except near the remains of some animals that died from sporadic cases of anthrax. Turnbull *et al.* (1991) believe that in order for an enzootic area to be maintained, it would be necessary for the etiologic agent to multiply in animals. However, a fact to be noted is the long survival of *B. anthracis* on the Scottish island of Gruinard, which was abundantly seeded with *B. anthracis* during the Second World War for purposes of experimentation with biological weapons. Some 40 years later, viable spores of *B. anthracis* were still detected. It is speculated that this long survival is due to the island's acidic soil and cold, moist climate, which are unfavorable to the activity of microbial flora.

For man, the source of infection is always infected animals, contaminated animal products, or environmental contamination by spores from these sources.

Cutaneous anthrax is contracted by inoculation during the process of skinning or butchering an animal or by contact with infected leather, pelts, wool, or fur. Broken

Figure 2. Anthrax. Transmission cycle.

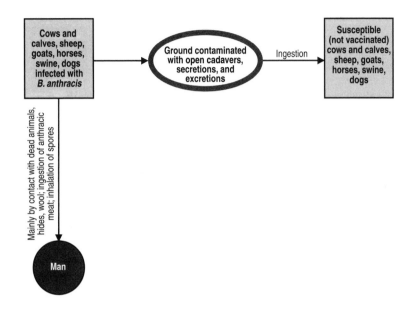

skin favors transmission. Products made from contaminated hair (e.g., shaving brushes), skins (e.g., drums), and bone meal (e.g., fertilizer) may continue to be sources of infection for many years. Transmission from animals to man is possible by means of insects acting as mechanical vectors, but reliably documented cases are few. A recent case occurred in a Croatian villager who was probably stung by a horsefly and developed a case of cutaneous anthrax on the back of her neck. The presumed source of infection was a cow close to her home that had died of anthrax (Braderic and Punda-Polic, 1992).

Pulmonary anthrax comes from inhaling spores released from contaminated wool or animal hair.

The source of infection for the gastrointestinal form is domestic and wild animals that died from anthrax. The pathway of transmission is through the digestive tract. Cases have been observed in Asia, Africa, and Latin America.

Animals contract the infection mainly by ingestion of pasture or water contaminated with *B. anthracis* spores, especially in places near anthrax-infected carcasses. An animal dying of anthrax produces an enormous quantity of *B. anthracis* in its tissues, and if the carcass is opened, the bacilli sporulate, contaminating the soil, grass, and water. Animals that graze in the contaminated area become infected themselves and produce new foci of infection. Animals and birds that feed on carrion can transport the infection some distance. The most serious outbreaks occur during dry summers after heavy rains. The rain washes spores loose and concentrates them in low spots, forming so-called "cursed fields," that are usually damp areas with glacial calcareous soils containing abundant organic material and having a pH above 6 (Van Ness, 1971). Nevertheless, outbreaks of anthrax may occur in acidic soil, as happened in the 1974 epizootic in Texas (USA), during which 218 cattle, 6 horses, and 1 mule died. Eighty-three percent of the fields where the outbreak took place had acid pH soil and 94% had subsoil with an alkaline pH (Whitford, 1979).

Contaminated animal by-products, especially bone meal and blood meal used as food supplements, can also give rise to distant foci of infection.

Another mode of transmission is cutaneous entry through insect bites, but this is considered of minor epidemiologic importance.

Role of Animals in the Epidemiology of the Disease: Animals are essential. Anthrax is transmitted to humans by animals or animal products. Transmission between humans is exceptional.

Diagnosis: The presence of the etiologic agent must be confirmed by microscopic examination of stained smears of vesicular fluid (in man), edemas (in swine), and blood (in other animals); by culturing the microorganism from the liquid aspirated from malignant pustules or from blood samples of a dead or dying animal; and by inoculation of laboratory animals (guinea pigs and mice). If the material is contaminated, cutaneous inoculation (by scarification) should be used. The use of antibiotics quickly reduces the possibility of isolating the etiologic agent.

The fluorescent antibody technique applied to fresh stains or blood smears can prove useful for presumptive diagnosis. Smears of blood or other bodily fluids can also be stained using the Giemsa or Wright method to make the pink capsule that surrounds the bacillus stand out. The Ascoli precipitation test has limited value due to its limited specificity, but is still used in some laboratories for animal products, from which the agent cannot be isolated.

The ELISA and Western Blot tests can be used to detect antibodies to the protective antigen in individuals who have had anthrax and from whom the agent cannot be isolated, i.e., in retrospective studies (Thurnbull *et al.*, 1986; Sirisanthana *et al.*, 1988; Harrison *et al.*, 1989). Antibodies have also been found in people living near animal reserves in Africa who have been exposed to anthrax in wild animals without becoming ill themselves (Thurnbull *et al.*, 1991).

Control: In man, the prevention of anthrax is based mainly on: (a) control of the infection in animals; (b) prevention of contact with infected animals and contaminated animal products; (c) environmental and personal hygiene in places where products of animal origin are handled (adequate ventilation and work clothing); (d) medical care for cutaneous lesions; and (e) disinfection of fur and wool with hot formaldehyde. Occupational groups at risk may benefit from vaccination with the protective antigen.

The human vaccine used in the US and Great Britain is acellular and consists of a filtrate of *B. anthracis* culture from a nonencapsulated strain that is adsorbed with aluminum hydroxide. This vaccine is not very potent and may not protect against all field strains. In the countries of Eastern Europe and in China, a live attenuated spore vaccine is administered by scarification.

In animals, anthrax control is based on systematic vaccination in enzootic areas. Sterne's avirulent spore vaccine is indicated because of its effectiveness and safety. The vaccine consists of spores from the nonencapsulated 34F2 strain with an adjuvant—usually a saponin—and is currently used worldwide, with a few exceptions. It is suitable for all domestic animal species. However, goats sometimes have severe reactions and the recommendation is thus to administer the vaccine in two doses in this species, with a month between doses (administer one-fourth of the dose in the first month and the full dose the following month). Pregnant females of any species should not be vaccinated unless they are at high risk of contracting anthrax. Antibiotics should not be administered a few days before or a few days after vaccination. In general, annual vaccination is sufficient; only in hyperenzootic areas is vaccination at shorter intervals recommended. Immunity is established in approximately one week in cattle, but takes longer in horses. In regions where anthrax occurs sporadically, mass vaccination is not justified and should be limited to affected herds. Rapid diagnosis, isolation, and treatment of sick animals with antibiotics (penicillin) are important.

Autopsies should not be performed on animals that have died from anthrax. An unopened carcass decomposes rapidly and the vegetative form of *B. anthracis* is destroyed in a short time. To make the diagnosis, it is recommended that blood be taken from a peripheral vessel with a syringe and sent to the laboratory in a sterile container. Dead animals should be destroyed where they lie as quickly as possible, preferably by incineration. The alternative is to bury them two meters deep and cover them with a layer of lime.

In areas where these procedures are not possible, the dead animal should be left intact so that it will start to decompose and, as much as possible, natural orifices and the surrounding soil should be treated with 10% formol (25% formalin).

Affected herds should be placed in quarantine, which should last until two weeks after the last case is confirmed, with no animal or animal product allowed out.

If anthrax is suspected at a slaughterhouse, all operations should be halted until the diagnosis is confirmed. If positive, all exposed carcasses should be destroyed and the premises carefully disinfected (with a 5% caustic lye solution for eight hours) before operations are resumed.

Bibliography

Abdenour D., B. Larouze, D. Dalichaouche, M. Aouati. Familial occurrence of anthrax in Eastern Algeria [letter]. *J Infect Dis* 155:1083–1084, 1987.

Brachman, P.S. Anthrax. *In*: Warren, K.S., A.A.F. Mahmoud, eds. *Tropical and Geographical Medicine*. New York: McGraw-Hill Book Co.; 1984.

Braderic N., V. Punda-Polic. Cutaneous anthrax due to penicillin-resistant *Bacillus anthracis* transmitted by an insect bite [letter]. *Lancet* 340:306–307, 1992.

Ebedes, H. Anthrax epizootics in wildlife in the Etosha Park, South West Africa. *In*: Page, L.A., ed. *Wildlife Diseases*. New York: Plenum Press; 1976.

Fragoso Uribe, R., H. Villicaña Fuentes. Antrax en dos comunidades de Zacatecas, México. *Bol Oficina Sanit Panam* 97:526–533, 1984.

Harrison, L.H, J.W. Ezzel, T.G. Abshire, *et al.* Evaluation of serologic tests for diagnosis of anthrax after an outbreak of cutaneous anthrax in Paraguay. *J Infect Dis* 160:706–710, 1989.

Hunter, L., W. Corbett, C. Grinden. Anthrax. Zoonoses update. *J Am Vet Med Assoc* 194:1028–1031, 1989.

La Force, F.M. Informe a la Oficina Sanitaria Panamericana. Haiti, 1978.

Little, S.F., G.B. Knudson. Comparative efficacy of *Bacillus anthracis* live spore vaccine and protective antigen vaccine against anthrax in the guinea pig. *Infect Immun* 52: 509–512, 1986.

Marshall, E. Sverdlovsk: Anthrax capital? [news and comments]. *Science* 240:383–385, 1988.

Ngampochjana, M., W.B. Baze, A.L Chedester. Human anthrax [letter]. *J Am Vet Med Assoc* 195:167, 1989.

Okolo, M.I. Studies on anthrax in food animals and persons occupationally exposed to the zoonoses in Eastern Nigeria. *Int J Zoonoses* 12:276–282, 1985.

Okolo, M.I. Prevalence of anthrax in emergency slaughtered food animals in Nigeria. *Vet Rec* 122:636, 1988.

World Health Organization. *Joint FAO/WHO Expert Committee on Zoonoses. Third Report.* Geneva: WHO; 1967. (Technical Report Series 378).

Rey, J.L., M. Meyran, P. Saliou. Situation épidémiologique de charbon human en Haute Volta. *Bull Soc Pathol Exot* 75:249–257, 1982.

Simaga, S.Y., E. Astorquiza, M. Thiero, R. Baylet. Un foyer de charbon humain et animal dans le cercle de Kati (République du Mali). *Bull Soc Pathol Exot* 73:23–28, 1980.

Sirisanthana, T., M. Navachareon, P. Tharavichitkul, *et al.* Outbreak of oral-pharyngeal anthrax: An unusual manifestation of human infection with *Bacillus anthracis. Am J Trop Med Hyg* 33:144–150, 1984.

Sirisanthana, T., K.E. Nelson, J.W. Ezzell, T.G. Abshire. Serological studies of patients with cutaneous and oral-orophangyngeal anthrax from northern Thailand. *Am J Trop Med Hyg* 39:575–581, 1988.

Sirol, J., Y. Gendron, M. Condat. Le charbon humain en Afrique. *Bull WHO* 49:143–148, 1973.

Sterne, M. Anthrax. *In*: Stableforth, A.W., I.A. Galloway, eds. *Infectious Diseases of Animals.* London: Butterworths; 1959.

Turnbull, P.C., R.H. Bell, K. Saigawa, *et al.* Anthrax in wildlife in the Luangwa Valley, Zambia. *Vet Rec* 128:399–403, 1991.

Turnbull, P.C., M.G. Broster, A. Carman, *et al.* Development of antibodies to protective antigen and lethal factor components of anthrax toxin in humans and guinea pigs and their relevance to protective immunity. *Infect Immun* 52:356–363, 1986.

Van Ness, G.B. Ecology of anthrax. *Science* 172:1303–1307, 1971.

Wade, N. Death at Sverdlovsk: A critical diagnosis. *Science* 209:1501–1502, 1980.

Whitford, H.W. Anthrax. *In*: Steele, J.H., H. Stoenner, W. Kaplan, M. Torten, eds. Vol I, Section A: *CRC Handbook Series in Zoonoses.* Boca Raton: CRC Press; 1979.

Wright, G.G. Anthrax. *In*: Hubbert, W.T., W.F. McCulloch, P.R. Schnurrenberger, eds. *Diseases Transmitted from Animals to Man.* 6th ed. Springfield: Thomas; 1975.

BOTULISM

ICD-10 A05.1

Synonyms: Allantiasis; "lamziekte" (bovine botulism in South Africa); "limberneck" (botulism in fowl).

Etiology: Toxins produced by *Clostridium botulinum*, which are the most potent known. *C. botulinum* is an obligate, spore-forming anaerobe. It has been sub-classified (Smith, 1977) into four groups (I to IV), according to culture and serological characteristics. Seven different types of botulinum antigens have been identified (A–G), according to their serological specificity. Classical botulism results from preformed toxins ingested with food. In wound botulism, the toxin forms by contamination of the injured tissue. In 1976, a new clinical type, infant botulism, was identified. It is caused by colonization of the infant's intestinal tract by *C. botulinum* and the resultant production and absorption of toxins.

The species *C. botulinum* is very heterogeneous. The different groups (I to IV) are differentiated according to their ability to digest proteins and break down sugars. Group I is highly proteolytic and saccharolytic and includes all the type A strains as well as various type B and F strains. Group II includes all the type E strains and the nonproteolytic type B and F strains that are highly saccharolytic. Group III consists of the type C and D strains, which are not proteolytic (except that they digest gelatin). Group IV contains only type G, which is proteolytic but not saccharolytic (Sakaguchi *et al.*, 1981; Concon, 1988).

Despite the metabolic and DNA differences among them, these groups of clostridia have until now been classified in a single species because they all produce a botulinum neurotoxin that acts similarly in animal hosts (Cato *et al.*, 1986). However, not all researchers agree with this scheme and one argument of those favoring a reclassification is the recent discovery of neurotoxigenic strains in *Clostridium baratii* and *C. butyricum*.

In effect, two cases of type E infant botulism in Rome, Italy, caused by *C. butyricum* (Aureli *et al.*, 1986) have been described and another case was described in New Mexico (USA) in a child suffering from a neurotoxigenic type F botulism produced by a clostridium that was later identified as *C. baratii* (Hall *et al.*, 1985). These clostridia were identified on the basis of their phenotype characteristics and were later confirmed through DNA hybridization (Suen *et al.*, 1988a). The neurotoxin isolated from *C. baratii* was similar in structure and amino acid sequence to *C. botulinum* types A, B, and E (Giménez *et al.*, 1992). The proponents of reclassification, such as Suen *et al.* (1988b), have suggested renaming group IV, which contains the single toxigenic type G, as *Clostridium argentinense*. Arnon (1986) agrees that reclassification would be justified based on logical criteria and taxonomic purity, but questions whether this would improve clinical, microbiological, and epidemiological knowledge.

Geographic Distribution: Occurs on all continents, with a marked regional distribution that probably reflects the presence in the soil of the microorganism and its different types of toxins.

Occurrence in Man: The disease occurs more frequently in the northern hemisphere than in the southern hemisphere, and can appear sporadically and among groups of people who ingest the same food with the preformed toxin. From 1950 to 1973, an average of 15.1 outbreaks occurred annually in the US, with 2.4 cases per outbreak. In that period, there were only three outbreaks affecting more than 10 people, but in 1977, an outbreak of 59 cases involving type B botulinum toxin was described, caused by food eaten in a restaurant (Terranova *et al.*, 1978). Figure 3 illustrates the reported cases and deaths by year in the US during the period 1960–1980 (PAHO, 1982). More than half of the cases reported since 1899 from 45 states occurred in five western states. Table 1 shows the foods and type of botulinum toxin that caused the illness. In the United States, only 4% of the outbreaks originated in restaurants, but they represent 42% of the 308 cases occurring between 1976 and 1984. The most widespread outbreak recorded in the United States

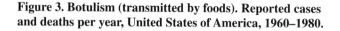

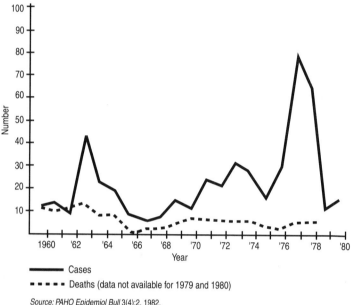

Figure 3. Botulism (transmitted by foods). Reported cases and deaths per year, United States of America, 1960–1980.

occurred in Michigan in 1977, when 59 people became sick after eating restaurant food that had been home-canned and contained botulinum toxin B (MacDonald *et al.*, 1986). In Canada, between 1979 and 1980, 15 incidents were investigated (PAHO, 1982). In Argentina, during the period 1967–1981, 139 cases were reported (Figure 4). In 1958, several suspected cases of botulism occurred in Brazil when six members of the same family died and others became ill after eating home-canned boiled fish. In 1981, two other suspected cases occurred in Rio de Janeiro, caused by ingestion of an industrially processed food.

In Europe and Asia, the occurrence of the illness varies from one country to another. In Poland, which seems to be the country hardest hit by botulism, the majority of cases have occurred in rural areas, as they have in other countries. From 1979 to 1983, there were a total of 2,390 cases and 45 deaths, with an average of 478 cases per year (Hauschild, 1989). The largest outbreak known to date took place in Dniepropetrovsk (former USSR), in 1933, with 230 cases and 94 deaths. More recently, about 14 outbreaks per year have occurred. In France, botulism is infrequent, with about four outbreaks annually. However, during World War II, 500 outbreaks were recorded with more than 1,000 cases in that country. Germany is second to Poland in the incidence of the illness. In the rest of Europe botulism is rare. During the period 1958–1983, there were 986 outbreaks, 4,377 cases, and 548 deaths in China; most of the cases (81%) occurred in the northwest province of Xinjiang (Ying *et al.*, 1986). During the period 1951–1984, there were 96 outbreaks,

Table 1. Foods giving rise to botulism, and number of outbreaks, United States of America, 1899–1977.[a, b]

Type of botulinum toxin	Vegetables	Fish and fish products	Fruits	Condi-ments[c]	Beef[d]	Milk and milk products	Pork	Fowl	Others[e]	Unknown[e]	Total
A	115	11	22	17	6	3	2	2	8	9	195
B	31	4	7	5	1	2	1	2	3	3	59
E	1	25	—	—	1	—	—	—	3	1	30
F	—	—	—	—	—	—	—	—	—	—	1
A and B	2	—	—	1	—	—	—	—	—	—	2
Unknown[e]	2	1	—	1	—	—	—	—	—	6	10
Total	151	41	29	23	8	5	3	4	14	19	297

[a]For the period 1899–1973, only outbreaks in which the type of toxin was confirmed are included; for 1974–1977, all outbreaks are included.
[b]Prepared by the Centers for Disease Control and Prevention, Atlanta, Georgia, USA.
[c]Includes outbreaks caused by tomato condiments, hot sauces, and salad dressings.
[d]Includes one type F outbreak caused by venison, and one type A outbreak caused by mutton.
[e]Categories added for the period 1974–1977.

Source: PAHO Epidemiol Bull 3(4):2, 1982.

Figure 4. Reported cases of botulism per year, Argentina, 1967–1981.

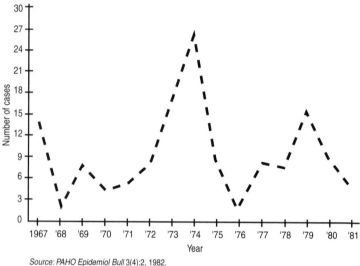

Source: PAHO Epidemiol Bull 3(4):2, 1982.

478 cases, and 109 deaths in Japan (Hauschild, 1989). In the rest of Asia and in Africa, few cases have been identified (Smith, 1977).

Infant botulism was recognized for the first time in the United States, and then in Canada, several European countries, and Australia. From 1976 to 1980, 184 cases were recorded in the United States, 88 of which occurred in California and 96 in 25 other states. Currently, infant botulism is the predominant form in the United States, with approximately 100 cases reported each year (Suen *et al.*, 1988). The disease has also been described in Argentina, Australia, Canada, the former Czechoslovakia, Great Britain, and Italy. Almost all cases occurred in children under 6 months of age (Morris, 1983) though some occurred in children up to 1 year.

The first case of wound botulism was recognized in the United States in 1943. By 1982, 27 cases were recorded, 20 of them in states west of the Mississippi River (CDC, 1982). In 1986, MacDonald *et al.* reported on the incidence of botulism in the United States between 1976 and 1984, including 16 cases of wound botulism (two of these in drug addicts using intravenous drugs).

Occurrence in Animals: Botulism in animals, including birds, is caused by types C (C alpha and C beta) and D, but there are also outbreaks due to A, E, and B. Botulism in bovines is becoming economically important in some areas, where it can affect a large number of animals. Such areas, generally poor in phosphorus, are found in the southwestern United States, in Corrientes province in Argentina, and in Piaui and Matto Grosso in Brazil. However, bovine botulism occurs even more frequently in South Africa ("lamziekte") and Australia. It is also important in Senegal, where it is believed to cause more cattle loss than any other disease. In other countries, sporadic outbreaks and cases occur, primarily caused by ingestion of fodder and silage containing the preformed toxins (Smith, 1977). Recently, various important outbreaks have been recorded due to consumption of bedding silage and bird droppings. In Great Britain, 80 out of 150 stabled cattle became sick and 68 died. Type C toxin was detected in 18 of the 22 sera examined and the same toxin was confirmed in the remains of dead chickens found in the silage (McLoughlin *et al.*, 1988). Similar outbreaks also occurred in Brazil and Canada because the bird bedding used to feed the cattle contained the type C toxin (Bienvenue *et al.*, 1990; Schocken-Iturrino *et al.*, 1990). Animal remains are usually found when botulism outbreaks occur in cattle, especially due to silage; however, no animal remains could be found in the fodder in various cases in the United States and Europe.

Bovine poisoning by type B is rare; outbreaks have occurred in Europe (Blood *et al.*, 1983), the United States (Divers *et al.*, 1986), and Brazil (Lobato *et al.*, 1988).

Botulism in sheep is due to type C and has been identified only in western Australia and South Africa.

In horses, botulism cases are sporadic and for the most part are caused by *C. botulinum* type C. It has been diagnosed in various European countries, the US, Israel, Australia, and South Africa. A special form occurs in colts at 6 to 8 weeks old ("shaker foal syndrome"); it is due to the type B neurotoxin and its pathogenesis is similar to botulism in children, since apparently *C. botulinum* has to colonize first in the intestine and other sites in order to produce the neurotoxin later. Outbreaks of this form have been described in the United States and Australia (Thomas *et al.*, 1988).

Botulism in swine is rare because of the natural high resistance of this species to botulinum toxin. Outbreaks diagnosed in Senegal and Australia were caused by type C beta and one in the United States was caused by type B.

Botulism in mink can be an important problem owing to their eating habits, if they are not vaccinated as recommended. Mink are highly susceptible to type C, which causes almost all the outbreaks.

Botulism in fowl occurs practically worldwide and is caused principally by type C alpha. Outbreaks of types A and E have been recorded in waterfowl. In the western United States, type C is responsible for massive outbreaks in wild ducks during the summer and early fall. Many other species of wild fowl are susceptible to botulism and outbreaks also occur in domestic chickens and farm-bred pheasants (Smith, 1977). Botulism in domestic fowl has been related to cannibalism and the ingestion of maggots in decomposing carcasses. The explanation is that the body temperature of fowl (41°C) favors the type C toxin, which would be produced and absorbed in the caecum, whose pH of 7.4 also favors the toxin (Castro *et al.*, 1988).

Botulism in dogs is rare and is caused primarily by ingesting bird carcasses, with type C being responsible for the disease (Hatheway and McCroskey, 1981).

The Disease in Man: (a) Botulism poisoning by foods is produced primarily by types A, B, and E and rarely by F or G. Outbreaks in man described as type C have not been confirmed, as the toxin has not been found in the patients' blood or feces nor in foods they ate. An outbreak of type D was identified in Chad, Africa, among people who had eaten raw ham (Smith, 1977). A new toxicogenic type, *C. botulinum* type G, was isolated from the soil in Argentina in 1969 (Giménez and Ciccarelli, 1970). The first human cases were recognized in Switzerland (Sonnabend *et al.*, 1981). The microorganism was isolated in autopsy specimens from four adults and an 18-week-old child. In addition, the presence of the toxin could be confirmed in the blood serum of three of these persons who died suddenly at home. The symptoms were similar to those of classic botulism. Nine additional cases of sudden and unexpected death were described (Sonnabend *et al.*, 1985).

The incubation period is usually from 18 to 36 hours, but the illness can show up within a few hours or as long as eight days after ingestion of the contaminated food. The clinical signs of the different types vary little, although the mortality rate seems to be higher for type A. The disease is afebrile, and gastrointestinal symptoms, such as nausea, vomiting, and abdominal pain, precede neurological symptoms. Neurological manifestations are always symmetrical, with weakness or descending paralysis. Diplopia, dysarthria, and dysphagia are common. Consciousness and sensibility remain intact until death. The immediate cause of death is usually respiratory failure. The mortality rate in botulinum poisonings is high. The highest rate is recorded in patients with short incubation periods, i.e., those who have ingested a high dose of the toxin. In the United States, the fatality rate has been reduced from 60% in 1899–1949 to 15.7% in 1970–1977, by means of early and proper treatment. In patients who survive, complete recovery, especially of ocular movement, may take as long as six to eight months.

Treatment should be initiated as soon as possible through administration of the trivalent botulinum antitoxin (A, B, and E). The patient must be hospitalized in intensive care in order to anticipate and treat respiratory distress, which is the immediate cause of death (Benenson, 1990).

(b) Infant botulism is an intestinal infection caused by the ingestion of *C. botulinum* spores, which change in the intestine into the vegetative form, multiply, and produce toxins. Of 96 cases studied (Morris *et al.*, 1983) in the United States, excluding California, 41 were caused by *C. botulinum* type A, 53 by type B, one by type F, and another by type B together with F. Type A appeared almost exclusively in the western states, while type B predominated in the East. This distribution is similar to that of the spores in the environment (see the section on source of poisoning or infection and mode of transmission). In addition, two cases in Italy due to type E produced by *Clostridium butyricum* and one case in New Mexico (USA) due to type F produced by *Clostridium baratii* have been described; i.e., by two species other than *C. botulinum* (see section on etiology). The case of a girl under age 6 months with paroxystic dyspnea due to *C. botulinum* type C toxin was also described. The child survived the illness, but may have been left with a cerebral lesion probably caused by hypoxia (Oguma *et al.*, 1990). Sonnabend *et al.* (1985) had previously identified the bacteria and C toxin in the colon of a child who died suddenly in Switzerland.

The fact that *C. botulinum* primarily colonizes the caecum and colon, and that 96% of patients with infant botulism are under 6 months of age led to research on the characteristics of the intestinal microflora that allow the clostridium to multiply. Using a normal mouse as a model, it was established that the microflora in adults prevent the establishment of *C. botulinum*; however, if adult "germ-free" mice are used, the clostridium multiplies in their intestines. The same thing happens to conventional mice from 7 to 13 days old, which are very susceptible. In addition, breastfed infants have feces with a lower pH (5.1–5.4) than those fed with formula (pH 5.9–8.0). This difference may be significant, because the multiplication of *C. botulinum* declines as pH falls and ceases below 4.6. In addition, breast-feeding has the advantage of transferring immunogenic factors to the infant (Arnon, 1986). Another important factor seems to be the frequency of defecation: of 58 patients who were at least 1 month old, 37 (64%) had a usual pattern of one defecation per day, as compared to 17 (15%) of the 115 in the control group (Spika *et al.*, 1989).

In adults, botulism may occur without the presence of preformed toxin in food: it may occur through colonization of the large intestine by *C. botulinum*, the production of toxins, and their absorption. Such cases are rare and primarily affect those who have alterations in intestinal structure and microflora.

The disease in infants begins with constipation, followed by lethargy and loss of appetite, ptosis, difficulty swallowing, muscular weakness, and loss of head control. Neuromuscular paralysis may progress from the cranial nerves to the peripheral and respiratory muscles, resulting in death. The severity of the illness varies from moderate to life-threatening, causing sudden death of the child. It has been estimated that infant botulism is responsible for at least 5% of the cases of sudden infant death syndrome (Benenson, 1990).

(c) Wound botulism is clinically similar to classic botulism in its neurological syndrome. It is a toxin infection produced as the result of a contaminated wound that creates anaerobic conditions where *C. botulinum* can become established, reproduce, and develop a neurotoxin that is absorbed by the vessels. Of the 27 known cases, 15 were associated with type A, 5 with type B, 1 with both A and B, and one was undetermined.

The Disease in Animals: Botulism in domestic mammals is caused primarily by types C and D, and in fowl, by type C. Outbreaks in bovines are usually associated with a phosphorus deficiency and the resultant osteophagea and compulsive consumption ("pica") of carrion containing botulinum toxins. In locations where types C beta and D are found, such as South Africa, *C. botulinum* spores multiply rapidly in carrion and produce toxins to which bovines are very susceptible. The main symptom is the partial or complete paralysis of the locomotor, masticatory, and swallowing muscles. The animals have difficulty moving, stay motionless or recumbent for long periods of time, and, as the illness progresses, cannot hold their heads up and so bend their necks over their flanks. The mortality rate is high.

In sheep, botulism is associated with protein and carbohydrate deficiencies, which lead the animals to eat the carcasses of small animals they find as they graze.

In horses, as in other mammals, the incubation period varies widely according to the amount of toxin ingested. In very acute cases, death may ensue in one or two days. When the course is slower, the disease generally begins with paralysis of the hind quarters and progresses to other regions of the body until it produces death due to respiratory failure. A toxin infection similar to infant botulism and wound botulism has been described in young colts. The neuromuscular paralytic syndrome affects colts from 2 to 8 weeks old; they show signs of progressive motor paralysis that includes muscular tremors (shaker foal syndrome), dysphagia with flaccid paralysis of the tongue, difficulty remaining on their feet, a tendency to collapse, dyspnea, mydriasis, and constipation (Thomas *et al.*, 1988). Sometimes they die without signs of disease ("sudden death"). The disease is produced by the type B toxin that requires prior colonization of *C. botulinum* in gastric, intestinal, umbilical, hepatic (necrosis), muscular, or subcutaneous lesions. Necrotic lesions seem to be necessary for toxicity, as in wound botulism in man (Swerczek, 1980).

Outbreaks with high death rates have been observed on mink farms. Food poisoning in these animals is due primarily to type C beta.

In ducks and other waterfowl, the first symptom of poisoning is paralysis of the wings, which then extends to other muscles, and finally to those of the neck. The birds drown when they can no longer hold their heads above water. An outbreak due to type E occurred in waterfowl on Lake Michigan (USA).

The illness in chickens is produced mainly by type C alpha. It has been given the name "limberneck" because flaccid paralysis is frequently observed in afflicted birds.

Treatment with botulinum antitoxin produced variable results in bovines. Better results were obtained from antitoxin C in mink and ducks, but the cost can be excessive. Control and prevention must be the principal tools for combating losses due to animal botulism.

Source of Poisoning or Infection and Mode of Transmission: The reservoir of *C. botulinum* is the soil, river and sea sediments, vegetables, and the intestinal tracts of mammals and birds. The spores formed by the bacteria are very resistant to heat and desiccation. The etiologic agent is distributed on all continents, though irregularly. The distribution of the toxicogenic types also varies according to region. In a study (Smith, 1978) carried out across the United States, subdividing it into four transverse sections, *C. botulinum* was found in 23.5% of 260 soil samples. Type A was most prevalent in the western states with neutral or alkaline soil. Type B had a more uniform distribution, but predominated in the East, a pattern which seems to be associated with highly organic soils. Type C was found in acid soils on the Gulf Coast, type D in some alkaline soils in the West, and type E in the humid soils of several states. In the former Soviet Union, *C. botulinum* was isolated from 10.5% of 4,242 soil samples, with type E accounting for 61% of all positive cultures. The greatest concentration of spores was found in the European section of the country south of 52° N latitude (Kravchenko and Shishulina, 1967).

The wide distribution of *C. botulinum* in nature explains its presence in food. Vegetables are contaminated directly from the soil. Foods of animal origin are probably contaminated via the animals' intestinal tract and by spores in the environment. The main source of botulinum poisoning for man and animals is food in which the microorganism has multiplied and produced the powerful toxin. After ingestion, the toxin is absorbed through the intestine, primarily the upper portion, and carried by the bloodstream to the nerves. It acts upon the presynaptic union of cholinergic nerve endings by inhibiting the release of acetylcholine.

Any food, whether of vegetable or animal origin, can give rise to botulism if conditions favor the multiplication of *C. botulinum* and, consequently, the production of toxins. The main requirements for the multiplication of *C. botulinum* are anaerobiosis and a pH above 4.5, but once the toxin is formed an acid medium can be favorable. Home-canned foods are generally responsible for the disease, although incorrectly sterilized or preserved commercial products are sometimes the cause. Poisoning ensues after eating a raw or insufficiently cooked product that was preserved some time earlier. The types of food responsible for poisoning vary according to regional eating habits.

The most common sources of types A and B botulism in the United States and Canada are home-canned fruits and vegetables. In Europe, on the other hand, meat and meat products seem to play the most important role. In Japan, the former Soviet Union, the northern United States, Alaska, and northern Canada, type E, which is associated with foods of marine origin, predominates.

Ethnic customs and food habits often favor food poisoning. In 1992, a family of Egyptian origin living in New Jersey (USA) became sick from type E botulism after consuming "moloha," an uneviscerated salt-cured fish (CDC, 1992). There had been an earlier outbreak in which two Russian immigrants in New York and five people in Israel became ill with type E botulism; all of them had eaten uneviscerated salt-cured, air-dried fish ("ribyetz") from the same source (CDC, 1989). A preserved regional dish that is popular in the Orient, a soft cheese prepared with soy milk, led to 705 (71.5%) of the 986 outbreaks of botulism recorded in China (Ying and Shuan, 1986).

In contrast to classic botulism (acquired through foods), infant botulism begins as an intestinal infection caused by C. botulinum, where the spores germinate, multiply, and produce the toxin that is absorbed through the intestinal wall. Honey has been implicated as a source of infection, since it is frequently a supplementary food for the nursing child. However, results of research on the presence of botulinum spores in this food, as well as epidemiological investigations, are inconclusive. In any case, there is no doubt that the infection is caused by ingestion.

The source of wound botulism is environmental. Botulism in bovines results from grazing ("lamziekte") or the consumption of bailed fodder or silage. Poisoning contracted while grazing usually occurs in areas lacking or deficient in phosphorus. Many species of animals in the area contain C. botulinum in their intestinal flora; when an animal dies, these bacteria invade the whole organism and produce great quantities of toxin. Bovines suffering from pica ingest animal remains containing the preformed toxin and contract botulism. After dying, these same bovines are a source of poisoning for the rest of the herd. Mortality in cattle has also been ascribed to drinking water that contained the decomposed bodies of small animals. Botulism contracted through the consumption of fodder or silage is produced by the accidental presence of a small animal's body (usually a cat) or the remains of birds and the diffusion of the botulinum toxin around them into the food (Smith, 1977). The sources of poisoning for other mammalian species are similar.

For wild ducks, the source of poisoning is insect larvae that invade the bodies of ducks that died from various causes. If a duck had C. botulinum in its intestinal flora, the bacteria invades the whole organism after its death. The larvae then absorb the toxin produced, constituting a source of toxin for birds. It is estimated that a duck need only ingest a few such larvae for death by botulism to ensue.

Research on outbreaks among pheasants has found that they ate maggots from the bodies of small animals.

Role of Animals in the Epidemiology of the Disease: No epidemiological relationship between human and animal botulism has been established. C. botulinum type A spores have been isolated from animal feces, and types A and B botulism microorganisms have been found in the intestine and liver of bovines that died from other causes. The microorganism has also been isolated from the intestine and bone marrow of healthy dogs. Thus the possibility exists that these animals are carriers of the microorganism and serve to transport and disseminate C. botulinum from one place to another.

Diagnosis: Clinical diagnosis should be confirmed with laboratory tests. The most conclusive evidence is the presence of botulinum toxin in the serum of the patient. Stomach contents and fecal material of persons exposed to the suspected food should also be examined for the toxin. The food in question should be cultured to isolate and identify the microorganism. In infant botulism, the attempt is made to isolate the agent and the toxin from the infant's feces, since the toxin is rarely detected in serum. An enzyme-linked immunosorbent assay (ELISA) test has been developed for the detection of A and B toxin in children's fecal samples; this may be useful as a screening test in clinical specimens (Dezfulian *et al.*, 1984). When a wound is the suspected origin of the poisoning, fluid is aspirated from the wound and biopsies are performed for bacteriological examination.

Control: With regard to man, control measures include: (a) regulation and inspection of industrial bottling, canning, and food-preserving processes, and (b) health education to point out the dangers of home canning and to make the public aware of important factors in the preservation of home products, such as duration, pressure, and temperature of sterilization. Home-canned foods should be boiled before being served to destroy the toxins that are thermolabile. Foods from swollen cans or food altered in taste, smell, or appearance should not be eaten even after cooking. Any food that is bottled, canned, or prepared in some other way (salted, dried, etc.) and has led to a case or outbreak should be seized.

Immediate epidemiological investigation and prompt diagnosis of an outbreak are essential to both the prevention of new cases and the recovery of the patient.

In areas where botulism in animals is a problem, the diet of livestock should be supplemented with feed rich in phosphorus to avoid osteophagia or pica; vaccination of animals with the appropriate toxoid can yield good results. When bird bedding is used as silage for cattle or for pasture fertilizer, any remains of birds or other animals should be carefully eliminated. When an outbreak occurs in a fowl facility, carcasses must be removed as soon as possible to prevent its progression.

Bibliography

Arnon, S.S. Infant botulism: Anticipating the second decade. *J Infect Dis* 154:201–206, 1986.

Aureli, P.L., F.B. Pasolini, M. Gianfranceschi, *et al.* Two cases of type E infant botulism caused by neurotoxigenic *Clostridium butyricum* in Italy. *J Infect Dis* 154:207–211, 1986.

Benenson, A.S., ed. *Control of Communicable Diseases in Man.* 15th ed. An official report of the American Public Health Association. Washington, D.C.: American Public Health Association; 1990.

Bienvenue, J.G., M. Morin, S. Forget. Poultry litter associated botulism (type C) in cattle. *Can Vet J* 31:711, 1990.

Blood, D.C., O.M. Radostits, J.A. Henderson. *Veterinary Medicine.* 6th ed. London: Baillière Tindall; 1983.

Castro, A.G.M., A.M. Carvalho, L. Baldassi, *et al.* Botulismo em aves de postura no estado de São Paulo. *Arq Inst Biol* 55:1–4, 1988.

Cato, E.P., W.L. George, S.N. Finegold. Clostridium. *In:* Sneath, P.H.A., N.S. Mair, M.E. Sharpe, J.G. Holt, eds. *Bergey's Manual of Systemic Bacteriology.* Vol 2. Baltimore: Williams & Wilkins; 1986.

Ciccarelli, A.S., D.F. Giménez. Clinical and epidemiological aspects of botulism in Argentina. *In:* Lewis, G.E., Jr., ed. *Biomedical Aspects of Botulism.* New York: Academic Press; 1981.

Concon, J.M. Part B: Contaminants and additives. *In: Food Toxicology*. New York: Marcel Dekker; 1988.

Dezfulian, M., C.L. Hatheway, R.H. Yolken, J.G. Bartlett. Enzyme-linked immunosorbent assay for detection of *Clostridium botulinum* type A and type B toxins in stool samples of infants with botulism. *J Clin Microbiol* 20:379–383, 1984.

Divers, T.J., R.C. Bartholomew, J.B. Messick, *et al. Clostridium botulinum* type B toxicosis in a herd of cattle and a group of mules. *J Am Vet Med Assoc* 188:382–386, 1986.

Giménez, D.F., A.S. Ciccarelli. Another type of *Clostridium botulinum*. *Zentralbl Bakteriol* 215:221–224, 1970.

Giménez, D.F., A.S. Ciccarelli. *Clostridium botulinum* en Argentina: presente y futuro. *Rev Asoc Argent Microbiol* 8:82–91, 1976.

Giménez, J.A., M.A. Giménez, B.R. Dasgupta. Characterization of the neurotoxin from a *Clostridium baratii* strain implicated in infant botulism. *Infect Immun* 60:518–522, 1992.

Hall, J.D., L.M. McCroskey, B.J. Pincomb, C.L. Hatheway. Isolation of an organism resembling *Clostridium barati* which produces type F botulinal toxin from an infant with botulism. *J Clin Microbiol* 21(4):654–655, 1985.

Hatheway, C.L., L.M. McCroskey. Laboratory investigation of human and animal botulism. *In*: Lewis, G.E., Jr., ed. *Biomedical Aspects of Botulism*. New York: Academic Press; 1981.

Hauschild, A.H. *Clostridium botulinum*. *In*: Doyle, M.P., ed. *Foodborne Bacterial Pathogens*. New York: Marcel Dekker; 1989.

Ingram, M., T.A. Roberts. *Botulism 1966*. London: Chapman & Hall; 1967.

Kravchenko, A.T., L.M. Shishulina. Distribution of *C. botulinum* in soil and water in the USSR. *In*: Ingram, M., T.A. Roberts, eds. *Botulism 1966*. London: Chapman & Hall; 1967.

Lobato, F.C.F., M.A. de Melo, N. de Silva, J.M. Diniz. Botulismo em bovinos causado pelo *Clostridium botulinum* tipo B [letter]. *Arq Brasil Med Vet Zootec* 40:445–446, 1988.

MacDonald, K.L., M.L. Cohen, P.A. Blake. The changing epidemiology of adult botulism in the United States. *Am J Epidemiol* 124:794–799, 1986.

McLoughlin, M.F., S.G. McIlroy, S.D. Neill. A major outbreak of botulism in cattle being fed ensiled poultry litter. *Vet Rec* 122:579–581, 1988.

Morris, J.G., J.D. Snyder, R. Wilson, R.A. Feldman. Infant botulism in the United States: An epidemiological study of cases occurring outside of California. *Am J Public Health* 73:1385–1388, 1983.

Oguma, K., K. Yokota, S. Hyashi, *et al.* Infant botulism due to *Clostridium botulinum* type C toxin. *Lancet* 336:1449–1450, 1990.

Pan American Health Organization (PAHO). Botulism in the Americas. *Epidemiol Bull* 3(4):1–3, 1982.

Prévot, A.R., A. Turpin, P. Kaiser. *Les bactéries anaérobies*. Paris: Dunod; 1967.

Riemann, H. Botulism: Types A, B, and F. *In*: Riemann, H., ed. *Food-borne Infections and Intoxications*. New York: Academic Press; 1969.

Sakaguchi, G., I. Ohishi, S. Kozaki. Purification and oral toxicities of *Clostridium botulinum* progenitor toxins. *In*: Lewis, G.E., Jr., ed. *Biomedical Aspects of Botulism*. New York: Academic Press; 1981.

Schocken-Iturrino, R.P., F.A. Avila, S.C.P. Berchielli, *et al.* Cama de frango contaminada con toxina botulínica. *Ciencia Vet Jaboticabal* 4:11–12, 1990.

Smith, L.D. Clostridial diseases of animals. *Adv Vet Sci* 3:463–524, 1957.

Smith, L.D. *Botulism: The Organism, its Toxins, the Disease*. Springfield: Thomas; 1977.

Smith, L.D. The occurrence of *Clostridium botulinum* and *Clostridium tetani* in the soil of the United States. *Health Lab Sci* 15:74–80, 1978.

Sonnabend, O., W. Sonnabend, R. Heinzle, T. Sigrist, R. Dirnohofer, U. Krech. Isolation of *Clostridium botulinum* type G and identification of type G botulinal toxin in humans: Report of five sudden unexpected deaths. *J Infect Dis* 143:22–27, 1981.

Sonnabend, O.A., W.F. Sonnabend, U. Krech, *et al.* Continuous microbiological and pathological study on 70 sudden and unexpected infant deaths: Toxigenic intestinal *Clostridium botulinum* infection in 9 cases of sudden infant death syndrome. *Lancet* 2:237–241, 1985.

Spika, J.S., N. Schaffer, N. Hargrett-Bean, *et al.* Risk factors for infant botulism in the United States. *Am J Dis Child* 143:828–832, 1989.

Suen, J.C., C.L. Hatheway, A.G. Steigerwalt, D.J. Brenner. Genetic confirmation of identities of neurotoxigenic *Clostridium baratii* and *Clostridium butyricum* implicated as agents of infant botulism. *J Clin Microbiol* 26:2191–2192, 1988a.

Suen, J.C., C.L. Hatheway, A.G. Steigerwalt, D.J. Brenner. *Clostridium argentinense* sp nov; a genetically homogenous group of all strains of *Clostridium botulinum* toxin type G and some nontoxigenic strains previously identified as *Clostridium subterminale* and *Clostridium hastiforme*. *Int J Syst Bacteriol* 38:375–381, 1988b.

Swerczek, T.W. Toxicoinfectious botulism in foals and adult horses. *J Am Vet Med Assoc* 176:217–220, 1980.

Terranova, W., J.G. Breman, R.P. Locey, S. Speck. Botulism type B: Epidemiologic aspects of an extensive outbreak. *Am J Epidemiol* 180:150–156, 1978.

Thomas, R.J., D.V. Rosenthal, R.J. Rogers. A *Clostridium botulinum* type B vaccine for prevention of shaker foal syndrome. *Aust Vet J* 65:78–80, 1988.

United States of America, Department of Health and Human Services, Centers for Disease Control and Prevention (CDC). *Botulism in the United States 1899–1973. Handbook for Epidemiologists, Clinicians, and Laboratory Workers.* Atlanta: CDC; 1974.

United States of America, Department of Health and Human Services, Centers for Disease Control and Prevention (CDC). Wound botulism associated with parenteral cocaine abuse. *MMWR Morb Mortal Wkly Rep* 31:87–88, 1982.

United States of America, Department of Health and Human Services, Centers for Disease Control and Prevention (CDC). International outbreak of type E botulism associated with ungutted, salted whitefish. *MMWR Morb Mortal Wkly Rep* 36:812–813, 1987.

United States of America, Department of Health and Human Services, Centers for Disease Control and Prevention (CDC). Outbreak of type E botulism associated with an uneviscerated, salt-cured fish product—New Jersey, 1992. *MMWR Morb Mortal Wkly Rep* 41:521–522, 1992.

Ying, S., C. Shuan. Botulism in China. *Rev Infec Dis* 8:984–990, 1986.

BRUCELLOSIS

ICD-10 A23.0 brucellosis due to *Brucella melitensis*; A23.1 brucellosis due to *Brucella abortus*; A23.2 brucellosis due to *Brucella suis*; A23.3 brucellosis due to *Brucella canis*

Synonyms: Melitococcosis, undulant fever, Malta fever, Mediterranean fever (in man); contagious abortion, infectious abortion, epizootic abortion (in animals); Bang's disease (in cattle).

Etiology: Six species are presently known in the genus *Brucella*: *B. melitensis*, *B. abortus*, *B. suis*, *B. neotomae*, *B. ovis*, and *B. canis*.

The first three species (called "classic brucella") have been subdivided into biovars that are distinguished by their different biochemical characteristics and/or reactions to the monospecific *A.* (*abortus*) and *M.* (*melitensis*) sera. Thus, *B. melitensis* is subdivided into three biovars (1–3); *B. abortus*, into seven (1–7)—biovars 7 and 8 were discarded and the current biovar 7 corresponds to 9 in the old classification; and *B. suis*, into five (1–5). From an epidemiological viewpoint, the taxonomic system of the genus *Brucella* has eliminated confusion arising from the naming of new species or subspecies that did not agree with epidemiological reality. Moreover, typing by biovars constitutes a useful research tool in that field. The characteristics of *B. abortus* determined by conventional methods vary greatly, such as sensitivity or tolerance to aniline dyes, production of H_2S, and CO_2 requirements for growth. Less plasticity is shown by *B. melitensis* or *B. suis* (Meyer, 1984). In various parts of the world, strains of *B. abortus* and, to a lesser extent, of *B. suis* or *B. melitensis* have been discovered that are difficult to place within the current scheme, in that they differ in some characteristics (Ewalt and Forbes, 1987; Corbel *et al.*, 1984; Banai *et al.*, 1990).

However, the genome of the genus *Brucella* is very homogeneous as shown by Verger *et al.* (1985) in a DNA:DNA hybridization study. These researchers propose maintaining a single species, *B. melitensis*, subdivided into six biogroups, which would correspond to the six previous species. For all practical purposes, and especially for epidemiological purposes, the previous scheme that divides the genus into species and biovars is still in effect.

Geographic Distribution: Worldwide. The distribution of the different species of *Brucella* and their biovars varies with geographic areas. *B. abortus* is the most widespread; *B. melitensis* and *B. suis* are irregularly distributed; *B. neotomae* was isolated from desert rats (*Neotoma lepida*) in Utah (USA), and its distribution is limited to natural foci, as the infection has never been confirmed in man or domestic animals. Infection by *B. canis* has been confirmed in many countries on several continents, and its worldwide distribution can be asserted. *B. ovis* seems to be found in all countries where sheep raising is an important activity.

Occurrence in Man: Each year about a half million cases of brucellosis occur in humans around the world (WHO, 1975). The prevalence of the infection in animal reservoirs provides a key to its occurrence in humans. *B. abortus* and *B. suis* infections usually affect occupational groups, while *B. melitensis* infections occur more frequently than the other types in the general population. The greatest prevalence in man is found in those countries with a high incidence of *B. melitensis* infection among goats, sheep, or both species. The Latin American countries with the largest number of recorded cases are Argentina, Mexico, and Peru. The same pattern holds true for Mediterranean countries, Iran, the former Soviet Union, and Mongolia.

In Saudi Arabia, 7,893 human cases of brucellosis were recorded in 1987 (74 per 100,000 inhabitants). Brucellosis probably became very important in public health because during the period 1979 to 1987, Saudi Arabia imported more than 8 million sheep, more than 2 million goats, more than 250,000 cattle, and other animals (buffalo, camels). In Iran, 71,051 cases (13 per 100,000) were recorded in 1988 and it is estimated that 80,000 cases have occurred each year since 1989. In Turkey, 5,003 cases (9 per 100,000) were recorded in 1990, an incidence three times higher than during the period 1986–1989 (3 per 100,000).

Programs for the control and eradication of bovine brucellosis markedly reduce the incidence of disease in humans. For example, in the United States, 6,321 cases were recorded in 1947, while in the period 1972–1981, the annual average was 224 cases (CDC, 1982). In Denmark, where some 500 cases per year were reported between 1931 and 1939, human brucellosis had disappeared by 1962 as a result of the eradication of the infection in animals. In Uruguay, where there is no animal reservoir of *B. melitensis* and where the few foci of *B. suis* had been eliminated (although they have recently been reintroduced through importation), the disease in humans has almost disappeared since compulsory vaccination of calves was begun in 1964. China and Israel have been able to significantly reduce the incidence of human brucellosis thanks to vaccination campaigns for sheep and goats. In the western Mediterranean area, there has also been a marked reduction of human brucellosis cases caused by *B. melitensis* due to vaccination of the small ruminants with the Rev. 1 vaccine. In Spain, for example, the incidence fell from 4,683 cases in 1988 to 3,041 in 1990.

Occurrence in Animals: Bovine brucellosis is found worldwide, but it has been eradicated in Finland, Norway, Sweden, Denmark, the Netherlands, Belgium, Switzerland, Germany, Austria, Hungary, the former Czechoslovakia, Rumania, and Bulgaria, as well as other countries (Timm, 1982; Kasyanov and Aslanyan, 1982). Most European countries are free of bovine brucellosis (García-Carrillo and Lucero, 1993). The large meat-producing countries, such as France, Great Britain, Australia, New Zealand, Canada, and the United States, among others, are free of bovine brucellosis or close to being so. Three important cattle-raising countries, Argentina, Brazil, and Mexico, still have limited control programs. A country-by-country analysis can be found in a monograph on bovine brucellosis (García-Carrillo and Lucero, 1993). In the rest of the world, rates of infection vary greatly from one country to another and between regions within a country. The highest prevalence is seen in dairy cattle. In many countries, including most of those Latin American countries that have no control programs, the data are unreliable. Nevertheless, available information indicates that it is one of the most serious diseases in cattle in Latin America as well as in other developing areas. Official estimates put annual losses from bovine brucellosis in Latin America at approximately US$ 600 million, which explains the priority given by animal health services to control of this disease.

Swine brucellosis is infrequent and occurs sporadically in most of Europe, Asia, and Oceania. In China, *B. suis* biovar 3 was introduced with breeding stock from Hong Kong in 1954 and spread rapidly through the southern part of the country (Lu and Zhang, 1989). In many European countries, swine brucellosis shows an epidemiological relationship to brucellosis caused by *B. suis* biovar 2 in hares (*Lepus europaeus*). With the new swine-breeding technology, swine have little access to hares and outbreaks have thus shown a marked decline. The disease has never been present in Finland, Norway, Great Britain, and Canada. Many predominantly Muslim countries and Israel are probably free of *B. suis* infection as a result of religious beliefs that have limited swine raising (Timm, 1982).

In most of Latin America, swine brucellosis is enzootic and, while the available data have little statistical value, this region is thought to have the highest prevalence in the world. However, recent surveys of breeding operations for purebreds and hybrids in Argentina and Rio Grande do Sul (Brazil) have shown the percentage of infected herds to be low. The problem is possibly rooted in commercial operations where animals of different origins are brought together. Thus far, only *B. suis* biovar 1, which predominates worldwide, has been confirmed from Latin America. Biovar 2 is limited to pigs and hares in central and western Europe, while biovar 3 is limited to the corn belt of the United States and to some areas of Asia and Africa. The US and Cuba have successful national eradication programs.

Goat and sheep brucellosis constitute a significant problem in the Mediterranean basin of Europe and Africa, in the southeastern part of the former Soviet Union, in Mongolia, in the Middle East, and Saudi Arabia. In Latin America, the prevalence of *B. melitensis* infection in goats is high in Argentina, Mexico, and Peru. To date, sheep infection with *B. melitensis* in Argentina has been identified only in flocks living with infected goats in the north of the country (Ossola and Szyfres, 1963). In Venezuela's goat-raising region, a serological and bacteriological examination was conducted in 1987. *B. abortus* biovar 1 was isolated from milk and lymph nodes. *B. melitensis* was not isolated (De Lord *et al.*, 1987). Goat brucellosis does not appear to exist in Brazil, which has a sizable number of goats. In Chile, where the rate of infection in Cajón de Maipo was significant, the Government reported that the disease had been eradicated (Chile, Ministerio de Agricultura, 1987). Other American countries, including the US, are free of goat brucellosis at the present time.

Ram epididymitis caused by *B. ovis* is widespread. It has been confirmed in New Zealand, Australia, Africa, and Europe. It is present in Argentina, Brazil (Rio Grande do Sul), Chile, Peru, Uruguay, and the US, i.e., in all American countries where sheep are raised on a large scale. Prevalence is high.

Infection of dogs with *B. canis* has been found in almost every country in the world where it has been studied. Prevalence varies according to region and diagnostic method used. It constitutes a problem for some dog breeders, since it causes abortions and infertility, but the infection is also found in family dogs and strays. In the latter, the incidence of infection is usually higher. In a study carried out in Mexico City, for example, 12% of 59 stray dogs were positive in the isolation of the etiologic agent (Flores-Castro *et al.*, 1977).

The Disease in Man: Man is susceptible to infection caused by *B. melitensis*, *B. suis*, *B. abortus*, and *B. canis*. No human cases caused by *B. ovis*, *B. neotomae*, or *B. suis* biovar 2 have been confirmed. The most pathogenic and invasive species for man is *B. melitensis*, followed in descending order by *B. suis*, *B. abortus*, and *B. canis*.

In general, the incubation period is one to three weeks, but may sometimes be several months. The disease is septicemic, with sudden or insidious onset, and is accompanied by continued, intermittent, or irregular fever. The symptomatology of acute brucellosis, like that of many other febrile diseases, includes chills and profuse sweating. Weakness is an almost constant symptom, and any exercise produces pronounced fatigue. Temperature can vary from normal in the morning to 40°C in the afternoon. Sweating characterized by a peculiar odor occurs at night. Common symptoms are insomnia, sexual impotence, constipation, anorexia, headache, arthralgia, and general malaise. The disease has a marked effect on the nervous system, evidenced by irritation, nervousness, and depression. Many patients have enlarged peripheral lymph nodes or splenomegaly and often hepatomegaly, but rarely jaundice. Hepatomegaly or hepatosplenomegaly is particularly frequent in patients infected by *B. melitensis* (Pfischner *et al.*, 1957). *Brucella* organisms localize intracellularly in tissues of the reticuloendothelial system, such as lymph nodes, bone marrow, spleen, and liver. Tissue reaction is granulomatous. The duration of the disease can vary from a few weeks or months to several years. Modern therapy has considerably reduced the disease's duration as well as the incidence of relapses. At times, it produces serious complications, such as encephalitis, meningitis, peripheral neuritis, spondylitis, suppurative arthritis, vegetative endocarditis, orchitis, seminal vesiculitis, and prostatitis. A chronic form of the disease occurs in some patients and may last many years, with or without the presence of localized foci of infection. The symptoms are associated with hypersensitivity. Diagnosis of chronic brucellosis is difficult.

Separate mention should be made of human infection caused by the *B. abortus* strain 19 vaccine, which is the vaccine used most often to protect cattle. Cases have been described of accidents among those administering the vaccine (veterinarians and assistants) who have pricked a finger or hand with the syringe needle or have gotten aerosol in their eyes. If someone has no prior exposure to brucellae and has no antibodies to the agent, the disease sets in abruptly after a period of 8 to 30 days. The course of the disease is usually shorter and more benign than that caused by the field strains of *B. abortus*, but there are severe cases that require hospitalization. In individuals who have been exposed to brucellae, as is usually the case with veterinarians and vaccinators, a different, allergic-type syndrome appears that is characterized by painful swelling at the inoculation site. After some hours, the patient may experience systemic symptoms similar to those described in individuals infected by strain 19 without prior exposure. The symptoms usually abate in a few days with or without treatment. Local and general symptoms may recur if the person has another accident (Young, 1989). Considering the millions of doses of strain 19 vaccine used each year throughout the world, the rate of incidence of the disease due to this strain is insignificant.

Another strain that is used to vaccinate small ruminants, *B. melitensis* Rev. 1, can also infect the vaccinator. Under the aegis of the World Health Organization (WHO) and its collaborative centers, Rev. 1 vaccine was administered to 6 million animals in Mongolia between 1974 and 1977. Six trained vaccinators inoculated themselves accidentally; four of them showed clinical symptoms but recovered after immediate hospital treatment.

There are many infections that occur asymptomatically in areas with enzootic brucellosis, particularly the bovine form.

The recommended treatment for acute brucellosis is a daily dose of 600 mg to 900 mg of rifampicin, combined with 200 mg per day of doxycycline for at least six weeks. Relapses are very rare with this treatment. If there is a Jarisch-Herxheimer reaction upon starting antibiotic treatment, intravenous administration of cortisol is recommended. Sometimes various series of treatment are needed. If antibiotic therapy is not successful, a chronic focus of infection should be sought, particularly in infections caused by *B. melitensis* and *B. suis* (WHO, 1986). In the event of a relapse, the treatment indicated above should be restarted. Steroids may be administered to counteract toxicity in patients who are very ill (Benenson, 1992).

The Disease in Animals: The principal symptom in all animal species is abortion or premature expulsion of the fetus.

CATTLE: The main pathogen is *B. abortus*. Biovar 1 is universal and predominant among the seven that occur in the world. The distribution of the different biovars varies geographically. In Latin America, biovars 1, 2, 3, 4, and 6 have been confirmed, with biovar 1 accounting for more than 80% of the isolations. In the United States, biovars 1, 2, and 4 have been isolated. In eastern Africa and China, biovar 3 predominates and affects both native cattle and buffalo (Timm, 1982). Biovar 5, which occurred in cattle in Great Britain and Germany, has biochemical and serological characteristics similar to *B. melitensis*. This similarity was a source of confusion for years until new methods of species identification (oxidative metabolism and phagocytolysis) established the biovar as *B. abortus*. The other biovars also have a more or less marked geographic distribution. Cattle can also become infected by *B. suis* and *B. melitensis* when they share pasture or facilities with infected pigs, goats, or sheep. The infection in cattle caused by heterologous species of *Brucella* are usually more transient than that caused by *B. abortus*. However, such cross-infections are a serious public health threat, since these brucellae, which are highly pathogenic for man, can pass into cow's milk. Infection caused by *B. suis* is not very common. By contrast, infections caused by *B. melitensis* have been seen in several countries, with a course similar to those caused by *B. abortus*.

In natural infections, it is difficult to measure the incubation period (from time of infection to abortion or premature birth), since it is not possible to determine the moment of infection. Experiments have shown that the incubation period varies considerably and is inversely proportional to fetal development: the more advanced the pregnancy, the shorter the incubation period. If the female is infected orally during the breeding period, the incubation period can last some 200 days, while if she is exposed six months after being bred, incubation time is approximately two months. The period of "serologic incubation" (from the time of infection to the appearance of antibodies) lasts several weeks to several months. The incubation period varies according to such factors as the virulence and dose of bacteria, the route of infection, and the susceptibility of the animal.

The predominant symptom in pregnant females is abortion or premature or full-term birth of dead or weak calves. In general, abortion occurs during the second half of the pregnancy, often with retention of the placenta and resultant metritis, which may cause permanent infertility. It is estimated that the infection causes a 20% to 25% loss in milk production as a result of interrupted lactation due to abortion and delayed conception. Cows artificially inseminated with infected semen may come into estrus repeatedly, as happens in cases of vibriosis or trichomoniasis. Nonpregnant females show no clinical symptoms and, if infected prior to breeding, often do not abort.

In bulls, brucellae may become localized in the testicles and adjacent genital glands. When the clinical disease is evident, one or both testicles may become enlarged, with decreased libido and infertility. Sometimes a testicle may atrophy due to adhesions and fibrosis. Seminal vesiculitis and ampullitis are common. Occasionally, hygromas and arthritis are observed in cattle.

Brucellae entering the animal's body multiply first in the regional lymph nodes and are later carried by the lymph and blood to different organs. Some two weeks after experimental infection, bacteremia can be detected and it is possible to isolate the agent from the bloodstream. Brucella organisms are most commonly found in the lymph nodes, uterus, udder, spleen, liver, and, in bulls, the genital organs. Large quantities of erythritol, a carbohydrate that stimulates the multiplication of brucellae, have been found in cow placentas. This could explain the high susceptibility of bovine fetal tissues.

Once an infected cow aborts or gives birth normally, the pathogen does not remain long in the uterus. The infection becomes chronic and the brucellae are harbored in the cow's lymph nodes and mammary glands. Brucellae may remain in the udder for years (García-Carrillo and Lucero, 1993).

Individual animals within a herd manifest different degrees of susceptibility to infection depending on their age and sex. Male and female calves up to 6 months of age are not very susceptible and generally experience only transitory infections. A bull calf fed milk containing brucella organisms can harbor the agent in its lymph nodes, but after six to eight weeks without ingesting the contaminated food, the animal usually rids itself of the infection.

Heifers kept separate from cows, as is routine in herd management, often have lower infection rates than adult cows. Heifers exposed to infection before breeding can become infected, but generally do not abort. In view of this, at the beginning of the century heifers were inoculated before breeding with virulent strains or with strains of unknown virulence to prevent abortion. This practice had to be abandoned, however, when it was found that a large number of animals remained infected.

Cows, especially when pregnant, are the most susceptible; infection is common and abortion frequently results.

Bulls are also susceptible, although some researchers maintain that they are more resistant to infection than females. This conclusion may reflect herd management practices more than natural resistance in males, however, since bulls are usually kept separate from cows. On the other hand, neutered males and females do not play a role in the epizootiology of brucellosis, since they cannot transmit brucellae to the exterior environment.

In addition to age and sex, it is important to take individual susceptibility into account. Even in the most susceptible categories—cows and heifers—some animals never become infected, or if they do, their infection is transient. Some less susceptible cows have generalized infections and suffer losses in reproductive function and milk production for one or more years, but then gradually recover. In such animals, the agglutination titer becomes negative, the shedding of brucellae may cease, and both reproductive function and milk production return to normal. However, most cows become infected, and their agglutination titers remain positive for many years or for life; although after one or two abortions they may give birth normally and resume normal production of milk, many continue to carry and shed brucellae. Other cows remain totally useless for breeding and milk production.

In a previously uninfected herd, brucellosis spreads rapidly from animal to animal, and for one or two years there are extensive losses from abortions, infertility, decreased milk production, and secondary genital infections. This acute or active phase of the disease is characterized by a large number of abortions and a high rate of reactors in serological tests. Because of individual differences in susceptibility to the infection, not all animals become infected and not all those that are serologically positive abort. After a year or two, the situation stabilizes and the number of abortions decreases. It is estimated that only between 10% and 25% of the cows will abort a second time. In this stabilization phase, it is primarily the heifers—not previously exposed to the infection—that become infected and may abort. A final, decline phase can be observed in small and self-contained herds. In this phase, the infection rate gradually decreases, and most of the cows return to normal reproductive function and milk production. Nevertheless, when a sufficient number of susceptible animals accumulates—either heifers from the same herd or newly introduced animals—a second outbreak can occur. In large herds, there are always enough susceptible animals to maintain the infection, and abortions continue. Trading and movement of animals also help maintain active infection.

SWINE: The main etiologic agent of brucellosis in swine is *B. suis*. In Latin America, only biovar 1 infection has been confirmed, while in the United States both 1 and 3 have been involved. Biovar 2 is found only in Europe. Infection by biovars 1 and 3 is spread directly or indirectly from pig to pig. In contrast, biovar 2 (or Danish biovar) is transmitted to pigs when they ingest European hares (*Lepus europaeus*). Pigs can also be infected by *B. abortus*, although it is less pathogenic for pigs and apparently not transmitted from one animal to another; the infection is generally asymptomatic, with the affected organisms limited to the lymph nodes of the head and neck.

When brucellosis is introduced into a previously healthy herd, the symptoms are those of acute disease: abortions, infertility, birth of weak piglets, orchitis, epididymitis, and arthritis. In small herds, the infection tends to die out or decrease in severity because of a lack of susceptible animals owing to the normal sale of some pigs and to the spontaneous recovery of others. In large herds, the infection is persistent and transmitted from one generation to the next.

Early abortions, which occur when the female is infected during coitus, generally go unnoticed under free-range conditions. The aborted fetuses are eaten by the pigs, and the only abnormality that may be noted by the owner is the sows' repeated estrus. Abortions occur in the second half of gestation when the females are infected after one or two months of pregnancy. Affected sows rarely have a second abortion, and females infected before sexual maturity rarely abort.

Infection is usually temporary in suckling pigs. However, a few may retain the infection and become carriers. It rarely results in recognizable clinical symptoms. Occasionally, arthritis is observed, but transient bacteremia and low agglutination titers may be found.

In infected pigs, abscesses of different sizes frequently occur in organs and tissues. Spondylitis is often found.

Infection of the genital organs lasts for a shorter period of time in the female than in the male. In the latter it may last for the life of the animal.

GOATS: The main etiologic agent of brucellosis in goats is *B. melitensis* with its three biovars. All types of goats are susceptible to infection by *B. melitensis*. Infection by *B. suis* and *B. abortus* has occasionally been found.

The symptomatology is similar to that observed in other species of animals and the main symptom is abortion, which occurs most frequently in the third or fourth month of pregnancy. In natural infections occurring in the field, other symptoms, such as arthritis, mastitis, spondylitis, and orchitis, are rarely found. These symptoms can be seen when the animals are inoculated experimentally with large doses of the agent. Sexually mature female goats that are not pregnant are susceptible and suffer from a chronic infection that may have no clinical symptoms, but that represents a risk for the other animals in the flock. Infection of the mammary gland is common (Alton, 1985). In chronically infected flocks, the signs of the disease are generally not very apparent. Gross pathological lesions are also not usually evident, though the pathogen can frequently be isolated from a large number of tissues and organs.

Several researchers have observed that young goats can be born with the infection or become infected shortly after birth. Most of them recover spontaneously before reaching reproductive age, but in some the infection may persist longer.

The primitive conditions under which goats are raised constitute one of the most important factors in the maintenance and spread of the infection in Latin America (Argentina, Mexico, and Peru) and in the rest of the developing world. In goat-raising areas, it is common to find community-shared pastures, a lack of hygiene in makeshift corrals, nomadic flocks, and owners with little understanding of herd management.

SHEEP: Two disease entities are distinguishable in sheep: classic brucellosis and ram epididymitis. Classic brucellosis is caused by *B. melitensis* and constitutes a public health problem equally or even more important than goat brucellosis in areas where the agent is found outside the American continent. In Latin America, the infection in sheep has been confirmed only in some mixed goat and sheep flocks raised far away from intensive sheep-raising areas.

While sheep brucellosis is similar in its symptomatology to the disease in goats, sheep appear to be more resistant to infection and, in mixed flocks, fewer sheep than goats are found to be infected. Susceptibility varies from breed to breed. Maltese sheep are very resistant, while Middle Eastern Awassi (fat tail) sheep are very susceptible (Alton, 1985). Abortions are also less common. The infection tends to disappear spontaneously, and the high prevalence of the disease in some areas can best be attributed to poor herd management.

Occasionally, sheep have been found to be infected by *B. suis* (biovar 2 in Germany) and *B. abortus* (in various parts of the world). These agents are not very pathogenic for sheep; they are acquired through contact with infected animals of other species, and are usually not transmitted from sheep to sheep. However, transmission can occur, as in the case described in an outbreak occurring on a ranch in the US (Luchsinger and Anderson, 1979).

Ram epididymitis is caused by *B. ovis*. The clinical signs consist of genital lesions in rams, associated with varying degrees of sterility. Sometimes the infection in pregnant ewes can cause abortion or neonatal mortality. Epididymitis is generally unilateral but can be bilateral and the tail of the organ is most commonly affected. Adhesions may occur in the tunica vaginalis testis, and the testicle may be atrophied with varying degrees of fibrosis. Lesions cannot be seen or palpated in many infected rams, even though *B. ovis* may be isolated from their semen. Some of these animals develop lesions in more advanced stages of the disease. Early in the infection, the semen contains many brucellae, but with time the number decreases, and eventually the semen may be free of the infectious agent. When localized in the kidneys, *B. ovis* is also shed through the urine.

HORSES: *B. abortus* and *B. suis* have been isolated from this species. The disease usually manifests itself in the form of fistulous bursitis, "poll evil" and "fistulous withers." Abortions are rare but they do occur (Robertson *et al.*, 1973). *B. abortus* has been isolated from horse feces, but this is uncommon. Horses acquire the infection from cattle or swine, but transmission from horses to cattle has also been proven. Man can contract the infection from horses that have open lesions. In general, horses are more resistant to the infection. Cases of horse-to-horse transmission are unknown. In areas where there is a high rate of infection, it is common to find horses with high agglutination titers.

DOGS AND CATS: Sporadic cases of brucellosis caused by *B. abortus*, *B. suis*, and *B. melitensis* occur in dogs. They acquire the infection primarily by eating contaminated material, especially fetuses, afterbirth, and milk. The course of the infection is usually subclinical, but sometimes the symptomatology can be severe, with fever, emaciation, orchitis, anestrus, arthritis, and sometimes abortion. Cases of dog-to-dog transmission are rare. In some cases, the infection may last for more than 150 days. Although it is rare, dogs can eliminate brucellae in their urine, vaginal secretions, feces, and aborted fetuses. A study conducted in Canada collected 14 dogs from 10 cattle properties with bovine brucellosis. Positive cultures were obtained from vaginal mucus and from the bladder of a single dog. The final positive vaginal secretion sample was obtained 464 days after the probable date when the dog was infected. In other dogs, *Brucella* was isolated from organs that do not discharge to the environment (Forbes, 1990). Several human cases have been described in which the source of infection was dogs (especially fetuses).

A canine disease that occurs worldwide and can reach epizootic proportions is that caused by *B. canis*. This form of brucellosis is characterized by a prolonged afebrile bacteremia, embryonic death, abortions, prostatitis, epididymitis, scrotal dermatitis, lymphadenitis, and splenitis. Abortion occurs about 50 days into gestation. The pups may be stillborn at full term or die a few days after birth. Survivors usually have enlarged lymph nodes and often have bacteremia.

In an experimental treatment, minocycline (27.5 mg/kg twice a day) was administered to 18 infected dogs. Fifteen of them had positive cultures in autopsies conducted between 6 and 28 weeks after treatment ended (WHO, 1986).

Man is susceptible to *B. canis*, though less so than to classic brucellae. Several cases have been confirmed in the United States, Mexico, Brazil, and Argentina in laboratory and kennel personnel as well as in members of families with infected dogs.

Cats are resistant to *Brucella* and no cases of natural disease occurrence are known.

OTHER DOMESTIC MAMMALS: Brucellosis caused by *B. abortus* occurs in domestic buffalo (*Bubalus bubalis*) and in yaks (*Bos grunniens*) with symptomatology similar to that in cattle. The disease has also been observed in Old World camels (*Camelus bactrianus*), in dromedaries (*Camelus dromedarius*), and in American Camelidae. Infection in Camelidae is caused primarily by *B. melitensis*, although *B. abortus* has been isolated (Al-Khalaf and El-Khaladi, 1989). An outbreak of brucellosis caused by *B. mellitus* biovar 1, accompanied by abortions and neonatal mortality, occurred on an alpaca (*Lama pacos*) ranch in the high plateau (altiplano) region of Peru; a serious outbreak also occurred in the human population of that ranch (Acosta *et al.*, 1972).

WILD ANIMALS: Natural infections caused by *Brucella* occur in a wide range of wild species. There are natural foci of infection, for example, among the desert rats of the United States (*Neotoma lepida*), which are the reservoir of *B. neotomae*. In Kenya, *B. suis* biovar 3 has been isolated from two species of rodents (*Arvicanthis niloticus* and *Mastomys natalensis*). In Australia, there are as yet unclassified biovars of *Brucella* in various species of rodents. In the Caucasus, rodents infected by *Brucella* were found; it was initially classified as *B. muris* and later as *B. suis* biovar 5. In Europe, the infection of hares (*Lepus europaeus*), which are the reservoir of *B. suis* biovar 2, is transmitted to domestic swine. Caribou (*Rangifer caribou*), which is the reservoir of *B. suis* biovar 4 in Alaska, can transmit the infection to man and to sled dogs. The infection can also be transmitted in the opposite direction, from domestic animals to wild animals. This is the case in Argentina, where infection in foxes (*Dusicyon gymnocercus, D. griseus*) (Szyfres and González Tomé, 1966) and grisons (*Galictis furax-huronax*) is caused by *B. abortus* biovar 1, infection in European hares (*Lepus europaeus*) is caused by *B. suis* biovar 1 (Szyfres *et al.*, 1968), and that in opossums (*Didelphis azarae*), by *B. abortus* biovar 1 and *B. suis* biovar 1 (De la Vega *et al.*, 1979). Carnivores acquire the infection by eating fetuses and afterbirth. There is no evidence that the infection is transmitted from one individual to another among carnivores, and it probably dies out when brucellosis is controlled in domestic animals. The situation is different when domestic animals transmit the infection to wild ruminants, such as the steppe antelope (*Saiga tatarica*) or the American bison (*Bison bison*), in which brucellosis persists.

Fur-bearing animals, such as minks and silver foxes, may contract brucellosis when fed viscera of infected animals, and they may in turn transmit this infection to man.

The etiologic agent has been isolated from many species of arthropods. Ticks can harbor the organism for lengthy periods and transmit the infection through biting. They also eliminate the bacteria in their coxal gland secretions. Nevertheless, the number of ticks harboring brucellae is insignificant (in one study done in the former Soviet Union, eight strains of *Brucella spp.* were isolated from 20,000 ticks) and there are few brucellae per tick. The species that have been isolated from arthropods are *B. melitensis* and *B. abortus*. In Brazil, *B. canis* was isolated from specimens of *Rhipicephalus sanguineus* attached to a bitch suffering from brucellosis (Peres *et al.*, 1981). There is consensus that arthropods play only a small role, if any, in the epidemiology of brucellosis.

FOWL: In a few cases, *Brucella* has been isolated from naturally infected domestic fowl. The symptomatology described is quite varied, and there is no certainty that it always involves brucellosis. The infection may not be evident, with symptoms such as weight loss, reduction in egg production, and diarrhea. Fowl do not play a role in maintaining the infection in nature. *Brucella* has been isolated from some wild bird species such as ravens (*Corvus corvix*) and crows (*Tripanscorax fragilecus*).

Source of Infection and Mode of Transmission: The natural reservoirs of *B. abortus, B. suis*, and *B. melitensis* are, respectively, cattle, swine, and goats and sheep. The natural host of *B. canis* is the dog and that of *B. ovis* is the sheep.

INFECTION IN HUMANS: Man is infected by animals through direct contact or indirectly by ingestion of animal products and by inhalation of airborne agents. The relative importance of the etiologic agent's mode of transmission and pathway of penetration varies with the epidemiological area, the animal reservoirs, and the occupational groups at risk. Fresh cheese and raw milk from goats and sheep infected with *B. melitensis* are the most common vehicles of infection and can cause multiple cases of human brucellosis. Sometimes more widespread outbreaks occur when infected goat's milk is mixed with cow's milk. Cow's milk infected by *B. melitensis* or *B. suis* has also been known to produce outbreaks of epidemic proportions. Cow's milk and milk products containing *B. abortus* may give rise to sporadic cases. The organisms rarely survive in sour milk, sour cream and butter, or fermented cheese (aged over three months).

In arctic and subarctic regions, there have been confirmed cases that resulted from eating bone marrow or raw meat from reindeer or caribou infected with *B. suis* biovar 4. Brucellae are resistant to pickling and smoke curing, therefore some meat products thus prepared could possibly cause human infection; however, this mode of transmission has never been verified.

It is also possible for raw vegetables and water contaminated with the excreta of infected animals to serve as sources of infection.

Transmission by contact predominates in areas where bovine and porcine brucellosis are enzootic. Human brucellosis is, for the most part, an occupational disease of stockyard and slaughterhouse workers, butchers, and veterinarians. The infection is usually contracted by handling fetuses and afterbirth, or by contact with vaginal secretions, excreta, and carcasses of infected animals. The microorganism enters through skin abrasions as well as through the conjunctiva by way of the hands. In slaughterhouses, prevalence of the disease is higher among recently employed staff. The practice in some companies of employing workers with negative serology is misguided, since an individual who is asymptomatic but has a positive serology is less likely to become sick.

In areas where goat and sheep brucellosis is enzootic, transmission by contact also occurs when shepherds handle newborn animals or fetuses. In some countries with hard winters, goats share the beds of goatherds and their families for protection against the cold, which results in infection of the whole family (Elberg, 1981).

Airborne transmission has been proved by experimentation and research. In laboratories, centrifugation of brucellosis suspensions poses a special risk when done in centrifuges that are not hermetically sealed. An epidemic outbreak of 45 cases occurred among students at Michigan State University (USA) in 1938–1939. The 45 students were attending classes on the second and third floors of a building that housed a brucellosis research laboratory in the basement. In the ensuing investigation, it was shown that the only possible means of transmission was by aerosol particles. Subsequent epidemiological studies have supplied proof that airborne transmission in meat lockers and slaughterhouses plays an important role, and perhaps is more frequent than transmission by direct contact with infected tissue. When air in the killing area is allowed to disperse, it leads to high rates of infection among workers in adjoining areas. The minimum infective dose for man by way of the respiratory passages seems to be small. When the killing area is completely separate, or maintained at a negative air pressure, the risk to surrounding areas is reduced (Kaufmann *et al.*, 1980; Buchanan *et al.*, 1974).

Some cases of possible human-to-human transmission of brucellosis have been described. One of them occurred in Kuwait due to transmission of *B. melitensis* to a 30-day-old girl through her mother's milk. The mother had experienced fever, discomfort, and arthralgia for at least two weeks prior to the child's becoming sick. *B. melitensis* biovar 1 was repeatedly isolated from the blood of both mother and child (Lubani *et al.*, 1988). In a hospital laboratory in the US, eight microbiologists were exposed to accidental dispersion of a clinical specimen in aerosol and *B. melitensis* biovar 3 was isolated from five of them. The spouse of one of the patients became ill six months after her husband had been admitted to the hospital and *B. melitensis* of the same biovar was isolated from her blood; it is suspected that the infection was sexually transmitted (Ruben *et al.*, 1991). A probable case of transmission during childbirth occurred in Israel. The mother had a fever on the first day postpartum and

Figure 5. Bovine brucellosis (*Brucella abortus*). Mode of transmission.

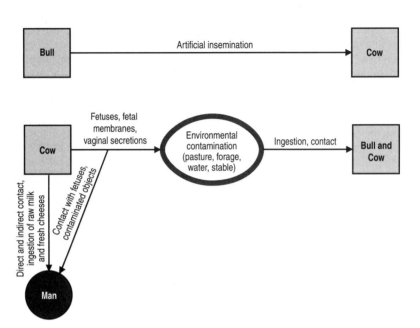

B. melitensis biovar 3 was identified in a cervical culture. Cervical and blood cultures continued to be positive. Although the child was asymptomatic, a positive blood culture of the same biovar and an agglutinating titer of 1:100 were obtained. Splenomegaly was the only abnormality found in the child at 13 days. Prior to these cases, there were descriptions of human-to-human transmission due to transfusion or bone marrow transplants.

INFECTION IN CATTLE **(Figure 5):** The main sources of infection for cattle are fetuses, afterbirth, and vaginal discharges containing large numbers of brucellae. To a lesser extent, farm areas can be contaminated by fecal matter of calves fed on contaminated milk, since not all the organisms are destroyed in the digestive tract.

The most common route of transmission is the gastrointestinal tract following ingestion of contaminated pasture, feed, fodder, or water. Moreover, cows customarily lick afterbirth, fetuses, and newborn calves, all of which may contain a large number of the organisms and constitute a very important source of infection. Cows' habit of licking the genital organs of other cows also contributes to transmission of the infection.

It has been shown experimentally that the organism may penetrate broken and even intact skin. The extent to which this mode of transmission is involved in natural infection is unknown.

Bang and others experimentally reproduced infection and disease via the vaginal route. The results of those experiments indicate that a large number of brucellae are necessary to infect a cow by this means. However, there is no doubt that the intrauterine route used in artificial insemination is very important in transmitting the infection. The use of infected bulls for artificial insemination constitutes an important risk, since the infection can thus be spread to many herds.

In closed environments, it is likely that infection is spread by aerosols; airborne infection has been demonstrated experimentally.

Congenital infection and the so-called latency phenomenon have also been described. An experiment was carried out in France (Plommet *et al.*, 1973) in which calves born to cows artificially infected with a high dose of *B. abortus* were separated from their mothers and raised in isolation units. At 16 months of age, the heifers were artificially inseminated. In six experiments (Fensterbank, 1980) using 55 heifers born to infected cows, 5 were infected and brucellae were isolated during calving and/or after butchering six weeks later. At 9 and 12 months of age, two of these animals had serologic titers that were unstable until pregnancy. The other three heifers did not have serological reactions until the middle or end of pregnancy (latency). The authors of the experiment admit that under natural range conditions the frequency of the latency phenomenon could be much lower. In herds in which vaccination of calves is systematically carried out, the phenomenon may go unnoticed. In a similar vein, other research projects (Lapraik *et al.*, 1975; Wilesmith, 1978) have been undertaken on the vertical transmission of brucellosis accompanied by a prolonged and serologically unapparent phase of the infection. In a retrospective study of highly infected herds (Wilesmith, 1978), it was found that 8 of 317 heifers (2.5%) born to reactive cows tested serologically positive. One study conducted on 150 calves born to naturally infected mothers (with positive culture for *B. abortus*), taken from 82 herds in three southern states in the US, suggests that the latency phenomenon does not occur very frequently. The calves were raised in isolation until sexual maturity and breeding. *Brucella* was not isolated from the progeny of 105 infected cows, nor from the 95 fetuses and newborns of these heifers (second generation). Two heifers from the first generation had positive and persistent serological reactions from an undetermined source (Ray *et al.*, 1988). The extent of the latency phenomenon is still not known, but it has not prevented the eradication of bovine brucellosis in vast areas and many countries. On the other hand, it has undeniably slowed its eradication in some herds.

INFECTION IN SWINE **(Figure 6):** In swine, the sources of infection are the same as in cattle. The principal routes of transmission are digestive and venereal. Contrary to the situation in cattle, natural sexual contact is a common and important mode of transmission. The infection has often been introduced into a herd following the acquisition of an infected boar. Pigs, because of their eating habits and the conditions in which they are raised, are very likely to become infected through the oral route. It is also probable that they become infected by aerosols entering via the conjunctiva or upper respiratory tract.

INFECTION IN GOATS AND SHEEP **(Figure 7):** Goats and sheep are infected with *B. melitensis* in a manner similar to cattle. The role of the buck and ram in transmission of the infection is not well established. Infection of goats *in utero* is not unusual, and kids can also become infected during the suckling period; such infection may persist in some animals.

In ram epididymitis caused by *B. ovis*, semen is the main and possibly the only source of infection. The infection is commonly transmitted from one ram to another by rectal or preputial contact. Transmission may also occur through the ewe when an infected ram deposits his semen and another ram breeds her shortly thereafter. The infection is not very common in ewes, and when it occurs it is contracted by sexual contact. *B. ovis* does not persist very long in ewes and is generally eliminated before the next lambing period.

**Figure 6. Swine brucellosis (*Brucella suis*).
Mode of transmission.**

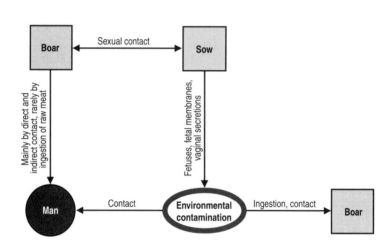

**Figure 7. Caprine and ovine brucellosis (*Brucella melitensis*).
Mode of transmission.**

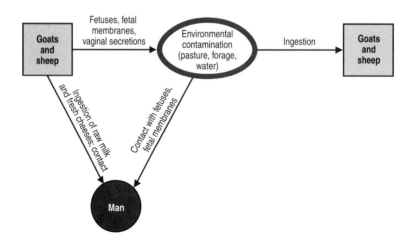

INFECTION IN DOGS: The transmission of *B. canis* occurs as a result of contact with vaginal secretions, fetuses, and fetal membranes. Infected males may transmit the infection to bitches during coitus. The milk of infected bitches is another possible source of infection. Human cases recorded in the literature amount to several dozen, many resulting from contact with bitches that had recently aborted.

Role of Animals in the Epidemiology of the Disease: The role of animals is essential. Cases of human-to-human transmission are exceptional. Brucellosis is a zoonosis par excellence.

Diagnosis: In man, a clinical diagnosis of brucellosis based on symptoms and history should always be confirmed in the laboratory. Isolation and typing of the causal agent is definitive and may also indicate the source of the infection. Blood or marrow from the sternum or ileal crest taken while the patient is febrile is cultured in appropriate media. Culture material may also be taken from lymph nodes, cerebrospinal fluid, and abscesses. It is recommended that the cultures be repeated several times, especially in enzootic areas of *B. abortus*. Due to the widespread use of antibiotics before diagnosis in febrile patients, bacteriologic examinations, particularly of blood, often yield negative results, and serologic tests become increasingly necessary. The serum agglutination test, preferably in tubes, is the simplest and most widely used procedure. A high titer (more than 100 international units, IU) and increasing titers in repeated serum samples provide a good basis for diagnosis. Cross-reactions in serum agglutination have been observed in cases of cholera or tularemia (or as a result of vaccination against these diseases) and in infections caused by *Yersinia enterocolitica* 0:9, as well as *Escherichia coli* 0:157 and 0:116, *Salmonella* serotypes of Kauffmann-White group N, and *Pseudomonas maltophila* (Corbel *et al.*, 1984). The serum agglutination test reveals both M and G immunoglobulins. It is generally accepted that in an active stage of brucellosis IgG is always present. Thus, when low serum agglutination titers are found, tests to detect the presence of IgG must be performed, such as the 2-mercaptoethanol (ME) and complement fixation (CF) test (in man, IgGs fix complement but often lack agglutinating power). These tests are of special interest in chronic brucellosis, where active infection may continue even though agglutination titers return to low levels. The intradermal test with noncellular allergens is useful for epidemiological studies, but not for clinical diagnosis.

The 2-mercaptoethanol test is also useful in following the treatment and cure of the patient. In one study (Buchanan and Faber, 1980), the titers of 92 brucellosis patients were followed for 18 months with tube agglutination and ME tests. Despite antibiotic treatment, the tube agglutination test continued positive for 18 months in 44 (48%) of the patients, but the ME titers were positive in only 8 (9%) of the patients at the end of one year and in 4 (4%) at 18 months. None of the 84 patients testing negative by ME at the end of a year of treatment had signs or symptoms of brucellosis and none acquired chronic brucellosis. By contrast, four of the eight patients testing positive by ME after a year continued to have symptoms of brucellosis and had to continue treatment. Thus, a negative result by ME provides good evidence that a patient does not have chronic brucellosis and that the antibiotic treatment was successful. If effective treatment is begun early, it is possible that IgG antibodies (resistant to ME) never develop. This was probably the case in three patients who acquired brucellosis in the laboratory and in whom infection was confirmed by blood culture. Diagnosis and treatment were done early enough that at no time during the two-year follow-up did these patients show ME-resistant antibodies (García-Carrillo and Coltorti, 1979). However, other researchers dispute the usefulness of this test in the diagnosis of brucellosis (Díaz and Moriyon, 1989).

Other useful methods for the diagnosis of human brucellosis are the rose bengal test and counterimmunoelectrophoresis. The rose bengal test is easily performed and is recommended over the plate agglutination test or the Huddleson method. In a study of 222 cases (Díaz et al., 1982), rose bengal was the most sensitive test, with 98.3% positive results. Counterimmunoelectrophoresis was positive in 84.9% of the acute cases and in 91.6% of the chronic cases.

The indirect enzyme-linked immunosorbent assay (ELISA) test has been used for some years with good results in terms of specificity and sensitivity in research (Díaz and Moriyón, 1989). It is a very versatile test and, once it is introduced in a laboratory, it can be adapted for use with many other diseases.

The Joint FAO/WHO Expert Committee on Brucellosis (WHO, 1986) calls attention to the limited value of serological tests in individuals who are repeatedly exposed to brucellae because they can be serologically positive in the absence of symptoms. This category would include veterinarians, vaccinators, and laboratory personnel involved in the production of antigens, vaccines, and cultures of clinical specimens.

In serologic diagnosis of humans or animals, it is necessary to bear in mind that at the outset of the infection only IgM antibodies are produced; consequently, the agglutination test will provide the best standard for diagnosis, since ME will yield negative results. As the infection progresses, IgG antibodies resistant to the ME test will appear and will increase unless appropriate treatment is begun.

Diagnosis of infection caused by *B. melitensis*, *B. suis*, and *B. abortus* is carried out with a properly standardized antigen of *B. abortus* (Alton et al., 1976). However, this antigen does not permit diagnosis of infection caused by *B. canis*, since this species of *Brucella* (as well as *B. ovis*) is found in a rugose (R) phase, lacking the lipopolysaccharidic surface that characterizes "classic brucellae" (for diagnosis of *B. canis* and *B. ovis*, see below).

In cattle, the diagnosis is based primarily on serology. A great many serologic tests are presently available, all of which are useful when applied with judgment. Both a serologic test reaction and the test's usefulness in each circumstance are a result of the sensitivity it shows to antibodies of different immunoglobulin types and of the seric concentration of each type of antibody (Chappel et al., 1978). The most thoroughly studied immunoglobulins in bovine brucellosis are IgM and IgG. Although available tests are not qualitative enough to identify an individual immunoglobulin, they do indicate which one predominates. In the diagnosis of bovine brucellosis, the evolution of immunoglobulins during infection and vaccination is of special interest. In both cases, the IgMs appear first, followed by the IgGs. The difference is that in infected animals, the IgGs tend to increase and persist, while in calves vaccinated at between three and eight months, the IgGs tend to disappear about six months after vaccination. Based on this fact, complementary tests are used to distinguish infection from the agglutination titer, which may persist after vaccination with strain 19, and also from heterospecific reactions caused by bacteria that share surface antigens with the brucellae and that give rise to antibodies that, in general, are the IgM type.

According to their use in different countries, serologic tests may be classified as follows: (1) routine or operative, (2) complementary, (3) epidemiological surveillance, and (4) screening tests. A single test might serve as operative, as diagnostically definitive, as a screen, or as complementary, depending on the program employing it.

Serum agglutination tests (tube and plate) have been and continue to be widely used. They contributed greatly to the reduction of infection rates in Europe, Australia, and the Americas. Nevertheless, when the proportion of infected herds and world-wide prevalence is reduced, their limitations become apparent in so-called "problem" herds and it becomes necessary to use other tests to help eradicate the infection. The tests are internationally standardized, easy to carry out, and allow the examination of a great many samples. In agglutination tests, the IgM reaction predominates. In animals classified as suspect or marginally positive, complementary tests are used to clarify their status. However, it is necessary to keep in mind that low agglutination titers could be due to recent infection and it is thus advisable to repeat the test.

The rose bengal test (with buffered antigen) is fast, easy, and allows processing of many samples per day. It is qualitative and classifies animals as positive or negative. In regions where incidence of infection is low or where systematic vaccination of calves is practiced, the rose bengal test gives many "false positives," and so is unspecific if used as the only and definitive test. In many countries, such as Great Britain and Australia, it is used as a preliminary or screening test. Animals showing a negative test result are so classified and those testing positive are subjected to other tests for confirmation. In regions of high incidence, results are very satisfactory. Rose bengal may also be used as a complementary test for those animals classified as suspect by agglutination. Many suspect sera test negative to rose bengal, and since this test is very sensitive (there are few "false negatives") and detects the infection early, there is little risk of missing infected animals.

The principal complementary tests are complement fixation, 2-mercaptoethanol, and rivanol. Other tests have been developed, such as indirect hemolysis, ELISA for different types of immunoglobulins, and radial immunodiffusion with a polysaccharide antigen. All these tests are used to distinguish antibodies caused by the infection from those left by vaccination or stimulated by heterospecific bacteria.

Both the direct and the competitive ELISA tests are appropriate for diagnosis of brucellosis in all species according to the consensus of groups of experts that have met several times in Geneva. WHO, with the collaboration of FAO, the International Organization of Epizootics, the International Atomic Energy Agency, and these organizations' reference laboratories, is coordinating a project to evaluate and standardize these assays as well as the antigens and other technical variables.

In Australia, the ELISA technique and the complement fixation test have been very useful in recent phases in the eradication of bovine brucellosis, when many "problem herds" occur with "latent carrier animals." In comparison with the CF test, ELISA revealed a significantly higher number of reactive animals in infected herds, both vaccinated (with strain 19) and unvaccinated, but gave negative results in herds free of brucellosis, whether vaccinated or not. The specificity of ELISA in the group of infected herds was less than that of CF, but sensitivity—which is what was needed—was greater (Cargill et al., 1985). It costs less to eliminate some false positive animals in the final phase of eradication than to allow the infection to reassert itself and spread in the herd because one or more infected animals remained (Sutherland et al., 1986). The competitive enzymatic immunoassay also lends itself to differentiating the reactions of animals vaccinated with strain 19 and animals naturally infected, using the O polysaccharide antigen (Nielsen et al., 1989).

The complement fixation test is considered the most specific, but it is laborious, complicated, and involves many steps and variables. Moreover, it is not standardized internationally. Other, simpler tests can take its place, such as 2-mercaptoethanol and rivanol, which measure the IgG antibodies.

Animal health laboratories in the US and various laboratories in Latin America have successfully used the BAPA (buffered antigen plate agglutination) or BPA (buffered plate antigen) screening test, which is performed on a plate with a buffered antigen at pH 3.65 (Angus and Barton, 1984). BAPA greatly simplifies the work when numerous blood samples must be examined, because it eliminates the negative samples and many of the sera with nonspecific reactions. The test results classify the samples as negative (which are definitively discarded) and presumably positive; the latter are submitted to one or more definitive and/or complementary tests, such as tube agglutination, complement fixation, or 2-mercaptoethanol. This test was also evaluated in Canada (Stemshorn *et al.*, 1985) and Argentina (González Tomé *et al.*, 1989) with very favorable results.

Epidemiological surveillance of brucellosis is carried out separately on dairy and meat-producing herds, at strategic checkpoints and using different diagnostic tests. The principal objective is to identify infected herds and monitor healthy ones. For beef cattle, screening tests or other tests of presumed high sensitivity are used, such as BAPA, and the checkpoints for collecting samples are cattle markets and slaughterhouses. The sera that test positive are then subjected to standard tests and the animals are traced back to their points of origin. For dairy cattle, the milk-ring test is used. It is very simple and allows the examination of many herds in a short time. The composite samples are gathered from milk cans or tanks at collection points and dairy plants or on the dairy farm itself. If a positive sample is found, individual serologic examinations of the animals belonging to the source herd must then be carried out.

Bacteriologic examinations are of more limited use. The samples most often tested in this way are taken from fetuses, fetal membranes, vaginal secretions, milk, and semen. Infected cows may or may not abort, but a high percentage will eliminate brucellae from the genital tract beginning a few days before parturition and continuing some 30 days afterwards. It is estimated that 85% of recently infected cows and more than 15% of chronically infected cows eliminate brucellae during calving. Since elimination through milk may be constant or intermittent, milk can be an excellent material for the isolation of *Brucella* if examinations are repeated. Serologic testing of bulls should be done using blood serum and seminal fluid. Bacteriologic examination of semen should be repeated if results are negative, since brucellae may be shed intermittently.

In swine, serologic tests are not indicated for individual diagnosis but rather to reveal the presence of herd infection. Agglutination (tube or plate), complement fixation, buffered-acid antigen (rose bengal), or BAPA tests may be used. The latter is preferable because it is negative in herds having only low and nonspecific agglutination (tube or plate) titers. For a herd to be classified as positive with the agglutination test (tube or plate), there must be one or more animals with titers of 100 IU or more.

In goats, serologic tests are also applied on a flock basis and not on individual animals. In infected flocks, one or more individuals are found with titers of 100 IU or more; in such cases, titers of 50 IU should be adopted as indicative of infection. The complement fixation test is considered superior to the agglutination test, especially in herds vaccinated with *B. melitensis* Rev. 1, where agglutinating antibodies persist for long periods. The 2-mercaptoethanol test has also given very good results in vaccinated flocks. The results from the buffered-acid antigen (rose bengal) test are promising, but experience with it is limited and definitive conclusions cannot be drawn at this time. The ELISA test is the most promising.

In diagnosing infections caused by *B. melitensis* in sheep, the Coombs' test (antiglobulin test) modified by Hajdu can reveal 70% of infected animals. The other tests (agglutination, complement fixation) give less satisfactory results. In using the agglutination and complement fixation tests, adoption of significant titer levels lower than those for other animal species is recommended. Counterimmunoelectrophoresis would detect antibodies against intracellular antigens that appear late in the serum but which remain a long time. Consequently, its use would be appropriate for sheep with chronic brucellosis that test negative by agglutination, rose bengal, and complement fixation (Trap and Gaumont, 1982). Experts agree that the diagnostic methods for brucellosis caused by *B. melitensis* in goats and sheep leave much to be desired and that more attention should be given to this problem given its public health importance.

In diagnosing ram epididymitis caused by *B. ovis*, antigen prepared with this agent must be used. The preferred tests are gel diffusion, complement fixation, and ELISA. A study conducted in Australia in flocks infected by *B. ovis* and flocks free of infection showed that this enzyme immunoassay detected more reactive animals and that the complement fixation test failed to detect some rams that excreted *B. ovis*. In infection-free flocks, both ELISA and CF produced false positives at a rate of 0.5% (Lee *et al.*, 1985). Bacteriologic examination of semen is an appropriate diagnostic method, but it should be kept in mind that the shedding of brucellae can be intermittent.

For dogs infected by *B. canis*, the surest diagnostic method is isolation of the etiologic agent from blood, vaginal discharges, milk, or semen, or from fetal tissue and placenta. Bacteremia can last from one to two years, but after the initial phase it may become intermittent; thus, a negative blood culture does not exclude the possibility of brucellosis.

The most common serologic tests are plate and tube agglutination using *B. canis* antigen, immunodiffusion in agar gel with antigens extracted from the cell wall, 2-mercaptoethanol plate agglutination, and the modified 2 ME tube agglutination test. Possibly the most specific test to date, but also the least sensitive, is the immunodiffusion test in agar gel that utilizes antigens extracted from the cytoplasm of *B. canis*. To a greater or lesser degree, all these tests give nonspecific reactions. Zoha and Carmichael (1982) showed that the immunodiffusion test using sonicated antigens (internal cellular antigens) is satisfactory shortly after the onset of bacteremia and can detect infected animals for up to six months after it disappears, i.e., when other tests give equivocal results. A new test has been developed that uses a nonmucoid (M–) variant of *B. canis* as the antigen in tube agglutination, after treating the sera with 2 ME. The test is more specific without reducing sensitivity (Carmichael and Joubert, 1987).

Control: The most rational approach for preventing human brucellosis is the control and elimination of the infection in animal reservoirs, as has been demonstrated in various countries in Europe and the Americas. Some human populations may be protected by mandatory milk pasteurization. In many goat- and sheep-herding regions, pasteurization of milk is an unattainable goal for the time being. Prevention of the infection in occupational groups (cattlemen, abattoir workers, veterinarians, and others who come into contact with animals or their carcasses) is more difficult and should be based on health education, the use of protective clothing whenever possible, and medical supervision.

Protecting refrigerator plant and slaughterhouse workers against brucellosis is particularly important because they constitute the occupational group at highest risk. Protection is achieved by separating the slaughter area from other sections and controlling air circulation. In countries with eradication programs, slaughter of reactive animals is limited to one or more designated slaughterhouses (cold storage plants) with official veterinary inspection in each region. These animals are butchered at the end of the workday with special precautions and proper supervision to protect the workers. Employees should be instructed in personal hygiene and provided with disinfectants and protective clothing. A 5% solution of chloramine or an 8% to 10% solution of caustic soda should be used to disinfect installations after slaughter (Elberg, 1981). Instruments should be sterilized in an autoclave or boiled for 30 minutes in a 2% solution of caustic soda. Clothes may be disinfected with a 2% solution of chloramine or a 3% solution of carbolic acid soap followed by washing. Hands should be soaked for five minutes in a solution of 1% chloramine or 0.5% caustic soda, and then washed with soap and water.

The immunization of high-risk occupational groups is practiced in the former Soviet Union and China. In the former Soviet Union, good results have apparently been obtained with the use of a vaccine prepared from strain 19-BA of *B. abortus* (derived from strain 19 used for bovine brucellosis), applied by skin scarification. Annual revaccination is carried out for those individuals not reacting to serologic or allergenic tests. To avoid the discomfort caused by the vaccine in man, a vaccine was recently developed that consists of chemically defined fractions of the lipid-polysaccharide (LPS) component of the strain 19-BA (Drannovskaia, 1991). In China, an attenuated live vaccine made from *B. abortus* strain 104M is applied percutaneously. These vaccines are not used in other countries because of possible side effects. Promising trials have also been conducted in France with antigenic fractions of *Brucella*.

Vaccination is recommended for control of bovine brucellosis in enzootic areas with high prevalence rates. The vaccine of choice is *B. abortus* strain 19, confirmed by its worldwide use, the protection it gives for the useful lifetime of the animal, and its low cost. To avoid interference with diagnosis, it is recommended that vaccination be limited (by legislation) to young animals (calves of 3 to 8 months), as these animals rapidly lose the antibodies produced in response to the vaccine. It is estimated that 65% to 80% of vaccinated animals remain protected against the infection. The antiabortive effect of the vaccine is pronounced, thus reducing one of the principal sources of infection, the fetuses. In a systematic vaccination program, the best results are obtained with 70% to 90% annual coverage in calves of the proper age for vaccination. Male calves and females over 8 months of age should not be vaccinated. Where possible, the upper limit should be 6 months. Revaccination is not recommended. The main objective of systematic and mandatory vaccination of calves in a given area or country is to reduce the infection rate and obtain herds

resistant to brucellosis, so that eradication of the disease may then begin. It is estimated that 7 to 10 years of systematic vaccination are necessary to achieve this
objective.

In regions or countries with a low prevalence of the disease, an eradication program can be carried out by repeated serologic diagnostic tests applied to the entire
herd, and elimination of reactors until all foci of infection have disappeared. This
procedure can be used alone (in countries with a low prevalence) or in combination
with the vaccination of calves. Epidemiological surveillance and control of animal
transport are very important in such programs. Countries that are close to eradication may suspend vaccination with strain 19 or any other vaccine.

Until a few years ago, the vaccination of adult cows with strain 19 was inadvis-
able because of the prolonged resistance of antibodies that could interfere with
diagnosis. In the 1950s, several researchers proved that vaccination of adult animals
with a smaller dose could impart an immunity comparable to that of a full dose,
while at the same time agglutination titers stayed lower and disappeared faster. In
1975, Nicoletti (1976) began a series of studies in the US using a reduced dose in
highly infected herds; he concluded that vaccination decreases the spread of the
infection within the herd, that antibodies disappear approximately six months after
vaccination, and that less than 1% of the females remained infected by the vaccine
strain from three to six months after vaccination. Complementary tests were very
useful in distinguishing between reactions due to infection and those due to vaccination. Other studies, done under both controlled and natural conditions, confirmed
these findings (Nicoletti *et al.*, 1978; Alton *et al.*, 1980; Viana *et al.*, 1982; Alton *et
al.*, 1983). Vaccination of adult females may be considered in herds suffering acute
brucellosis characterized by abortions and rapidly spreading infections, as well as in
large herds where chronic brucellosis has proven hard to eradicate. The recommended dose is one to three billion cells of strain 19 *Brucella* administered subcutaneously. Only animals testing negative should be vaccinated and they should be
indelibly marked under government supervision. At the beginning of the operation,
reactors should be eliminated immediately. Vaccinated animals should be examined
serologically 6 months later, using tests such as rivanol, mercaptoethanol, and complement fixation, and those that have become infected should be slaughtered. Using
periodic serologic examination, it is estimated that a problem herd can be free of
infection in 18 to 24 months (Barton and Lomme, 1980).

The control of swine brucellosis consists of identifying and certifying brucellosis-
free herds. If infection is diagnosed in an establishment where pigs are raised for
market, it is advisable to send the entire herd to the abattoir and reestablish it with
animals from a brucellosis-free herd. If the infected pigs are valuable for breeding
or research, suckling pigs should be weaned at 4 weeks and raised in facilities separate from the main herd. Periodic serologic tests (such as rose bengal) are recommended to eliminate any reactor. Finally, when no brucellosis is found in the new
herd and it is well established, the original herd should be sent to slaughter. There
are no effective vaccines for swine.

Control of the infection caused by *B. melitensis* in goats and sheep is based
mainly on vaccination. The preferred vaccine is *B. melitensis* Rev. 1, which is
administered to 3- to 6-month-old females. Adult females can receive a smaller dose
(20,000 times fewer bacterial cells than in the dose for young females) of the same
vaccine (Alton *et al.*, 1972).

As goats are generally raised in marginal areas where socioeconomic conditions are very poor, it is difficult to carry out eradication programs. In these areas, reinfection occurs constantly, flocks are often nomadic, and animal-raising practices make sanitary control difficult. Another important factor is that diagnostic methods for small ruminants are deficient. Experience with Rev. 1 vaccine in Italy, Turkey, Iran, Mongolia, Peru, and the Caucasian Republics of the former Soviet Union has proven it to be an excellent means of control. In Mongolia, 6 million animals were vaccinated between 1974 and 1977; as a result, the prevalence of from 3 to 4 per 10,000 animals was reduced by half or more, as was the incidence of human cases. In Malta, after seven years of vaccination of small ruminants with Rev. 1, the number of human cases per year fell from 260 to 29. The same thing happened in Italy, although there are no reference data (Alton, 1987). However, the control procedure of diagnosing and sacrificing reactor animals has produced satisfactory results in areas of low prevalence.

Rev. 1 vaccine has some limitations, such as residual virulence, the possibility of abortions when pregnant females are vaccinated, and the limited stability of the vaccine, which necessitates constant monitoring. These disadvantages should not eliminate use of the vaccine as the basis for control of brucellosis in small ruminants, at least until there is a better vaccine. A Chinese strain of *B. suis* biovar 1, known as *B. suis* strain 2, is considered reliable. This strain was isolated from a swine fetus and its virulence was attenuated by continuous and repeated replications in culture media over years, reaching an attenuation that remains stable. Vaccine *B. suis* strain 2 has been used in China with very good results for more than 20 years, not only in small ruminants but in cattle and swine as well. Its use began in the semiarid regions of northern China, where vaccination operations were very difficult due to the lack of fetters and traps, and thus the vaccine was administered in the drinking water (Xin, 1986). Various research institutes have conducted tests on conjunctive, oral (with syringes of the type used to administer antiparasitic agents), and subcutaneous vaccines in small ruminants; it has generally been possible to confirm the results obtained in China. Elimination of the vaccine strain in milk or through the vagina has not been confirmed and studies continue on this vaccine.

Ram epididymitis can be successfully controlled by a combination of the following measures: elimination of rams with clinically recognizable lesions, elimination of clinically normal rams positive to the gel diffusion or the complement fixation test, and separation of young rams (those not yet used for breeding) from adult males. In some countries, such as New Zealand and the US, a bacterin prepared from *B. ovis* and adjuvants is used. Animals are vaccinated when weaned, revaccinated one or two months later and annually thereafter. This vaccine produces antibodies against *B. ovis* but not *B. abortus*. The *B. melitensis* Rev. 1 vaccine is effective against epididymitis, but also produces *B. abortus* antibodies, which could be confused with infection by *B. melitensis*. The *B. suis* strain 2 vaccine does not provide protection against ram epididymitis.

Brucellosis caused by *B. canis* in dog kennels can be controlled by repeated serologic tests and blood cultures, followed by elimination of reactor animals. No vaccines are available yet. Veterinary clinics should advise owners of the risk of keeping a dog with brucellosis and should recommend that the dog be put to sleep.

Bibliography

Acosta, M., H. Ludueña, D. Barreto, M. Moro. Brucellosis en alpacas. *Rev Invest Pec* 1:37–49, 1972.

Al-Khalaf, S., A. El-Khaladi. Brucellosis in camels in Kuwait. *Com Immun Microbiol Infect Dis* 12:1–4, 1989.

Alton, G.G. The epidemiology of *Brucella melitensis* infection in sheep and goats. *In*: Verger, J.M., M. Plommet, eds. *Brucella melitensis*. Seminar held in Brussels, 14–15 November 1984. Dordrecht: Martinus Nijhoff; 1985.

Alton, G.G. Control of *Brucella melitensis* infection in sheep and goats—A review. *Trop Anim Health Prod* 19:65–74, 1987.

Alton, G.G., L.A. Corner, P.P. Plackett. Vaccination of pregnant cows with low doses of *Brucella abortus* strain 19 vaccine. *Aust Vet J* 56:369–372, 1980.

Alton, G.G., L.A. Corner, P.P. Plackett. Vaccination of cattle against brucellosis. Reduced doses of strain 19 compared with one and two doses of 45/20 vaccine. *Aust Vet J* 60:175–177, 1983.

Alton, G.G., L.M. Jones, C. García-Carrillo, A. Trenchi. *Brucella melitensis* Rev. 1 and *Brucella abortus* 45/20 vaccines in goats: Immunity. *Am J Vet Res* 33:1747–1751, 1972.

Alton, G.G., L.M. Jones, D.E. Pietz. *Laboratory techniques in brucellosis*. 2nd ed. Geneva: World Health Organization; 1975. (Monographs Series 55).

Anczykowski, F. Further studies on fowl brucellosis. II. Laboratory experiments. *Pol Arch Wet* 16:271–292, 1973.

Angus, R.D., C.E. Barton. The production and evaluation of a buffered plate antigen for use in a presumptive test for brucellosis. *In*: *Third International Symposium on Brucellosis, Algiers, Algeria, 1983. Developments in Biological Standardization*. Basel: Karger; 1984.

Banai, M., I. Mayer, A. Cohen. Isolation, identification, and characterization in Israel of *Brucella melitensis* biovar 1 atypical strains susceptible to dyes and penicillin, indicating the evolution of a new variant. *J Clin Microbiol* 28:1057–1059, 1990.

Barg, L. Isolamento de *Brucella canis* em Minas Gerais, Brazil. Pesquisa de aglutininas em soros caninos e humanos [thesis]. Belo Horizonte: Universidad Federal de Minas Gerais, 1975.

Barton, C.E., J.R. Lomme. Reduced-dose whole herd vaccination against brucellosis: A review of recent experience. *J Am Vet Med Assoc* 177:1218–1220, 1980.

Benenson, A.S., ed. *Control of Communicable Diseases in Man*. 15th ed. An official report of the American Public Health Association. Washington, D.C.: American Public Health Association; 1990.

Buchanan, T.M., L.C. Faber. 2-mercaptoethanol brucella agglutination test: Usefulness for predicting recovery from brucellosis. *J Clin Microbiol* 11:691–693, 1980.

Buchanan, T.M., S.L. Hendricks, C.M. Patton, R.A. Feldman. Brucellosis in the United States. An abattoir-associated disease. Part III. Epidemiology and evidence for acquired immunity. *Medicine* 53:427–439, 1974.

Cargill, C., K. Lee, I. Clarke. Use of an enzyme-linked immunosorbent assay in a bovine brucellosis eradication program. *Aust Vet J* 62:49–52, 1985.

Carmichael, L.E., J.C. Joubert. A rapid agglutination test for the serodiagnosis of *Brucella canis* infection that employs a variant (M–) organism as antigen. *Cornell Vet* 77:3–12, 1987.

Chappel, R.J., D.J. McNaught, J.A. Bourke, G.S. Allen. Comparison of the results of some serological tests for bovine brucellosis. *J Hyg* 80:365–371, 1978.

Chile, Ministerio de Agricultura, Servicio Agrícola and Ganadero. *Brucellosis bovina, ovina and caprina. Diagnóstico, control, vacunación*. Paris: Office International des Epizooties; 1987. (Technical Series 6).

Corbel, M.J. The serological relationship between *Brucella* spp., *Yersinia enterocolitica* serotype IX and Salmonella serotypes of Kauffman-White group. *J Hyg* 75:151–171, 1975.

Corbel, M.J., F.A. Stuart, R.A. Brewer. Observations on serological cross-reactions between smooth *Brucella* species and organisms of other genera. *In: Third International Symposium on Brucellosis, Algiers, Algeria, 1983. Developments in Biological Standardization.* Basel: Karger; 1984.

Corbel, M.J., E.L. Thomas, C. García-Carrillo. Taxonomic studies on some atypical strains of *Brucella suis. Br Vet J* 140:34–43, 1984.

De Lord, V., S. Nieto, E. Sandoval *et al.* Brucellosis en caprinos: estudios serológicos and bacteriológicos en Venezuela. *Vet Trop* 12:27–37, 1987.

De la Vega, E., C. García-Carrillo, C. Arce. Infección natural por *Brucella* en comadrejas *Didelphis marsupialis* en la República Argentina. *Rev Med Vet* 60:283–286, 1979.

Díaz, R., E. Maravi-Poma, J.L. Fernández, S. García-Merlo, A. Rivero-Puente. Brucellosis: estudio de 222 casos. Parte IV: Diagnóstico de la brucellosis humana. *Rev Clin Esp* 166:107–110, 1982.

Díaz, R., I. Moriyon. Laboratory techniques in the diagnosis of human brucellosis. *In:* Young, E.J., M.J. Corbel, eds. *Brucellosis: Clinical and Laboratory Aspects.* Boca Raton: CRC Press; 1989.

Drannovskaia, E. Brucella and brucellosis in man and animals. Izmir, Turkey, 1990. *Turkish Microbiol Soc* 16:87–100, 1991.

Elberg, S.S. The Brucellae. *In:* Dubos, R.J., J.G. Hirsch, eds. *Bacterial and Mycotic Infections of Man.* 4th ed. Philadelphia and Montreal: Lippincott; 1965.

Elberg, S.S. Immunity to *Brucella* infection. *Medicine* 52:339–356, 1973.

Elberg, S.S. A guide to the diagnosis, treatment and prevention of human brucellosis. Geneva: World Health Organization; 1981. VPH/81.31 Rev.1. (Unpublished document).

Ewalt, D.R., L.B. Forbes. Atypical isolates of *Brucella abortus* from Canada and the United States characterized as dye sensitive with M antigen dominant. *J Clin Microbiol* 25:698–701, 1987.

Fensterbank, R. Congenital brucellosis in cattle. Geneva: World Health Organization; 1980. WHO/BRUC/80.352. (Unpublished document).

Flores-Castro, R., F. Suárez, C. Ramírez-Pfeiffer, L.E. Carmichael. Canine brucellosis: Bacteriological and serological investigation of naturally infected dogs in Mexico City. *J Clin Microbiol* 6:591–597, 1977.

Forbes, L.B. *Brucella abortus* infection in 14 farm dogs. *J Am Vet Med Assoc* 196: 911–916, 1990.

Fredickson, L.E., C.E. Barton. A serologic survey for canine brucellosis in a metropolitan area. *J Am Vet Med Assoc* 165:987–989, 1974.

García-Carrillo, C. Métodos para el diagnóstico de la brucellosis. *Gac Vet* 32:661–667, 1970.

García-Carrillo, C. *Programa de erradicación de la brucellosis en California.* Buenos Aires: Centro Panamericano de Zoonosis, 1975. (Scientific and Technical Monographs 9).

García-Carrillo, C., E.A. Coltorti. Ausencia de anticuerpos resistentes al 2-marcaptoetanol en tres pacientes de brucellosis. *Medicina* 39:611–613, 1979.

García-Carrillo, C., N.E. Lucero. *Brucellosis bovina.* Buenos Aires: Hemisferio Sur; 1993.

García-Carrillo, C., B. Szyfres, J. González Tomé. Tipificación de brucelas aisladas del hombre y los animales en Latin America. *Rev Latinoam Microbiol* 14:117–125, 1972.

George, L.W., L.E. Carmichael. A plate agglutination test for the rapid diagnosis of canine brucellosis. *Am J Vet Res* 35:905–909, 1974.

Gilman, H.L. Brucellosis. *In:* Gibbons, W.J., ed. *Diseases of Cattle, a text and reference work. The work of 54 authors.* Wheaton: American Veterinary Publication; 1963.

González Tomé, J.S., L.J. Villa, E. del Palacio, R. Gregoret. El test de Angus and Barton (BPA) como prueba tamiz en el diagnóstico de la brucellosis bovina. *Rev Med Vet* 70:34–36, 1989.

Hendricks, S.L., M.E. Meyer. Brucellosis. *In:* Hubbert, W.T., W.F. McCulloch, P.R. Schnurrenberger, eds. *Diseases Transmitted from Animals to Man.* 6th ed. Springfield: Thomas; 1975.

Kasyanov, A.N., R.G. Aslanyan. Epizootiology and clinical appearance of animal brucellosis. *In*: Lisenko, A., ed. *Zoonoses Control*. Moscow: VII Centre Projects; 1982.

Kaufmann, A.F., M.D. Fox, J.M. Boyce, D.C. Anderson, M.E. Potter, W.J. Martone, *et al.* Airborne spread of brucellosis. *Ann NY Acad Sci* 353:105–114, 1980.

Lapraik, R.D., D.D. Brown, H. Mann. Brucellosis. A study of five calves from reactor dams. *Vet Rec* 97:52–54, 1975.

Lee, K., C. Cargill, H. Atkinson. Evaluation of an enzyme-linked immunosorbent assay for the diagnosis of *Brucella ovis* infection in rams. *Aust Vet J* 62:91–93, 1985.

Lu, S-L., J-L. Zhang. Brucellosis in China. *In*: Young, E.J., M.J. Corbel, eds. *Brucellosis: Clinical and Laboratory Aspects*. Boca Raton: CRC Press; 1989.

Lubani, M., D. Sharda, I. Helin. Probable transmission of brucellosis from breast milk to a newborn. *Trop Geogr Med* 40:151–152, 1988.

Luchsinger, D.W., R.K. Anderson. Longitudinal studies of naturally acquired *Brucella abortus* infection in sheep. *Am J Vet Med Res* 40:1307–1312, 1979.

Manthei, C.A. Brucellosis as a cause of abortion today. *In*: Faulkner, L.C., ed. *Abortion Diseases of Livestock*. Springfield: Thomas; 1968.

Manthei, C.A. Brucellosis. *In*: Dunne, H.W., ed. *Diseases of Swine*. 3rd ed. Ames: Iowa State University Press; 1970.

McCaughey, W.J. Brucellosis in wildlife. *In*: Diarmid, A., ed. *Diseases in Free-living Wild Animals*. New York: Academic Press; 1969.

McCullough, N.B. Microbial and host factors in the pathogenesis of brucellosis. *In*: Mudd, S., ed. *Infectious Agents and Host Reactions*. Philadelphia: Saunders; 1970.

Meyer, M.E. Inter- and intra-strain variants in the *Genus Brucella*. *In*: *Third International Symposium on Brucellosis, Algiers, Algeria, 1983. Developments in Biological Standardization*. Basel: Karger; 1984.

Morgan, W.J.B. Brucella classification and regional distribution. *In*: *Third International Symposium on Brucellosis, Algiers, Algeria, 1983. Developments in Biological Standardization*. Basel: Karger; 1984.

Myers, D.M., L.M. Jones, V.M. Varela-Díaz. Studies of antigens for complement fixation and gel diffusion tests in the diagnosis of infections caused by *Brucella ovis* and other *Brucella*. *Appl Microbiol* 23:894–902, 1972.

Nicoletti, P. A preliminary report on the efficacy of adult cattle vaccination using strain 19 in selected dairy herds in Florida. *Proc Annu Meet US Livest Sanit Assoc* 80:91–106, 1976.

Nicoletti, P., L.M. Jones, D.T. Berman. Adult vaccination with standard and reduced doses of *Brucella abortus* strain 19 in a dairy herd infected with brucellosis. *J Am Vet Med Assoc* 173:1445–1449, 1978.

Nicoletti, P., F.W. Milward. Protection by oral administration of *Brucella abortus* strain 19 against an oral challenge exposure with a pathogenic strain of *Brucella*. *Am J Vet Res* 44:1641–1643, 1983.

Nielsen, K., J.W. Cherwonogrodzky, J.R. Duncan, D.R. Bundle. Enzyme-linked immunosorbent assay for differentiation of the antibody response of cattle naturally infected with *Brucella abortus* or vaccinated with strain 19. *Am J Vet Res* 50:5–9, 1989.

Ossola, A.L., B. Szyfres. Natural infection of sheep by *Brucella melitensis* in Argentina. *Am J Vet Res* 24:446–449, 1963.

Pacheco, G., M.T. De Mello. *Brucelose*. Rio de Janeiro: Instituto Brasileiro de Geografia e Estatística; 1956.

Pan American Health Organization. Guía para la preparación and evaluación de proyectos de lucha contra la brucellosis bovina. Buenos Aires: Centro Panamericano de Zoonosis; 1972. (Technical Note 14).

Peres, J.N., A.M. Godoy, L. Barg, J.O. Costa. Isolamento de *Brucella canis* de carrapatos (*Rhipicephalus sanguineus*). *Arq Esc Vet UFMG* 33:51–55, 1981.

Pfischner, W.C.E., K.G. Ishak, E. Neptune, *et al.* Brucellosis in Egypt: A review of experience with 228 patients. *Am J Med* 22:915, 1957. Cited in: Young, E.J. Clinical manifestations of human brucellosis. *In*: Young, E.J., M.J. Corbel, eds. *Brucellosis: Clinical and Laboratory Aspects.* Boca Raton: CRC Press; 1989.

Plommet, M., R. Fensterbank. Vaccination against bovine brucellosis with a low dose of strain 19 administered by the conjunctival route. III.—Seriological response and immunity in the pregnant cow. *Ann Rech Vét* 7:9–23, 1976.

Plommet, M., R. Fensterbank, G. Renoux, J. Gestin, A. Philippon. Brucellose bovine expérimentale. XII. Persistance a l'age adulte de l'infection congénitale de la génisse. *Ann Rech Vét* 4:419–435, 1973.

Ramacciotti, F. *Brucelosis.* Córdoba, Argentina: Edición del Autor; 1971.

Ray, W.C., R.B. Brown, D.A. Stringfellow, *et al.* Bovine brucellosis: An investigation of latency in progeny of culture-positive cows. *J Am Vet Med Assoc* 192:182–185, 1988.

Robertson, F.J., J. Milne, C.L. Silver, H. Clark. Abortion associated with *Brucella abortus* (biovar 1) in the T.B. mare. *Vet Rec* 92:480–481, 1973.

Ruben, B., J.D. Band, P. Wong, J. Colville. Person-to-person transmission of *Brucella melitensis. Lancet* 337:14–15, 1991.

Schwabe, C.W. *Veterinary Medicine and Human Health.* 2nd ed. Baltimore: Williams & Wilkins; 1969.

Spink, W.W. *The Nature of Brucellosis.* Minneapolis: University of Minnesota Press; 1956.

Spink, W.W. Brucellosis (Undulant fever, Malta fever). *In*: Wyngaarden, I.B., L.H. Smith, Jr., eds. *Cecil Textbook of Medicine.* 16th ed. Philadelphia: Saunders; 1982.

Stemshorn, B.W., L.B. Forbes, M.D. Eaglesome, *et al.* A comparison of standard serological tests for the diagnosis of bovine brucellosis in Canada. *Can J Comp Med* 49: 391–394, 1985.

Sutherland, S.S., R.J. Evans, J. Bathgate. Application of an enzyme-linked immunosorbent assay in the final stages of a bovine brucellosis eradication program. *Aust Vet J* 63:412–415, 1986.

Szyfres, B. La situación de la brucellosis en Latin America. *Bol Hig Epidemiol* 5:400–409, 1967.

Szyfres, B. Taxonomía del género *Brucella. Gac Vet* 33:28–40, 1971.

Szyfres, B., J. González Tomé. Natural *Brucella* infection in Argentine wild foxes. *Bull World Health Organ* 34:919–923, 1966.

Szyfres, B., J. González Tomé, T. Palacio Mendieta. Aislamiento de *Brucella suis* de la liebre europea (*Lepus europaeus*) en la Argentina. *Bol Oficina Sanit Panam* 65:441–445, 1968.

Timm, B.M. *Brucellosis. Distribution in Man, Domestic and Wild Animals.* Berlin: Springer; 1982.

Trap, D., R. Gaumont. Comparaison entre electrosynerèse et épreuves serologiques classiques dans le diagnostic de la brucellose ovine. *Ann Rech Vét* 13:33–39, 1982.

United States, Department of Health and Human Services, Centers for Disease Control and Prevention (CDC). Annual summary 1981: Reported morbidity and mortality in the United States. *MMWR Morb Mort Wkly Rep* 30:14, 1982.

Van der Hoeden, J. Brucellosis. *In*: Van der Hoeden, J., ed. *Zoonoses.* Amsterdam: Elsevier; 1964.

Verger, J.M., F. Grimont, P.A.D. Grimont, M. Grayon. *Brucella*: a monospecific genus as shown by deoxyribonucleic acid hybridization. *Int J Syst Bacteriol* 35:292–295, 1985.

Viana, F.C., J.A. Silva, E.C. Moreira, L.G. Villela, J.G. Mendez, T.O. Dias. Vacinação contra brucelose bovina com dose reduzida (amostra B_{19}) por via conjuntival. *Arq Esc Vet UFMG* 34:279–287, 1982.

Wilesmith, J.W. The persistence of *Brucella abortus* infection in calves: A retrospective study of heavily infected herds. *Vet Rec* 103:149–153, 1978.

Witter, J.F., D.C. O'Meara. Brucellosis. *In*: Davis, J.W., L.H. Karstady, D.O. Trainer. *Infectious Diseases of Wild Mammals*. Ames: Iowa State University Press; 1970.

World Health Organization (WHO). *Fifth Report on the World Health Situation, 1969–1972*. Geneva: WHO; 1975. (Official Records 225).

World Health Organization (WHO). *Joint FAO/WHO Expert Committee on Brucellosis, Sixth Report*. Geneva: WHO; 1986. (Technical Report Series 740).

Xin, X. Orally administrable brucellosis vaccine: *Brucella suis* strain 2 vaccine. *Vaccine* 4:212–216, 1986.

Young, E.J. Clinical manifestations of human brucellosis. *In*: Young, E.J., M.J. Corbel, eds. *Brucellosis: Clinical and Laboratory Aspects*. Boca Raton: CRC Press; 1989.

Zoha, S.J., L.E. Carmichael. Serological response of dogs to cell wall and internal antigens of *Brucella canis* (*B. canis*). *Vet Microbiol* 7:35–50, 1982.

CAMPYLOBACTERIOSIS

ICD-10 A04.5 campylobacter enteritis

The genus Campylobacter *(heretofore* Vibrio*) contains several species of importance for both public and animal health. The principal pathogenic species are* C. jejuni *and* C. fetus *subsp.* fetus *(previously subsp.* intestinalis*) and* C. fetus *subsp.* venerealis. *Occasionally* C. coli, C. laridis, *and* C. upsaliensis *cause enteritis in man and animals. These bacteria are gram-negative, microaerophilic, thermophilic, catalase positive (with the exception of* C. upsaliensis*), and have a curved or spiral shape.*

The importance of campylobacteriosis as a diarrheal disease became evident when better knowledge was gained about its requirements for culture and isolation, particularly oxygen pressure (strictly microaerophilic) and an optimum temperature of 42°C (thermophilic).

Increased medical interest since 1977 in enteritis caused by C. jejuni *and the enormous bibliography on this new zoonosis make it advisable to discuss this disease separately from those caused by* C. fetus *and its two subspecies. Furthermore, the disease caused by* C. jejuni *and those caused by* C. fetus *are clinically different.*

1. Enteritis caused by *Campylobacter jejuni*

Synonym: Vibrionic enteritis.

Etiology: *Campylobacter jejuni* and occasionally *C. coli*. Two principal schemes have been proposed for serotyping *C. jejuni*. The scheme proposed by Penner uses somatic antigens and includes 60 serotypes, which are identified using the passive hemagglutination method (Penner and Hennessy, 1980; McMyne *et al.*, 1982). The scheme proposed by Lior uses a flaggelar antigen and identifies 90 serotypes with the slide plate agglutination method (Lior, 1982). Patton *et al.* (1985) compare both schemes in 1,405 isolates of human, animal, and environmental origin, and find that

96.1% could be typed using the Penner system and 92.1% could be typed using the Lior system. They also conclude that these schemes complement each other and are useful for epidemiological research.

Geographic Distribution: Worldwide.

Occurrence in Man: At present, *C. jejuni* is considered to be one of the principal bacterial agents causing enteritis and diarrhea in man, particularly in developed countries. In these countries, the incidence is similar to that of enteritis caused by *Salmonella.* As culture media and isolation methods have been perfected, the number of recorded cases caused by *C. jejuni* has increased. In Great Britain, the 200 public health and hospital laboratories had been reporting isolations of salmonellas exceeding those of *Campylobacter*, but beginning in 1981, the proportions were reversed: 12,496 isolations of *Campylobacter* as opposed to 10,745 of *Salmonella* (Skirrow, 1982). According to Benenson (1990), campylobacteriosis causes 5% to 14% of diarrhea cases worldwide. Based on records from private medical practice, it has been estimated that 20% of office consultations for enteritis in Great Britain were associated with campylobacteriosis and that there are a projected 600,000 cases annually at the national level (Skirrow, 1982). It is harder to establish the incidence in developing countries; because of deficiencies in hygiene, *C. jejuni* is isolated from 5% to 17% of persons without diarrhea (Prescott and Munroe, 1982) and from 8% to 31% of persons with diarrhea. Thus, it is likely that *Campylobacter* is an important cause of infantile diarrhea in the Third World (Skirrow, 1982).

The illness affects all age groups. In developing countries, it particularly affects children under the age of 2 years; in developed countries, children and young adults become ill more frequently. Campylobacteriosis is also an important cause of "travellers' diarrhea" (Benenson, 1990). The disease is primarily sporadic, although there are also epidemic outbreaks. The largest known epidemics originated from common sources, such as unpasteurized milk or contaminated water from the municipal supply of two European cities. In countries with a temperate climate, the disease is most prevalent in the warm months.

In Great Britain, the US, Canada, and Switzerland, consumption of unpasteurized milk or products prepared with raw milk has caused campylobacteriosis outbreaks. The largest outbreak in Great Britain affected approximately 3,500 people (Jones *et al.*, 1981). Outbreaks may be due to milk contaminated by fecal matter or, less frequently, to milk from udders with mastitis caused by *C. jejuni.* Another outbreak affected more than 30 people in a small town in Great Britain. The ensuing investigation showed that the source of infection was two cows with mastitis caused by *C. jejuni* that contaminated the bulk milk of 40 cows (Hutchinson *et al.*, 1985). The same serotypes of *C. jejuni* were isolated from the cows, patients' feces, milk filters, and bulk milk.

It is estimated that *C. jejuni* causes more than 90% of human cases of the disease (Karmali and Skirrow, 1984) and only 10% in other species.

Occurrence in Animals: Domestic and wild mammals and birds constitute the large reservoir of *C. jejuni*, but it is difficult to implicate this agent as a cause of diarrheal disease because a high rate of infection is found in clinically healthy animals.

The Disease in Man: Enteritis caused by *C. jejuni* is an acute illness. In general, the incubation period is from two to five days. The principal symptoms are diarrhea, fever, abdominal pain, vomiting (in one-third of the patients), and visible or occult blood (50% to 90% of patients). Fever is often accompanied by general malaise, headache, and muscle and joint pain. The feces are liquid and frequently contain mucus and blood. The course of the illness is usually benign, and the patient recovers spontaneously in a week to 10 days; acute symptoms often fade in two to three days. Symptoms may be more severe in some patients, similar to those of ulcerative colitis and salmonellosis, and may lead to suspicion of appendicitis and an exploratory laparatomy. In some cases, septicemia has been confirmed, either simultaneous to the diarrheic illness or afterward. Complications are rare and consist of meningitis and abortions.

Enteric campylobacteriosis is a self-limiting disease and does not usually require medication, except for electrolyte replacement. In cases that require medication, erythromycin is the antibiotic of choice.

The Disease in Animals: *C. jejuni* has been identified as an etiologic agent in several illnesses of domestic animals (Prescott and Munroe, 1982).

CATTLE: Enteritis caused by *C. jejuni* in calves is clinically similar to that in man. Calves suffer a moderate fever and diarrhea that may last as long as 14 days. It is also possible that this agent causes mastitis in cows, as demonstrated by the fact that experimental inoculation of the udder with a small number of bacteria causes acute mastitis (see outbreaks due to raw milk in the section on occurrence in man).

SHEEP: *C. jejuni* is a major cause of abortions in sheep. In the number of outbreaks, it is assigned a role similar to that of *C. fetus* subsp. *fetus* (*intestinalis*). Sheep abort toward the end of their pregnancy or give birth at term to either dead or weak lambs that may die within a few days.

DOGS AND CATS: Puppies with diarrhea constitute a source of infection for their owners. Diarrhea is the predominant symptom and vomiting seems to be frequent. The disease is more frequent in puppies, but may occur in adult animals as well. Fox *et al.* (1984) described an outbreak caused by *C. jejuni* in nine of 10 young beagles that had diarrheal feces with traces of bile and occasionally blood. In England, a study of dogs treated at various veterinary clinics isolated *C. jejuni* from 59 (11.6%) of the 505 dogs with diarrhea and from only 2 (1.6%) of the 122 dogs without diarrhea. In another study (Fleming, 1983), 39 dogs had either persistent or intermittent chronic diarrhea.

Burnens and Nicolet (1992) cultured 241 samples of fecal matter from dogs and 156 from cats with diarrhea. The cultures were positive for *Campylobacter* spp. in 20% of the dog samples and in 13% of the cat samples. The frequency of *C. upsaliensis* among the positive cultures was approximately equal in dogs and cats. However, the authors present no conclusions regarding the pathogenic role of *C. upsaliensis* in dogs and cats because they did not examine animals without diarrhea.

OTHER MAMMALS: Enteritis caused by *C. jejuni* probably occurs in many other animal species. It has been described in monkeys and in one outbreak in young horses.

FOWL: Fowl are an important reservoir of *C. jejuni*. Although it was possible to cause diarrhea in 3-day-old chicks with orally administered *C. jejuni*, it is not known if the illness occurs naturally, since a high proportion of healthy birds harbor the bacteria in their intestines.

Figure 8. Campylobacteriosis (*Campylobacter jejuni*).
Mode of transmission.

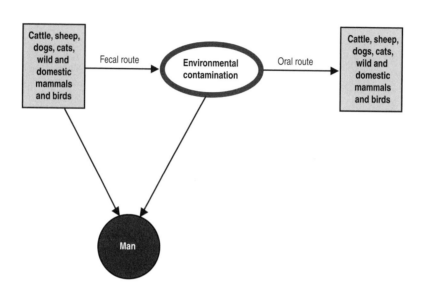

Source of Infection and Mode of Transmission (Figure 8): Mammals and birds, both domestic and wild, are the principal reservoir of *C. jejuni*. In studies by various authors (Skirrow, 1982; Prescott and Munroe, 1982), *C. jejuni* was found in the ceca of 100% of 600 turkeys and in the droppings of 38 out of 46 chickens and 83 out of 94 ducks that had large numbers of the bacteria in their intestines prior to slaughter. The organism has been found in several species of wild birds, for example, in 35% of migratory birds, 50% of urban pigeons, and 20% to 70% of seagulls. The agent has been isolated from the feces of 2.5% to 100% of healthy cows, from the gallbladder of 20 out of 186 sheep, from the feces of 0% to 30% of healthy dogs, and also from a wide variety of wild mammal species.

C. jejuni is commonly found in natural water sources, where it can survive for several weeks at low temperatures. However, it is interesting to note that it has always been found in the presence of fecal coliforms, and therefore the contamination presumably stems from animals (mammals and fowl) and, in some circumstances, from man. The source of infection is almost always food, although it is sometimes difficult to identify the immediate source. Given the common occurrence of *C. jejuni* and *C. coli* in the intestines of mammals and fowl *(C. jejuni* can survive for several weeks at 4°C on the moist surface of chickens), it can easily be assumed that contamination of bird and animal meat is a frequent occurrence. One study conducted by various laboratories in the US demonstrated that approximately 30% of the 300 chickens included in the sample had *C. jejuni* and that 5.1% of the 1,800 samples of red meat were contaminated. *C. coli* was isolated from pork and *C. jejuni* was isolated from other meats (Stern *et al.*, 1985).

The infection in man may be caused by cross contamination in the kitchen of meats with *C. jejuni* and other foods that do not require cooking, or that are under-cooked (Griffith and Park, 1990). Other sources of infection are unpasteurized milk and milk products, river water, and inadequately treated municipal water. In some cases, the infection is acquired directly from animals, especially from puppies and cats with diarrhea. The victims are almost always children who play with these animals and come in contact with the animal's feces.

In peripheral urban areas of Lima (Peru), Grados *et al.* (1988) studied 104 children under the age of 3 years who had diarrhea and compared them to the same number of children without gastrointestinal disorders (control group) in order to identify the various risk factors. The authors concluded that the presence of chickens and hens in the home environment constitutes an important risk factor. Children become infected by contact with the droppings of birds in the household environment. Another interesting fact is that slaughterhouse workers—particularly those who come into direct contact with animals and their by-products—have a much higher rate of positive reactions to *Campylobacter* spp. than the blood donors who served as controls (Mancinelli *et al.*, 1987).

Person-to-person transmission may occur, but is unusual. Among the few cases described was a nosocomial infection of children in Mexico (Flores-Salorio *et al.*, 1983). Untreated patients may eliminate *C. jejuni* for six weeks, and a few for a year or more. As in the case of other enteric infections, entry is through the digestive tract.

Diagnosis: Consists mainly of isolating the agent from the patient's feces. Diagnosis is made using selective media that are incubated in an atmosphere of 5% oxygen, 10% carbon dioxide, and 85% nitrogen, preferably at a temperature of 43°C. Serologic diagnosis may be done using direct immunofluorescence or other tests on paired sera.

In animals, because of the high rate of healthy carriers, isolation of the agent is inadequate proof that it is responsible for the illness, and it is advisable to confirm an increase in titers with serologic testing.

Control: According to present knowledge of the epidemiology of the illness, preventive measures can be only partial in scope. In a study of risk factors in Colorado (USA), where sporadic cases of infection were caused by *C. jejuni*, it was estimated that approximately one-third of the cases could have been prevented by such measures as avoiding the consumption of untreated water, unpasteurized milk, or under-cooked chicken (Hopkins *et al.*, 1984). People in contact with dogs and cats with diarrhea should follow personal hygiene rules, such as thorough handwashing. Sick animals should not be in contact with children. The same recommendations on personal hygiene apply to homemakers. In the kitchen, care should be taken to separate raw animal products from other foods, particularly in the case of fowl. Control of the infection in animals is clearly desirable, but is not presently feasible, given the wide diffusion of the agent and its presence in wild animal reservoirs.

Bibliography

Benenson, A.S., ed. *Control of Communicable Diseases in Man*. 15th ed. An official report of the American Public Health Association. Washington, D.C.: American Public Health Association; 1990.

Burnens, A.P., J. Nicolet. Detection of *Campylobacter upsaliensis* in diarrheic dogs and cats, using a selective medium with cefoperazone. *Am J Vet Res* 53:48–51, 1992.

Fleming, M.P. Association of *Campylobacter jejuni* with enteritis in dogs and cats. *Vet Rec* 113:372–374, 1983.

Flores-Salorio, S.G., V. Vázquez-Alvarado, L. Moreno-Altamirano. *Campylobacter* como agente etiológico de diarrea en niños. *Bol Med Hosp Infant Mex* 40:315–319, 1983.

Fox, J.G., K.O. Maxwell, J.I. Ackerman. *Campylobacter jejuni* associated diarrhea in commercially reared beagles. *Lab Animal Sci* 34:151–155, 1984.

Grados, O., N. Bravo, R.E. Black, J.P. Butzler. Paediatric campylobacter diarrhoea from household exposure to live chickens in Lima, Peru. *Bull World Health Organ* 66:369–374, 1988.

Griffiths, P.L., R.W. Park. Campylobacters associated with human diarrhoeal disease. A review. *J Appl Bacteriol* 69:281–301, 1990.

Hopkins, R.S., R. Olmsted, G.R. Istre. Endemic *Campylobacter jejuni* infection in Colorado: Identified risk factors. *Am J Public Health* 74:249–250, 1984.

Hutchinson, D.N., F.J. Bolton, P.M. Hinchliffe, *et al.* Evidence of udder excretion of *Campylobacter jejuni* as the cause of milk-borne campylobacter outbreak. *J Hyg* 94: 205–215, 1985.

Jones, P.H., A.T. Willis, D.A. Robinson, *et al. Campylobacter* enteritis associated with the consumption of free school milk. *J Hyg* 87:155–162, 1981.

Karmali, M.A., M.B. Skirrow. Taxonomy of the genus *Campylobacter*. *In*: Butzler, J.P., ed. *Campylobacter Infection in Man and Animals*. Boca Raton: CRC Press; 1984.

Lior, H., D.L. Woodward, J.A. Edgar, *et al.* Serotyping of *Campylobacter jejuni* by slide agglutination based on heat-labile antigenic factors. *J Clin Microbiol* 15:761–768, 1982.

Mancinelli, S., L. Palombi, F. Riccardi, M.C. Marazzi. Serological study of *Campylobacter jejuni* infection in slaughterhouse workers [letter]. *J Infect Dis* 156:856, 1987.

McMyne, P.M.S., J.L. Penner, R.G. Mathias, W.A. Black, J.N. Hennessy. Serotyping of *Campylobacter jejuni* isolated from sporadic cases and outbreaks in British Columbia. *J Clin Microbiol* 16:281–285, 1982.

Patton, C.M., T.J. Barrett, G.K. Morris. Comparison of the Penner and Lior methods for serotyping *Campylobacter* spp. *J Clin Microbiol* 22:558–565, 1985.

Penner, J.L., J.N. Hennessy. Passive hemagglutination technique for serotyping *Campylobacter fetus* subsp. *jejuni* on the basis of soluble heat-stable antigens. *J Clin Microbiol* 12:732–737, 1980.

Prescott, J.M., D.L. Munroe. *Campylobacter jejuni*. Enteritis in man and domestic animals. *J Am Vet Med Assoc* 181:1524–1530, 1982.

Sandstedt, K., J. Ursing. Description of *Campylobacter upsaliensis* sp.nov. previously known as CNW group. *System Appl Microbiol* 14:39–45, 1989.

Skirrow, M.B. *Campylobacter* enteritis. The first five years. *J Hyg* 89:175–184, 1982.

Stern, N.J., M.P. Hernández, L. Blakenship, *et al.* Prevalence and distribution of *Campylobacter jejuni* and *Campylobacter coli* in retail meats. *J Food Protect* 48:595–599, 1985.

2. Diseases caused by *Campylobacter fetus*

Synonyms: Vibriosis, vibrionic abortion, epizootic infertility, bovine genital vibriosis, epizootic ovine abortion.

Etiology: *Campylobacter* (*Vibrio*) *fetus* subsp. *fetus* (*intestinalis*) and *C. fetus* subsp. *venerealis*. *C. fetus* develops in such media as blood agar and *Brucella* agar; it is microaerophilic, but is unlike *C. jejuni* in that it grows at 25°C but not at 42°C.

Geographic Distribution: Worldwide.

Occurrence in Man: Uncommon. Up to 1981, the literature recorded at least 134 confirmed cases (Bokkenheuser and Sutter, 1981), most of them occurring in the US and the rest in various parts of the world. The incidence is believed to be much higher than that recorded.

Occurrence in Animals: The disease is common in cattle and sheep and occurs worldwide.

The Disease in Man: The strains isolated from man have characteristics similar to those of *C. fetus* subsp. *fetus* (*intestinalis*), which causes outbreaks of abortion among sheep and sporadic cases in cattle. Two cases caused by *C. fetus* subsp. *venerealis* have also been described (Veron and Chatelain, 1973). Campylobacteriosis is generally recognized when accompanied by predisposing debilitating factors, such as pregnancy, premature birth, chronic alcoholism, neoplasia, and cardiovascular disease. The majority of isolations are from pregnant women, premature babies, and men and women over 45 years of age. The proportion of cases is higher in men than in women.

Infection by *C. fetus* causes septicemia in man. In more than half of the cases, bacteremia is secondary and follows different localized infections. Between 17% and 43% of septicemic patients die (Morrison *et al.*, 1990). Most cultures have been obtained from the bloodstream during fever, but the etiologic agent has also been isolated from synovial and spinal fluid, and sometimes from the feces of patients with acute enteritis.

In pregnant women, the illness has been observed from the fifth month of pregnancy, accompanied by a sustained fever and often by diarrhea. Pregnancy may terminate in miscarriage, premature birth, or full-term birth. Premature infants and some full-term infants die from the infection, which presents symptoms of meningitis or meningoencephalitis. The syndrome may begin the day of birth with a slight fever, cough, and diarrhea; after two to seven days, the signs of meningitis appear. The case fatality rate is approximately 50%. Malnourished children, and at times apparently healthy ones, can develop bacteremia along with vomiting, anorexia, diarrhea, and fever. The patient usually recovers spontaneously or after antibiotic treatment. In adults, often those already weakened by other illness, the disease appears as a generalized infection with extremely variable symptomatology (Bokkenheuser and Sutter, 1981). *C. fetus* subsp. *fetus* is above all an opportunistic pathogen that gives rise to a systemic infection but rarely causes enteritis, in contrast to *C. jejuni*. Some cases of gastroenteritis caused by *C. fetus* subsp. *fetus* have been noted in men without a compromised immune system (Devlin and McIntyre, 1983; Harvey and Greenwood, 1983).

Gentamicin is the recommended antibiotic in the case of bacteremia and other clinical forms of nonenteric infection. Chloramphenicol is recommended when the central nervous system is involved. Prolonged antibiotic treatment is necessary to prevent relapses (Morrison *et al.*, 1990).

The Disease in Animals: In cattle and sheep, vibriosis is an important disease that causes considerable losses due to infertility and abortions.

CATTLE: In this species, the principal etiologic agent is *C. fetus* subsp. *venerealis* and, to a lesser degree, subsp. *fetus*. Genital vibriosis is a major cause of infertility, causing early embryonic death. The principal symptom is the repetition of estrus after service. During an outbreak, a high proportion of cows come into heat repeatedly for three to five months, but only 25% to 40% of them become pregnant after being bred twice. Of the cows or heifers that finally become pregnant, 5% to 10% abort five months into gestation. An undetermined proportion of females harbor *C. fetus* subsp. *venerealis* during the entire gestation period and become a source of infection for the bulls in the next breeding season. After the initial infection, cows acquire resistance to the disease and recover their normal fertility, i.e., the embryo develops normally. However, immunity to the infection is only partial and the animals may become reinfected even though the embryos continue to develop normally. Resistance decreases substantially after three to four years.

The infection is transmitted by natural breeding or artificial insemination. Bulls are the normal, though in most cases temporary, carriers of the infection. They play an important role in its transmission to females. The etiologic agent is carried in the preputial cavity. Bulls may become infected while servicing infected cows, as well as by contaminated instruments and equipment used in artificial insemination. The etiologic agent is sensitive to antibiotics that are added to the semen used in artificial insemination.

C. fetus subsp. *fetus* is responsible for sporadic abortions in cattle. Some females are carriers of the infection, house the infectious agent in the gallbladder, and eliminate it in fecal matter.

SHEEP: The principal agents of epizootic abortion in sheep are *C. fetus* subsp. *fetus* and *C. jejuni* and, to a lesser extent, *C. fetus* subsp. *venerealis*. The disease is characterized by fetal death and abortions in the final months of gestation, or by full-term birth of dead lambs or lambs that die shortly thereafter. The infection also gives rise to metritus and placentitis, both of which may result in septicemia and death of the ewe. Losses of 10% to 20% of the lambs and 5% of the ewes that abort are common. The rate of abortions varies and depends on the proportion of susceptible ewes. Infected animals acquire immunity. Ewes do not abort again for about three years. If the infection is recent in the flock, the abortion rate can be quite high, at times up to 70% of the pregnant ewes. The infection is transmitted orally; venereal transmission apparently plays no role.

Source of Infection and Mode of Transmission (Figure 9): The reservoir of *C. fetus* is animals, but it is not clear how man contracts the infection. It is presumed that he can become infected by direct contact with infected animals, by ingestion of contaminated food (unpasteurized milk, raw liver) or water, by transplacental transmission, exposure during birth, or sexual contact. It should be noted, however, that some patients have denied any contact with animals or even with products of animal origin. It is also suspected that the infection may be endogenous. The etiologic agent would be an oral commensal parasite that could penetrate the bloodstream during a dental extraction. Another hypothesis is that *C. fetus* could be harbored in the human intestine without becoming evident until the host loses resistance due to some illness. It would then invade through the mucosa, causing a generalized infection. In summary, the source and pathogenesis of *C. fetus* in man continue to be unknown (Morrison *et al.*, 1990).

The sources of infection in cattle are carrier bulls and also cows that remain infected from one parturition to the next. The mode of transmission is sexual contact.

For sheep, the source of infection is environmental contamination. The placentas of infected sheep that abort or even of those that give birth normally, as well as

**Figure 9. Campylobacteriosis (*Campylobacter fetus*).
Probable mode of transmission.**

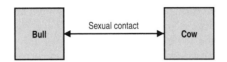

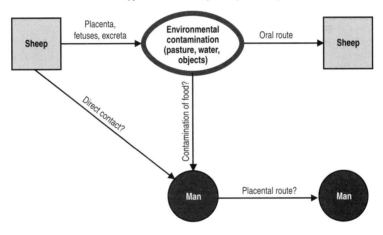

NOTE: It is not known how the disease is transmitted to humans; transmission is assumed to occur through direct contact, contamination of foods, or transplacental passage.

aborted fetuses and vaginal discharges, contain a large number of *Campylobacter*. A few infected ewes become carriers by harboring the infection in the gallbladder and shedding the agent in fecal matter. Contaminated grass, tools, and clothing are the vehicles of infection. Transmission is oral. Sexual transmission has not been demonstrated, but knowledge on this subject is inadequate.

Role of Animals in the Epidemiology of the Disease: Animals are the natural reservoir of *C. fetus*. The agent has been observed to lodge in the human gallbladder, but it is not known how often man may become a carrier and give rise to human foci of infection. It is probably an exceptional occurrence. The mechanism of transmission from animals to humans is unclear.

Diagnosis: So far, diagnosis of campylobacteriosis in man has been largely fortuitous, when *C. fetus* is discovered in hemocultures of patients in whom the etiology was not suspected. During the febrile period, repeated blood samples should be taken for culture. In cases of meningitis, cultures of cerebrospinal fluid should also be made. For isolation from vaginal fluid, repeated cultures on antibiotic media are recommended.

In cattle, diagnosis of epizootic infertility is based on the history of the herd, on the culture of the preputial secretion and semen from bulls and of vaginal mucus from nonpregnant cows and heifers, and also on culture of fluid from the abomasum and from the liver of aborted fetuses. All samples should be cultured within six hours of collection. The highest rate of isolation of *C. fetus* from the cervicovaginal mucus is obtained in the two days immediately before or after estrus.

When the infection is suspected in a herd of beef cattle, bacteriologic examination of the cervicovaginal mucus of about 20 heifers that were bred but remained barren is recommended. Samples should be taken six months after the start of the breeding season.

A good diagnostic technique for herd infection, though not for individual infection, is the agglutination test using cervicovaginal mucus. Another test in use is indirect hemagglutination, also employing vaginal mucus. Immunofluorescence is nonspecific in cows, since *C. fetus* subsp. *venerealis* gives cross-reactions with *C. fetus* subsp. *fetus*.

Individual diagnosis is difficult in bulls. An isolation obtained from the preputial secretion is conclusive if the culture is positive but not if it is negative. It is accepted that before a bull is introduced into an artificial insemination center, he must pass four consecutive bacteriological tests at one-week intervals or four immunofluorescence tests. An excellent test is to have him service virgin heifers and subsequently culture their cervicovaginal mucus.

In sheep, diagnosis is carried out primarily by culture of fetal tissue, afterbirths, and vaginal fluid. Fluid from the abomasum and liver of the fetus is preferable for isolation.

Control: The few facts available at present on the epidemiology of the human infection are insufficient to determine control measures.

The best method for preventing epizootic infertility in cattle is to use semen from infection-free bulls in artificial insemination. In herds where this procedure is not practical, cows and heifers can be vaccinated annually some two or three months before breeding using commercial bacterins with an adjuvant. Several trials offer evidence that vaccination with bacterins can also eliminate the carrier state in bulls and cows. The curative properties of the vaccines provide a new perspective in control. Nevertheless, it must be borne in mind that while this method can reduce the infection in bulls under range conditions, vaccination of infected animals will not eliminate the infection from the herd. In one experiment (Vázquez *et al.*, 1983), *C. fetus* subsp. *venerealis* was isolated from 2 out of 10 artificially infected bulls five weeks after administration of the recommended two doses one month apart.

In sheep, good control can be obtained based on the vaccination of females with both monovalent (with the subsp. *fetus*) and bivalent (*fetus* and *venerealis*) bacterins with adjuvants, although the combined product is preferable. In flocks where adult females have acquired natural immunity, good results have been obtained by vaccinating only the yearly replacement ewes. Proper sanitary management is important, especially such measures as immediate removal of fetuses and afterbirths, isolation of sheep that have aborted, and protection of water from contamination.

Bibliography

Andrews, P.J., F.W. Frank. Comparison of four diagnostic tests for detection of bovine genital vibriosis. *J Am Vet Med Assoc* 165:695–697, 1974.

Bokkenheuser, V. *Vibrio fetus* infection in man. I. Ten new cases and some epidemiologic observations. *Am J Epidemiol* 91:400–409, 1970.

Bokkenheuser, V.D., V.L. Sutter. *Campylobacter* infections. *In*: Balows, A., W.Y. Hausler, Jr., eds. *Bacterial Mycotic and Parasitic Infections*. 6th ed. Washington, D.C.: American Public Health Association; 1981.

Bouters, R., J. De Keyser, M. Fandeplassche, A. Van Aert, E. Brone, P. Bonte. *Vibrio fetus* infection in bulls. Curative and preventive vaccination. *Brit Vet J* 129:52–57, 1973.

Bryner, J.H. Vibriosis due to *Vibrio fetus*. *In*: Hubbert, W.T., W.F. McCulloch, P.R. Schnurrenberger, eds. *Diseases Transmitted from Animals to Man*. 6th ed. Springfield: Thomas; 1975.

Bryner, J.H., P.C. Estes, J.W. Foley, P.A. O'Berry. Infectivity of three *Vibrio fetus* biotypes for gallbladder and intestines of cattle, sheep, rabbits, guinea pigs, and mice. *Am J Vet Res* 32:465–470, 1971.

Bryner, J.H., P.A. O'Berry, A.H. Frank. *Vibrio* infection of the digestive organs of cattle. *Am J Vet Res* 25:1048–1050, 1964.

Carroll, E.J., A.B. Hoerlein. Diagnosis and control of bovine genital vibriosis. *J Am Vet Med Assoc* 161:1359–1364, 1972.

Clark, B.L. Review of bovine vibriosis. *Aust Vet J* 47:103–107, 1971.

Clark, B.L., J.H. Duffy, M.J. Monsbourgh, I.M. Parsonson. Studies on venereal transmission of *Campylobacter fetus* by immunized bulls. *Aust Vet J* 51:531–532, 1975.

Devlin, H.R., L. McIntyre. *Campylobacter fetus* subsp. *fetus* in homosexual males. *J Clin Microbiol* 18:999–1000, 1983.

Firehammer, B.D., W.W. Hawkings. The pathogenicity of *Vibrio fetus* isolated from ovine bile. *Cornell Vet* 54:308–314, 1964.

Harvey, S.M., J.R. Greenwood. Probable *Campylobacter fetus* subsp. *fetus* gastroenteritis. *J Clin Microbiol* 18:1278–1279, 1983.

Hoerlein, A.B. Bovine genital vibriosis. *In*: Faulkner, L.C., ed. *Abortion Diseases of Livestock*. Springfield: Thomas; 1968.

Hoerlein, A.B., E.J. Carroll. Duration of immunity to bovine genital vibriosis. *J Am Vet Med Assoc* 156:775–778, 1970.

Laing, J.A. Vibrio fetus *Infection of Cattle*. Rome: Food and Agriculture Organization; 1960. (Agricultural Studies 51).

Miller, V.A. Ovine genital vibriosis. *In*: Faulkner, L.C., ed. *Abortion Diseases of Livestock*. Springfield: Thomas; 1968.

Miner, M.L., J.L. Thorne. Studies on the indirect transmission of *Vibrio fetus* infection in sheep. *Am J Vet Res* 25:474–477, 1964.

Morrison, V.A., B.K. Lloyd, J.K.S. Chia, C.U. Tuazon. Cardiovascular and bacteremic manifestations of *Campylobacter fetus* infection: Case report and review. *Rev Infect Dis* 12:387–392, 1990.

Osburn, B.I., R.K. Hoskins. Experimentally induced *Vibrio fetus* var. *intestinalis* infection in pregnant cows. *Am J Vet Res* 31:1733–1741, 1970.

Schurig, G.G.D., C.E. Hall, K. Burda, L.B. Corbeil, J.R. Duncan, A.J. Winter. Infection patterns in heifers following cervicovaginal or intrauterine instillation of *Campylobacter* (*Vibrio*) *fetus venerealis*. *Cornell Vet* 64:533–548, 1974.

Schurig, G.G.D., C.E. Hall, L.B. Corbeil, J.R. Duncan, A.J. Winter. Bovine venereal vibriosis. Cure genital infection in females by systemic immunization. *Infect Immun* 11:245–251, 1975.

Storz, J., M.L. Miner, A.E. Olson, M.E. Marriott, Y.Y. Elsner. Prevention of ovine vibriosis by vaccination: Effect of yearly vaccination of replacement of ewes. *Am J Vet Res* 27:115–120, 1966.

Vásquez, L.A., L. Ball, B.W. Bennett, G.P. Rupp, R. Ellis, J.D. Olson, *et al.* Bovine genital campylobacteriosis (vibriosis): Vaccination of experimentally infected bulls. *Am J Vet Res* 44:1553–1557, 1983.

Véron, M., R. Chatelain. Taxonomic study of the genus *Campylobacter* Sebald and Véron and designation of the neotype strain for the type species, *Campylobacter fetus* (Smith and Taylor) Sebald and Véron. *Int J Syst Bacteriol* 23:122–134, 1973.

White, F.H., A.F. Walsh. Biochemical and serologic relationships of isolants of *Vibrio fetus* from man. *J Infect Dis* 121:471–474, 1970.

CAT-SCRATCH DISEASE

ICD-10 A28.1

Synonyms: Cat-scratch fever, benign inoculation lymphoreticulosis, cat-scratch syndrome.

Etiology: For many years, microbiologists were unable to identify the etiologic agent. Various microbes considered the etiologic agent at one time or another were isolated; these included viruses, chlamydiae, and various types of bacteria. In 1983, Wear *et al.* conducted a histopathologic examination of the lymph nodes of 39 patients and demonstrated in 34 of them the presence of small, gram-negative, pleomorphic bacilli located in capillary walls or near areas of follicular hyperplasia and inside microabscesses. The observed bacilli were intracellular in the affected areas; they increased in number as lesions developed and diminished as they disappeared. The sera of three convalescent patients and human anti-immunoglobulin conjugated with peroxidase resulted in a precipitate with bacilli from the histological sections of different patients, demonstrating that they were serologically related (Wear *et al.*, 1983). This finding was later confirmed by other researchers during the period 1984–1986 in skin lesions, lymph nodes, and conjunctiva.

Researchers managed to culture and isolate the bacillus in a biphasic medium of brain-heart infusion broth, as well as in tissue cultures (English *et al.*, 1988; Birkness *et al.*, 1992). It is a bacillus that is difficult to isolate and its dimensions are at the light microscope's limit of resolution. A polar flagellum could be seen in electron microscope images. Depending on the temperature at which cultures are incubated, vegetative forms (at 32°C) or forms with defective walls (at 37°C) are seen. There are more vegetative bacilli in lesions of the skin and conjunctiva (at 32°C), and fewer in lymph node lesions (37°C). This would also explain why cat-scratch disease (CSD) could only be reproduced in armadillos and not in guinea pigs and other common laboratory animals.

This bacillus, for which the name *Afipia felis* was suggested (Birkness *et al.*, 1992), satisfies Koch's postulates for being the etiologic agent of CSD, according to English *et al.* (1988). Birkness *et al.* were very cautious about considering *A. felis* the etiologic agent of CSD. This caution appears to be well-founded, as a microorganism belonging to the rickettsiae, *Bartonella* (formerly *Rochalimaea*) *henselae*, was recently detected, which could be the agent responsible for most cases of cat-scratch disease and which also causes other diseases in man (see Infections caused by *Rochalimaea henselae*, in Volume 2: Chlamydioses, Rickettsioses, and Viroses).

Geographic Distribution: Worldwide (Benenson, 1990). It occurs sporadically. According to Heroman and McCurley (1982), more than 2,000 cases occur each year. Approximately 75% of the cases occurred in children. Small epidemic outbreaks and familial clustering have been reported in several countries. When an outbreak occurs in a family, there are usually several familial contacts in whom intracutaneous tests will be positive to the Hanger-Rose antigen. It is possible, but questionable, that several endemic areas exist around Toronto (Canada), New York City (USA), and Alfortville (France). Positive intracutaneous tests have been obtained in 10% of the population living in the vicinity of Alfortville, a result that is difficult to interpret.

The Disease in Man: Seven to twenty days or more can elapse between the cat scratch or bite (or other lesion caused by some inanimate object) and the appearance of symptoms. The disease is characterized by a regional lymphadenopathy without lymphangitis. In about 50% of the cases, primary lesions are seen at the point of inoculation. These consist of partially healed ulcers surrounded by an erythematous area, or of erythematous papules, pustules, or vesicles. Lymphadenitis is generally unilateral and commonly appears in the epitrochlear, axillary, or cervical lymph nodes, or in the femoral and inguinal lymph glands. Swelling in the lymph glands, which is generally painful and suppurates in about 25% of patients, persists for periods ranging from a few weeks to a few months. A high proportion of patients show signs of systemic infection, which consist of a low, short-lived fever and, less frequently, chills, anorexia, malaise, generalized pain, vomiting, and stomach cramps. Morbilliform cutaneous eruptions sometimes occur.

In general, the disease is benign and heals spontaneously without sequelae. Complications have been observed in a small proportion of the patients. The most common is Parinaud's oculoglandular syndrome; encephalitis, osteolytic lesions, and thrombocytopenic purpura are less frequent. The lymph gland lesions are not pathognomonic, but they follow a certain pattern, which helps in diagnosis. Histopathologic studies have shown that alterations begin with hyperplasia of the reticular cells, followed by an inflammatory granulomatous lesion. The center of the granuloma degenerates and becomes a homogenous eosinophilic mass, in which abscesses and microabscesses later appear.

In a study of 76 cases with neurological complications (51 with encephalopathy and 15 with disorders of the cranial or peripheral nerves), 50% of the patients had a fever, but only 26% had temperatures above 30°C. Forty-six percent of the patients had convulsions and 40% displayed aggressive behavior. Lethargy, with or without coma, was accompanied by various neurological symptoms. Of the other 15 patients without encephalopathy, 10 had neuroretinitis, two children had facial paresis, and three women had peripheral neuritis. Seventy-eight percent of the patients recovered without sequelae within a period of 1 to 12 weeks and the rest recovered within a year. Treatment consisted of controlling the convulsions and support measures. Commonly used antibiotics were apparently ineffective (Carithers and Margileth, 1991). Infection of the viscera is rare, but has been reported as well (Delahoussaye and Osborne, 1990).

Most cases have occurred in children, who have more contact with cats.

In temperate climates, the disease tends to be seasonal, with most cases occurring in fall and winter. In hot climates, there are no seasonal differences.

Source of Infection and Mode of Transmission: The most salient fact in the epidemiology of this disease is its causal relation with a cat scratch. It is estimated that about 65% of patients were scratched or bitten by cats and that 90% of the cases had some contact with these animals. Nevertheless, cases have been observed in which the skin lesion was inflicted by such inanimate objects as splinters, thorns, or pins.

Cats undoubtedly play an important role in the epidemiology, but there is doubt about whether it is as host for the etiologic agent or simply as a mechanical vector. Another possibility is that the etiologic agent is part of the normal flora of the cat's mouth and is transferred to the nails when the cat grooms itself (Hainer, 1987). Several observations—among them the fact that some cases were caused by inanimate agents—suggest that cats could be mechanical transmitters. Cats implicated in human cases were healthy animals, almost always young, that did not react to the Hanger-Rose intradermal test. It is also interesting to note that cats inoculated with material from the lymph nodes of human patients did not become ill. In summary, it has not yet been possible to show that cats are infected with the disease or are carriers of its causal agent, despite the many attempts made. According to Margileth (1987), cats are only able to transmit the infection for a short time (two to three weeks). CSD is usually transmitted from cats to man through a scratch and, less frequently, through a bite or licking. In Parinaud's oculoglandular syndrome, the point of entry for the agent is the conjunctiva or eyelids when a person rubs his or her eyes after picking up a cat (August, 1988).

Diagnosis: CSD can be clinically confused with other diseases that cause regional lymphadenopathies, such as tularemia, brucellosis, tuberculosis, pasteurellosis, infectious mononucleosis, Hodgkin's disease, venereal lymphogranuloma, lymphosarcoma, and lymphoma. All these diseases must be excluded before considering a diagnosis of CSD. The symptoms described above, a history of a skin lesion caused by a cat scratch or bite, the histopathology of biopsy material taken from the affected lymph node, and the Hanger-Rose intradermal test constitute the basis for diagnosis. The Hanger-Rose antigen is prepared by suspending pus taken from an abscessed lymph node in a 1:5 saline solution and heating it for 10 hours at 60°C. The antigen is very crude and difficult to standardize. The test is carried out by intradermal inoculation with 0.1 ml of the antigen. The reaction may be read in 48 hours. Edema measuring 0.5 cm and erythema of 1 cm are considered a positive reaction. The test is very useful, since 90% of 485 clinically diagnosed cases gave positive results, while only 4.1% out of 591 controls tested positive.

There is a danger of transmitting viral hepatitis with this antigen; therefore, the preparation should be heat-treated for a lengthy period, as indicated above. It may be very useful to demonstrate the presence of the putative etiologic agent, *A. felis*, using Warthin-Starry stain on histological sections from the skin or lymph nodes.

Control: Prevention is limited to avoiding cat scratches and bites. Cutting the cat's nails, washing and disinfecting any scratch or bite, and washing one's hands after petting or handling a cat are also recommended (August, 1988).

Bibliography

Andrews, C., H.G. Pereira. *Viruses of Vertebrates*. 3rd ed. Baltimore: Williams & Wilkins; 1972.

August, J.R. Cat-scratch disease. Zoonosis update. *J Am Vet Med Assoc* 193:312–315, 1988.

Benenson, A.S., ed. *Control of Communicable Diseases in Man*. 15th ed. An official report of the American Public Health Association. Washington, D.C.: American Public Health Association; 1990.

Birkness, K.A., V.G. George, E.H. White, *et al.* Intracellular growth of *Afipia felis*, a putative etiologic agent of cat-scratch disease. *Infect Immun* 60:2281–2287, 1992.

Carithers, H.A. Cat-scratch disease. An overview based on a study of 1,200 patients. *Am J Dis Child* 139:1124–1133, 1985.

Carithers, H.A., A.M. Margileth. Cat-scratch disease. Acute encephalopathy and other neurologic manifestations. *Am J Dis Child* 145:98–101, 1991.

Delahoussaye, P.M., B.M. Osborne. Cat-scratch disease presenting as abdominal visceral granulomas. *J Infect Dis* 161:71–78, 1990.

Emmons, R.W., J.L. Riggs, J. Schachter. Continuing search for the etiology of cat-scratch disease. *J Clin Microbiol* 4:112–114, 1976.

English, C.K, D.J. Wear, A.M. Margileth, *et al.* Cat-scratch disease. Isolation and culture of the bacterial agent. *JAMA* 259:1347–1352, 1988.

Euseby, J.B. Le genre *Afipia* et la maladie de griffes du chat. *Revue Med Vet* 143:95–105, 1992.

Gerber, M.A., A.K. Sedgwick, T.J. MacAlister, K.B. Gustafson, M. Ballow, R.C. Tilton. The aetiological agent of cat-scratch disease. *Lancet* 1:1236–1239, 1985.

Griesemer, R.A., L.G. Wolfe. Cat-scratch disease. *J Am Vet Med Assoc* 158:1008–1012, 1971.

Hainer, B.L. Cat-scratch disease. *J Fam Pract* 25:497–503, 1987.

Heroman, V.M, W.S. McCurley. Cat-scratch disease. *Otolaryngol Clin North Am* 15:649–658, 1982. Cited in: Delahoussaye, P.M., B. Osborne. Cat-scratch disease presenting as abdominal visceral granulomas. *J Infect Dis* 161:71–78, 1990.

Macrae, A.D. Cat-scratch fever. *In*: Graham-Jones, O., ed. *Some Diseases of Animals Communicable to Man in Britain*. Oxford: Pergamon Press; 1968.

Margileth, A.M. Cat-scratch disease. A therapeutic dilemma. *Vet Clin North Am Small Anim Pract* 17:91–103, 1987. Cited in: August, J.R. Cat-scratch disease. Zoonosis update. *J Am Vet Med Assoc* 193:312–315, 1988.

Rose, H.M. Cat-scratch disease. *In*: Wyngaarden, J.B., L.H. Smith, Jr., eds. *Cecil Textbook of Medicine*. 16th ed. Philadelphia: Saunders; 1982.

Warwick, W.J. The cat-scratch syndrome, many diseases or one disease. *Progr Med Virol* 9:256–301, 1967.

Wear, D.J., A.M. Margileth, T.L. Hadfield, *et al.* Cat-scratch disease: A bacterial infection. *Science* 221:1403–1404, 1983.

CLOSTRIDIAL FOOD POISONING

ICD-10 A05.2 foodborne *Clostridium perfringens* [*Clostridium welchii*] intoxication

Synonyms: Clostridial gastroenteritis, clostridial toxicosis.

Etiology: *Clostridium perfringens* (*C. welchii*) is an anaerobic, gram-positive, sporogenic, nonmotile, encapsulated bacillus that produces extracellular toxins. The optimum temperature for its growth is between 41°C and 45°C. At these temperatures, *C. perfringens* reproduces at what is considered record speed for most bacteria. This growth potential is very important in food protection. A temperature of 60°C is lethal for the vegetative form of *C. perfringens* in culture media. It is more resistant to heat when found in foods (Labbe, 1989). Five different toxigenic types are known, designated by the letters A through E; these produce four principal toxins. The vegetative forms produce large quantities of enterotoxins during sporulation in the intestine. The optimum temperature for sporulation is between 35°C and 40°C.

Geographic Distribution: *C. perfringens* type A is ubiquitous in the soil and in the intestinal tract of humans and animals worldwide. The other types are found only in the intestinal tract of animals. Types B and E have a marked regional distribution.

Occurrence in Man: Outbreaks of food poisoning due to *C. perfringens* type A probably occur the world over, but most of the information comes from developed countries.

In Great Britain, where food poisoning is a notifiable disease, clostridial poisoning is estimated to cause 30% of all cases, as well as many general and familial outbreaks; an average of 37 people are affected per outbreak.

In the United States, during the period 1976–1980, 62 outbreaks affecting 6,093 persons were reported, representing 7.4% of all outbreaks of food toxicoses with known etiology and 14.8% of the total number of known cases in the country over the same period. The median number of cases per outbreak was 23.5, but six outbreaks affected more than 200 persons (Shandera *et al.*, 1983).

Even in developed countries, cases are greatly underreported, because the disease is mild and usually lasts no more than 24 hours. Moreover, laboratory diagnosis cannot always be performed, as it depends on obtaining food and patient stool samples that are not always available.

Outbreaks affecting large numbers of people are usually reported. These are caused by meals prepared in restaurants or institutions. An outbreak occurred in Argentina at the farewell ceremony for 60 participants in an international course. The food served included meat pies, canapés, and sweet cakes provided by a restaurant. Of the 41 people who were still in the country during the epidemiological investigation, 56% reported having developed symptoms typical of gastroenteritis. The meat pies were considered the source of the poisoning (Michanie *et al.*, 1993).

In New Guinea, necrotic enteritis in man caused by *C. perfringens* type C has been confirmed.

Occurrence in Animals: In domesticated ruminants, several types of exterotoxemias due to *C. perfringens* types B, C, D, and E are known. Enterotoxemia results from the absorption into the bloodstream of toxins produced in the intestine by the various types of *C. perfringens* that form part of the normal intestinal flora.

The Disease in Man: The disease is contracted upon ingestion of foods (especially red meat and fowl) in which *C. perfringens* type A has multiplied. It is now known that illness is caused by thermoresistant strains, which can survive at 100°C for more than an hour, as well as by thermolabile and hemolytic strains, which are inactivated after approximately 10 minutes at 100°C.

The incubation period is from 6 to 24 hours after ingestion, but has been as short as two hours in a few people, which indicates that the food ingested contained preformed toxin. The disease begins suddenly, causing abdominal cramps and diarrhea, but usually not vomiting or fever. It lasts a day or less and its course is benign, except in debilitated persons, in whom it may prove fatal. Food poisoning caused by *C. perfringens* type A does not usually require medical treatment.

In recent years, an intestinal infection with diarrhea not associated with food consumption has been described. The disease is due to an infection caused by colonization of *C. perfringens* in the intestine and the production of enterotoxin. Its clinical picture is very different from that of clostridial food poisoning and more closely resembles an infection caused by *Salmonella* or *Campylobacter*. In England, a series of cases was described involving 50 elderly patients (ages 76 to 96) who were hospitalized with diarrhea not associated with food consumption. The diarrhea lasted for an average of 11 days, but lasted for a shorter period in two-thirds of the patients. Sixteen of 46 patients had bloody stools (Larson and Borriello, 1988).

Necrotic enteritis produced by the ingestion of food contaminated with *C. perfringens* type C is characterized by a regional gangrene in the small intestine, especially the jejunum.

A rare type of necrotizing enteritis caused by *C. perfringens* type A was described in the Netherlands in a 17-year-old girl. The patient recovered after resection of three meters of her intestine and intravenous treatment with gentamicin, cefotaxime, and metronidazole for seven days. Counterimmunoelectrophoresis of blood samples indicated the presence of antibodies for the alpha toxin that is predominant in type A. A similar illness appeared in Germany and Norway after the Second World War. Currently, necrotic enteritis is rare in the Western world, though some cases among adolescents and the elderly have been described (Van Kessel *et al.*, 1985).

On rare occasions, gastroenteritis due to *C. perfringens* type D has been confirmed in man. This type causes enterotoxemia in sheep and goats.

The Disease in Animals: *C. perfringens* type A is part of the normal flora of the intestine, where it does not usually produce its characteristic alpha toxin. Few cases of illness caused by type A have been confirmed in cattle. In California and Oregon (USA), a disease produced by type A in nursing lambs ("yellow lamb disease") has been described. The disease occurs in spring, when there is a large population of nursing animals. The lambs suffer depression, anemia, jaundice, and hemoglobinuria. They die 6 to 12 hours after the onset of clinical symptoms (Gillespie and Timoney, 1981).

Type B is the etiologic agent of "lamb dysentery," which occurs in Great Britain, the Middle East, and South Africa. It usually attacks lambs less than 2 weeks old. It is characterized by hemorrhagic enteritis, and is frequently accompanied by ulceration of the mucosa. It also affects calves and colts.

Type C causes hemorrhagic enterotoxemia ("struck") in adult sheep in Great Britain, as well as necrotic enteritis in calves, lambs, suckling pigs, and fowl in many parts of the world (Timoney *et al.*, 1988).

Type D is the causal agent of enterotoxemia in sheep. It is distributed worldwide and attacks animals of all ages. The disease is associated with abundant consumption of food, whether milk, pasture, or grains. Outbreaks have also been described in goats and, more rarely, in cattle.

Type E causes dysentery or enterotoxemia in calves and lambs, and has been confirmed in the US, England, and Australia (Timoney *et al.*, 1988).

Source of Infection and Mode of Transmission: The natural reservoir of *C. perfringens* type A is the soil and the intestine of man and animals. Some studies (Torres-Anjel *et al.*, 1977) have shown that man harbors higher numbers of *C. perfringens* than fowl or cattle and that some people excrete great quantities of these bacteria, making man the most important reservoir of clostridial food poisoning. The amount of *C. perfringens* type A in the intestine varies with the animal species and location. *C. perfringens* is found in large numbers in the small intestine of pigs, in small amounts in sheep, goats, and cattle, and is practically nonexistent in horses (Smith, 1965).

Type A enterotoxemia is caused primarily by the alpha toxin, which forms in the intestine and is released during sporulation, for which the small intestine is a favorable environment. The source of poisoning for man is food contaminated by spores that survive cooking. Heat (heat shock) activates the spores, which then germinate. The vegetative forms multiply rapidly if the prepared food is left at room temperature, and can reach very high concentrations if the temperature is high for a sufficient amount of time (see the section on etiology). The vegetative forms carried to the intestine by the food sporulate, releasing the enterotoxin in the process. The food vehicle is almost always red meat or fowl, since they provide *C. perfringens* with the amino acids and vitamins it needs. Less frequently, other foods, such as pigeon peas, beans, mashed potatoes, cheeses, seafood, potato salad, noodles, and olives have given rise to the disease (Craven, 1980). Immersing meat in broth or cooking it in large pieces creates anaerobic conditions that favor the multiplication of the bacteria during cooling or storage. The foods that cause poisoning are usually prepared in large quantities by restaurants or dining halls and are served later that day or the next. The spores of some strains of *C. perfringens* can be destroyed by adequate cooking, but other spores are heat-resistant. Reheating food before serving it can stimulate the multiplication of bacteria if the heating temperature is not high enough. It is now known that high concentrations of the vegetative form of *C. perfringens* in food cannot be destroyed by stomach acid, and thus pass into the intestine. The enterotoxin synthesized in the intestine when the bacteria sporulate is resistant to intestinal enzymes, has a cytotoxic effect on the intestinal epithelium, affects the electrolyte transport system, and thus causes diarrhea (Narayan, 1982).

It should be borne in mind that not all strains of *C. perfringens* are toxigenic. One study of strains implicated in food poisonings found that 86% were toxigenic, while another study found that 2 strains out of 174 isolated from other sources produced the enterotoxin (Narayan, 1982).

In lamb dysentery caused by *C. perfringens* type B, the animals are infected during the first days of life, apparently from the mother or the environment. Young lambs that receive a lot of milk are particularly likely to fall ill. The bacteria multiply and produce beta toxin when they sporulate (Timoney *et al.*, 1988).

In hemorrhagic enteritis or "struck" caused by *C. perfringens* type C in adult sheep in England, the agent is found in the soil of areas of Romney Marsh and it is possible that most of the sheep in the region are infected. Beta toxin predominates. The soil and the intestinal tract of healthy sheep are the reservoir for type D, which is the agent of enterotoxemia in sheep. Epsilon toxin is the most important (Timoney *et al.*, 1988).

The intestines of 75 animals with diarrhea of unknown origin were examined postmortem to detect the presence of *C. perfringens* enterotoxins. Positive results were found in 8 of 37 swine, 4 of 10 sheep, 1 of 3 goats, 1 of 16 cattle, and none of 9 horses (Van Baelen and Devriese, 1987).

In animals, *C. perfringens* seems to multiply primarily in the intestine, where it sporulates and produces toxins. The types of *C. perfringens* (B, C, D, E) that produce enterotoxemia in animals multiply rapidly in the intestine and produce toxins when animals are suddenly released to rich pastures, are given too much fodder, or consume large quantities of milk.

Role of Animals in the Epidemiology of the Disease: Human food poisoning is caused by foods contaminated by *C. perfringens* type A, usually foods consisting mainly of red meat or fowl. The animals themselves do not play a direct role in the epidemiology, since the etiologic agent is ubiquitous and can be found in the soil or in dust. Foods of animal origin are important as substrates for the multiplication of the bacteria and as vehicles for the disease. The soil and the intestines of humans and animals are the reservoir of the etiologic agent. *C. perfringens* type A is found in the muscles and organs of animals a few hours after slaughter, unless they are rapidly refrigerated.

Heat-resistant strains of *C. perfringens* may be found in the mesenteric lymph nodes of some animals after slaughter. Strains are isolated at a lower rate in animals allowed to rest 24 to 48 hours before butchering.

Diagnosis: The incubation period and clinical picture make it possible to distinguish clostridial food poisoning, which is afebrile, from salmonellosis, shigellosis, or colibacillosis, which produce fever. Staphylococcal intoxication usually results in vomiting, while this symptom is rare with clostridial poisoning. Laboratory confirmation is based on the *C. perfringens* count in the implicated food and in the patient's stool (within 48 hours of onset of illness). The existence of 10^5 cells per gram of food and 10^6 per gram of fecal material is considered significant. Serotyping of strains from food and feces with a battery of 70 sera has provided good results in epidemiological research in Great Britain, but not in the United States, where only 40% of the strains received by the Centers for Disease Control and Prevention could be typed. There is no proof that only certain serotypes are related to the disease (Shandera, 1983).

Laboratory diagnosis of animal enterotoxemias is performed by mouse inoculation to demonstrate the presence of specific toxins. Some mice are inoculated only with intestinal contents and others are inoculated with both intestinal contents and antitoxin. Tests to directly detect the toxin can also be performed and are currently preferred. These include reverse passive latex agglutination, enzyme immunoassay, or culturing of Vero cells with neutralizing antibodies to inhibit the cytopathic effects (Bartlett, 1990).

Control: In man, the control measures are as follows. Meat dishes should be served hot and as soon as possible after cooking. If food must be kept for a while before eating, it should be rapidly refrigerated. If possible, meat should be cut into small pieces for cooking. Broth should be separated from the meat. The use of pressure cookers is a good preventive measure. If necessary, food should be reheated at a temperature high enough to destroy the agent's vegetative cells.

Educating those who prepare meals in restaurants or at home is very important, since it is impossible to avoid the presence of *C. perfringens* in red meats and raw chicken (Michanie *et al.*, 1993).

In animals, enterotoxemia control consists of good herd management, avoidance of a sudden change from poor to rich pasture, and active immunization with specific toxoids. Two doses of toxoid a month apart, followed by a booster at six months (type D) or a year (type C), are recommended.

To protect lambs, ewes should be vaccinated with two doses, with the second dose administered two weeks before lambing. To prevent lamb dysentery (type B), ewes can be vaccinated with the specific toxoid or lambs can be passively immunized with antiserum at birth. In *C. perfringens* types B and C, the beta toxin predominates, and therefore a toxoid or antiserum from one type will give cross-immunity.

Bibliography

Bartlett, J.G. Gas gangrene (other clostridium-associated diseases). *In*: Mandell, G.L., R.G. Douglas, Jr., J.E. Bennett, eds. *Principles and Practice of Infectious Diseases.* 3rd ed. New York: Churchill Livingstone, Inc.; 1990.

Craven, S.E. Growth and sporulation of *Clostridium perfringens* in foods. *Food Techn* 34:80–87, 1980.

Dobosch, D., R. Dowell. Detección de enterotoxina de *Clostridium perfringens* en casos de intoxicación alimentaria. *Medicina* 43:188–192, 1983.

Faich, G.A., E.J. Gangarosa. Food poisoning, bacterial. *In*: Top, F.M., P.F. Wehrle, eds. *Communicable and Infectious Diseases.* 7th ed. Saint Louis: Mosby; 1972.

Gillespie, J.H., J.F. Timoney. *Hagan and Bruner's Infectious Diseases of Domestic Animals.* 7th ed. Ithaca: Cornell University Press; 1981.

Hobbs, B.C. *Clostridium perfringens* and *Bacillus cereus* infections. *In*: Riemann, H., ed. *Food-borne Infections and Intoxications.* New York: Academic Press; 1969.

Labbe, R. *Clostridium perfringens*. *In*: Doyle, M.P., ed. *Food-borne Bacterial Pathogens.* New York: Marcel Dekker; 1989.

Larson, H.E., S.P. Borriello. Infectious diarrhea due to *Clostridium perfringens*. *J Infect Dis* 157:390–391, 1988.

Michanie, S., A. Vega, G. Padilla, A. Rea Nogales. Brote de gastroenteritis provocado por el consumo de empanadas de carne. *Alimentacion Latinoamer* 194:49–54, 1993.

Narayan, K.G. Food-borne infection with *Clostridium perfringens* Type A. *Int J Zoonoses* 9:12–32, 1982.

Roberts, R.S. Clostridial diseases. *In*: Stableforth, A.W., I.A. Galloway, eds. *Infectious Diseases of Animals.* London: Butterworths; 1959.

Rose, H.M. Diseases caused by Clostridia. *In*: Wyngaarden, J.B., L.H. Smith, Jr., eds. *Cecil Textbook of Medicine.* 16th ed. Philadelphia: Saunders; 1982.

Shandera, W.X., C.O. Tacket, P.A. Blake. Food poisoning due to *Clostridium perfringens* in the United States. *J Infect Dis* 147:167–170, 1983.

Smith, H.W. Observations on the flora of the alimentary tract of animals and factors affecting its composition. *J Path Bact* 89:95–122, 1965. Cited in: Van Baelen, D., L.A. Devriese.

Presence of *Clostridium perfringens* enterotoxin in intestinal samples from farm animals with diarrhoea of unknown origin. *J Vet Med B* 34:713–716, 1987.

Smith, L.D.S. Clostridial diseases of animals. *Adv Vet Sci* 3:463–524, 1957.

Timoney, J.F., J.H. Gillespie, F.W. Scott, J.E. Barlough. *Hagan and Bruner's Microbiology and Infectious Diseases of Domestic Animals.* 8th ed. Ithaca: Comstock; 1988.

Torres-Anjel, M.J., M.P. Riemann, C.C. Tsai. *Enterotoxigenic* Clostridium perfringens *Type A in Selected Humans: A Prevalence Study.* Washington, D.C.: Pan American Health Organization; 1977. (Scientific Publication 350).

Van Baelen, D., L.A. Devriese. Presence of *Clostridium perfringens* enterotoxin in intestinal samples from farm animals with diarrhoea of unknown origin. *J Vet Med B* 34:713–716, 1987.

Van Kessel, L.J.P., H.A. Verbugh, M.F. Stringer, *et al.* Necrotizing enteritis associated with toxigenic Type A *Clostridium perfringens* [letter]. *J Infect Dis* 151:974–975, 1985.

CLOSTRIDIAL WOUND INFECTIONS

ICD-10 A48.0 gas gangrene

Synonyms: Gas gangrene, clostridial myonecrosis, histotoxic infection, anaerobic cellulitis; malignant edema (in animals).

Etiology: Wound infection is characterized by mixed bacterial flora. The most important species are *Clostridium perfringens* (*welchii*), *C. novyi*, *C. septicum*, *C. sordelli*, *C. histolyticum*, and *C. fallax*. Like all clostridia, these bacteria are gram-positive, anaerobic, sporogenic bacilli. These species produce potent exotoxins that destroy tissue. In human gas gangrene, the most important etiologic agent is *C. perfringens*, toxigenic type A. Infection by *C. septicum* predominates in animals.

Geographic Distribution: Worldwide.

Occurrence in Man: Gas gangrene used to be more prevalent in wartime than in peacetime. It has been estimated that during World War I, 100,000 German soldiers died from this infection. However, its incidence has decreased enormously during more recent wars. During the eight years of the Vietnam War, there were only 22 cases of gas gangrene out of 139,000 wounds, while in Miami (USA), there were 27 cases in civilian trauma patients over a 10-year period (Finegold, 1977). The disease is relatively rare and occurs mainly in traffic- and occupational accident victims. However, in natural disasters or other emergencies, it constitutes a serious problem. Gas gangrene also occurs after surgery, especially in older patients who have had a leg amputated. It may also develop in patients receiving intramuscular injections, especially of medications suspended in an oil base. Gas gangrene can occur in soft tissue lesions in patients with vascular insufficiency, such as diabetics (Bartlett, 1990).

Occurrence in Animals: The frequency of occurrence in animals is not known.

The Disease in Man: Pathogenic species of *Clostridium* may be found as simple contaminants in any type of traumatic lesion. When infection occurs, the microorganisms multiply and produce gas in the tissues. Gas gangrene is an acute and serious condition that produces myositis as its principal lesion. The incubation period lasts from six hours to three days after injury. The first symptoms are increasing pain around the injured area, tachycardia, and decreased blood pressure, followed by fever, edematization, and a reddish serous exudate from the wound. The skin becomes taut, discolored, and covered with vesicles. Crepitation is felt upon palpation. Stupor, delirium, and coma develop in the final stages of the disease. The infection may also begin in the uterus following an abortion or difficult labor. These cases show septicemia, massive hemolysis, and acute nephrosis, with shock and anuria.

C. perfringens type A, alone or in combination with other pathogens, caused 60% to 80% of gas gangrene cases in soldiers during the two world wars.

Treatment consists primarily of debridement with extensive removal of the affected muscle. Amputation of the limb affected by gas gangrene should be considered. Penicillin G is generally the preferred antibacterial. However, better results have been obtained with clindamycin, metronidazole, rifampicin, and tetracycline (Bartlett, 1990). Mortality is still very high.

The Disease in Animals: *C. septicum* is the principal agent of clostridial wound infection, known as "malignant edema." *C. septicum* produces four toxins that cause tissue damage. The incubation period lasts from a few hours to several days. This disease is characterized by an extensive hemorrhagic edema of the subcutaneous tissue and intermuscular connective tissue. The muscle tissue turns dark red; little or no gas is present. The infected animal exhibits fever, intoxication, and lameness. Swellings are soft and palpation leaves depressions. The course of the disease is rapid and the animal can die a few days after symptoms appear. Cattle are the most affected species, but sheep, horses, and swine are also susceptible. The infection is rare in fowl.

C. perfringens type A is sometimes responsible for infection of traumatic wounds in calves, lambs, and goats. As in man, the infection gives rise to gas gangrene. Edema with a large amount of gas develops around the injury site, spreads rapidly, and causes death in a short time.

In animals, as in man, other clostridia (e.g., *C. novyi*, *C. sordelli*, and *C. histolyticum*) can cause wound infection and the wound's bacterial flora may be mixed.

Treatment with high doses of penicillin or broad-spectrum antibiotics may yield results if administered at the onset of disease.

Source of Infection and Mode of Transmission: Clostridia are widely distributed in nature, in the soil, and in the intestinal tract of man and most animals. The sources of infection for man and animals are the soil and fecal matter. Transmission is effected through traumatic wounds or surgical incisions. Gas gangrene can also occur without any wound or trauma (endogenous or spontaneous gas gangrene) in patients weakened by malignant disease and those with ulcerative lesions in the gastrointestinal or urogenital tract or in the bile ducts (Finegold, 1977). In animals, the infection may originate in minor wounds, such as those produced by castration, tail docking, and shearing.

Role of Animals in the Epidemiology of the Disease: Wound clostridiosis is a disease common to man and animals, not a zoonosis.

Diagnosis: Diagnosis is based primarily on clinical manifestations, such as the color around the lesion or wound, swelling, toxemia, and muscle tissue destruction. The presence of gas is not always indicative of clostridial infection. A smear of exudate from the wound or a gram-stained muscle tissue sample may be helpful in diagnosis if numerous large gram-positive bacilli are found. The culture of anaerobic bacilli from human cases is generally of little value because of the time required and the urgency of diagnosis. Moreover, isolation of a potentially pathogenic anaerobe from a wound may only indicate contamination and not necessarily active infection (penetration and multiplication in the human or animal organism). In animals, culture can be important in distinguishing infection caused by *C. chauvoei* (symptomatic anthrax, blackleg, or emphysematous gangrene) from infections caused by *C. septicum.* The latter bacterium rapidly invades the animal's body after death; thus, the material used for examination should be taken before or very shortly after death.

The fluorescent antibody technique permits identification of the pathogenic clostridia in a few hours and can be very useful in diagnosis.

Control: Prevention of the infection consists of prompt treatment of wounds and removal of foreign bodies and necrotic tissue. Special care must be taken to ensure that tourniquets, bandages, and casts do not interfere with circulation and thus create conditions favorable to the multiplication of anaerobic bacteria by reducing local oxidation-reduction potential.

Combined vaccines of *C. chauvoei* and *C. septicum* are used for active immunization of calves and lambs. Vaccination with bacterins or alpha toxoid must be carried out prior to castration, tail docking, shearing, or removal of horns. Calves can be vaccinated at 2 months of age.

Bibliography

Bartlett, J.G. Gas gangrene (other clostridium-associated diseases). *In*: Mandell, G.L., R.G. Douglas, Jr., J.E. Bennett, eds. *Principles and Practice of Infectious Diseases*. 3rd ed. New York: Churchill Livingstone, Inc.; 1990.

Bruner, D.W., J.H. Gillespie. *Hagan's Infectious Diseases of Domestic Animals*. 6th ed. Ithaca: Comstock; 1973.

Finegold, S.M. *Anaerobic Bacteria in Human Disease*. New York: Academic Press; 1977.

Joklik, W.K., D.T. Smith. *Zinsser's Microbiology*. 15th ed. New York: Meredith; 1972.

MacLennan, J.D. The histotoxic clostridial infections of man. *Bact Rev* 26:177–274, 1962.

Prévot, A.R., A. Turpin, P. Kaiser. *Les bactéries anaerobies*. Paris: Dunod; 1967.

Rose, H.M. Disease caused by clostridia. *In*: Wyngaarden, J.B., L.H. Smith, Jr., eds. *Cecil Textbook of Medicine*. 16th ed. Philadelphia: Saunders; 1982.

Rosen, M.M. Clostridial infections and intoxications. *In*: Hubbert, W.T., W.F. McCulloch, P.R. Schnurrenberger, eds. *Diseases Transmitted from Animals to Man*. 6th ed. Springfield: Thomas; 1975.

Smith, D.L.S. Clostridial diseases of animals. *Adv Vet Sci* 3:465–524, 1957.

Smith, L.D., L.V. Holderman. *The Pathogenic Anaerobic Bacteria*. Springfield: Thomas; 1968.

COLIBACILLOSIS

ICD-10 A04.0 enteropathogenic *Escherichia coli* **infection;**
A04.1 enterotoxigenic *Escherichia coli* **infection;**
A04.2 enteroinvasive *Escherichia coli* **infection;**
A04.3 enterohemorrhagic *Escherichia coli* **infection**

Synonyms: Colibacteriosis, colitoxemia, enteropathogenic diarrhea.

Etiology and Physiopathogenesis: *Escherichia coli* belongs to the family *Enterobacteriaceae*. *E. coli* is a normal component of the flora in the large intestine of warm-blooded animals, including man. It is a gram-negative, motile or nonmotile, facultatively anaerobic bacillus.

It is classified into different serotypes according to the scheme originally developed by Kauffmann, which is based primarily on the somatic O antigens (polysaccharide and thermostable) that differentiate *E. coli* into more than 170 serogroups. The flagellar H antigen, which is thermolabile and proteinic, distinguishes the serotypes (56 to date) of each serogroup. The K (capsular) and F (fimbrial) antigens are also important (Doyle and Padhye, 1989). The pathogenic strains, which cause enteric disease, are grouped into six categories: (a) enterohemorrhagic (EHEC), (b) enterotoxigenic (ETEC), (c) enteroinvasive (EIEC), (d) enteropathogenic (EPEC), (e) enteroaggregative (EAggEC), and (f) diffuse-adherent (DAEC). The last two categories are not yet well defined, and the last category is not dealt with here. These categories differ in their pathogenesis and virulence properties, and each comprises a distinct group of O:H serotypes. Their clinical symptoms and epidemiological patterns may also differ (Chin, 2000).

In terms of the zoonoses, the most important category is the enterohemorrhagic, which is also the most severe.

a) Enterohemorrhagic *E. coli* **(EHEC).** The principal etiologic agent of this colibacillosis is *E. coli* O157:H7. Since it was first recognized in 1983 (Riley *et al.*, 1983), this category has been a public health problem in Europe and the US, which became more serious with an outbreak that occurred in the latter between November 15, 1992 and February 28, 1993. In Washington State and other western US states, 470 people fell ill and four died—three in Washington and one in San Diego, California (Spencer, 1993; Dorn, 1993). Griffin and Tauxe (1991) conclude that O157:H7 is an emerging and new pathogen, because they feel that such a distinctive illness—which often has serious consequences (hemolytic uremic syndrome)—would have attracted attention in any period. Later, O26:H11, O45:H2, and three nonmotile *E. coli*—O4, O111, and O145—were added to this serotype. This group is characterized by a 60-megadalton virulence plasmid and by its secretion of Shiga-like toxins or verotoxins. The Shiga-like toxin was thus named because it is similar in structure and activity to the toxin produced by *Shigella dis-enteriae* type 1, and is neutralized by the Shiga toxin antiserum. There are actually two toxins, Shiga-like toxin I and Shiga-like toxin II (or verotoxins I and II). Both are cytotoxic (lethal to Vero and HeLa cells), cause fluid accumulation in rabbit ligated ileal loops, and paralysis and death in mice and rabbits (O'Brien and Holmes, 1987). Verotoxin II produces hemorrhagic colitis in adult rabbits. The two toxins are antigenically different.

Geographic Distribution and Occurrence in Man: Worldwide. Serotype O157:H7 has been isolated in outbreaks in Canada, Great Britain, and the United States. It has also been isolated in Argentina, Australia, Belgium, the former Czechoslovakia, China, Germany, Holland, Ireland, Italy, Japan, and South Africa (Griffin and Tauxe, 1991). These isolates were obtained from fecal samples taken from sporadic cases of hemorrhagic diarrhea submitted to public health or hospital laboratories for examination.

From 1982 to 1992, 17 outbreaks occurred in the US; the smallest affected 10 people and the largest 243. In November 1992, an outbreak occurred among people who had eaten undercooked hamburgers at a fast food restaurant chain. The same *E. coli* serotype was isolated from the ground beef found in these restaurants (CDC, 1993). Seventeen more outbreaks occurred in 1993. Case-reporting is now compulsory in 18 US states. It is estimated that there are 8 cases each year per 100,000 inhabitants in Washington State (approximately the same incidence as for salmonellosis).

During the same period (1982–1992), there were three outbreaks in Canada and two in Great Britain (Griffin and Tauxe, 1991).

Occurrence in Animals: Based on outbreaks in the US, studies were conducted to evaluate the infection rate in cattle. The agent was isolated from only 25 suckling calves of the approximately 7,000 examined in 28 states. This study indicated that the agent is widely distributed in the US, but that the rate of animals harboring this serotype is low. The prevalence of infected herds is estimated at approximately 5%. In Washington State, between 5% and 10% of herds harbor *E. coli* O157:H7 (Spencer, 1993). This serotype was also isolated from cattle in Argentina, Canada, Egypt, Germany, Great Britain, and Spain. In Argentina and Spain, there was an association between serotype O157:H7 and a diarrheal disease in cattle, whereas in the other countries the isolates were produced from apparently normal cattle (Dorn, 1993).

The Disease in Man: The incubation period is from two to nine days. The appearance of the disease ranges from a slight case of diarrhea to severe hemorrhagic colitis, with strong abdominal pains and little or no fever. At the outset, diarrhea is watery but later becomes hemorrhagic, either with traces of blood or highly hemorrhagic stools. Diarrhea lasts an average of four days and about 50% of patients experience vomiting. Hemorrhagic diarrhea was present in more than 95% of a large number of sporadic cases recorded. In some outbreaks in nursing homes, where stricter surveillance was possible, it was shown that between 56% and 75% of affected patients had hemorrhagic stools and the rest had diarrhea without blood; asymptomatic infections were also confirmed (Griffin and Tauxe, 1991). *E. coli* O157:H7 infection is feared primarily because of its complications. One of these is hemolytic uremic syndrome, which is the principal cause of acute renal deficiency in children and frequently requires dialysis and transfusions. Another complication is thrombotic thrombocytopenic purpura, which is characterized by thrombocytopenia, hemolytic anemia, azotemia, fever, thrombosis in the terminal arterioles and capillaries, and neurological symptoms that dominate the clinical picture. Depending on the population, cases involving hemolytic uremic syndrome probably represent between 2% and 7% of the total number of cases due to *E. coli* O157:H7 (Griffin and Tauxe, 1991).

Although *E. coli* O157:H7 is susceptible to many commonly used antibiotics, they should not be used as a preventive measure. During an outbreak in a nursing home, antibiotics were considered a risk factor for contracting infection (Carter *et al.*, 1987). It is believed that antibiotics may increase the risk of infection and complications, probably by stimulating the production of toxin and altering the normal intestinal flora, thus allowing greater growth of serotype O157:H7. There is also a risk of producing resistant strains (Dorn, 1993).

Source of Infection and Mode of Transmission: Of nine outbreaks in the US, six were caused by undercooked ground beef and three by roast beef. An outbreak in Canada was caused by raw milk. These facts point to cattle as the reservoir of the EHEC agent. Other foods, such as cold sandwiches and uncooked potatoes, were also investigated; calf feces was the suspected contaminant in the potatoes. A later study indicated that undercooked meat (especially from calves and heifers) was the source of infection in more than 75% of the outbreaks. Another outbreak that occurred in 1989 in Cabool, Missouri (USA) and affected 243 people (one of every 12 people in the town) was caused by city-supplied water. The water may have been contaminated by deer feces. Human-to-human transmission also occurs, as secondary cases, through the fecal-oral route. A baby-sitter contracted the infection while caring for a sick child. Secondary cases have also occurred in day-care centers (Dorn, 1993).

Diagnosis: Sorbitol-MacConkey (SMAC) agar is recommended for isolation of *E. coli* O157:H7 from fecal samples. Various enzyme immunoassay techniques can be used to detect Shiga-like toxins in fecal matter or cultures. Isolation becomes difficult beyond one week after the onset of symptoms.

Control and Prevention: Ground beef should be cooked until it is no longer pink. Meat from cattle, like that of other mammalian and avian species, can be contaminated by feces during slaughter and processing. Thus, all precautions should be taken to minimize this risk, and foods of animal origin should be well cooked before they are eaten. Personal hygiene, particularly handwashing after relieving oneself, is also important (Doyle and Padhye, 1989).

b) Enterotoxigenic *E. coli* (ETEC). Enterotoxigenic *E. coli* has been the category most intensely studied in recent years. Research has not only added knowledge about the physiopathogenic action mechanisms of these bacteria, but has also provided means to prevent diarrheal disease in several animal species. Enterotoxigenic strains synthesize various types of toxins—a heat-labile (LT) toxin that is immunologically related to the cholera toxin, a heat-stable (ST) toxin that is not antigenic, or both (LT/ST). The toxins are plasmid-dependent and may be transferable from one ETEC strain to other strains that lack them.

Enterotoxigenic strains are distributed heterogeneously among the different O:H serotypes. ETEC strains make use of fimbriae or pili (nonflagellar, proteinic, filamentous appendices) to adhere to the mucosa of the small intestine, multiply, and produce one or more toxins. These pili interact with epithelial cells, are very important virulence elements, and are called colonization factors. Since the toxins are plasmid-dependent, the antigenic characteristics of the pili differ in different animal species. In man, there are seven colonization factors: CFA-1 and CS1 through CS6 (WHO, 1991). In calves and lambs, the implicated pili are primarily F5 (formerly

K99). Although F4 (K88) and 987P have also been isolated, they are not believed to play a role in ETEC virulence in these animals. The pili associated with enterotoxigenic colibacillosis in suckling pigs are F4 (K88), F5 (K99), F41, and 987P.

In the developing countries, the enterotoxigenic *E. coli* group primarily affects children under 2 or 3 years of age. In unhygienic homes, children may frequently suffer from ETEC. The incidence of the disease declines after the age of 4 and remains low. In addition, ETEC is the most common cause of "traveller's diarrhea" in adults who visit endemic countries. This epidemiological characteristic suggests that the population in endemic countries acquires immunity, while in industrialized countries the population is little exposed to these agents and does not acquire immunity.

The disease in man produces symptoms that closely resemble those caused by *Vibrio cholerae*. After an incubation period of 12 to 72 hours, there is profuse, watery diarrhea; abdominal colic; vomiting; acidosis; and dehydration. The feces do not contain mucus or blood and there may be fever. The duration of the illness is short and the symptoms generally disappear in two to five days.

ETEC can be diagnosed in man by demonstrating the presence of enterotoxin TL, TS, or both through an enzyme immunoassay. DNA probes can also be used to identify the genes in the bacteria that encode the toxins.

Man is the main reservoir and source of infection is the feces of patients and carriers. The route of transmission is fecal-oral. The vehicle of infection may be food and water contaminated by human feces.

ETEC is the cause of some outbreaks that affected many people in the developed countries. Some occurred in children's hospitals in Great Britain and the US, although the source of infection was not definitively determined. There have been outbreaks among adults that affected hundreds of people and were attributed to specific foods and contaminated water. One of the largest outbreaks, affecting more than 2,000 people, occurred in 1975 in a national park in Oregon (USA). Other outbreaks were due to imported Brie cheese that caused enterocolitis in several US states as well as in Denmark, the Netherlands, and Sweden. A large outbreak affecting 400 people occurred among diners at a restaurant in Wisconsin (USA). In this case, the source of infection was believed to be an employee who had diarrhea two weeks prior to the outbreak. A passenger on a cruise ship suffered two episodes of gastroenteritis caused by ETEC, one of them due to the ship's contaminated water (Doyle and Padhye, 1989).

c) Enteroinvasive *E. coli* (EIEC). This category represents a small group of *E. coli*. Many components are nonmotile (lacking the H antigen) and they are slow to ferment lactose or are nonlactose fermenting. The disease they cause is very similar to bacillary dysentery caused by *Shigella*. Their somatic antigens may cross-react with those of *Shigella*. Enteroinvasive *E. coli* can invade and multiply in the cells of the intestinal mucosa, especially in the colon.

EIEC colitis begins with strong abdominal pains, fever, malaise, myalgia, headache, and watery feces containing mucus and blood. The incubation period is from 10 to 18 hours. If diarrhea is severe, the patient can be treated with ampicillin.

The reservoir seems to be man and the source of infection contaminated water or food. However, the source of infection is not always definitively identified.

EIEC is endemic in the developing countries and accounts for 1% to 5% of all patients with diarrhea who see a doctor (Benenson, 1990). Studies conducted with volunteers indicate that a very high bacterial load is needed to reproduce the disease. Some outbreaks due to contaminated water and food have occurred in the developed countries.

EIEC can be suspected when a large number of leukocytes is found in a preparation made from fecal mucus. The guinea pig-keratoconjunctivitis test (Sereny test) has diagnostic value. This test uses enteroinvasive *E. coli* cultures to demonstrate the capacity to invade epithelial cells. An enzyme immunoassay has been developed to detect a polypeptide in the surface membrane of the bacteria that determines virulence (invasive capacity).

d) Enteropathogenic *E. coli* (EPEC). The etiologic agents of the enteropathogenic disease belong to 15 O serogroups of *E. coli*. The disease occurs primarily in nursing babies under 1 year, in whom it can cause a high mortality rate.

The disease is characterized by watery diarrhea containing mucus but no visible blood; fever; and dehydration. The incubation period is short.

The disease occurs primarily in developing countries and has practically disappeared in Europe and the US. It occurs mostly in the warm seasons (summer diarrhea) and the sources of infection are formula milk and weaning foods that become contaminated due to poor cleaning of bottles and nipples, or deficient hygiene on the mother's part. Children in poor socioeconomic groups are frequently exposed to EPEC and generally acquire immunity after the first year of life. In epidemic diarrhea in newborns in nurseries, airborne transmission is possible through contaminated dust. Some outbreaks have also been described in adults.

E. coli isolated from feces must be serotyped. Once the EPEC serotype has been determined, a DNA probe should be used to try to identify the EPEC adherence factor (EAF), which is plasmid-dependent. EPEC strains also show localized adherence to HEp-2 cells.

In epidemics, hospitals and nurseries should have a separate room for sick babies. Treatment consists primarily of electrolyte replacement with oral saline solutions, or with intravenous solutions, if necessary. In most cases, no other treatment is needed. In serious cases, the child can be given oral cotrimoxazole, which reduces the intensity and duration of the diarrhea. Feeding, including breast-feeding, should continue (Benenson, 1990).

e) Enteroaggregative *E. coli* (EAggEC). This name is given to a group of *E. coli* that has an aggregative adherence pattern in an HEp-2 assay rather than a localized (as in EPEC) or diffuse one. This category is provisional until it is better defined. A study was done on 42 cultures—40 from children with diarrhea in Santiago (Chile), 1 from Peru, and 1 from a North American student who had visited Mexico. All these strains tested negative for enterohemorrhagic, enterotoxigenic, enteropathogenic, and enteroinvasive *E. coli* with DNA probes. They also failed to fit in one of these categories on the basis of serotyping. This group causes characteristic lesions in rabbit ligated ileal loops and mice (Vial *et al.*, 1988; Levine *et al.*, 1988).

EAggEC causes persistent diarrhea in nursing babies. The incubation period is estimated at one to two days (Benenson, 1990).

The Disease in Animals: In addition to sporadic cases of mastitis, urogenital infections, abortions, and other pathological processes, *E. coli* is responsible for several important diseases.

CATTLE: Calf diarrhea (white scours) is an acute disease that causes high mortality in calves less than 10 days old. It manifests as serious diarrhea, with whitish feces and rapid dehydration. It may last from a few hours to a few days. Colostrum-deprived calves are almost always victims of this disease. Colostrum, with its high IgM content, is essential in preventing diarrhea in calves. In the first 24 to 36 hours of life, the intestinal membrane is permeable to immunoglobulins, which pass quickly into the bloodstream and protect the animal against environmental microorganisms.

Enterotoxigenic strains that cause diarrhea in newborn calves are different from human strains. They generally produce a heat-stable toxin and the pili antigen is almost always type F5 (K99).

The septicemic form of colibacillosis in colostrum-deprived calves includes diarrhea as well as signs of generalized infection. Animals that survive longer usually suffer from arthritis and meningitis (Gillespie and Timoney, 1981).

Mastitis due to *E. coli* appears particularly in older cows with dilated milk ducts. In milk without leukocytes, coliforms multiply rapidly, causing an inflammatory reaction that destroys the bacteria and releases a large quantity of endotoxins. This produces acute mastitis, with fever, anorexia, cessation of milk production, and weight loss. In the next lactation period, the mammary glands return to normal function.

SHEEP: A disease with white diarrhea, similar to that in calves, has been reported in lambs in several countries. In South Africa, colipathogens were indicated as the cause of a septicemic illness in lambs, with neurological symptoms, ascites, and hydropericarditis, but without major gastrointestinal disorders.

HORSES: A long-term study of horse fetuses and newborn colts found that close to 1% of abortions and 5% of newborn deaths were due to *E. coli*.

SWINE: Neonatal enteritis in suckling pigs, caused by *E. coli*, begins 12 hours after birth with profuse, watery diarrhea and may end with fatal dehydration. Mortality is particularly high in suckling pigs from sows giving birth for the first time. About 50% of isolated strains are toxicogenic and some produce both thermostable (ST) and thermolabile (LT) toxins (Gillespie and Timoney, 1981). In newborn piglets, the colonization factors are F4 (K88), F5 (K99), F41, and 987P and there is probably one other factor. Diarrhea in weaned piglets is caused by hemolytic strains of ETEC that have the F4 (K88) colonization factor, but there are also some strains that express no known factor (Casey *et al.*, 1992). Diarrhea begins shortly after weaning and is a very common complication. The animals also suffer from anorexia and depression. Mortality is lower than in newborn suckling pigs and the pathogenesis may be similar.

Edema in suckling pigs is an acute disease that generally attacks between 6 and 14 weeks of age. It is becoming increasingly important in swine-producing areas. It is characterized by sudden onset, uncoordinated movement, and edema of the eyelids, the cardiac region of the stomach, and occasionally other parts of the body. Body temperature is usually normal. Neurological symptoms may be preceded by diarrhea (Nielsen, 1986). The disease usually occurs in winter. Morbidity ranges from 10% to 35% and mortality from 20% to 100%. The disease seems to be triggered by stress due to weaning, changes in diet, and vaccination against hog cholera. The disease mechanism could be an intestinal toxemia caused by specific strains of *E. coli*. A variant toxin similar to Shiga-like toxin II (see enterohemorrhagic *E. coli*) was identified as the principal factor in the edema. This variant is toxic for Vero cells, but not HeLa cells (Dobrescu, 1983; Marques *et al.*, 1987; Kausche *et al.*, 1992).

FOWL: Pathogenic serotypes of *E. coli* have been isolated in septicemic diseases of fowl, as well as in cases of salpingitis and pericarditis. Contamination of eggs by feces or through ovarian infection is the source of colibacillosis in newborn chicks. Colibacillosis in adult chickens and turkeys primarily affects the lungs, though it may also invade the circulatory system and cause septicemia and death (Timoney *et al.*, 1988). Another avian disease, "swollen head" syndrome, has also been described. It is characterized by swelling of the orbital sinuses, torticollis, opisthotonos, and a lack of coordination. The illness lasts two to three weeks, and mortality is between 3% and 4% (O'Brien, 1985). Its etiology is uncertain. Viruses, *E. coli*, and some other bacteria have been isolated. The viral infection (paramyxovirus, coronavirus, pneumovirus) is thought to cause acute rhinitis and prepare the way for *E. coli* to invade subcutaneous facial tissue. It was possible to reproduce the disease with some strains of *E. coli*; in contrast, the disease could not be reproduced with the viruses (White *et al.*, 1990; Pages Mante and Costa Quintana, 1987). A colibacillary etiology has also been attributed to Hjarre's disease (coligranuloma), which causes granulomatous lesions in the liver, cecum, spleen, bone marrow, and lungs of adult fowl. The lesions resemble those of tuberculosis and mucoid strains of *E. coli* have been isolated from them. The disease can be reproduced in laboratory animals and chickens by parenteral inoculation but not by oral administration.

Source of Infection and Mode of Transmission: Man is the reservoir for all categories except enterohemorrhagic *E. coli* (EHEC), for which there are strong indications that the reservoir is cattle.

Cattle and swine may occasionally harbor strains of enterotoxigenic *E. coli* (ETEC) in their intestines, as Doyle and Padhye (1989) point out. In Bangladesh, three ETEC cultures were isolated from healthy calves and cows; these were of the same serotype and toxin variety as those taken from patients with diarrhea who had been in contact with the animals (Black *et al.*, 1981). In the Philippines, an ETEC serotype (O78:H12, LT⁺ST⁺) was isolated from a rectal swab from a pig; this serotype was considered to be the agent of human diarrhea in many countries (Echeverría *et al.*, 1978, cited in Doyle and Padhye, 1989). However, volunteers were fed an ETEC strain isolated from a pig, but none of them had diarrhea (Du Pont *et al.*, 1971, cited in Doyle and Padhye, 1989). The source of infection is the feces of infected persons (primarily sick persons, secondarily carriers) and objects contaminated by them. The most common mode of transmission is the oral-fecal route. Contaminated foods, including those from animals (meat, milk, cheeses), are a common vehicle in various categories of human colibacillosis. In EHEC, beef is considered the principal source of human infection. In the case of epidemic diarrhea in newborn infants in nurseries, airborne transmission by contaminated dust is possible.

In animals, the source of infection and mode of transmission follow the same patterns as in human infection. Animals with diarrhea constitute the main source of infection.

Diagnosis: Diagnosis in man is based on isolation of the etiologic agent and on tests that can identify it as enterohemorrhagic, enterotoxigenic, enteroinvasive, or enteroaggregative (see each separate category for the most suitable diagnostic method).

In the case of diarrhea in newborn cattle, sheep, and swine, fresh feces or the intestinal contents of a recently dead or slaughtered animal can be cultured.

The immunofluorescence test is very useful for detecting colonization factors; sections of the ileal loop of a recently dead animal are stained with conjugate for this purpose (Timoney *et al.*, 1988).

Control: For man, control measures include: (a) personal cleanliness and hygienic practices, sanitary waste removal, and environmental sanitation; (b) provision of maternal and child hygiene services; (c) protection of food products, pasteurization of milk, and compulsory veterinary inspection of meat; and (d) special preventive measures in hospital nursery wards. These measures should include keeping healthy newborns separate from sick nursing infants or older children. Nurses who tend the nurseries should not have contact with other wards, and those in charge of feeding bottles should not change diapers. Special precautions should be taken in the laundry.

To prevent colibacillosis in animals, the commonly accepted rules of herd management should be followed. For calves, colostrum is important for the prevention of white scours, and for pigs, all unnecessary stress should be avoided during weaning in order to prevent edema.

In recent years, investigations of the factors that permit enterotoxigenic *E. coli* strains to colonize the small intestine have opened up new horizons in colibacillosis prevention in animals. Vaccines for cattle and swine have been developed based on fimbria (pili) antigens. These antigens inhibit *E. coli* from adhering to the mucosa of the small intestine. To this end, gestating cows and sows are vaccinated with vaccines based on F5 (K99) and F4 (K88) antigens, respectively. Newborns acquire passive immunity via colostrum and milk, which contain antibodies against these factors. In the same way, good results have been obtained in protecting newborn lambs by vaccinating ewes with F5 (K99). In addition, studies (Rutter *et al.*, 1976; Myers, 1978; Nagy, 1980) are being carried out with oral vaccines for humans using toxicogenic *E. coli* toxoids of both thermolabile and thermostable toxins as well as antiadherence factors (purified fimbriae). Genetic engineering is another approach being used to obtain vaccines with attenuated *E. coli* virulence (Levine and Lanata, 1983).

Bibliography

Benenson, A.S., ed. *Control of Communicable Diseases in Man.* 15th ed. An official report of the American Public Health Association. Washington, D.C.: American Public Health Association; 1990.

Biester, H.E., L.H. Schwarte, eds. *Diseases of Poultry.* 4th ed. Ames: Iowa State University Press; 1959.

Binsztein, N. Estudio de la diarrea. Factores de virulencia and mecanismos fisiopatogénicos. *Bacteriol Clin Argent* 1:138–142, 1982.

Black *et al.*, 1981. Cited in: Doyle, M.P., V.V. Padhye. *Escherichia coli. In:* Doyle, M.P., ed. *Foodborne Bacterial Pathogens.* New York: Marcel Dekker; 1989.

Carter, A.O., A.A. Borczyk, J.A. Carlson, *et al.* A severe outbreak of *Escherichia coli* O157:H7-associated hemorrhagic colitis in a nursing home. *N Engl J Med* 317:1496–1500, 1987.

Casey, T.A., B. Nagy, H.W. Moon. Pathogenicity of porcine enterotoxigenic *Escherichia coli* that do not express K88, K99, F41, or 987P adhesins. *Am J Vet Res* 53:1488–1492, 1992.

Chin, J., ed. *Control of Communicable Diseases Manual.* 17th ed. An official report of the American Public Health Association. Washington, D.C.: American Public Health Association; 2000.

Dobrescu, L. New biological effect of edema disease principle (*Escherichia coli* neurotoxin) and its use as an in vitro assay for this toxin. *Am J Vet Res* 44:31–34, 1983.

Dorn, C.R. Review of foodborne outbreak of *Escherichia coli* O157:H7 infection in the western United States. *J Am Vet Med Assoc* 203:1583–1587, 1993.

Doyle, M.P., V.V. Padhye. *Escherichia coli.* In: Doyle, M.P., ed. *Foodborne Bacterial Pathogens.* New York: Marcel Dekker; 1989.

Du Pont *et al.*, 1971. Cited in: Doyle, M.P., V.V. Padhye. *Escherichia coli.* In: Doyle, M.P., ed. *Foodborne Bacterial Pathogens.* New York: Marcel Dekker; 1989.

Echeverría *et al.*, 1978. Cited in: Doyle, M.P., V.V. Padhye. *Escherichia coli.* In: Doyle, M.P., ed. *Foodborne Bacterial Pathogens.* New York: Marcel Dekker; 1989.

Edwards, P.R., W.H. Ewing. Identification of *Enterobacteriaceae.* 3rd ed. Minneapolis: Burgess; 1972.

Ellens, D.J., P.W. de Leeuw, H. Rozemond. Detection of the K99 antigen of *Escherichia coli* in calf feces by enzyme-linked immunosorbent assay (ELISA). *Tijdschr Dieregeneedskd* 104:169–175, 1979.

Fraser, C.M., J.A. Bergeron, A. Mays, S.E. Aiello, eds. *The Merck Veterinary Manual.* 7th ed. Rahway: Merck; 1991.

Gay, C.C. *Escherichia coli* and neonatal disease of calves. *Bact Rev* 29:75–101, 1965.

Gillespie, J.H., J.F. Timoney. *Hagan and Bruner's Infectious Diseases of Domestic Animals.* 7th ed. Ithaca: Comstock; 1981.

Griffin, P.M., R.V. Tauxe. The epidemiology of infections caused by *Escherichia coli* O157:H7, other enterohemorrhagic *E. coli*, and the associated hemolytic uremic syndrome. *Epidemiol Rev* 13:60–98, 1991.

Kausche, F.M., E.A. Dean, L.H. Arp, *et al.* An experimental model for subclinical edema disease (*Escherichia coli* enterotoxemia) manifest as vascular necrosis in pigs. *Am J Vet Res* 53:281–287, 1992.

Levine, M.M., C. Lanata. Progresos en vacunas contra diarrea bacteriana. *Adel Microbiol Enf Infec* 2:67–118, 1983.

Levine, M.M, V. Prado, R. Robins-Browne, *et al.* Use of DNA probes and HEp-2 cell adherence assay to detect diarrheagenic *Escherichia coli. J Infect Dis* 158:224–228, 1988.

Marques, L.R.M., J.S.M. Peiris, S.J. Cryz, *et al. Escherichia coli* strains isolated from pigs produce a variant Shiga-like toxin II. *FEMS Microbiol Lett* 44:33–38, 1987.

Merson, M.H., R.H. Yolken, R.B. Sack, J.L. Froehlich, H.B. Greenberg, I. Huq, *et al.* Detection of *Escherichia coli* enterotoxins in stools. *Infect Immun* 29:108–113, 1980.

Mills, K.W., K.L. Tietze, R.M. Phillips. Use of enzyme-linked immunosorbent assay for detection of K88 pili in fecal specimens from swine. *Am J Vet Res* 44:2188–2189, 1983.

Myers, L.L. Enteric colibacillosis in calves: immunogenicity and antigenicity of *Escherichia coli* isolated from calves with diarrhea. *Infect Immun* 13:1117–1119, 1978.

Nagy, B. Vaccination of cows with a K99 extract to protect newborn calves against experimental enterotoxic colibacillosis. *Infect Immun* 27:21–24, 1980.

Nielsen, N.O. Edema disease. In: Leman, A.D., B. Straw, R.D. Glock, *et al.*, eds. *Diseases of Swine.* 6th ed. Ames: Iowa State University Press; 1986.

O'Brien, A.D., R.K. Holmes. Shiga and Shiga-like toxins. *Microbiol Rev* 51: 206–220, 1987.

O'Brien, J.D. Swollen head syndrome in broiler breeders. *Vet Rec* 117:619–620, 1985.

Pages Mante, A., L. Costa Quintana. Síndrome de cabeza hinchada (SH). Etiología and profilaxis. *Med Vet* 4:53–57, 1987.

Riley, L.W., R.S. Remis, S.D. Helgerson, *et al.* Hemorrhagic colitis associated with a rare *Escherichia coli* serotype. *N Engl J Med* 308:681–685, 1983.

Robins-Browne, R.M., M.M. Levine, B. Rowe, E.M. Gabriel. Failure to detect conventional enterotoxins in classical enteropathogenic (serotyped) *Escherichia coli* strains of proven pathogenicity. *Infect Immun* 38:798–801, 1982.

Rowe, B., J. Taylor, K.A. Bettelheim. An investigation of traveller's diarrhoea. *Lancet* 1:1–5, 1970.

Rutter, J.M., G.W. Jones, G.T. Brown, M.R. Burrows, P.D. Luther. Antibacterial activity in colostrum and milk associated with protection of piglets against enteric disease caused by K88-positive *Escherichia coli*. *Infect Immun* 13:667–676, 1976.

Ryder, R.W., R.A. Kaslow, J.G. Wells. Evidence for enterotoxin production by a classic enteropathogenic serotype of *Escherichia coli*. *J Infect Dis* 140:626–628, 1979.

Saltys, M.A. *Bacteria and Fungi Pathogenic to Man and Animals.* London: Baillière, Tindall and Cox; 1963.

Spencer, L. Escherichia coli O157:H7 infection forces awareness of food production and handling. *J Am Vet Med Assoc* 202:1043–1047, 1993.

Timoney, J.F., J.H. Gillespie, F.W. Scott, J.E. Barlough. *Hagan and Bruner's Microbiology and Infectious Diseases of Domestic Animals.* 8th ed. Ithaca: Comstock; 1988.

United States of America, Department of Health and Human Services, Centers for Disease Control and Prevention (CDC). Preliminary report: Foodborne outbreak of *Escherichia coli* O157:H7 infections from hamburgers—western United States, 1993. *MMWR Morb Mort Wkly Rep* 42:85–86, 1993.

Vial, P.A., R. Robins-Browne, H. Lior, *et al.* Characterization of enteroadherent-aggregative *Escherichia coli*, a putative agent of diarrheal disease. *J Infect Dis* 158:70–79, 1988.

White, D.G., R.A. Wilson, A. San Gabriel, *et al.* Genetic relationship among strains of avian *Escherichia coli* associated with swollen-head syndrome. *Infect Immun* 58: 3613–3620, 1990.

Williams, L.P., B.C. Hobbs. *Enterobacteriaceae* infections. *In*: Hubbert, W.T., W.F. McCulloch, P.R. Schnurrenberger, eds. *Diseases Transmitted from Animals to Man.* 6th ed. Springfield: Thomas; 1975.

World Health Organization (WHO). Research priorities for diarrhoeal disease vaccines: Memorandum from a WHO meeting. *Bull WHO* 69:667–676, 1991.

World Health Organization Scientific Working Group. *Escherichia coli* diarrhoea. *Bull WHO* 58:23–36, 1980.

CORYNEBACTERIOSIS

ICD-10 A48 other bacterial diseases, not elsewhere classified

Etiology: The genus *Corynebacterium* consists of slightly inflexed, gram-positive, non–acid-fast, nonmotile, nonsporogenic, nonencapsulated, facultatively aerobic or anaerobic, catalase-positive bacilli. The genus is related to *Nocardia*, *Rhodococcus*, and *Mycobacterium*.

The genus *Corynebacterium* includes species such as *C. diphtheriae* (type species), the agent of human diphtheria, and such animal pathogens as *C. pseudotuberculosis* (*C. bovis*) and *C. renale*. There are also species that are pathogenic for plants and others that are saprophytes. Corynebacteria, with the exception of the species *C. diphtheriae*, are often called diphtheroids.

The species that are animal commensals or pathogens and are transmitted to man are *C. pseudotuberculosis*, *C. ulcerans*, *C. bovis* (the latter two are still not recognized as species), *C. kutscheri*, and a group of three species: *C. renale*, *C. pilosum*, and *C. cystitidis*.

Geographic Distribution: Worldwide.

Occurrence in Man: Few cases have been recognized.

Occurrence in Animals: *C. pseudotuberculosis* (*C. ovis*) occurs in many parts of the world among sheep and goats. It is less frequent in horses and camels. *C. bovis* is a commensal bacteria in the udder and genital tract of bovines. It may occasionally cause mastitis (Gillespie and Timoney, 1981). *C. ulcerans* is found in the nose and throat of man and horses (Wiggins *et al.*, 1981). The species of the group *C. renale* are frequent etiological agents of cystitis, ureteritis, and pyelonephritis in bovines. *C. kutscheri* is a commensal and pathogen in rodents.

The Disease in Man: Twelve human cases caused by *C. pseudotuberculosis* (*C. ovis*) have been described. The common lesion in these patients was a suppurative granulomatous lymphadenitis. There was only one different clinical picture: a veterinary student who contracted eosinophilic pneumonia after exposure in a microbiology laboratory. The victims were treated with erythromycin or tetracycline for several weeks (Brown, 1990). Almost all strains of *C. pseudotuberculosis* produce a dermonecrotic toxin.

C. ulcerans has caused a variety of pathological symptoms in man, particularly pharyngitis, but also ulcers in the limbs, presumed cases of pneumonia, and a disease similar to diphtheria, with pseudomembranes and cardiac and neurological manifestations (Brown, 1990; Krech and Hollis, 1991).

C. bovis is a common commensal in cow's milk, whose fat it hydrolyzes. The literature describes seven human cases of disease caused by this agent. Three of these had CNS impairment and the others had prosthetic valve endocarditis, chronic otitis, and a persistent ulcer on one leg (Vale and Scott, 1977; Brown, 1990).

C. renale has caused rectal and chest abscesses.

C. kutscheri is an opportunistic pathogen in wild and laboratory rodents (rats and mice). There are only two known human cases of disease caused by this agent: one with septic arthritis and the other a premature infant with chorioamnionitis (Krech and Hollis, 1991). The species is not clearly defined in the human cases described in the literature.

The recommended treatment is simultaneous administration of rifampicin and erythromycin (Brown, 1990).

The Disease in Animals: The corynebacterioses are much more important in veterinary medicine. Some of the diseases are described briefly below (Timoney *et al.*, 1988).

C. pseudotuberculosis is the usual etiologic agent of caseous lymphadenitis in sheep and goats, which occurs in many parts of the world where these animal species are raised. The agent gains entry through wounds and localizes in the regional lymph nodes, where it forms a caseous greenish pus. Abscesses may also be found in the lungs, as well as in the mediastinal and mesenteric lymph nodes.

Two different pathological conditions have been found in horses. One is ulcerative lymphangitis, with metacarpal and metatarsophalangeal abscesses that contain a thick, greenish pus and at times leave an ulceration that is slow to heal. The other consists of large and painful abscesses on the chest and in the inguinal and abdominal regions. It may also affect camels, deer, mules, and bovines.

C. pseudotuberculosis has two serotypes. Serotype 1 predominates in sheep and goats, and serotype 2 in buffalo and cows. It produces an exotoxin, phospholipase D, which gives the bacteria much of its virulence by increasing vascular permeability. The other virulence factors are a thermostable pyogenous factor that attracts leukocytes and a surface lipid that is toxic to leukocytes.

C. renale is the most frequent agent in the group that causes pyelonephritis. It is also responsible for many cases of cystitis and ureteritis, particularly in cows. This bacteria produces diphtherial inflammation of the bladder, ureters, kidneys, and pelvis. It can be found in healthy cows in herds with sick animals. *C. renale* also affects horses and sheep sporadically. *C. pilosum* is not very virulent and is only occasionally the agent of pyelonephritis. *C. cystitidis* causes severe hemorrhagic cystitis, followed by pyelonephritis. *C. bovis* is usually a commensal in the udder and is only sometimes the primary agent of mastitis.

C. ulcerans is a commensal in bovines and horses. It has been isolated from milk and is presumed to occasionally cause mastitis in cows (Lipsky *et al.*, 1982). An outbreak of gangrenous dermatitis caused by *C. ulcerans* occurred in Richardson ground squirrels (*Spermophilus richardsonii*) captured within the city limits of Calgary (Canada). Between two and five months after capture, 63 (18%) of the animals fell ill with symptoms of dermatitis and cellulitis. Some of the 350 squirrels captured died, probably due to toxemia and/or septicemia, and had lesions from acute necrotic dermatitis over a large part of their bodies. Pharyngitis was found in 4 of the 10 that were examined (Olson *et al.*, 1988). The infection is assumed to have spread through bites, in a manner similar to that described in monkeys (May, 1972).

Most infections due to *C. kutscheri* in rodents are subclinical. Clinical cases show nasal and ocular secretion, as well as dyspnea, arthritis, and cutaneous abscesses that form gray nodules some 15 mm in diameter. Upon autopsy, abscesses are found in the liver, kidneys, lungs, and lymph nodes. Diagnosis can be performed through culture and isolation of the etiologic agent or serology (ELISA, complement fixation, agglutination). Treatment with penicillin can prevent the appearance of clinical symptoms in animals in an affected colony, but does not eliminate carrier status (Fraser *et al.*, 1991).

C. diphtheriae is an exclusively human pathogen. However, in an outbreak that occurred in a colony of 300 guinea pigs in Nigeria, 60 died with pneumonia lesions, endometritis, and slight intestinal congestion. *C. diphtheriae* was considered the cause of death, since it was isolated from the lungs and heart blood. The source of infection could not be determined (Okewole *et al.*, 1990).

Treatment with high doses of penicillin is effective if begun early in the course of the disease.

Source of Infection and Mode of Transmission: The corynebacteria described here are considered zoonotic, with the exception of *C. diphtheriae*, for which the reservoir is man and transmission is from human to human.

The reservoir of *C. pseudotuberculosis* is sheep and goats. Man acquires the infection through contact with sick animals, their organs, or products (skins, milk). Among sheep and goats, the infection is transmitted from an animal with an open abscess to another animal with abrasions, such as those produced during shearing. Sometimes *C. pseudotuberculosis* can penetrate through abrasions in the oral mucosa, or it can be inhaled and cause abscesses in the lungs (Timoney *et al.*, 1988).

C. ulcerans is a common commensal in bovines and horses. The bacteria is probably transmitted to man through raw milk. The infection may also be transmitted via the airborne route (Brown, 1990).

C. bovis is a commensal in the reproductive system of bovines and can frequently be found in milk; only occasionally does it cause mastitis. In a survey conducted in 74 dairy farms in Ontario (Canada), *C. bovis* was found in the milk of 36% of the cows (Brooks *et al.*, 1983).

The reservoir of *C. renale*, *C. pilosum*, and *C. cystitidis* is bovines. The mode of transmission from bovines to man is unclear. *C. renale* and *C. pilosum* are transmitted among bovines when the urine from a sick cow reaches the vulva of a healthy cow. *C. cystitidis* is a commensal of the prepuce of bulls and can be transmitted sexually. It can also be transmitted when drops of urine are sprinkled from one cow to another.

Diagnosis: A diagnosis of human corynebacteriosis can only be confirmed through isolation and identification of the species.

The same applies to animal corynebacteriosis, although in the case of caseous lymphadenitis in the surface lymph nodes of sheep and goats, the lesions, along with a gram-stained smear, are sufficiently characteristic for diagnosis. Several serological tests have been used to detect healthy carriers of *C. pseudotuberculosis*.

Control: The few human cases identified to date do not justify the establishment of special preventive measures. However, correct diagnosis is important for effective treatment.

To prevent caseous lymphadenitis due to *C. pseudotuberculosis*, it is essential to avoid lesions during shearing. When they do occur, they should be treated promptly and correctly.

Bibliography

Brooks, B.W., D.A. Barnum, A.H. Meek. An observational study of *Corynebacterium bovis* in selected Ontario dairy herds. *Can J Comp Med* 47:73–78, 1983.

Brown, A.E. Other corynebacteria. *In*: Mandell, G.L., R.G. Douglas, Jr., J.E. Bennett, eds. *Principles and Practice of Infectious Diseases.* 3rd ed. New York: Churchill Livingstone, Inc.; 1990.

Fraser, C.M., J.A. Bergeron, A. Mays, S.E. Aiello. *The Merck Veterinary Manual.* 7th ed. Rahway: Merck; 1991.

Gillespie, J.H., J.F. Timoney. *Hagan and Bruner's Infectious Diseases of Domestic Animals.* 7th ed. Ithaca: Comstock; 1981.

Krech, T., D.G. Hollis. *Corynebacterium* and related organisms. *In*: Balows, A., W.J. Hausler, K.L. Hermann, H.D. Isenberg, H.J. Shadomy, eds. *Manual of Clinical Microbiology.* 5th ed. Washington, D.C.: American Society for Microbiology; 1991.

Lipsky, B.A., A.C. Goldberger, L.S. Tompkins, J.J. Plorde. Infections caused by nondiphtheria corynebacteria. *Rev Infect Dis* 4:1220–1235, 1982. Cited in: Krech, T., D.G. Hollis.

Corynebacterium and related organisms. *In*: Balows, A., W.J. Hausler, K.L. Hermann, H.D. Isenberg, H.J. Shadomy, eds. *Manual of Clinical Microbiology*. 5th ed. Washington, D.C.: American Society for Microbiology; 1991.

May, B.D. *Corynebacterium ulcerans* infections in monkeys. *Lab Anim Sci* 22:509–513, 1972.

Meers, P.D. A case of classical diphtheria and other infections due to *Corynebacterium ulcerans*. *J Infect* 1:139–142, 1979.

Okewole, P.A., O.S. Odeyemi, E.A. Irokanulo, *et al. Corynebacterium diphtheriae* isolated from guinea pigs. *Indian Vet J* 67:579–580, 1990.

Olson, M.E., I. Goemans, D. Bolingbroke, S. Lundberg. Gangrenous dermatitis caused by *Corynebacterium ulcerans* in Richardson ground squirrels. *J Am Vet Med Assoc* 193:367–368, 1988.

Rountree, P.M., H.R. Carne. Human infection with an unusual corynebacterium. *J Pathol Bacteriol* 94:19–27, 1967.

Timoney, J.F., J.H. Gillespie, F.W. Scott, J.E. Barbough. *Hagan and Bruner's Microbiology and Infectious Diseases of Domestic Animals*. 8th ed. Ithaca: Comstock; 1988.

Vale, J.A., G.W. Scott. *Corynebacterium bovis* as a cause of human disease. *Lancet* 2:682–684, 1977.

Van Etta, L.L., G.A. Filice, R.M. Ferguson, D.N. Gerding. *Corynebacterium equi*: A review of 12 cases of human infection. *Rev Infect Dis* 5:1012–1018, 1983.

Wiggins, G.L., F.O. Sottnek, G.Y. Hermann. Diphtheria and other corynebacterial infections. *In*: Balows, A., W.J. Hausler, Jr., eds. *Diagnostic Procedures for Bacterial, Mycotic and Parasitic Infections*. 6th ed. Washington, D.C.: American Public Health Association; 1981.

Willet, H.P. *Corynebacterium*. *In*: Joklik, W.K., H.P. Willet, D.B. Amos, eds. *Zinsser Microbiology*. 17th ed. New York: Appleton-Century-Crofts; 1980.

DERMATOPHILOSIS

ICD-10 A48.8 other specified bacterial diseases

Synonyms: Streptothrichosis, mycotic dermatitis (in sheep).

Etiology: *Dermatophilus congolensis* (*D. dermatonomus*, *D. pedis*) is a bacterium belonging to the order *Actinomycetales*. It is facultatively anaerobic, grampositive, and non–acid-fast. *D. congolensis* is characterized by branched filaments with transverse and longitudinal septation. When the filaments mature, they fragment and release motile, flagellate spores, called zoospores, which constitute the infective agent. In turn, the zoospores germinate and form filaments that produce new zoospores, thus repeating the cycle.

Geographic Distribution: Worldwide. Dermatophilosis has been confirmed in many areas of Africa, Australia, Europe, and New Zealand, as well as in North and South America.

Occurrence in Man: The first known cases were identified in 1961 in New York (USA), where four people became ill after handling a deer with dermatophilosis lesions. Subsequently, several other cases were described: one in a student at the University of Kansas (USA), three cases in Australia, and two in Brazil (Kaplan, 1980; Portugal and Baldassi, 1980). A case was recorded in Costa Rica of a veterinarian who came into contact with infected cattle.

Occurrence in Animals: The disease has been observed in several species of domestic and wild animals. Those most frequently affected are cattle, sheep, goats, and horses. The disease is most prevalent in tropical and subtropical climates. The importance of dermatophilosis lies in the economic losses it causes, due to the damage to leather, wool, and pelts. In some African countries, from 16% (Kenya) to 90% (Tanzania) of cow hides have been damaged. In Great Britain, it has been estimated that affected fine wool loses 20% of its commercial value. Moreover, shearing is difficult in chronically sick woolbearing animals.

The Disease in Man: In the few known cases, the disease has been characterized by pimples and multiple pustules (2–25) on the hands and forearms, containing a serous or yellowish white exudate. Upon rupturing, they left a reddish crateriform cavity. The lesions healed in 3 to 14 days, leaving a purplish red scar.

The Disease in Animals: In dermatophilosis or streptotrichosis in bovines, sheep, horses, or goats, a serous exudate at the base of hair tufts dries and forms a scab. When the scab comes off, it leaves a moist alopecic area. The lesions vary in size; some may be very small and go unnoticed, but at times they are confluent and cover a large area. In general, they are found on the back, head, neck, and places where ticks attach. In sheep, the disease known as mycotic dermatitis (lumpy wool) begins with hyperemia and swelling of the affected area of skin, and an exudation that becomes hard and scablike. In chronic cases, conical hard crusts with a horny consistency form around tufts of wool. In mild cases, the disease is seen only during shearing, since it makes the operation difficult. Animals do not experience a burning sensation and are not seen to scratch themselves against posts or other objects. Secondary infections may cause death in lambs. Dermatophilosis is also a factor favoring semispecific myiases (see section on myiases in Volume III: Parasitic Diseases), caused in Australia by *Lucillia cuprina* (the principal agent of "body strike"). The fly not only prefers the moist areas affected by dermatophilosis above other moist areas in the fur for egg laying, but larval development is aided by the skin lesion caused by *D. congolensis* (Gherardi *et al.*, 1981).

In Great Britain, a localized form of the disease in the distal regions of the extremities of sheep has been confirmed and named proliferative hoof dermatitis. This form is characterized by extensive inflammation of the skin and formation of thick scabs. The scabs come loose, revealing small hemorrhagic dots that cause the lesion to resemble a strawberry, from which the disease's common name, "strawberry foot rot," is derived. In cases without complications and in the dry season, the lesions heal spontaneously in about three weeks.

In dermatophilosis cases described in domestic cats, the lesions differ from those of other domestic species in that they affect deeper tissues. In cats, granulomatous lesions due to *D. congolensis* have been found on the tongue, bladder, and popliteal lymph nodes (Kaplan, 1980).

Source of Infection and Mode of Transmission: The etiologic agent, *D. congolensis*, is an obligate parasite that has been isolated only from lesions in animals.

However, according to Bida and Dennis (1977), the agent can be found in the soil during the dry season.

Environmental humidity and moist skin are predisposing factors in the disease. The zoospore needs moisture to mobilize and be released. The rainy seasons in tropical climates are the most favorable to spread of the infection. Another important factor in sheep is malnutrition, which usually occurs during the dry season due to the lack of pasture. Malnourished animals have more persistent and chronic lesions than well-nourished animals. The difference is probably due to the reduced growth of wool and reduced production of lanoline in malnourished animals (Sanders *et al.*, 1990). Most researchers assign great importance to the level of tick infestation in cattle (Koney and Morrow, 1990) and other animal species, as well as to infestation by other insects.

Human cases have arisen from direct contact with animal lesions. Man is probably quite resistant to the infection, as the number of human cases is small despite the frequency of the disease in animals.

The most common means of transmission between animals seems to be mechanical transport by arthropod vectors, including ticks, flies, and mosquitoes. The infective element is the zoospore. Most infections occur at the end of spring and in summer, when insects are most abundant. An important factor in transmission is moisture, which allows the zoospore to detach from the mycelium.

The most serious outbreaks occur during prolonged humid seasons and during the rainy season in tropical areas. Sheep with long wool that retains moisture are most susceptible to the infection. During dry seasons, the agent can survive in moist spots on the body, such as the axilla or in skinfolds.

The infection may also be transmitted by means of objects, such as plant thorns or shears that cause lesions on the extremities or on the lips.

Role of Animals in the Epidemiology of the Disease: The infection is transmitted from one animal to another and only occasionally from animal to man. The only known reservoirs of the agent are domestic and wild animals.

Diagnosis: Clinical diagnosis is confirmed by microscopic examination of stained smears (Giemsa, methylene blue, or Wright's stain) made from exudates or scabs. This is the simplest and most practical method. Immunofluorescence may also be used on smears or tissue samples.

The isolation of the agent should be done in rich media such as blood agar. This culture method is often difficult due to contamination. To overcome this difficulty, passage through rabbits has been used.

Several serological methods have been used to detect antibodies to *D. congolensis*. In a study comparing passive hemagglutination, immunodiffusion in agar gel, and counterimmunoelectrophoresis, the last test gave the best results in terms of both sensitivity and specificity (Makinde and Majiyagbe, 1982).

Control: Given the few cases of dermatophilosis in man, special control measures to protect against infection are not justified. Nevertheless, it would be prudent not to handle animals with lesions with bare hands (especially if one has abrasions or skin wounds).

In Africa, tick control has been shown to be effective in preventing bovine dermatophilosis.

Sheep with mycotic dermatitis should be shorn last or, preferably, in a separate place. Affected wool should be burned. Satisfactory results have been obtained using

1% alum dips. In chronic cases, an intramuscular injection of 70 mg of streptomycin and 70,000 units of penicillin may be administered two months before shearing. This drug therapy seems to be very effective and prevents difficulties in shearing.

The use of antibiotics (streptomycin, penicillin, and others) was effective in producing clinical cure or improvement in affected animals, but did not always eliminate the causal agent.

The infection is controlled by isolating or eliminating chronically sick animals and combating ectoparasites. Externally applied insecticides are used to combat biting insects.

The study of a vaccine against animal dermatophilosis is in an experimental stage (Sutherland and Robertson, 1988; How *et al.*, 1990).

Bibliography

Ainsworth, G.C., P.K.C. Austwick. *Fungal Diseases of Animals.* 2nd ed. Farnham Royal, Slough, United Kingdom: Commonwealth Agriculture Bureau; 1973.

Bida, S.A., S.M. Dennis. Sequential pathological changes in natural and experimental dermatophilosis in Bunaji cattle. *Res Vet Sci* 22:18–22, 1977.

Carter, G.R. *Diagnostic Procedures in Veterinary Microbiology.* 2nd ed. Springfield: Thomas; 1973.

Dean, D.J., M.A. Gordon, C.W. Sveringhaus, E.T. Kroll, J.R. Reilly. Streptothricosis: A new zoonotic disease. *N Y State J Med* 61:1283–1287, 1961.

Gherardi, S.G., N. Monzu, S.S. Sutherland, K.G. Johnson, G.M. Robertson. The association between body strike and dermatophilosis of sheep under controlled conditions. *Aust Vet J* 57:268–271, 1981.

Gordon, M.A. The genus *Dermatophilus. J Bacteriol* 88:508–522, 1964.

How, S.J., D.H. Lloyd, A.B. Sanders. Vaccination against *Dermatophilus congolensis* infection in ruminants: Prospects for control. *In:* Tcharnev C., R. Halliwell, eds. *Advances in Veterinary Dermatology.* London: Baillière Tindall; 1990.

Kaplan, W. Dermatophilosis in man and lower animals: A review. *In: Proceedings of the Fifth International Conference on the Mycoses. Superficial, cutaneous, and subcutaneous infections. Caracas, Venezuela, 27–30 April 1980.* Washington, D.C.: Pan American Health Organization; 1980. (Scientific Publication 396).

Koney, E.B.M., A.N. Morrow. Streptothricosis in cattle on the coastal plains of Ghana: A comparison of the disease in animals reared under two different management systems. *Trop Anim Health Prod* 22:89–94, 1990.

Makinde, A.A., K.A. Majiyagbe. Serodiagnosis of *Dermatophilus congolensis* infection by counterimmunoelectrophoresis. *Res Vet Sci* 33:265–269, 1982.

Pier, A.C. Géneros *Actinomyces, Nocardia y Dermatophilus. In:* Merchant, I.A., R.A. Packer. *Bacteriología veterinaria.* 3.ª ed. Zaragoza, España: Acribia; 1970.

Portugal, M.A.C.S., L. Baldassi. A dermatofilose no Brasil. Revisão bibliográfica. *Arq Inst Biol* 47:53–58, 1980.

Roberts, D.S. *Dermatophilus* infection. *Vet Bull* 37:513–521, 1967.

Sanders, A.B., S.J. How, D.H. Lloyd, R. Hill. The effect of energy malnutrition in ruminants on experimental infection with *Dermatophilus congolensis. J Comp Pathol* 103:361–368, 1990.

Sutherland, S.S., G.M. Robertson. Vaccination against ovine dermatophilosis. *Vet Microbiol* 18:285–295, 1988.

DISEASES CAUSED BY NONTUBERCULOUS MYCOBACTERIA

ICD-10 A31.0 pulmonary mycobacterial infection; A31.1 cutaneous mycobacterial infection; A31.8 other mycobacterial infections

Synonyms: Mycobacteriosis, nontuberculous mycobacteriosis, nontuberculous mycobacterial infection.

Etiology: The etiologic agents of nontuberculous mycobacteriosis (NTM) form a group separate from those that cause tuberculosis in mammals, *Mycobacterium tuberculosis*, *M. bovis*, *M. africanum*, and *M. microti* (the agent of tuberculosis in rodents). Previously called anonymous, atypical, or unclassified mycobacteria, they have since been characterized and given specific names.

Mycobacteria potentially pathogenic for man and animals currently include some 15 species. The most important group among these species is *Mycobacterium avium* complex (MAC), replacing what was formerly called MAI (*M. avium-intracellulare*) or MAIS (*M. avium-intracellulare-scrofulaceum*). These mycobacteria are important pathogens for birds (avian tuberculosis) and some mammals (swine tuberculosis). MAC has become important as a human pathogen due to the AIDS epidemic.

There are both genetic and antigenic indications that *M. paratuberculosis*, the agent of chronic hypertrophic enteritis in cattle and sheep, should be included in the same complex as *M. avium* (Grange *et al.*, 1990). There are also data suggesting that the mycobacterial strains isolated from patients with Crohn's disease are genetically related to *M. paratuberculosis* (Sanderson *et al.*, 1992).

M. paratuberculosis is characterized by its requirement of mycobactin (a lipid that binds iron) for growth in culture media. There are also strains similar to MAC that are mycobactin-dependent to a greater or lesser degree, among them the strains isolated from the wild pigeon (*Palumba palumbus*), which through experimental inoculation in cattle produces a disease similar to paratuberculosis.

DNA:DNA hybridization studies demonstrated that *M. avium*, *M. paratuberculosis*, and the mycobacteria of the European wild pigeon (*Palumba palumbus*) belong to a single genomic species. Based on numerical taxonomy studies of mycobactin-dependent mycobacteria, DNA sequences, and genotype and other studies, Thorel *et al.* (1990) suggest dividing the species into *M. avium* subsp. *avium*, *M. avium* subsp. *paratuberculosis*, and *M. avium* subsp. *silvaticum*. The latter would correspond to the mycobacteria isolated from the wild pigeon.

MAC is composed of 28 serotypes (1–28); the first three belong to *M. avium*, and the rest to *M. intracellulare*. Serotyping has been valuable in research but is not applicable in routine laboratories and has been discontinued. Runyon's classification, developed in 1959, is still in use. It subdivides the mycobacteria into four large groups: photochromogens (Group 1), scotochromogens (Group 2), nonchromogens (Group 3), and rapid growers (Group 4). The different species of mycobacteria are distinguished by their phenotypic characteristics, such as optimum growth temperature, rapid or slow growth, utilization of niacin, nitrate reduction, and other biochemical properties (Wayne and Kubica, 1986).

The mycobacteria that are potentially pathogenic for man and animals include the slow-growing MAC, *M. kansasii*, *M. marinum*, *M. xenopi*, *M. szulgai*, and *M. simiae*; and the fast-growing *M. fortuitum* and *M. chelonae* (or *M. fortuitum* complex).

Geographic Distribution: Their presence, distribution, and relative importance as a cause of disease have been studied primarily in the more developed countries, where the prevalence of tuberculosis is also lower. Some species are distributed worldwide, while others predominate in certain areas. For example, the pulmonary disease in man caused by *M. kansasii* is prevalent in England and Wales (United Kingdom), and in Kansas City, Chicago, and the state of Texas (USA). On the other hand, the disease caused by MAC is more frequent in the southeastern United States, western Australia, and Japan (Wolinsky, 1979). The situation has changed radically with the advance of the AIDS epidemic.

Distribution is similar in animals, since the infection comes from an environmental source. These agents are believed to be more important in hot and humid areas than in temperate and cold climates.

Occurrence in Man: A distinction must be made between colonization and temporary sensitivity, infection, and cases of disease. Since diagnosis depends on the isolation and typing of the etiologic agent, most confirmations come from countries with a good system of laboratories. In Australia, the annual rate of pulmonary infection has been estimated at 1.7 to 4 cases per 100,000 inhabitants in Queensland and from 0.5 to 1.2 per 100,000 in the entire country. In the Canadian province of British Columbia, the annual rate for all nontuberculous mycobacterial diseases increased from 0.17 to 0.53 per 100,000 inhabitants between 1960 and 1972 (Wolinsky, 1979). The incidence of MAC in AIDS patients continues to increase. In the US, it was 5.7% in the period 1985–1988, while it reached 23.3% in 1989–1990 (Havlik *et al.*, 1992). Isolates of nontuberculous mycobacteria from 727 AIDS patients in the US (sample from the entire country) were sent to the Centers for Disease Control and Prevention for serotyping. It was possible to type 87% and almost all the isolates belonged to MAC serotypes 1 to 6 and 8 to 11. Most *M. avium* isolates and the isolates that could not be typed were taken from blood samples. *M. intracellulare* made up of only 3% of the isolates. More than 50% of all the cultures came from New York and California (Yakrus and Good, 1990).

A prospective study of AIDS patients was able to diagnose MAC only in those who had a CD4+ count of less than 100 cells/mm^3. These patients had fever, diarrhea, and weight loss (Havlik *et al.*, 1992).

In Zurich (Switzerland), a retrospective study covering the period 1983–1988 examined patients negative for human immunodeficiency virus (HIV). Nontuberculous mycobacteria were isolated from 513 cases, 34 of whom had an obvious disease. In 23 of the 34 cases, the disease was pulmonary; the soft tissues were affected in 10 cases and there was 1 case of disseminated infection (Debrunner *et al.*, 1992).

In Argentina, 8,006 cultures from 4,894 patients were studied. Of these cultures, 113 (1.4%) were identified as nontuberculous mycobacteria, belonging to 18 cases (0.37% of the total number of patients). The agents isolated were *M. kansasii* in eight cases, MAIS in another eight cases, *M. marinum* in one case, and an infection caused by both *M. tuberculosis* and *M. kansasii* in another case. Localization was pulmonary in 16 cases and cutaneous in 2 (Di Lonardo *et al.*, 1983). A study conducted by 15 laboratories in 6 regions of Argentina obtained 13,544 mycobacteria cultures from 7,662 patients. The etiologic agent was *Mycobacterium tuberculosis* in 99.17% of the patients, *M. bovis* in 0.47%, and MAIS in 0.35% (Barrera and De Kantor, 1987). Between June 1985 and December 1991, at the Muñiz Hospital (for infectious diseases) in Buenos Aires, the prevalence of nontuberculous mycobacterial diseases was 6.2% in HIV-positive or AIDS patients, and 0.5% in HIV-negative patients (Di Lonardo *et al.*, 1993).

In Mexico, 547 cultures were made from samples taken from patients diagnosed with tuberculosis using bacterioscopy. Of these cultures, 89.6% were identified as *M. tuberculosis* and 8.9% as potentially pathogenic nontuberculous mycobacteria, such as *M. fortuitum*, *M. chelonae*, *M. scrofulaceum*, and *M. kansasii*.

Occurrence in Animals: The same considerations that apply to man are also valid for animals. The disease has been confirmed in many mammalian and avian animal species, as well as poikilotherms. Among domestic animals, the disease is economically important in swine due to the losses it causes. MAC serotypes 1 and 2 are the most commonly isolated from swine. These two serotypes are also responsible for avian tuberculosis. Serotype 8 is an important pathogen for both man and animals (Thoen *et al.*, 1981). Serotypes 4 and 5 are also isolated from swine in the US.

Surveillance and identification of mycobacteriosis in animals is mainly carried out in countries where bovine tuberculosis has been controlled, as in the United States. Nontuberculous mycobacteria may interfere in the diagnosis of tuberculosis, causing unnecessary losses due to the slaughter of nontuberculous animals. There is little information on animal mycobacteriosis in other areas.

The Diseases in Man: The most common diseases in people with intact cellular immunity are: (a) pulmonary disease, (b) lymphadenitis, and (c) soft tissue lesions. Other organs and tissues may be affected and, in some cases, hematogenous dissemination occurs (Wolinsky, 1979).

a) Chronic pulmonary disease resembling tuberculosis is the most important clinical problem caused by nontuberculous mycobacteria. The most common etiologic agents of this disease are MAC and *M. kansasii*. *M. xenopi*, *M. scrofulaceum*, *M. szulgai*, *M. simiae*, and *M. fortuitum-chelonae* are found less frequently. As with tuberculosis, there is great variation in the clinical presentation of the disease, from minor lesions to an advanced disease with cavitation. Most cases occur in middle-aged persons who have preexisting pulmonary lesions (pneumoconiosis, chronic bronchitis, and others). Persons taking immunosuppressant drugs or with acquired immune deficiency are also susceptible. However, an appreciable percentage of patients have acquired the disease without having previous damage to the respiratory or immune systems (Wolinsky, 1979).

b) Mycobacterial lymphadenitis occurs in children from 18 months to 5 years of age. The affected lymph nodes are primarily those of the neck close to the jaw bone, and generally on one side only. They soften rapidly and develop openings to the outside. The child's general health is not affected. Calcification and fibrosis occur during the healing process.

In countries at low risk for tuberculous infection, lymphadenitis due to MAC is prevalent, unlike countries with a medium to high prevalence of tuberculosis. In

British Columbia (Canada), the case rate was 0.37 per 100,000 inhabitants, while for tuberculous lymphadenitis due to *M. tuberculosis*, it was only 0.04 per 100,000 inhabitants annually. In Great Britain, as in many other parts of the world, *M. tuberculosis* is prevalent in cases of lymphadenitis caused by *Mycobacterium* (Grange and Yates, 1990). The most common etiologic agents are different MAC serotypes, *M. scrofulaceum*, and *M. kansasii*. The proportion of each of these mycobacteria varies by region. Other mycobacteria are isolated from lesions less frequently (Wolinsky, 1979).

c) Diseases of the skin and subcutaneous tissue are caused by *M. marinum, M. ulcerans, M. fortuitum*, and *M. chelonae.*

Localized abscesses ensue, particularly after injections, surgical interventions, war wounds, thorn penetration, and various traumas.

Granulomas (swimming pool granuloma, fish tank granuloma) develop on the extremities as a group of papules that ulcerate and scab over. Lesions may persist for months. Healing is usually spontaneous. The etiologic agent is *M. marinum*, which inhabits and multiplies in fresh and salt water. *M. marinum* is a photochromogen also found in marine animals; it grows well at 32°C and little or not at all at 37°C (Sanders and Horowitz, 1990). In Glenwood Spring, Colorado (USA), 290 cases of granulomatous lesions were found among children who swam in a pool of tepid mineral water.

Infections caused by *M. ulcerans* occur in many tropical areas of the world, particularly in central Africa. They start as erythematous nodules on the extremities and gradually become large, indolent ulcers with a necrotic base. This lesion is known as "Buruli ulcer" in Africa and "Bairnsdale ulcer" in Australia.

Infections caused by nontuberculous mycobacteria have also been described in the joints, spinal column, and the urogenital tract, and as osteomyelitis of the sternum after heart operations. A generalized, highly lethal infection may occur mainly in leukemia patients or those undergoing treatment with immunosuppressants. Generalized infection with bacteremia detectable through hemoculture has been confirmed only in AIDS patients.

Many other species of mycobacteria generally considered saprophytes can cause pathological processes in man.

There has been much interest and much controversy over the possibility that *M. paratuberculosis*, or a similar MAC mycobacteria, is the agent of Crohn's disease. This chronic disease in man is of unknown etiology and causes a granulomatous process in the terminal ileum, although lesions are also found in other parts of the intestine as well as the skin, the liver, and the joints. A mycobacterium that is the agent of chronic enteritis in cattle, sheep, and occasionally nonhuman primates (with characteristics very similar to *M. paratuberculosis*) was isolated from a few patients. It is a mycobactin-dependent mycobacterium that has biochemical, genomic, and culturing characteristics similar to *M. paratuberculosis* (except in the arylsulfatase and niacin reactions). It is experimentally pathogenic and capable of producing a granulomatous disease in the intestine of goats. Further research is needed to determine whether this mycobacterium is actually the agent of Crohn's disease (McFadden *et al.*, 1987; Thorel, 1989; Sanderson *et al.*, 1992). A primary objective should be to improve culture media so that the mycobacterium can be isolated.

Treatment of the pulmonary forms caused by MAC is difficult due to the resistance of these mycobacteria to the antimicrobials commonly used in treating tuberculosis. It is generally advisable to treat with various medications, selecting them after conducting a sensitivity test on the isolated mycobacteria (Benenson, 1990). Such drugs would include isoniazid, rifampicin, and ethambutol, adding streptomycin at the start, and treatment must be sufficiently prolonged. Clarithromycin has proven to be highly active *in vitro* and *in vivo*. The intracellular activity of clarithromycin increases with ethambutol and rifampicin. An evaluation of the various drugs can be found in the article by Inderlied *et al.* (1993). In cases of serious or disseminated pulmonary disease, the patient may benefit from the addition of other medications (Sanders and Horowitz, 1990). If the disease is limited—such as a localized pneumopathy, a nodule, cervical lymphadenitis, or a subcutaneous abscess—surgical resection should be considered (Benenson, 1990).

The Diseases in Animals: Many species of mammals and birds are susceptible to nontuberculous mycobacteria. The various MAC serotypes are the most important etiological agents. The most frequent clinical form in mammals is lymphadenitis, but other tissues and organs may be affected (Thoen *et al.*, 1981).

CATTLE: In cattle, the most common nontuberculous mycobacterial infection affects the lymph glands. In the United States during the period 1973–1977, nontuberculous mycobacteria were isolated from more than 14% of specimens submitted to laboratories on suspicion of tuberculosis (Thoen *et al.*, 1979). More than 50% of the isolates corresponded to serotypes 1 and 2 of the *M. avium* complex; the rest primarily consisted of other serotypes from the same complex, and only 2.7% were other species, such as *M. fortuitum, M. paratuberculosis, M. kansasii, M. scrofulaceum,* and *M. xenopi.*

In São Paulo (Brazil), attempts at isolations from lesions in 28 cows and 62 caseous lesions in slaughterhouse carcasses yielded 18 isolations of *M. bovis* and one each of *M. tuberculosis, M. fortuitum,* and *M. kansasii* (Correa and Correa, 1973).

Although nontuberculous mycobacteria usually cause lesions only in lymph nodes, granulomas are sometimes found in other tissues.

The principal problem presented by nontuberculous mycobacteria in cattle lies in the paraspecific sensitization for mammalian tuberculin, which causes confusion in diagnosis as well as the unnecessary slaughter of animals. The comparative tuberculin test (mammalian and avian) carried out in several countries shows that sensitization to MAC is common in some countries and rare in others (Grange *et al.*, 1990).

SWINE: In swine, MAC infection causes serious economic losses in many parts of the world due to confiscations of animals from slaughterhouses and lockers. In countries that have carried out successful programs to eradicate bovine tuberculosis, swine confiscated for "tuberculosis" are primarily infected by MAC. Serotypes 1, 2, 4, 5, and 8 of this complex are the principal causes of mycobacterial infection in swine in the United States (Songer *et al.*, 1980). Serotype 8, in particular, has caused outbreaks with great losses for swine producers in several countries, including the United States, Japan, and South Africa. Lesions in these animals are usually restricted to cervical and mediastinal lymph glands, that is particularly near the digestive tract. Generalized lesions are usually due to *M. bovis,* but nontuberculous mycobacteria may sometimes be responsible. In addition to the various MAC serotypes, other nontuberculous mycobacteria have also been isolated from swine, including *M. kansasii* and *M. fortuitum*. Strains similar to *M. fortuitum*, but differing in several biochemical characteristics, were isolated from swine with lymphadenitis; the name *M. porcinum* has been proposed for these strains (Tsukamura *et al.*, 1983).

MAC bacteria can sometimes be isolated from the apparently healthy lymph nodes of a large percentage of animals inspected in slaughterhouses (Brown and Neuman, 1979).

In the US, any mycobacterial lesion is considered tuberculous for purposes of inspecting pork. Economic losses due to tuberculosis were US$ 2.3 million in 1976, but fell 73% in 1988 (Dey and Parham, 1993).

CATS AND DOGS: In cats, nodular lesions, with or without fistulation, are seen in the cutaneous and subcutaneous tissues, primarily on the venter. *M. fortuitum* is among the mycobacteria identified; on one occasion, *M. xenopi* was also found. This disease should be distinguished from "cat leprosy," whose etiologic agent is *M. lepraemurium* and which is probably transmitted by rat bite. The cutaneous or subcutaneous nodules of "leprosy" can localize in any part of the body (White *et al.*, 1983). Skin infections caused by nontuberculous mycobacteria also occur in dogs. Although dogs are resistant to MAC, 10 cases were confirmed in basset hounds; their susceptibility may be due to a genetic immunodeficiency (Carpenter *et al.*, 1988).

OTHER SPECIES: In addition to infections caused by the prevalent tuberculosis mycobacteria (*M. tuberculosis* and *M. bovis*), infections caused by nontuberculous mycobacteria, such as various MAC serotypes, also occur in nonhuman primates kept in captivity. The infection is predominantly intestinal and manifests as diarrhea and emaciation. Lesions in these animals differ from those caused by *M. tuberculosis* and *M. bovis* in that tubercles do not form and necrosis and giant cells are absent. The lamina propria of the intestine is infiltrated by epithelioid cells (Thoen *et al.*, 1981). In a cage of macaques (*Macaca arctoides*), MAC infection was prevalent among various diseases and caused the death of 44 of 54 animals over a period of two-and-a-half years. The lesions found upon autopsy indicated an enteric origin for the disease process. Histopathological examination and clinical laboratory examinations suggested that the common basis of the diseases was an immunologic abnormality (Holmberg *et al.*, 1985).

Infection due to nontuberculous mycobacteria also occurs in other animal species kept in captivity. In poikilotherms, the disease may be caused by various species of mycobacteria, such as *M. chelonae*, *M. marinum*, *M. fortuitum*, and *M. avium*.

An infection due to *M. ulcerans* was described in koalas (*Phascolarctos cinereus*) on Raymond Island (Australia). The animals had ulcers on the flexor muscles of their extremities. This is the first confirmation of infection due to *M. ulcerans* in animals other than man (Mitchell and Johnson, 1981).

Disease among aquarium or aquiculture fish may be caused by several mycobacteria, particularly *M. marinum* and *M. fortuitum*. The clinical symptoms are variable and may resemble other diseases, with emaciation, ascites, skin ulcerations, hemorrhages, exophthalmos, and skeletal deformities. Upon necropsy, grayish white necrotic foci are found in the viscera. Exposure to *M. marinum* in fish kept in aquariums may cause skin infections in man (Leibovitz, 1980; Martin, 1981).

Unculturable mycobacteria that can be confused with *M. leprae* have been found in several animal species, such as frogs in Bolivia (*Pleurodema cinera* and *P. marmoratus*) and water buffalo in Indonesia (*Bubalus bubalis*).

In the province of Buenos Aires (Argentina), the lymph nodes of 67 apparently normal armadillos were cultured. Potentially pathogenic mycobacterial strains were isolated from 22 (53.7%) of 41 hairy armadillos (*Chaetophractus villosus*) examined. These strains included *M. intracellulare, M. fortuitum,* and *M. chelonae.* Mycobacterial cultures were not obtained from 26 *Dasypus hybridus* armadillos ("mulitas") (De Kantor, 1978).

To avoid errors, leprologists doing experimental work with armadillos must take into account both identified mycobacteria from these animals as well as those insufficiently characterized to be identified (Resoagli *et al.*,1982).

FOWL: Avian tuberculosis is due to *M. avium* serotypes 1, 2, and 3. Serotype 2 is the most common in chickens, and serotype 1, in wild or captive birds in the US (Thoen *et al.*, 1981). *M. intracellulare* is usually not pathogenic for fowl (Grange *et al.*, 1990). The lesions are found mainly in the liver, spleen, intestine, and bone marrow, and, infrequently, in the lungs and kidneys. Avian tuberculosis is common; it has a high incidence on farms where chickens have been kept for many years and the enclosures and grounds are contaminated. *M. avium* can survive in the soil for several years. In industrial establishments, the infection is rare because of the rapid replacement of fowl, maintenance conditions, and hygienic measures.

Turkeys can contract tuberculosis by living in association with infected chickens. Ducks and geese are not very susceptible to *M. avium.*

The disease has been observed in several species of wild birds. It may affect any species kept in zoos. Among birds kept as family pets, tuberculosis infections have occasionally been found in parrots, with *M. tuberculosis* as the etiologic agent causing infections localized on the skin and in the natural orifices. This situation is exceptional among birds.

Source of Infection and Mode of Transmission: Man and animals contract the infection from environmental sources, such as water, soil, and dust. Human-to-human transmission has never been reliably demonstrated. *M. fortuitum* abounds in nature and the ability of this mycobacteria, as well as *M. chelonae*, to multiply in soil has been confirmed experimentally. The natural hosts of serotypes 1, 2, and 3 of *M. avium* are fowl, whose droppings help to contaminate the soil, which would be the real reservoir. Other MAC serotypes have been isolated repeatedly from water. In one study (Gruft *et al.*, 1981), MAIS complex mycobacteria were isolated from 25% of 250 water samples collected along the eastern coast of the United States, primarily from the warmer waters of the southeast coast. Similarly, isolations were more abundant from estuarine samples than from river or sea water. During this study, *M. intracellulare* was isolated from aerosols, which would explain the mechanism of transmission to man. Various MAC serotypes were also isolated from soil and house dust in research carried out in Australia and Japan. *M. kansasii* and *M. xenopi* were isolated from drinking water systems. The habitat of *M. marinum* is water, and it has been isolated from snails, sand, and infected aquarium fish.

Many nontuberculous mycobacteria are able to colonize the mucosa of the nasopharynx, bronchia, and intestines of immunocompetent people, who may experience mycobacterial disease when their defenses are low. However, colonization is generally temporary in normal people, as demonstrated by PPD-A (avian) and PPD-B (Battey bacillus or *M. intracellulare*) tuberculin tests that become negative over time. However, the more virulent MAC strains and serotypes that are able to establish themselves in normal subjects and immunodeficient individuals, such as AIDS patients, now constitute an important pathogen.

Nontuberculous mycobacteria are particularly abundant in soil contaminated by infected animals, such as in pigsties, from where they may be carried to surface waters (Kazda, 1983).

MAC and other mycobacteria can colonize drinking water. In a hospital in Boston (USA), MAC was cultured from 11 of 16 hot water faucets and shower heads, as well as from 3 of 18 cold water faucets. Serotype 4 was predominant (du Moulin *et al.*, 1988 cited in Grange *et al.*, 1990).

It is likely that the pulmonary disease in man is acquired through the respiratory system via aerosols. On the other hand, judging from the affected lymph nodes, lymphadenitis in man, cattle, and swine is possibly acquired through the intestine. Obviously, the mycobacteria that cause abscesses, cutaneous granulomas, and ulcers penetrate through skin lesions.

Tuberculosis in birds is transmitted by way of the intestine, through contaminated food, soil, and water.

Role of Animals in the Epidemiology of the Disease: Mycobacteriosis is not a zoonosis but rather a disease common to man and animals. Both acquire the infection from environmental sources. Animals help to contaminate the environment, as in the case of birds and swine with MAC.

Diagnosis: A reliable diagnosis can only be obtained through culture and identification of the causal agent. The possibility of environmental contamination of the culture media should be kept in mind, as well as the fact that sputum, gastric wash, and saliva may contain nontuberculous mycobacteria without these causing disease. Repeated cultures with abundant growth of a potentially pathogenic *Mycobacterium* species isolated from a patient with symptoms consistent with the disease should be considered significant. The diagnosis is certain when nontuberculous mycobacteria are isolated from surgical resection specimens. Differential diagnosis between tubercular pulmonary infections (*M. tuberculosis*, *M. bovis*, and *M. africanum*) and nontuberculous mycobacterial infections is important, since *M. avium-intracellulare* is naturally resistant to anti-tuberculosis medications, while *M. kansasii* is sensitive to rifampicin and slightly resistant to the other medications (Wolinsky, 1979). The other common forms of infection due to nontuberculous mycobacteria present fewer problems in diagnosis.

Infection in cattle and swine is generally diagnosed using lymph nodes obtained in the slaughterhouse or lockers and sent to the laboratory for culture.

Clinical diagnosis of avian tuberculosis can be confirmed through autopsy and laboratory techniques. The avian tuberculin test on the wattle is useful for diagnosing the disease on farms. The agglutination test with whole blood is considered more useful in birds than the tuberculin test (Thoen and Karlson, 1991).

The enzyme-linked immunosorbent assay (ELISA) has proven to be highly sensitive for detecting antibodies to mycobacteria in swine, fowl, cattle, and other animals (Thoen *et al.*, 1981).

Control: Prevention of the pulmonary disease in man would consist of removing the environmental sources of infection, which are difficult to recognize. Consequently, the recommended alternative is prevention and treatment of predisposing causes.

Specific measures for preventing lymphadenitis in children are not available either. On the other hand, proper skin care, proper treatment of wounds, and avoidance of contaminated swimming pools can prevent dermal and subcutaneous infections.

The source of infection in swine affected by lymphadenitis has been determined on several occasions, such as in cases described in Australia, the US, and Germany (Songer *et al.*, 1980). When other materials were substituted for sawdust and shavings used as bedding, the problem disappeared.

The control of avian tuberculosis should focus primarily on farms. Given the long-term survival of *M. avium* in the environment contaminated with the droppings of tubercular fowl, the only remedy is to eliminate all existing birds on a farm and repopulate with healthy stock in an area not previously inhabited by fowl.

Similar measures are needed to control mycobacteriosis in fish. Infected fish should be destroyed and the aquarium disinfected. In addition, the introduction of contaminated fish or products should be avoided.

Bibliography

Barrera, L., I.N. De Kantor. Nontuberculous mycobacteria and *Mycobacterium bovis* as a cause of human disease in Argentina. *Trop Geogr Med* 39:222–227, 1987.

Benenson, A.S., ed. *Control of Communicable Diseases in Man*. 15th ed. An official report of the American Public Health Association. Washington, D.C.: American Public Health Association; 1990.

Blancarte, M., B. Campos, S. Serna Villanueva. Micobacterias atípicas en la República Mexicana. *Salud Publica Mex* 24:329–340, 1982.

Brown, J., M.A. Neuman. Lesions of swine lymph nodes as a diagnostic test to determine mycobacterial infection. *Appl Environ Microbiol* 37:740–743, 1979.

Brown, J., J.W. Tollison. Influence of pork consumption on human infection with *Mycobacterium avium-intracellulare*. *Appl Environ Microbiol* 38:1144–1146, 1979.

Carpenter, J.L., A.M. Myers, M.W. Conner, *et al.* Tuberculosis in five basset hounds. *J Am Vet Med Assoc* 192:1563–1568, 1988.

Correa, C.N., W.M. Correa. Micobacterias isoladas de bovinos e suinos em São Paulo, Brasil. *Arq Inst Biol* 40:205–208, 1973.

Debrunner, M., M. Salfinger, O. Brandli, A. von Graevenitz. Epidemiology and clinical significance of nontuberculous mycobacteria in patients negative for human immunodeficiency virus in Switzerland. *Clin Infect Dis* 15:330–345, 1992.

De Kantor, I.N. Isolation of mycobacteria from two species of armadillos: *Dasypus hybridus* ("mulita") and *Chaetophractus villosus* ("peludo"). *In*: Pan American Health Organization. *The Armadillo as an Experimental Model in Biomedical Research*. Washington, D.C.: PAHO; 1978. (Scientific Publication 366).

Dey, B.P., G.L. Parham. Incidence and economics of tuberculosis in swine slaughtered from 1976 to 1988. *J Am Vet Med Assoc* 203:516–519, 1993.

Di Lonardo, M., J. Benetucci, M. Beltrán, *et al.* La tuberculosis and la infección por VIH/SIDA en Argentina. Un resumen de información. *Respiración* 8:60–62, 1993.

Di Lonardo, M., N.C. Isola, M. Ambroggi, G. Fulladosa, I.N. De Kantor. Enfermedad producida por micobacterias no tuberculosas en Buenos Aires, Argentina. *Bol Oficina Sanit Panam* 95:134–141, 1983.

Du Moulin, et al., 1988. Cited in: Grange, J.M., M.D. Yates, E. Boughton. The avian tubercle bacillus and its relatives. *J Appl Bacteriol* 68:411–431, 1990.

Grange, J.M., M.D. Yates, E. Boughton. The avian tubercle bacillus and its relatives. *J Appl Bacteriol* 68:411–431, 1990.

Gruft, H., J.O. Falkinham III, B.C. Parker. Recent experience in the epidemiology of disease caused by atypical mycobacteria. *Rev Infect Dis* 3:990–996, 1981.

Guthertz, L.S., B. Damsker, E.J. Bottone, *et al. Mycobacterium avium* and *Mycobacterium intracellulare* infections in patients with and without AIDS. *J Infect Dis* 160:1037–1041, 1989.

Havlik, J.A., Jr., C.R. Horsburgh, Jr., B. Metchock, *et al.* Disseminated *Mycobacterium avium* complex infection: Clinical identification and epidemiologic trends. *J Infect Dis* 165:577–580, 1992.

Holmberg, C.A., R. Henrickson, R. Lenninger, *et al.* Immunologic abnormality in a group of *Macaca arctoides* with high mortality due to atypical mycobacterial and other disease processes. *Am J Vet Res* 46:1192–1196, 1985.

Inderlied, C.B., C.A. Kemper, L.E. Bermúdez. The *Mycobacterium avium* complex. *Clin Microbiol Rev* 6:266–310, 1993.

Kazda, J. The principles of the ecology of mycobacteria. *In*: Ratledge C., J.L. Stanford, eds. Vol 2: *The Biology of the Mycobacteria*. London: Academic Press; 1983.

Leibovitz, L. Fish tuberculosis (mycobacteriosis). *J Am Vet Med Assoc* 176:415, 1980.

Martin, A.A. Mycobacteriosis: A brief review of a fish-transmitted zoonosis. *In*: Fowler, M.F., ed. Wildlife Diseases of the Pacific Basin and Other Countries. 4th International Conference of the Wildlife Diseases Association, Sydney, Australia, 1981.

McFadden, J.J., P.D. Butcher, R. Chiodini, J. Hermon-Taylor. Crohn's disease-isolated mycobacteria are identical to *Mycobacterium paratuberculosis*, as determined by DNA probes that distinguish between mycobacterial species. *J Clin Microbiol* 25:796–801, 1987.

Mitchell, P., D. Johnson. The recovery of *Mycobacterium ulcerans* from koalas in east Gippsland. *In*: Fowler, M.F., ed. Wildlife Diseases of the Pacific Basin and Other Countries. 4th International Conference of the Wildlife Diseases Association, Sydney, Australia, 1981.

Resoagli, E., A. Martínez, J.P. Resoagli, S.G. de Millán, M.I.O. de Rott, M. Ramírez. Micobacteriosis natural en armadillos, similar a la lepra humana. *Gac Vet* 44:674–676, 1982.

Runyon, E.H. Anonymous mycobacteria in pulmonary disease. *Med Clin North Am* 43:273–290, 1959.

Sanders, W.E., Jr., E.A. Horowitz. Other *Mycobacterium* species. *In*: Mandell, G.L., R.G. Douglas, Jr., J.E. Bennett, eds. *Principles and Practice of Infectious Diseases*. 3rd ed. New York: Churchill Livingstone, Inc.; 1990.

Sanderson, J.D., M.T. Moss, M.L. Tizard, J. Hermon-Taylor. *Mycobacterium paratuberculosis* DNA in Crohn's disease tissue. *Gut* 33:890–896, 1992.

Schaefer, W.B. Incidence of the serotypes of *Mycobacterium avium* and atypical mycobacteria in human and animal diseases. *Am Rev Respir Dis* 97:18–23, 1968. Cited in: Wolinsky, E. Non tuberculous mycobacteria and associated diseases. *Am Rev Resp Dis* 119:107–159, 1979.

Songer, J.G., E.J. Bicknell, C.O. Thoen. Epidemiological investigation of swine tuberculosis in Arizona. *Can J Comp Med* 44:115–120, 1980.

Thoen, C.O., E.M. Himes, W.D. Richards, J.L. Jarnagin, R. Harrington, Jr. Bovine tuberculosis in the United States and Puerto Rico: A laboratory summary. *Am J Vet Res* 40:118–120, 1979.

Thoen, C.O., A.G. Karlson. Tuberculosis. *In*: Calnek, B.W., H.J. Barnes, C.W. Beard, W.M. Reid, H.W. Yoder, Jr., eds. *Diseases of Poultry*. 9th ed. Ames: Iowa State University Press; 1991.

Thoen, C.O., A.G. Karlson, E.M. Himes. Mycobacterial infections in animals. *Rev Infect Dis* 3:960–972, 1981.

Thorel, M.F. Relationship between *Mycobacterium avium, M. paratuberculosis* and mycobacteria associated with Crohn's disease. *Ann Rech Vet* 20:417–429, 1989.

Thorel, M.F., M. Krichevsky, V.V. Levy-Frebault. Numerical taxonomy of mycobactin-dependent mycobacteria, emended description of *Mycobacterium avium*, and description of *Mycobacterium avium* subsp. *avium* subsp. nov., *Mycobacterium avium* subsp. *paratubercu-*

losis subsp. nov., and *Mycobacterium avium* subsp. *silvaticum* subsp. nov. *Int J Syst Bacteriol* 40:254–260, 1990.

Tsukamura, M., H. Nemoto, H. Yugi. *Mycobacterium porcinum* sp. nov. A porcine pathogen. *Int J Syst Bacteriol* 33:162–165, 1983.

Wayne, L.G., G.P. Kubica. Family Mycobacteriaceae. *In*: Sneath, P.A., M.S. Mair, M.E. Sharpe. Vol 2: *Bergey's Manual of Systemic Bacteriology*. Baltimore: Williams & Wilkins; 1986.

White, S.D., P.J. Ihrke, A.A. Stannard, C. Cadmus, C. Griffin, S.A. Kruth, *et al*. Cutaneous atypical mycobacteriosis in cats. *J Am Vet Med Assoc* 182:1218–1222, 1983.

Wolinsky, E. Nontuberculous mycobacteria and associated diseases. *Am Rev Resp Dis* 119:107–159, 1979.

Yakrus, M.A., R.C. Good. Geographic distribution, frequency, and specimen source of *Mycobacterium avium* complex serotypes isolated from patients with acquired immunodeficiency syndrome. *J Clin Microbiol* 28:926–929, 1990.

DISEASES IN MAN AND ANIMALS CAUSED BY NON-O1 *VIBRIO CHOLERAE*

ICD-10 A00.0 cholera due to *Vibrio cholerae* O1, biovar cholerae

Etiology: *Vibrio cholerae*, a slightly curved, comma-shaped, gram-negative, motile bacillus, 1.5 microns long by 0.4 microns in diameter. This species includes O1 *V. cholerae*, the etiologic agent of pandemic cholera, and non-O1 *V. cholerae*, which sometimes causes disease in man and animals.

V. cholerae is serologically divided on the basis of its somatic O antigen. The etiological agents of typical, Asiatic, or epidemic cholera belong to serogroup O1. All the rest that do not agglutinate with the O1 antigen are non-O1 *V. cholerae*, formerly called nonagglutinable vibrios (NAGs).

In March 1993, an epidemic strain of non-O1 *V. cholerae* was identified in South Asia and was designated as serogroup O139 (WHO, 1993). The first outbreak occurred in November 1992 in Madras (India) and quickly assumed epidemic proportions in India and Bangladesh, with thousands of cases and high mortality (Das *et al.*, 1993). Isolated strains of serogroup O139 produce a cholera toxin (CT) and hybridize with the CT's DNA probe (Nair and Takeda, 1993). *V. cholerae* O139 contains a large number of gene copies of the toxin and is capable of producing it in large quantities so as to produce a severe pathogenic reaction (Das *et al.*, 1993).

Non-O1 *Vibrio cholerae* has biochemical and culturing properties that are very similar to those of the El Tor biotype of *V. cholerae* that is currently causing the seventh cholera pandemic, which began in Indonesia in 1958 and spread to a large part of the Third World. Non-O1 *V. cholerae* does not agglutinate with a polyvalent serum against El Tor or against the Ogawa and Inaba subtypes. In addition, there is a great similarity between the O1 and non-O1 strains in numeric taxonomy, isoenzyme analysis, and DNA:DNA hybridization analysis (Benenson, 1991).

There are various schemes that classify non-O1 *V. cholerae* in serovars (or serotypes). One of them (currently used in the US) is the Smith scheme (Smith, 1977), which distinguishes more than 70 serovars. Serotyping is limited to reference laboratories for epidemiologic studies.

Geographic Distribution: Worldwide. The presence of non-O1 *V. cholerae* has been confirmed on all inhabited continents, either in the environment (particularly in bodies of water), or in man and animals. In Asia, serogroup O139 has spread from Bangladesh and India to China, Malaysia, Nepal, Pakistan, and Thailand, and may spread further. The first case introduced into the US was a California resident who had traveled to India. There was also a case in the UK.

Occurrence in Man: In man, it appears as sporadic cases or small outbreaks. In areas where cholera is endemic, patients have frequently suffered a disease similar to cholera, but caused by non-O1 *V. cholerae*. In India and Pakistan, nonagglutinable vibrios were isolated (i.e., non-O1 *V. cholerae*) from a small percentage of patients with choleriform symptoms. In 1968, an outbreak attributed to this agent occurred in Sudan and caused gastroenteritis in 544 people, 31 of whom died (Kamal, 1971). In the former Czechoslovakia, an outbreak of gastroenteritis affected 56 young people at a training center. NAGs were isolated from 42 of the 56, but not from 100 controls. The disease was attributed to this etiologic agent and the vehicle of infection was thought to be potatoes (possibly contaminated after cooking) that the patients ate. The disease was mild and short lived (Aldová *et al.*, 1968). There was also an outbreak on a flight from London to Australia that was attributed to an asparagus and egg salad (Dakin *et al.*, 1974). Sporadic cases are more common and have occurred in several countries.

The appearance of serogroup O139 completely changed the scenario. This serogroup is not distinguished from serogroup O1 as an epidemic agent of cholera. The epidemic it is causing has affected tens of thousands of people, with approximately a 5% mortality rate (WHO, 1993). The fear is that this new agent has the potential to cause a pandemic. The epidemic wave has already moved from India to Thailand, Bangladesh, and other countries.

Occurrence in Animals: Non-O1 *V. cholerae* has been isolated from many domestic and wild mammalian species, as well as from birds. In India, 14% of more than 500 dogs harbored "noncholeric vibrios" in their intestines. In the same geographic area, the same vibrios were found in ravens (Sack, 1973). In another area of India, far from the endemic cholera area, 195 domestic animals were examined (goats, cows, dogs, and birds) in a search for an animal reservoir for *V. cholerae*. Fifty-four strains were isolated, 8 of which were O1 *V. cholerae* and 46 of which were non-O1. Serotype O1 was found only during the months when cholera was highly prevalent in the population, whereas the other serotype was found throughout the year (Sanyal *et al.*, 1974).

The Disease in Man: It appears in two forms: intestinal, which is prevalent, and extraintestinal.

Gastroenteritis caused by non-O1 *V. cholerae* is usually of short duration and the symptoms are mild to moderate. The disease is only occasionally severe, as occurs in epidemic cholera (Morris, 1990). The clinical picture is usually variable. In a group of 14 patients in the US, 100% had diarrhea (25% of the patients had bloody diarrhea), 93% had abdominal pain, 71% had fever, and 21% had nausea and vomiting. Eight of the 14 patients required hospitalization (Morris, 1990). A severe disease was diagnosed in two young tourists who returned to Canada from the Dominican Republic (Girouard *et al.*, 1992).

Of three strains given to volunteers, only one reproduced the diarrheal disease with stool volumes of 140 ml to 5,397 ml (Morris *et al.*, 1990).

In contrast with epidemic *V. cholerae*, which is exclusively intestinal, non-O1 was isolated from different localizations, such as blood (20,8%), wounds (approximately 7%), the respiratory tract (5%), the ears (11.9%), and others (cystitis, cellulitis, peritonitis).

Septicemia caused by non-O1 *V. cholerae* occurs primarily in immunodeficient individuals (chronic hepatopathy, malignant hematological diseases, transplants), with a fatal outcome in more than 60% of cases. In other localizations, non-O1 is often found with other pathogens, and thus it is difficult to discern its true role (Morris, 1990). A case of spontaneous peritonitis and sepsis caused by non-O1 vibrio was described in Argentina. The underlying disease was hepatitis B and non-O1 *Vibrio cholerae* was isolated through blood culture as well as from ascitic fluid in a pure state (Soloaga *et al.*, 1991). In addition, serotype O139 was isolated from the blood of a hepatic patient in India, something that does not occur with patients suffering from cholera caused by O1 *V. cholerae*.

The disease caused by serogroup O139 is not distinguished from that caused by O1. Infection due to O1 *Vibrio cholerae* apparently does not confer cross immunity against O139, as the latter occurs in areas where people of all ages should have some level of immunity to cholera.

In severe cases, dehydration must be treated through fluid and electrolyte replacement. In addition, patients should be treated with tetracycline.

Treatment for patients infected by O139 is the same as for patients infected by O1 *V. cholerae*: rehydration and, in severe cases, administration of tetracycline.

The Disease in Animals: There are few records of the disease in animals; most species seem to be asymptomatic carriers.

In western Colorado (USA), there was an outbreak of the disease in which 7 of approximately 100 American bison (*Bison bison*) died in about three days. The sick bison were depressed and separated themselves from the rest of the herd. The principal symptoms were diarrhea, vomiting, serous nasal discharge, weepy eyes, and conjunctival congestion. Upon necropsy, lesions were found only in the digestive tract. Non-O1 *V. cholerae* was isolated from the abomasum, duodenum, and colon of one animal and from an intestinal swab from another animal. The agent had been isolated previously in the same region from a colt and a sheep (Rhodes *et al.*, 1985). Rhodes *et al.* (1986) studied several bodies of water, from freshwater to salt water (17 mmol of sodium/L). In western Colorado, 16 different serovars of non-O1 *V. cholerae* were found.

In Argentina, an outbreak occurred in young bulls, affecting 20% of 800 animals, with 50% mortality. The main symptom was diarrhea with dark green feces and weight loss. Upon necropsy, hypertrophy of the mesenteric lymph node chain was found. A bacterium with the characteristics of non-O1 *V. cholerae* was isolated from the lymph nodes (Fain Binda *et al.*, 1986).

In addition to these outbreaks, sporadic cases have been recorded in several countries.

Source of Infection and Mode of Transmission: Non-O1 *V. cholerae* is a natural inhabitant of the surface waters of estuaries, rivers, streams, lakes, irrigation channels, and the sea. It has also been isolated from wastewater from an Argentine city (Corrales *et al.*, 1989). Thus, water constitutes the principal reservoir of this etiologic agent.

Non-O1 *V. cholerae* has been isolated from many animal species in different parts of the world. However, their role as reservoirs is still in dispute (Morris, 1990).

Man can be a carrier of the agent and the source of infection for others. In a study conducted on Iranian pilgrims returning from Mecca, several of their contacts acquired the infection and had diarrhea (Zafarí *et al.*, 1973). The source of infection is different in each country. In the US, the main source of infection is raw oysters. Of 790 samples of fresh oysters, 14% contained non-O1 *V. cholerae*. The number of isolations was higher in the summer months, when there are more vibrios in the water (Twedt *et al.*, 1981). As expected, the highest number of human cases has also occurred in summer and autumn. A variety of contaminated foods have been implicated in other countries (see the section on occurrence in man). Surface water adjacent to a cistern was possibly the vehicle of infection for an outbreak in Sudan in 1968 (Kamal, 1971). In a refugee camp in Thailand, 16% of drinking water samples were contaminated by non-O1 *V. cholerae* (Taylor *et al.*, 1988).

A case of cystitis occurred in a woman after she swam in Chesapeake Bay (USA). Ear and wound infections have almost always been caused by exposure to seawater. It is more difficult to establish the source of infection in septicemias. Some are associated with diarrhea, which would indicate infection via the oral route. Shellfish have been suspected in several cases.

Only a minority of strains of non-O1 *V. cholerae* are pathogenic. At present, it can be stated that strains isolated from patients are more virulent than environmental strains. Strains are differentiated based on hemolysins, their ability to colonize the intestine (adherence factor), and the production of a toxin similar to cholera toxin, Shiga-like toxin, and a thermostable enterotoxin similar to that produced by enterotoxigenic *Escherichia coli*. In India and Bangladesh, non-O1 strains that produce cholera toxin were isolated, but this happens less frequently in other countries. In Thailand, only 2% of 237 environmental non-O1 strains and none of 44 strains isolated from clinical cases carried gene sequences homologous with the cholera toxin gene. In summary, strains of *V. cholerae* vary greatly in terms of the factors that could determine virulence and no single characteristic has been identified that could be used to differentiate pathogenic strains from avirulent strains (Morris, 1990).

Role of Animals in the Epidemiology of the Disease: Although the agent has been isolated from many animal species and many researchers consider such animals reservoirs or possible sources of infection for man (Sack, 1973; Sanyal *et al.*, 1974), their actual role is questionable.

Diagnosis: Culture, isolation, and characterization of the microorganism is the only irrefutable method for diagnosing the disease. Alkaline peptone water (APW) and Monsur broth with tellurite and bile salts are useful enrichment media. The recommended selective medium is thiosulfate citrate bile salts sucrose agar (TCBS) (Corrales et al., 1989).

The corresponding antiserum should be used for specific diagnosis of the O139 strain (WHO, 1993).

Control and Prevention: The few recommendations that can be made are not to eat raw or inadequately cooked shellfish and other seafood, and to drink only potable water.

To prevent infection by serogroup O139, the same recommendations as for classic cholera (serogroup O1) apply.

Bibliography

Aldová, E., K. Laznickova, E. Stepankova, J. Lietava. Isolation of nonagglutinable vibrios from an enteritis outbreak in Czechoslovakia. *J Infect Dis* 118:25–31, 1968. Cited in: Morris, J.G., Jr. Non-O group 1 *Vibrio cholerae*: A look at the epidemiology of an occasional pathogen. *Epidemiol Rev* 12:179–191, 1990.

Benenson, A.S. Cholera. *In*: Evans, A.S., P.S. Brachman, eds. *Bacterial Infections of Humans.* 2nd ed. New York: Plenum Medical Book Co.; 1991.

Corrales, M.T., G.B. Fronchkowsky, T. Eiguer. Aislamiento en Argentina de *Vibrio cholerae* no O1 en líquidos cloacales. *Rev Argent Microbiol* 21:71–77, 1989.

Dakin, W.P., D.J. Howell, R.G. Sutton, *et al.* Gastroenteritis due to non-agglutinable (non-cholera) vibrios. *Med J Aust* 2:487–490, 1974. Cited in: Morris, J.G., Jr. Non-O group 1 *Vibrio cholerae*: A look at the epidemiology of an occasional pathogen. *Epidemiol Rev* 12:179–191, 1990.

Das, B., R.K. Ghosh, C. Sharma, *et al.* Tandem repeats of cholera toxin gene in *Vibrio cholerae* O139. *Lancet* 342(8880):1173–1174, 1993.

Fain Binda, J.C., E.R. Comba, H. Sánchez, *et al.* Primer aislamiento de *Vibrio cholerae* no O1 en la Argentina de una enteritis bovina. *Rev Med Vet* 67:203–207, 1986.

Girouard, Y., C. Gaudreau, G. Frechette, M. Lorange-Rodriques. Non-O1 *Vibrio cholerae* enterocolitis in Quebec tourists returning from the Dominican Republic. *Can Commun Dis Rep* 18:105–107, 1992.

Kamal, A.M. Outbreak of gastroenteritis by nonagglutinable (NAG) vibrios in the Republic of the Sudan. *J Egypt Public Health Assoc* 46:125–173, 1971. Cited in: Benenson, A.S. Cholera. *In*: Evans, A.S., P.S. Brachman, eds. *Bacterial Infections of Humans.* 2nd ed. New York: Plenum Medical Book Co.; 1991.

Kaper, J., H. Lockman, R.R. Colwell, S.W. Joseph. Ecology, serology, and enterotoxin production of *Vibrio cholerae* in Chesapeake Bay. *Appl Environ Microbiol* 37:91–103, 1979.

Morris, J.G., Jr. Non-O group 1 *Vibrio cholerae*: A look at the epidemiology of an occasional pathogen. *Epidemiol Rev* 12:179–191, 1990.

Morris, J.G., Jr., T. Takeda, B.D. Tall, *et al.* Experimental non-O group 1 *Vibrio cholerae* gastroenteritis in humans. *J Clin Invest* 85:697–705, 1990.

Nair, G.B., Y. Takeda. *Vibrio cholerae* in disguise: A disturbing entity. *Wld J Microbiol Biotech* 9:399–400, 1993.

Rhodes, J.B., D. Schweitzer, J.E. Ogg. Isolation of non-O1 *Vibrio cholerae* associated with enteric disease of herbivores in western Colorado. *J Clin Microbiol* 22:572–575, 1985.

Rhodes, J.B., H.L. Smith, Jr., J.E. Ogg. Isolation of non-O1 *Vibrio cholerae* serovars from surface waters in western Colorado. *Appl Environ Microbiol* 51:1216–1219, 1986.

Sack, R.B. A search for canine carriers of *Vibrio*. *J Infect Dis* 127:709–712, 1973.

Sanyal, S.C., S.J. Singh, I.C. Tiwari, *et al.* Role of household animals in maintenance of cholera infection in a community. *J Infect Dis* 130:575–579, 1974.

Smith, H.L. Serotyping of non-cholera vibrios. *J Clin Microbiol* 30:279–282, 1977.

Soloaga, R., G. Martínez, A. Cattani, *et al.* Peritonitis bacteriana espontánea y sepsis por *Vibrio cholerae* no O1. *Infect Microbiol Clin* 3:58–62, 1991.

Taylor, D.N., P. Echeverría, C. Pitarangsi, *et al.* Application of DNA hybridization techniques in the assessment of diarrheal disease among refugees in Thailand. *Am J Epidemiol*

127:179–187, 1988. Cited in: Morris, J.G., Jr. Non-O group 1 *Vibrio cholerae*: A look at the epidemiology of an occasional pathogen. *Epidemiol Rev* 12:179–191, 1990.

Twedt, R.M., J.M. Madden, J.M. Hunt, *et al.* Characterization of *Vibrio cholerae* isolated from oysters. *Appl Environ Microbiol* 41:1475–1478, 1981.

World Health Organization (WHO). Epidemic diarrhoea due to *Vibrio cholerae* non-O1. *Wkly Epidemiol Rec* 68(20):141–142, 1993.

Zafarí, Y., S. Rahmanzadeh, A.Z. Zarifi, N. Fakhar. Diarrhoea caused by non-agglutinable *Vibrio cholerae* (non-cholera Vibrio). *Lancet* 2:429–430, 1973. Cited in: Morris, J.G., Jr. Non-O group 1 *Vibrio cholerae*: A look at the epidemiology of an occasional pathogen. *Epidemiol Rev* 12:179–191, 1990.

ENTEROCOLITIC YERSINIOSIS

ICD-10 A04.6 enteritis due to *Yersinia enterocolitica*

Etiology: *Yersinia enterocolitica* is a gram-negative coccobacillus that is motile at 25°C and belongs to the family *Enterobacteriaceae*. This species includes a very heterogeneous group of bacteria that differ greatly in their biochemical properties. Currently, the biochemically atypical strains have been classified as seven different additional species: *Y. aldovae, Y. bercovieri, Y. frederiksenii, Y. intermedia, Y. mollaretii, Y. kristensenii,* and *Y. rohdei.* These are generally environmental species, can be confused with *Y. enterocolitica*, and at times cause some extraintestinal infections (Farmer and Kelly, 1991). The suggestion has been made to subdivide the species *Y. enterocolitica* into biotypes and serotypes. Biotyping is based on biochemical characteristics, while serotyping is based on the O antigen. The species has been subdivided into more than 50 serotypes, but only some have proven to be pathogenic for man or animals. More recently, the use of ribotyping was suggested for serotype O:3, permitting the differentiation of four clones. Most O:3 isolates belong to clones I and II. These same ribotypes were isolated in Japan. Ribotype I was isolated in Canada and ribotypes II and IV were isolated in Belgium (Blumberg *et al.,* 1991).

A 40- to 50-megadalton plasmid is apparently responsible for the virulence of *Y. enterocolitica.* Strains with this plasmid are characterized by autoagglutination, calcium dependence (antigens V and W cause dependence on calcium for growth at 37°C), and absorption of Congo red. There are also strains that do not contain the plasmid; these are pathogenic and generally negative to pyrazinamide, salicin, and aesculin (Riley and Toma, 1989). Several researchers have found inconsistencies between virulence markers and disease. A study conducted in Santiago (Chile) on a cohort of children up to 4 years of age isolated *Y. enterocolitica* from the feces of 1.1% of children with diarrhea and from 0.2% of the controls. In a subgroup of this cohort, 6% of the children with weekly fecal cultures were bacteriologically positive without presenting clinical symptoms. The isolates of *Y. enterocolitica* from the asymptomatic children were serotype O:3, but did not have the virulence properties attributed to virulent strains (Morris *et al.*, 1991).

Geographic Distribution: Worldwide. The agent has been isolated from animals, man, food, and water. The human disease has been confirmed on five continents and in more than 30 countries (Swaminathan *et al.*, 1982). There are geographic differences in the distribution of serotypes. Serotypes 3, 5, 9, and 27 are found in Europe and many countries on other continents with temperate or cold climates. Serotypes 8, 13, 18, 20, and 21 appear primarily in the US. Serotype 8 has caused several epidemic outbreaks (Carniel and Mollaret, 1990). Outside the Americas, serotype 8 has been isolated from the fecal matter of a healthy dog and a piglet in Nigeria. None of these strains had virulence markers (Trimnell and Adesiyun, 1988).

The serotype pattern is changing in the US. In New York City and New York State, serotype 3 appears most frequently; this is also true in California. From 1972 to 1979, only two isolates of O:3 were confirmed in California, but the frequency of this serotype began to increase such that from 1986 to 1988 it was part of 41% of all isolates of *Y. enterocolitica* (Bissett *et al.*, 1990). This trend seems to be spreading as serotype O:3 in children has emerged in Atlanta, Georgia and in other US cities (Lee *et al.*, 1991).

Occurrence in Man: There are marked differences in disease incidence between different regions and even between neighboring countries. The highest incidence rates are observed in Scandinavia, Belgium, several eastern European countries, Japan, South Africa, and Canada. The disease is less common in the United States, Great Britain, and France. In Belgium, the agent was isolated from 3,167 patients between 1963 and 1978, with isolations increasing since then. Of the strains isolated, 84% belonged to serotype 3, but isolations of serotype 9 have risen since then (de Groote *et al.*, 1982). In Canada from 1966 to 1977, 1,000 isolations (serotype 3) were made from human patients, while in the US from 1973 to 1976, 68 cases occurred, with serotype 8 predominating. Approximately 1% to 3% of acute enteritis cases in Sweden, the former West Germany, Belgium, and Canada are caused by *Y. enterocolitica* (WHO Scientific Working Group, 1980). The lack of laboratory facilities hinders knowledge of disease incidence in developing countries. In tropical areas, *Y. enterocolitica* seems to be a minor cause of diarrhea (Mata and Simhon, 1982).

Most cases are sporadic or appear as small, familial outbreaks, but several epidemics have also been described. Three of these outbreaks occurred in Japan in 1972 and affected children and adolescents, with 189 cases in one epidemic, 198 in another, and 544 in the third. The source of infection could not be determined. In 1976, an outbreak in the state of New York affected 218 school children. The source of the infection was thought to be chocolate milk (possibly made with contaminated chocolate syrup). An outbreak in 1982 in the US affected three states (Tennessee, Arkansas, and Mississippi), and caused 172 patients to be hospitalized. Serotypes 13 and 18 of *Y. enterocolitica*, which are rare in the US, were isolated from these patients. Statistical association indicated milk from a single processing plant as the source of infection (Tacket *et al.*, 1984). An outbreak was reported in 1973 in Finland that affected 94 conscripts (Lindholm and Visakorpi, 1991). A study conducted in a hospital in the Basque country of Spain on 51 cases of yersiniosis recorded during the period 1984–1989 found that most of the patients were urban, 62% were male, their average age was 16–19 years, and the hospital stay was 6 to 12 days for adults and less for children (Franco-Vicario *et al.*, 1991). However, this scenario varies from country to country. In many industrialized countries, *Y. enterocolitica* is one of the principal causes of gastroenteritis in children and sometimes is second to *Salmonella* in isolates taken from the pediatric population (Cover and Aber, 1989). In late 1989 and early 1990, an outbreak occurred in Atlanta, Georgia (USA) among black children. *Y. enterocolitica* serotype 3 was isolated from 38 (0.78%) of 4,841 fecal samples from seven hospitals in different American cities. Twenty of the 38 children had eaten pig intestines ("chitterlings"), which were probably undercooked. Other intestinal pathogens isolated were *Shigella* (1.01%), *Campylobacter* (1.24%), and *Salmonella* (2.02%) (Lee *et al.*, 1991). An outbreak affecting 80 children was recorded in Rumania (Constantiniu *et al.*, 1992).

Most cases occur in fall and winter in Europe and from December to May in South Africa.

Occurrence in Animals: *Y. enterocolitica* has been isolated from many domestic and wild mammals, as well as from some birds and cold-blooded animals. The serotypes isolated from most animal species differ from those in man. Important exceptions are swine, dogs, and cats, from which serotypes 3 and 9, the most prevalent causes of human infection in many countries, have been isolated. In addition, serotype 5 was found in swine and is common in people in Japan (Hurvell, 1981).

In some countries, the rate of isolations from animals is very high. In Belgium, serotypes that affect man were isolated from 62.5% of pork tongues collected from butchers (de Groote *et al.*, 1982). Studies done in Belgium and Denmark revealed that 3% to 5% of swine carry the agent in their intestines.

The Disease in Man: *Y. enterocolitica* is mainly a human pathogen that usually affects children. The predominant symptom in small children is an acute enteritis with watery diarrhea lasting 3 to 14 days; blood is present in the stool in 5% of cases. In older children and adolescents, pseudoappendicitis syndrome predominates, with pain in the right iliac fossa, fever, moderate leukocytosis, and a high rate of erythrosedimentation. The syndrome's great similarity to acute appendicitis has frequently led to surgery. In adults, especially in those over 40 years of age, an erythema nodosum may develop one to two weeks after enteritis. The prognosis is favorable for almost all those affected, 80% of whom are women. Reactive arthritis of one or more joints is a more serious complication. About 100 cases of septicemia have been described, mainly in Europe. Other complications may be present, but are much rarer.

Of 1,700 patients with *Y. enterocolitica* infection in Belgium, 86% had gastroenteritis, nearly 10% had the pseudoappendicitis syndrome, and less than 1% had septicemia and hepatic abscesses (Swaminathan *et al.*, 1982).

An epidemic with 172 cases occurred in the United States in 1982 and was attributed to pasteurized milk: 86% had enteritis and 14% had extraintestinal infections localized in the throat, blood, urinary tract, peritoneum, central nervous system, and wounds. Extraintestinal infections were more common in adults. In patients with enteritis (mostly children), the disease caused fever (92.7%), abdominal pain (86.3%), diarrhea (82.7%), vomiting (41.4%), sore throat (22.2%), cutaneous eruptions (22.2%), bloody stool (19.7%), and joint pain (15.1%). The last symptom was seen only in patients 3 years of age or older (Tacket *et al.*, 1984).

Although extraintestinal complications are rare, they can be fatal (mortality is estimated at 34% to 50%) (Marasco *et al.*, 1993). Complications, such as hepatic or splenic abscesses, occur in adults and generally in immunodeficient patients. Mortality is very high in septicemia caused by transfusion of red blood cells contaminated by *Y. enterocolitica*. Of 35 cases counted, 23 were fatal. Fever and hypotension are the principal symptoms and appear in less than one hour (see the section on source of infection and mode of transmission).

In Norway during the period 1974–1983, 458 cases of yersiniosis were diagnosed and patients were followed up for 10 years. Upon admission to the hospital, 184 patients had abdominal pain, 200 had diarrhea, 45 experienced vomiting, and 36 experienced weight loss. Mesenteric lymphadenitis or ileitis was found in 43 of 56 who underwent laparotomy. Four to 14 years after discharge, 38 were readmitted with abdominal pain, and 28 with diarrhea. High mortality was confirmed in 16 of 22 patients who suffered from chronic hepatitis as a result of the infection (Saebo and Lassen, 1992a and 1992b).

Treatment may be useful in the case of gastrointestinal symptoms and is highly recommended for septicemia and complications from the disease (Benenson, 1992). *Y. enterocolitica* is susceptible to commonly used antimicrobials, except for ampicillin and cephalothin. There are indications that there is no good correlation between *in vitro* assays and clinical efficacy (Lee *et al.*, 1991). Aminoglycosides are the antibiotics recommended most often in cases of septicemia. Other indicated antimicrobials are cotrimoxazole and ciprofloxacin.

The Disease in Animals: In the 1960s, several epizootics in chinchillas occurred in Europe, the United States, and Mexico, with many cases of septicemia and high mortality. These outbreaks were originally attributed to *Y. pseudotuberculosis*, but the agent was later determined to be *Y. enterocolitica* serotype 1 (biotype 3), which had never been isolated from man. The principal clinical symptoms consisted of sialorrhea, diarrhea, and weight loss. In the same period, cases of septicemia were described in hares, from which serotype 2 (biotype 5) was isolated; this serotype also does not affect man. *Y. enterocolitica* has been isolated from several species of wild animals, in some of which intestinal lesions or hepatic abscesses were found. In the former Czechoslovakia and the Scandinavian countries, *Y. enterocolitica* was isolated from 3% to 26% of wild rodents, but necropsy of these animals revealed no lesions. Similar results were obtained in southern Chile, where the agent was isolated from 4% of 305 rodents of different species and from different habitats (Zamora *et al.*, 1979). Serotypes isolated from rodents are generally not those pathogenic for man. Among wild animals in New York State, serotype O:8 has been isolated from a gray fox (*Urocyon cinereoargenteus*) and from a porcupine (*Erethizon dorsatum*); serotype O:3 has been isolated from another gray fox. Both serotypes are pathogenic for man (Shayegani *et al.*, 1986).

Studies carried out on swine, dogs, and cats are of particular interest, since these animals harbor serotypes that infect man. The agent has been isolated from clinically healthy swine and from animals destined for human consumption. In one study, a much higher rate of isolations was obtained from swine with diarrhea than from apparently healthy animals. In another study, however, the agent was isolated from 17% of healthy swine and from 5.4% of swine tested because of various symptoms (Hurvell, 1981). *Y. enterocolitica* has been isolated from swine during outbreaks of diarrhea, with no other pathogen detected. Blood or mucus do not generally appear in the feces, but may be found in the stool of some animals. Diarrhea is accompanied by a mild fever (Taylor, 1992). Swine that are carriers of *Y. enterocolitica* serotypes that infect man have been noted primarily in countries where the incidence of human disease is higher, such as in the Scandinavian countries, Belgium, Canada, and Japan. The rate of isolation from swine varies from one herd to another and depends on the level of contamination in each establishment. On one farm the agent may be isolated only sporadically and at a low rate, while on another, isolations may be continuous and reach 100% of the groups examined (Fukushima *et al.*, 1983).

Y. enterocolitica has been isolated from young sheep with enterocolitis in New Zealand and also in southern Australia. The sheep from 14 herds in New South Wales from which the agent (serotypes 2, 3) was isolated had diarrhea and some showed delayed growth and died (Philbey *et al.*, 1991). In Great Britain, *Y. enterocolitica* was thought to have caused abortions in sheep. The etiologic agent was isolated from sheep fetuses and most of the serotypes were 6,30 and 7, which did not have the plasmid that determines the markers to which virulence is attributed (Corbel *et al.*, 1990). An O:6,30 strain isolated from the liver of an aborted sheep fetus was inoculated intravenously in a group of sheep that had been pregnant for approximately 90 days; the infection produced a necrotizing placentitis and abortions (Corbel *et al.*, 1992).

Abortions have been described in association with *Y. enterocolitica* in cattle in the former Soviet Union and Great Britain and in buffalo in India. In the latter country, serotype O:9 was isolated from nine buffaloes that aborted; this serotype shares common antigens with *Brucella* and gives serologic cross reactions with that bacterial species (Das *et al.*, 1986).

Serotypes of *Y. enterocolitica* were isolated from 5.5% of 451 dogs in Japan (Kaneko *et al.*, 1977) and from 1.7% of 115 dogs in Denmark (Pedersen and Winblad, 1979). In contrast, the incidence of canine carriers in the US and Canada is low. The disease seems to occur rarely in dogs, but it should be borne in mind that many clinical cases are not diagnosed because isolation is not attempted. In two cases of enteritis described in Canada, the dogs manifested neither fever nor abdominal pains, but they had frequent defecations covered with mucous and blood (Papageorges and Gosselin, 1983). *Y. enterocolitica* has also been isolated from apparently healthy cats. Serotypes O:8 and O:9 are among the types isolated from dogs and cats.

Infection caused by *Y. enterocolitica* has been confirmed in several monkey species. In one colony of patas monkeys (*Erythrocebus patas*) in Missouri (USA), two monkeys died less than one month apart from a generalized infection caused by *Y. enterocolitica*. The remaining 20 monkeys were examined and the agent was isolated from rectal swabs taken from five of the clinically normal monkeys (Skavlen *et al.*, 1985).

Source of Infection and Mode of Transmission (Figure 10): The epidemiology of enterocolitic yersiniosis is not entirely clear. The agent is widespread in water, food, many animal species, and man. Of interest is the fact that the serotypes isolated from water and food often do not correspond to the types that produce disease in man. This is also true of the serotypes found in the majority of animal species,

**Figure 10. Enterocolitic yersiniosis (*Yersinia enterocolitica*).
Supposed mode of transmission.**

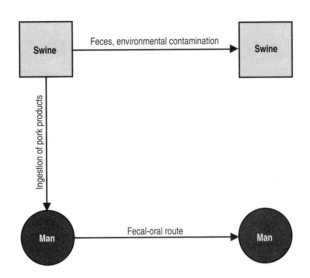

with the exception of pigs and, to some extent, dogs and cats. In countries with the highest incidence of human disease, pigs are frequently carriers of serotypes pathogenic for man. In contrast, in those countries where the incidence of human disease is low, such as the US or Great Britain, serotypes pathogenic for man are rarely isolated from pigs (Wooley *et al.*, 1980; Brewer and Corbel, 1983).

Research conducted in Scandinavia, Canada, and South Africa strongly suggests that the probable reservoir of the agent is swine. In other countries, however, the reservoir is still unknown. Serotype 8, which predominated in the United States, was isolated from 2 of 95 asymptomatic individuals after an outbreak in New York State due to chocolate milk and caused by the same serotype. Serotype 8 was isolated from water and foods in the former Czechoslovakia, but no human cases were seen (Aldova *et al.*, 1981). Some nosocomial outbreaks indicate that human-to-human transmission is possible. A study was conducted in a university hospital in the United States between 1987 and 1990 to evaluate nosocomial transmission of the infection. Of 18 patients from whom *Y. enterocolitica* was isolated, 8 acquired the infection outside the hospital, 5 were infected in the hospital 18 to 66 days after being admitted for causes other than gastroenteritis, and in 5 cases, the origin could not be identified (Cannon and Linnemann, 1992). Some familial outbreaks have been attributed to exposure to dogs. Nevertheless, dogs and cats are not considered important reservoirs.

At present, serotype O:3 predominates throughout the world as a human pathogen. Swine are the primary reservoir and source of infection. In Denmark, where there are approximately 2,000 human cases each year, it was demonstrated that more than 80% of swine herds are infected. Healthy pigs show a high prevalence of *Y. enterocolitica* serotype O:3. A study conducted at a slaughterhouse in

Denmark examined 1,458 pigs; serotype O:3 was isolated from the feces of 360 (24.7%) animals. Fecal contamination of the carcass varied with the evisceration technique. In the manual procedure, which is the traditional technique, frequency was 26.3%, while in the mechanical procedure—suggested along with plugging the anus and rectum with a plastic bag—it fell by 1% to 2.2%, depending on the region of the carcass (Andersen, 1988). The clinically important serotypes, O:3, O:5,27, and O:8, have been isolated from chopped pork, pig tongue, and from chicken.

Swine slaughterhouse workers are an occupational group at risk of being infected. Enzyme-linked immunosorbent assay (ELISA) was used to examine serum samples from 146 workers in Finland; antibodies were found for serotype O:3 in 19% of them and in 10% of blood donors used as controls. The tonsils of 31 of 120 pigs from the same slaughterhouse yielded positive cultures for serotype O:3 (Merilahti-Palo et al., 1991). In a similar study conducted in Norway, 25 (11.1%) of 316 slaughterhouse workers and 9.9% of 171 veterinarians were positive for IgG antibodies to serotype O:3. Counter to expectations, of 813 army recruits, prevalence was higher among those from urban areas (15.2%) than from rural areas (Nesbakken et al., 1991).

Milk and water are vehicles of infection, among others. An outbreak in 1976 was attributed to pasteurized chocolate milk. Another outbreak occurred in New York in 1981, when 239 people became ill. The largest outbreak of all occurred in several U.S. states and affected 1,000 people who drank recontaminated pasteurized milk. Unlike other outbreaks, the infection was caused by very rare serotypes (O:13a, O:13b). Pasteurization is effective in destroying the agent, and thus it is assumed that contamination occurred afterward. Water contaminated by animal fecal matter has been assumed to be the common source of infection in various Nordic countries in Europe and in the US. A small familial outbreak occurred in Canada; it was caused by serotype O:3, which is responsible for about 75% of all human cases in that country. The agent was isolated from two family members and from water from a shallow well that may have been contaminated by dog feces swept in by heavy rains. The strains from the patients and the water had the same characteristics (Thompson and Gravel, 1986).

It is often difficult to identify the source of infection. Foods may contain a small number of pathogenic Y. enterocolitica within a large population of other bacteria, primarily environmental species of Yersinia spp. and nonpathogenic serotypes of Y. enterocolitica. Isolation and enrichment procedures are not always able to detect the etiologic agent (Schiemann, 1989).

Blood transfusion is another route for human-to-human transmission. Although rare, the consequences of such cases are usually serious. From April 1987 to February 1991, there were 10 cases in the US of bacteremia caused by transfusion of red blood cells. The final six of these patients showed fever and hypotension within 50 minutes of transfusion. One patient suffered explosive diarrhea within 10 minutes of transfusion. Four of the six died within a period of 12 hours to 37 days. The serotypes isolated were O:5,27 (4 cases), O:3 (one case), and O:20 (one case) (CDC, 1991). Blood donors were interviewed and some acknowledged having had diarrhea in the 30 days prior to donating blood; one had diarrhea the same day and two indicated they had had no gastrointestinal complaints. In Great Britain, four of a total of six cases were fatal in 1988. Two cases occurred in Scotland in four months alone and both people died (Prentice, 1992; Jones et al., 1993). Prentice (1992) estimates that outside Great Britain there have been 27 cases of septicemia caused by blood transfusion, 17 of them fatal. One case of autologous transfusion has also been described (Richards *et al.*, 1992).

The mode of transmission is not well known either, but it is widely accepted that the infection is contracted by ingestion of contaminated foods, as in the case of other enterobacterial diseases, as well as by contact with carrier animals and by human-to-human transmission. It is known that *Y. enterocolitica* can multiply at refrigeration temperature. It is believed that this led to the 1982 epidemic in the US (see the section on occurrence in man) produced by recontaminated pasteurized milk. This epidemic also reveals that serotypes other than 3, 5, 8, and 9 can give rise to the disease, although less commonly.

Role of Animals in the Epidemiology of the Disease: Although not providing definitive proof, the accumulated data in countries with a high incidence of the human disease indicate that swine are probably an important reservoir of *Y. enterocolitica*, particularly serotype O:3, which is currently the prevalent type, and type O:9, which is also frequent in swine. The disease caused by a dish prepared with pig intestines ("chitterlings") in various American cities is good evidence that the infection is transmitted through food.

Diagnosis: In cases of enteritis, appendicitis, erythema nodosum, and reactive arthritis, the possibility of *Y. enterocolitica* infection should be considered. The agent can be isolated from the patients' feces. MacConkey agar and a selective agar called cefsulodina irgasan novobiocin (CIN), created specifically for *Yersinia*, can be used for this purpose. Both biotype and serotype should be identified. The cold enrichment technique is useful, particularly in the case of carriers that may excrete few *Y. enterocolitica* cells. Samples are suspended in peptone culture broth or a buffered phosphate solution for 3 to 7 days at 4°C to encourage the growth of *Y. enterocolitica* and suppress that of other bacteria. However, routine diagnosis is an impractical procedure, takes a long time (about 1 month), and does not exclude non-pathogenic *Yersinia*.

Tube serum agglutination and the ELISA test can be used with good results as additional diagnostic techniques. Active infections produce high titers that decline over time. Serum agglutination titers of 1/40 to 1/80 are rare in healthy individuals, but common in yersiniosis patients and can rise to very high titers. Positive cultures without clear evidence of gastroenteritis are not always accompanied by a high serum agglutination titer.

Very high titers are common in patients with acute appendicitis (Schiemann, 1989). In countries where serotype 9 is a frequent pathogen for man and is also harbored by swine, cross-reaction between *Brucella* and that serotype may cause difficulties.

Antibodies in swine against serotype 9 of *Y. enterocolitica* can be differentiated from those against *Brucella* by flagellar antigens, which *Y. enterocolitica* has and brucellae do not. *Y. enterocolitica* also possesses the common enterobacterial antigen, which *Brucella* does not have and which therefore may also be used to distinguish them (Mittal *et al.*, 1984). Other animals that have been exposed to serotype 9 can also show cross-reactions with *Brucella*.

A comparison of three tests for serum diagnosis of type O:3 (immunoelectrophoresis, ELISA, and agglutination) produced similar results in terms of sensitivity and specificity (Paerregaard *et al.*, 1991).

A method has been developed for direct identification of *Yersinia enterocolitica* in blood using polymerase chain reaction (PCR). This procedure can detect the agent in 500 bacteria per 100 microliters of blood (Feng *et al.*, 1992).

Control: Currently recommended measures are to observe food hygiene rules; to ensure that animal products, particularly pork, are well cooked; and to not drink raw milk or water of doubtful purity.

An important step in prevention is to avoid contaminating swine carcasses with fecal matter (see the section on source of infection and mode of transmission). Given the possibility of interhuman infection in hospitals, generally recommended measures for nosocomial infections should be implemented.

A practical method for preventing transmission through transfusions is to screen with hematology stains (Wright, Wright-Giemsa) any blood bank unit that has been refrigerated for 25 days or more. Testing has shown that when the contamination is from a single colony forming unit (CFU) of *Y. enterocolitica*, the bacterial count at 26 days rises to 10^7–10^8 CFU and ≥ 1 ng/mL of endotoxin is detected (CDC, 1991).

Bibliography

Aldova, E., J. Sobotková, A. Brezinova, J. Cerna, M. Janeckova, J. Pegrimkova, *et al. Yersinia enterocolitica* in water and foods. *Zbl Bakt Mikrobiol Hyg [B]* 173:464–470, 1981.

Andersen, J.K. Contamination of freshly slaughtered pig carcasses with human pathogenic *Yersinia enterocolitica*. *Int J Food Microbiol* 7:193–202, 1988.

Benenson, A.S., ed. *Control of Communicable Diseases in Man.* 15th ed. An official report of the American Public Health Association. Washington, D.C.: American Public Health Association; 1990.

Bissett, M.L., C. Powers, S.L. Abbott, J.M. Janda. Epidemiologic investigations of *Yersinia enterocolitica* and related species: Sources, frequency and serogroup distribution. *J Clin Microbiol* 28:910–912, 1990.

Blumberg, H.M., J.A. Kiehlbauch, I.K. Wachsmuth. Molecular epidemiology of *Yersinia enterocolitica* O:3 infections: Use of chromosomal DNA restriction fragment length polymorphisms of rRNA genes. *J Clin Microbiol* 29:2368–2374, 1991.

Brewer, R.A., M.J. Corbel. Characterization of *Yersinia enterocolitica* strains isolated from cattle, sheep and pigs in the United Kingdom. *J Hyg* 90:425–433, 1983.

Cannon, C.G., C.C. Linnemann. *Yersinia enterocolitica* infections in hospitalized patients: The problem of hospital-acquired infections. *Infect Control Hosp Epidemiol* 13:139–143, 1992.

Carniel, E., H.H Mollaret. Yersiniosis. *Comp Immunol Microbiol Infect Dis* 13(2):51–58, 1990.

Constantiniu, S., C. Naciu, A. Romaniuc, *et al.* Serological diagnosis in human *Yersinia* infections. *Roum Arch Microbiol Immunol* 51:225–232, 1992.

Corbel, M.J., R.A. Brewer, D. Hunter. Characterisation of *Yersinia enterocolitica* strains associated with ovine abortion. *Vet Rec* 127:526–527, 1990.

Corbel, M.J., B. Ellis, C. Richardson, R. Bradley. Experimental *Yersinia enterocolitica* placentitis in sheep. *Brit Vet J* 148:339–349, 1992.

Cover, T.L., R.C. Aber. *Yersinia enterocolitica. N Engl J Med* 321:16–24, 1989.

Das, A.M., V.L. Paranjape, S. Winblad. *Yersinia enterocolitica* associated with third trimester abortion in buffaloes. *Trop Anim Health Prod* 18:109–112, 1986.

de Groote, G., J. Vandepitte, G. Wauters. Surveillance of human *Yersinia enterocolitica* infections in Belgium: 1963–1978. *J Infect* 4:189–197, 1982.

Farmer, J.J., III., M.T. Kelly. Enterobacteriaceae. *In*: Ballows, A., W.J. Hausler, Jr., K.L. Hermann, H.D. Isenberg, H.J. Shadomy. *Manual of Clinical Microbiology*. 5th ed. Washington, D.C.: American Society for Microbiology; 1991.

Feng, P., S.P. Keasler, W.E. Hill. Direct identification of *Yersinia enterocolitica* in blood by polymerase chain reaction amplification. *Transfusion* 32:850–854, 1992.

Franco-Vicario, R., P. Echevarria Villegas, P. Martínez-Olaizola, *et al.* Yersiniosis en un hospital general del País Vasco (1984–1989). Aspectos clínicos and epidemiológicos. *Med Clin* 97:241–244, 1991.

Fukushima, H., R. Nakamura, Y. Ito, K. Saito, M. Tsubokura, K. Otsuki. Ecological studies of *Yersinia enterocolitica*. I. Dissemination of *Y. enterocolitica* in pigs. *Vet Microbiol* 8:469–483, 1983.

Hurvell, B. Zoonotic *Yersinia enterocolitica* infection: Host-range, clinical manifestations, and transmission between animals and man. *In*: Bottone, E.J., ed. *Yersinia enterocolitica*. Boca Raton: CRC Press; 1981.

Jones, B.L., M.H. Saw, M.F. Hanson, *et al. Yersinia enterocolitica* septicaemia from transfusion of red cell concentrate stored for 16 days. *J Clin Pathol* 46:477–478, 1993.

Kaneko, K., S. Hamada, E. Kato. Ocurrence of *Yersinia enterocolitica* in dogs. *Jpn J Vet Sci* 39:407–414, 1977.

Lee, L.A., J. Taylor, G.P. Carter, *et al. Yersinia enterocolitica* O:3: An emerging cause of pediatric gastroenteritis in the United States. The *Yersinia enterocolitica* Collaborative Study Group. *J Infect Dis* 163:660–663, 1991.

Lindholm, H., R. Visakorpi. Late complications after a *Yersinia enterocolitica* epidemic: A follow up study. *Ann Rheum Dis* 50:694–696, 1991.

Marasco, W.J., E.K. Fishman, J.E. Kuhlman, R.H. Hruban. Splenic abscess as a complication of septic yersinia: CT evaluation. *Clin Imaging* 17:33–35, 1993.

Mata, L., A. Simhon. Enteritis y colitis infecciosas del hombre. *Adel Microbiol Enf Infec* (Buenos Aires) 1:1–50, 1982.

Merilahti-Palo, R., R. Lahesmaa, K. Granfors, *et al.* Risk of *Yersinia* infection among butchers. *Scand J Infect Dis* 23:55–61, 1991.

Mittal, K.R., I.R. Tizard, D.A. Barnum. Serological cross-reactions between *Brucella abortus* and *Yersinia enterocolitica* 09. International Symposium on Human and Animal Brucellosis. Taipei, Taiwan, 1984.

Morris, J.G., V. Prado, C. Ferreccio, *et al. Yersinia enterocolitica* isolated from two cohorts of young children in Santiago, Chile: Incidence of and lack of correlation between illness and proposed virulence factors. *J Clin Microbiol* 29:2784–2788, 1991.

Nesbakken, T., G. Kapperud, J. Lassen, E. Skjerve. *Yersinia enterocolitica* O:3 antibodies in slaughterhouse employees, veterinarians, and military recruits. Occupational exposure to pigs as a risk factor for yersiniosis. *Contr Microbiol Immunol* 12:32–39, 1991.

Paerregaard, A., G.H. Shand, K. Gaarslev, F. Espersen. Comparison of crossed immunoelectrophoresis, enzyme-linked immunosorbent assays, and tube agglutination for serodiagnosis of *Yersinia enterocolitica* serotype O:3 infection. *J Clin Microbiol* 29:302–309, 1991.

Papageorges, M., R. Higgins, Y. Gosselin. *Yersinia enterocolitica* enteritis in two dogs. *J Am Vet Med Assoc* 182:618–619, 1983.

Pedersen, K.B., S. Winblad. Studies on *Yersinia enterocolitica* isolated from swine and dogs. *Acta Path Microbiol Scand [B]* 87B:137–140, 1979.

Philbey, A.W., J.R. Glastonbury, I.J. Links, L.M. Mathews. *Yersinia* species isolated from sheep with enterocolitis. *Aust Vet J* 68:108–110, 1991.

Prentice, M. Transfusing *Yersinia enterocolitica*. *Brit Med J* 305:663–664, 1992.

Richards, C., J. Kolins, C.D. Trindade. Autologous transfusion-transmitted *Yersinia enterocolitica* [letter]. *JAMA* 268:154, 1992.

Riley, G., S. Toma. Detection of pathogenic *Yersinia enterocolitica* by using Congo red-magnesium oxalate agar medium. *J Clin Microbiol* 27:213–214, 1989.

Saebo, A., J. Lassen. Acute and chronic liver disease associated with *Yersinia enterocolitica* infection: A Norwegian 10-year follow-up study of 458 hospitalized patients. *J Intern Med* 231:531–535, 1992a.

Saebo, A., J. Lassen. Acute and chronic pancreatic disease associated with *Yersinia enterocolitica* infection: A Norwegian 10-year follow-up study of 458 hospitalized patients. *J Intern Med* 231:537–541, 1992b.

Schiemann, D.A. *Yersinia enterocolitica* and *Yersinia pseudotuberculosis*. *In*: Doyle, M.P., ed. *Foodborne Bacterial Pathogens*. New York: Marcel Dekker; 1989.

Shayegani, M., W.B. Stone, I. DeForge, *et al. Yersinia enterocolitica* and related species isolated from wildlife in New York State. *Appl Environ Microbiol* 52:420–424, 1986.

Skavlen, P.A., H.F. Stills, E.K. Steffan, C.C. Middleton. Naturally ocurring *Yersinia enterocolitica* septicemia in patas monkeys (*Erythrocebus patas*). *Lab Anim Sci* 35:488–490, 1985.

Swaminathan, B., M.C. Harmon, I.J. Mehlman. *Yersinia enterocolitica*. *J Appl Bacteriol* 52:151–183, 1982.

Tacket, C.O., J.P. Narain, R. Sattin, J.P. Lofgren, C. Konigsberg, R.C. Rendtorff, *et al.* A multistate outbreak of infections caused by *Yersinia enterocolitica* transmitted by pasteurized milk. *J Am Med Assoc* 251:483–486, 1984.

Taylor, D.J. Infection with *Yersinia*. *In*: Leman, A.D., B.E. Straw, W.L. Mengeling, S. D'Allaire, D.J. Taylor, eds. *Diseases of Swine*. 7th ed. Ames: Iowa State University Press; 1992.

Thompson, J.S., M.J. Gravel. Family outbreak of gastroenteritis due to *Yersinia enterocolitica* serotype O:3 from well water. *Can J Microbiol* 32:700–701, 1986.

Trimnell, A.R., A.A. Adesiyun. Characteristics of the first isolate of *Yersinia enterocolitica* serogroup O:8 from a dog in Nigeria. *Isr J Vet Med* 44:244–247, 1988.

United States of America, Department of Health and Human Services, Centers for Disease Control and Prevention (CDC). Update: *Yersinia enterocolitica* bacteremia and endotoxin shock associated with red blood cell transfusions—United States, 1991. *MMWR Morb Mortal Wkly Rep* 40(11):176–178, 1991.

WHO Scientific Working Group. Enteric infections due to *Campylobacter, Yersinia, Salmonella,* and *Shigella*. *Bull World Health Organ* 58:519–537, 1980.

Wooley, R.E., E.B. Shotts, J.W. McConnell. Isolation of *Yersinia enterocolitica* from selected animal species. *Am J Vet Res* 41:1667–1668, 1980.

Zamora, J., O. Alonso, E. Chahuán. Isolement et caracterisation de *Yersinia enterocolitica* chez les rongeurs sauvages du Chili. *Zentralbl Veterinarmed [B]* 26:392–396, 1979.

ENTEROCOLITIS DUE TO *CLOSTRIDIUM DIFFICILE*

ICD-10 A04.7

Synonyms: Pseudomembranous enterocolitis, antibiotic-associated diarrhea, hemorrhagic necrotizing enterocolitis.

Etiology: *Clostridium difficile* is an anaerobic, gram-positive bacillus 3–16 microns long and 0.5–1.9 microns in diameter that forms oval, subterminal spores.

Some strains produce chains of two to six cells. *C. difficile* is generally motile in broth cultures.

C. difficile produces two types of toxins: enterotoxin A and cytotoxin B. Toxin A is lethal to hamsters when administered orally. Toxin B is cytotoxic for cultured cells of all types. A picogram of toxin B is enough to produce the cytotoxic effect (Cato *et al.*, 1986). Not all strains produce toxins. Another virulence factor is a substance that affects intestinal motility.

Various subclassification schemes have been devised for a better understanding of the pathogenicity of *C. difficile* as well as for epidemiological purposes. One of them is based on electrophoretic patterns of proteins on the cellular surface due to the different protein profiles produced by SDS-PAGE (polyacrylamide gel electrophoresis with sodium dodecyl sulphate), staining and autoradiography of radiomarked proteins. This method has made it possible to distinguish 15 types of *C. difficile* (Tabaqchali, 1990). In addition, 15 serogroups were distinguished using the plate serotyping system. Six of these serogroups proved to be cytotoxigenic. The cultures were isolated from patients who had pseudomembranous colitis or antibiotic-associated diarrhea (Toma *et al.*, 1988).

Geographic Distribution: Probably worldwide. The agent has been isolated from several sources, such as soil; marine sediment; and fecal matter from dogs, cats, cattle, camels, horses and other animals; as well as from people without diarrhea (Cato *et al.*, 1986). The number of animals and environmental samples (non-nosocomial) studied to determine *C. difficile* carriage was very limited (Levett, 1986).

Occurrence in Man: The disease appears sporadically and in nosocomial outbreaks. Most cases of pseudomembranous colitis are nosocomial infections (Lyerly *et al.*, 1988). It is estimated that more than 90% of pseudomembranous colitis cases are due to *C. difficile* and that about 20% of diarrhea cases are associated with antibiotics.

Occurrence in Animals: Outbreaks of enterocolitis have occurred in horses, rabbits, hamsters, guinea pigs, and dogs.

In Australia, a study was done of dogs and cats treated in two veterinary clinics. *C. difficile* was successfully cultured in 32 of 81 fecal samples (39.5%). Of the 29 animals that received antibiotics, 15 (52%) tested positive in cultures for *C. difficile*. There was no difference in carriage rate between dogs and cats. The environment of both clinics was also surveyed for contamination. In one clinic, 15 of 20 sites were contaminated; in the other, 6 of 14 sites were contaminated. There were both cytotoxigenic and noncytotoxigenic isolates. Fifty percent of the animal isolates and 71.4% of the environmental isolates were not cytotoxigenic. Both dogs and cats may be potential reservoirs (Riley *et al.*, 1991).

The Disease in Man: *C. difficile* produces pseudomembranous colitis or antibiotic-associated diarrhea in man. The clinical symptoms range from watery diarrhea, with varying degrees of abdominal pain, to pseudomembranous hemorrhagic necrotizing colitis. Infections outside the intestine caused by *C. difficile* are less important and occur less frequently. Abscesses, wound infections, pleurisy, and other organic effects have been described. Arthritis may also occur as a complication of acute colitis caused by *C. difficile* (Limonta *et al.*, 1989).

Forty to fifty percent of infants have a high load of *C. difficile* in their intestines, with a high rate of A and B toxins; despite this, they do not become ill. There is no satisfactory explanation for this phenomenon yet (Lyerly *et al.*, 1988). Children who suffer from other diseases or have undergone surgery are at risk of developing pseudomembranous colitis (Adler *et al.*, 1981). In contrast, *C. difficile* is part of the normal flora in a very small percentage (approximately 3%) of adults (Limonta *et al.*, 1989).

Pseudomembranous colitis was described in the late 1800s, but its importance was established in the 1970s with the use of antibiotics against anaerobes. Pseudomembranous colitis emerged as reports began to appear on the death of patients treated with clindamycin, a derivative of lincomycin that had proven effective against serious anaerobe infections. Diarrhea had already been observed in patients treated with lincomycin, but with the new antibiotic a severe inflammation of the mucosa of the colon with pseudomembranes occurred as well. The mortality rate among patients treated sometimes reached 10%, but was generally less (Lyerle *et al.*, 1988). It was soon seen that other antibiotics, such as ampicillin and cephalosporins, could cause enterocolitis as well (George, 1984). In essence, antibiotics altered the normal flora of the intestine, disturbing the balance among the different bacterial species and allowing *C. difficile* to multiply.

The first step in treatment should be to stop treatment with the antibiotic that may have caused the disease. The most common treatment is with vancomycin, which is not absorbed in the intestine and can reach high concentrations. The patient recovers rapidly. Metronidazole, which is less expensive and widely used in Europe, is also effective. It should be kept in mind that vancomycin and metronidazole may, in turn, cause the disease if their concentration in the colon is below an inhibitory level (Lyerly *et al.*, 1988). Relapses occur in approximately 20% of the patients treated. One study compared the efficacy of vancomycin and teicoplanin. Clinical cure was achieved in 100% of 20 patients treated with vancomycin; 96.2% of 25 patients treated with teicoplanin were cured. After treatment, five (25%) of those treated with vancomycin and two (7.7%) of those treated with teicoplanin were carriers of *C. difficile* (de Lalla *et al.*, 1992).

The Disease in Animals: The difference between the disease in humans and animals lies in the different sites affected. While the disease appears primarily as enterocolitis in man, in animals the disease may be cecitis or ileocecitis. Typhlocolitis also occurs.

In the state of Missouri (USA), an outbreak of colitis associated with the possibly accidental contamination of feed by lincomycin was described. Seven horses developed diarrhea. Autopsy of a stallion revealed that the cecum was black and contained some 20–30 L of a serosanguineous fluid; the abdominal cavity contained some 5 L of a clear liquid. Two other outbreaks affecting 15 horses occurred in the same state (Raisbeck *et al.*, 1981).

An outbreak of diarrhea in colts 2 to 5 days old occurred in Colorado (USA). *C. difficile* was isolated from the feces of 27 of 43 neonates with diarrhea (63%) and the cytotoxin was detected in the feces of 65% of the animals. *C. difficile* could not be isolated from healthy foals and adults. This outbreak was not associated with antimicrobial treatment. One foal that died had hemorrhagic necrotizing enteritis; an abundant culture was obtained from the contents of the small intestine (Jones *et al.*,

1987). Hemorrhagic necrotizing enteritis in neonate foals is usually caused by other clostridia, such as *C. perfringens* types B and C, and *C. sordelli*. Some cases may be due to *C. difficile*. *C. difficile* was isolated from four foals that died at three ranches, and the presence of the cytotoxin was also confirmed (Jones *et al.*, 1988). A case of typhlocolitis was also described in an adult horse (Perrin *et al.*, 1993). Traub-Dargatz and Jones (1993) recently reviewed the literature on the disease in horses.

Chronic diarrhea due to *C. difficile* was described in dogs; it was successfully treated with metronidazole (Berry and Levett, 1986).

A rabbit breeder observed green, watery diarrhea in approximately 25% of his 130 animals. Upon autopsy, lesions (of varying intensity) were found only in the cecum. The total loss was 40 rabbits. A study confirmed that the feed was contaminated by a food meant for swine, to which lincomycin had been added (permitted only in feed for pigs and fowl). The situation returned to normal when the feed was changed (Thilsted *et al.*, 1981).

Hamsters (*Mesocricetus auratus*) are very susceptible to *C. difficile* and are used as model animals. Proliferative ileitis is seen in young animals; in adult hamsters, the disease is characterized by chronic typhlocolitis with hyperplasia of the mucosa (Rehg and Lu, 1982; Chang and Rohwer, 1991; Ryden *et al.*, 1991).

Outbreaks of typhlitis not induced by antibiotics also occur in guinea pigs. An outbreak occurred in a colony of 400 female specific-pathogen free guinea pigs, maintained gnotobiologically with mice; 123 animals became ill, died, or were sacrificed. The disease was attributed to deficient intestinal flora (Boot *et al.*, 1989).

Source of Infection and Mode of Transmission: Diarrhea due to *C. difficile* occurs in both man and animals absent any association with antibiotics. However, the use of antibiotics and the resulting imbalance in the normal intestinal flora is a predominant factor inducing pseudomembranous enteritis or diarrhea varying from slight to profuse and hemorrhagic. The implicated antibiotics are, in particular, clindamycin and lincomycin, but other antimicrobials may also be responsible (ampicillin and cephalosporins). An intraperitoneal injection of ampicillin given to mice increased the rate of *C. difficile* fecal isolates from 19.4% to 63.6% (Itoh *et al.*, 1986).

The main reservoir of *C. difficile* seems to be infants in the first months of life. The carriage and excretion of cytotoxigenic strains in diarrheal dogs may also be an additional zoonotic source of infection (Berry and Levett, 1986; Weber *et al.*, 1989; Riley *et al.*, 1991).

Another aspect to consider is that *C. difficile* forms spores that are resistant to environmental factors. Environmental contamination by *C. difficile* plays an important role in the epidemiology of the disease, in both hamsters and man. *C. difficile* was isolated from 31.4% of the environmental samples from a hospital ward (Kaatz *et al.*, 1988). Studies conducted with epidemiological markers demonstrate cross infection between nosocomial patients and hospital acquisition of the infection, as well as a direct relationship between symptoms and the type of *C. difficile* (Tabaqchali, 1990). A recent study on nosocomial transmission is illustrative in this regard. Rectal swabs taken from 49 chronic-care patients in a geriatric hospital confirmed the presence of *C. difficile* in 10 of them (20.4%). A prospective study took samples from 100 consecutive patients admitted to an acute care ward in the same hospital, upon admission and every two weeks thereafter. Two patients (2%) were positive upon admission and 12 of the initial 98 negatives became colonized by *C. difficile*, representing a 12.2% nosocomial acquisition rate. The length of hospitalization was the most important determinant in colonization (Rudensky *et al.*, 1993).

Role of Animals in the Epidemiology of the Disease: Animals play a limited role in the transmission of the infection.

Diagnosis: Clinical diagnosis of pseudomembranous enterocolitis can be obtained through endoscopy to detect the presence of pseudomembranes or microabscesses in the colon of diarrheal patients with *C. difficile* toxins in their feces (Lyerly *et al.*, 1988).

Laboratory diagnosis consists of culturing the patient's feces in CCFA medium (cycloserine cefoxitin fructose egg yolk agar), which is a selective and differential medium. Patients generally have an elevated number (10^7 or more) of *C. difficile* in their feces (Bartlett *et al.*, 1980). The medium can be improved by substituting sodium taurocholate for egg yolk.

Since not all strains are toxigenic, detection of the toxin in the feces confirms the diagnosis. One of the assays used most often is tissue culture, which is extremely sensitive: it can detect a picogram of toxin B (cytotoxin). The mouse lethality test can also be used. Currently, a commercially available system containing a monolayer of preputial fibroblasts in a 96-well microdilution plate is used (Allen and Baron, 1991).

Prevention: Avoid abuse of antibiotics. This factor is particularly acute in the developing countries, where antibiotics can often be obtained without a prescription.

Hypochlorite solutions have been recommended for disinfection of surfaces in hospital settings (Kaatz *et al.*, 1988); glutaraldehyde-based disinfectants have been recommended for instruments, particularly endoscopes (Rutala *et al.*, 1993).

Bibliography

Adler, S.P., T. Chandrika, W.F. Berman. *Clostridium difficile* associated with pseudomembranous colitis. Occurrence in a 12 week-old infant without prior antibiotic therapy. *Am J Dis Child* 135:820–822, 1981.

Allen, S.D., E.J. Baron. *Clostridium*. *In*: Ballows, A., W.J. Hausler, K.L. Hermann, H.D. Isenberg, H.J. Shadomy, eds. *Manual of Clinical Microbiology*. 5th ed. Washington, D.C.: American Society for Microbiology; 1991.

Bartlett, J.G., N.S. Taylor, T. Chang, J. Dzink. Clinical and laboratory observations in *Clostridium difficile* colitis. *Am J Clin Nutr* 33:2521–2526, 1980.

Berry, A.P., P.N. Levett. Chronic diarrhoea in dogs associated with *Clostridium difficile*. *Vet Rec* 118:102–103, 1986.

Boot, R., A.F. Angulo, H.C. Walvoort. *Clostridium difficile*-associated typhlitis in specific pathogen free guineapigs in the absence of antimicrobial treatment. *Lab Anim* 23:203–207, 1989.

Cato, E.P., W.L. George, S.M. Finegold. Genus *Clostridium* Prazmowski 1880. *In*: Sneath, P.H.A., N.S. Mair, M.E. Sharpe, J.G. Holt. Vol 2: *Bergey's Manual of Systemic Bacteriology*. Baltimore: Williams & Wilkins; 1986.

Chang, J., R.G. Rohwer. *Clostridium difficile* infection in adult hamsters. *Lab Anim Sci* 41:548–552, 1991.

de Lalla, F., R. Nicolin, E. Rinaldi, *et al.* Prospective study of oral teicoplanin versus oral vancomycin for therapy of pseudomembranous colitis and *Clostridium difficile*-associated diarrhea. *Antimicrob Agents Chemother* 36:2192–2196, 1992.

George, W.L. Antimicrobial agent-associated colitis and diarrhea: Historical background and clinical aspects. *Rev Infect Dis* 6(Suppl 1):S208–S213, 1984.

Itoh, K., W.K. Lee, H. Kawamura, *et al.* Isolation of *Clostridium difficile* from various colonies of laboratory mice. *Lab Anim* 20:266–270, 1986.

Jones, R.L., W.S. Adney, A.F. Alexander, *et al.* Hemorrhagic necrotizing enterocolitis associated with *Clostridium difficile* infection in four foals. *J Am Vet Med Assoc* 193:76–79, 1988.

Jones, R.L., W.S. Adney, R.K. Shidaler. Isolation of *Clostridium difficile* and detection of cytotoxin in the feces of diarrheic foals in the absence of antimicrobial treatment. *J Clin Microbiol* 25:1225–1227, 1987.

Kaatz, G.W., S.D. Gitlin, D.R. Schaberg, *et al.* Acquisition of *Clostridium difficile* from the hospital environment. *Am J Epidemiol* 127:1289–1294, 1988.

Limonta, M., A. Arosio, D. Salvioni, A. De Carli. Due casi di artralgia associati ad infezione da *Clostridium difficile*. *Boll Ist Sieroter Milan* 68:142–144, 1989.

Levett, P.N. *Clostridium difficile* in habitats other than the human gastrointestinal tract. *J Infect* 12:253–263, 1986.

Lyerly, D.M., H.C. Krivan, T.D. Wilkins. *Clostridium difficile*: Its disease and toxins. *Clin Microbiol Rev* 1:1–18, 1988.

Perrin, J., I. Cosmetatos, A. Galluser, *et al. Clostridium difficile* associated with typhlocolitis in an adult horse. *J Vet Diagn Invest* 5:99–101, 1993.

Raisbeck, M.F., G.R. Holt, G.D. Osweiler. Lincomycin-associated colitis in horses. *J Am Vet Med Assoc* 179:362–363, 1981.

Rehg, J.E., Y.S. Lu. *Clostridium difficile* typhlitis in hamsters not associated with antibiotic therapy. *J Am Med Vet Assoc* 181:1422–1423, 1982.

Riley, T.V., J.E. Adams, G.L. O'Neill, R.A. Bowman. Gastrointestinal carriage of *Clostridium difficile* in cats and dogs attending veterinary clinics. *Epidemiol Infect* 107:659–665, 1991.

Rudensky, B., S. Rosner, M. Sonnenblick, *et al.* The prevalence and nosocomial acquisition of *Clostridium difficile* in elderly hospitalized patients. *Postgrad Med J* 69:45–47, 1993.

Rutala, W.A., M.F. Gergen, D.J. Weber. Inactivation of *Clostridium difficile* spores by disinfectants. *Infect Control Hosp Epidemiol* 14:36–39, 1993.

Ryden, E.B., N.S. Lipman, N.S. Taylor, *et al. Clostridium difficile* typhlitis associated with cecal mucosal hyperplasia in Syrian hamsters. *Lab Anim Sci* 41:553–558, 1991.

Tabaqchali, S. Epidemiologic markers of *Clostridium difficile*. *Rev Infect Dis* 12(Suppl 2):S192–S199, 1990.

Thilsted, J.P., W.M. Newton, R.A. Crandell, R.F. Bevill. Fatal diarrhea in rabbits resulting from the feeding of antibiotic-contaminated feed. *J Am Vet Med Assoc* 179:360–362, 1981.

Toma, S., G. Lesiak, M. Magus, *et al.* Serotyping of *Clostridium difficile*. *J Clin Microbiol* 26:426–428, 1988.

Traub-Dargatz, J.L., R.L. Jones. Clostridia-associated enterocolitis in adult horses and foals. *Vet Clin North Am Equine Pract* 9:411–421, 1993.

Weber, A., P. Kroth, G. Heil. Untersuchungen zum Vorkommen von *Clostridium difficile* in Kotproben von Hunden und Katzen. *Zentralbl Veterinarmed* 36:568–576, 1989.

FOOD POISONING CAUSED BY
VIBRIO PARAHAEMOLYTICUS

ICD-10 A05.3 foodborne *Vibrio parahaemolyticus* intoxication

Etiology: *Vibrio parahaemolyticus*, belonging to the family *Vibrionaceae*, is a gram-negative, motile, curved or straight bacillus that does not produce spores. It is a halophile that develops best in media with 2% to 3% sodium chloride but can multiply in an 8% concentration of this salt. In most cases, isolated strains are urease negative, but urease-positive strains are also found; this difference may serve as an epidemiological marker.

Based on O (somatic) and K (capsular) antigens, 20 O groups and 65 K serotypes are serologically distinguished. Most clinical strains can be typed, but environmental strains cannot.

Many clinical strains of *V. parahaemolyticus* cultured in Wagatsuma agar (which contains human red blood cells) are beta-hemolytic, while environmental isolates from water are not. This has been called the Kanagawa phenomenon or test. Given the difference in hemolytic capacity between clinical and environmental strains, it was assumed that hemolysin is a virulence factor. This toxin is called thermostable direct hemolysin (TDH). However, it has been demonstrated that TDH-negative strains can cause disease and produce an immunologically related toxin, thermostable related hemolysin (TRH), with very similar properties. The two hemolysins are coded by two different genes. In some strains, it was possible to find both hemolysins. Of 112 *V. parahaemolyticus* strains studied, 52.3% had the TDH gene alone, 24.3% had the TRH gene, and 11.2% had both genes (TDH and TRH). It can thus be stated that TDH and TRH are important factors in virulence (Shirai *et al.*, 1990). In addition, strains from diarrhea patients producing TRH were compared with environmental strains of *V. parahaemolyticus* (isolated from seawater or seafood) producing TRH. The results show that they were indistinguishable (Yoh *et al.*, 1992).

Pili are another important factor in intestinal colonization and thus in virulence. Various researchers have shown that pili attach to rabbit intestinal epithelium and that adhesive capacity is blocked by treating the vibrios with anti-pilus antibodies (Fab fraction). This does not produce an antihemolysin serum (Nakasone and Iwanaga, 1990 and 1992; Chakrabarti *et al.*, 1991).

Geographic Distribution: *V. parahaemolyticus* has been isolated from sea and estuary waters on all continents. The agent's distribution shows marked seasonal variations in natural reservoirs. During cold months, it is found in marine sediment; during warm months, it is found in coastal waters, fish, and shellfish (Benenson, 1990). There have been a few reports of the isolation of *V. parahaemolyticus* from continental waters and fish in rivers or lakes. It is assumed that these waters had a high concentration of sodium chloride, which would allow the agent to survive (Twedt, 1989). The factors that determine the abundance of the bacteria include water temperature, salinity, and plankton, among other factors.

The countries most affected by the disease are Japan, Taiwan, and other Asian coastal regions, though cases of disease have been described in many countries and on many continents.

Occurrence in Man: Food poisoning caused by this agent occurs sporadically or in outbreaks. Much of the knowledge about this disease is due to researchers in Japan, where the disease was first described in 1953. Subsequent studies showed that during the summer months, 50% to 70% of food poisoning cases and outbreaks were caused by *V. parahaemolyticus* (Snydman and Gorbach, 1991).

It is difficult to estimate the number of sporadic cases that occur. Many of those who fall ill do not see a doctor, and if they do, diagnosis is limited to a clinical examination without laboratory confirmation. Outbreaks can affect few or many people. During an outbreak that occurred in 1978, two-thirds of the 1,700 people who attended a dinner in Port Allen, Louisiana (USA) fell ill. The source of the outbreak was probably undercooked shrimp (CDC, 1978). The attack rate of people exposed during outbreaks in the US varied from 24% to 86% and the number of those affected ranged from 6 to 600. In the four years between 1983 and 1986, there was an outbreak that affected two people (Snydman and Gorbach, 1991).

Another outbreak that affected several hundred people occurred in the Bahamas in 1991. At the most critical point in the outbreak, 348 cases were treated in a hospital on the island. The outbreak was attributed to a gastropod (*Strombus gigas*), commonly called "conch," that the population usually eats raw or partially cooked. Kanagawa-positive *V. parahaemolyticus* was isolated from 5 of 14 patients' stool samples; two positive cultures were also isolated from eight conch samples. Although the number of cultures was limited, it is thought that *V. parahaemolyticus* was the causative agent of the diarrheal disease, which during the entire course of the outbreak affected more than 800 people, most of them adults.

In British Columbia (Canada), *V. parahaemolyticus* cultures were isolated from 13 patients as well as from 221 environmental samples; 23% and 1.4%, respectively, were Kanagawa positive. The cases of infection contracted locally were urease positive and Kanagawa negative; the patients who were infected during a trip abroad were urease negative and Kanagawa positive. Eight percent of the environmental samples were also urease positive and Kanagawa negative. These results suggest that the hemolysin identified by the Kanagawa test is not the only hemolysin involved in the pathogenesis of the infection (Kelly and Stroh, 1989. Also see the section on etiology).

In Recife, in northeastern Brazil, in 8 (38%) of 21 fecal samples from adult patients with gastroenteritis, cultures were also isolated that were urease positive and Kanagawa negative (Magalhães *et al.*, 1991b). Also in Recife, *V. parahaemolyticus* was isolated from 14 (1.3%) of 1,100 diarrheal fecal samples. If only adult samples are taken into account, the isolation rate would be 7.1%. It was also possible to show that the cultures belonged to seven different K antigen serovars (Magalhães *et al.*, 1991a).

Occurrence in Animals: *V. parahaemolyticus* is frequently isolated from fish, mollusks, and crustaceans in coastal waters, throughout the year in tropical climates and during the summer months in cold or temperate climates.

The Disease in Man: The incubation period is from 12 to 24 hours, but may vary from 6 to more than 90 hours. The most prominent symptom is watery diarrhea, which becomes bloody in some cases, as has been seen in Bangladesh, the US, and India. The other common symptoms are abdominal pains, nausea, vomiting, cephalalgia, and sometimes fever and chills (Twedt, 1989).

The disease is usually mild and lasts from one to seven days, but there have been fatal cases (Klontz, 1990). Some extraintestinal cases have occurred, such as infection of wounds, ears, and eyes, and there have also been isolates from blood. In some of these latter cases, there is doubt as to whether they were caused by *V. parahaemolyticus* or other halogenous *Vibrios*. Sautter *et al.* (1988) described the case of a foot wound infected by Kanagawa-negative *V. parahaemolyticus*. A hospital employee suffered a superficial abrasion and a small bruise on the ankle and traveled the following day to the eastern coast of the US. The abrasion began to ulcerate, edema and erythema formed around the ulcer, and the area became painful. By the sixth day, the erythema had grown to 18 cm and a 4 cm ulcer appeared. The patient was treated with dicloxacillin for 14 days. After two days of treatment, the ulcer began to leak a serosanguineous fluid, from which *V. parahaemolyticus* was isolated. Treatment was completed, the patient recovered, and the cultures were negative.

Generally no treatment other than rehydration is required for food poisoning caused by *V. parahaemolyticus*. The use of antibiotics should be reserved for prolonged or severe cases.

The Disease in Animals: *V. parahaemolyticus* causes only an inapparent contamination or infection in fish, mollusks, and crustaceans.

Source and Mode of Transmission: The major reservoir is seawater. Fish, mollusks, and crustaceans acquire the infection from seawater. When humans eat them raw or insufficiently cooked, they act as a source of infection. Humans need a load of 10^5–10^7 of *V. parahaemolyticus* to become infected (Twedt, 1989).

Recently caught fish have a *V. parahaemolyticus* load of only 1,000 per gram or less and recently harvested mollusks have a load of some 1,100 per gram; i.e., a load lower than that needed to infect humans (Twedt, 1989). It is thus assumed that the higher load is caused by handling of these seafoods, permitting multiplication of *V. parahaemolyticus* in the food. *V. parahaemolyticus* reproduces in a very short time (approximately 12 minutes) and exposure of the food to room temperature for a few hours is enough to allow the bacterial load to produce poisoning in man.

A very important factor in the epidemiology of the disease in many countries is the custom of eating raw seafood. Japan is one of the countries with the most outbreaks of food poisoning caused by *V. parahaemolyticus* because raw fish, shellfish, and crustaceans are consumed there. In the US, the most common source of poisoning is the consumption of raw oysters and even some uncooked or undercooked crustaceans.

Carrier status lasts for a few days and there are no known cases of secondary infection.

Role of Animals: The role is indirect and transmission is through food. The only vertebrates involved in the chain of transmission to man are fish, along with mollusks and crustaceans.

Diagnosis: A diarrheal disease occurring during the warm months and in association with the ingestion of seafood should lead one to suspect the possibility of food poisoning caused by *V. parahaemolyticus*. Certain diagnosis is obtained through isolation and characterization of the etiologic agent.

The medium most often used for culturing feces is thiosulfate citrate bile salts sucrose (TCBS) agar. The colonies in this medium take on a green or bluish color, with a darker green center. As a pre-enrichment medium, water with 1% peptone and 3% salt can be used. Wagatsuma medium is used to determine whether the culture is Kanagawa-positive or negative.

Prevention: The main recommendation is to cook shellfish, crustaceans, and fish at a sufficiently high temperature (15 minutes at 70°C) to destroy *V. parahaemolyticus*, with particular attention to the volume of the seafood in order to achieve the appropriate temperature.

However, the well-established custom in some countries of eating raw seafood makes it very difficult to enforce the recommendation to inactivate *V. parahaemolyticus* in fish, crustaceans, and mollusks by sufficiently cooking these foods.

An experiment conducted to study the increase of hemolysin in comparison with the bacterial count reached the conclusion that the toxin appears when *V. parahaemolyticus* reaches the level of 10^6 per gram and continues to increase with multiplication of the microbe. At 35°C it reached 32 units of hemolysin per gram after 24 hours; at 25°C it reached this level after 48 hours. Once formed, hemolysin is quite stable. Hemolysin showed its maximum heat resistance at a pH of between 5.5 and 6.5. The Kanagawa hemolysin in shrimp homogenate proved to be stable for 17 days when kept at 4°C; at temperatures between 115°C and 180°C, it took between 48.1 and 10.4 minutes for thermal inactivation as demonstrated in rats (Bradshaw *et al.*, 1984).

The results of this and other experiments indicate that from the outset it is necessary to prevent the load of *V. parahaemolyticus* in seafood as much as possible. A contra-indicated practice is washing fish or other seafood in contaminated estuarine water. Cold storage is recommended as soon as possible after cooking. Table surfaces where these products are processed should be waterproof and must be completely cleaned with fresh water (without salt) as there may be cross contamination, particularly from salted foods.

Bibliography

Benenson, A.S., ed. *Control of Communicable Diseases in Man.* 15th ed. An official report of the American Public Health Association. Washington, D.C.: American Public Health Association; 1990.

Bradshaw, J.G., D.B. Shah, A.J. Wehby, *et al.* Thermal inactivation of the Kanagawa hemolysin of *Vibrio parahaemolyticus* in buffer and shrimp. *J Food Sci* 49:183–187, 1984.

Chakrabarti, M.K., A.K. Sinha, T. Biswas. Adherence of *Vibrio parahaemolyticus* to rabbit intestinal epithelial cells *in vitro*. *FEMS Microbiol Lett* 68:113–117, 1991.

Doyle, M.P. Pathogenic *Escherichia coli, Yersinia enterocolitica*, and *Vibrio parahaemolyticus*. *Lancet* 336(8723):1111–1115, 1990.

Kelly, M.T., E.M. Stroh. Urease-positive, Kanagawa-negative *Vibrio parahaemolyticus* from patients and the environment in the Pacific Northwest. *J Clin Microbiol* 27:2820–2822, 1989.

Klontz, K.C. Fatalities associated with *Vibrio parahaemolyticus* and *Vibrio cholerae* non-O1 infections in Florida (1981 to 1988). *South Med J* 83:500–502, 1990.

Magalhães, V., R.A. Lima, S. Tateno, M. Malgahães. Gastroenterites humanas associadas a *Vibrio parahaemolyticus* no Recife, Brasil. *Rev Inst Med Trop Sao Paulo* 33:64–68, 1991a.

Magalhães, M., V. Malgahães, M.G. Antas, S. Tateno. Isolation of urease-positive *Vibrio parahaemolyticus* from diarrheal patients in northeast Brasil. *Rev Inst Med Trop Sao Paulo* 33:263–265, 1991b.

Nakasone, N., M. Iwanaga. Pili of a *Vibrio parahaemolyticus* strain as a possible colonization factor. *Infect Immun* 58:61–69, 1990.

Nakasone, N., M. Iwanaga. The role of pili in colonization of the rabbit intestine by *Vibrio parahaemolyticus* Na2. *Microbiol Immunol* 36:123–130, 1992.

Sautter, R.L., J.S. Taylor, J.D. Oliver, C. O'Donnell. *Vibrio parahaemolyticus* (Kanagawa-negative) wound infection in a hospital dietary employee. *Diagn Microbiol Infect Dis* 9:41–45, 1988.

Shirai, H., H. Ito, T. Hirayama, *et al.* Molecular epidemiologic evidence for association of thermostable direct hemolysin (TDH) and TDH-related hemolysin of *Vibrio parahaemolyticus* with gastroenteritis. *Infect Immun* 58:3568–3573, 1990.

Snydman, D.R., S.L. Gorbach. Bacterial food poisoning. *In*: Evans, A.S., P.S. Brachman, eds. *Bacterial Infections of Humans.* 2nd ed. New York: Plenum Medical Book Co.; 1991.

Spriggs, D.R., R.B. Sack. From the National Institute of Allergy and Infectious Diseases. Summary of the 25th United States-Japan Joint Conference on Cholera and Related Diarrheal Diseases. *J Infect Dis* 162:584–590, 1990.

Twedt, R.M. *Vibrio parahaemolyticus. In*: Doyle, M., ed. *Foodborne Bacterial Pathogens.* New York: Marcel Dekker; 1989.

United States of America, Department of Health and Human Services, Centers for Disease Control and Prevention (CDC). *Vibrio parahaemolyticus* foodborne outbreak—Louisiana. *MMWR Morb Mortal Wkly Rep* 27:345–346, 1978.

Yoh, M., T. Miwatani, T. Honda. Comparison of *Vibrio parahaemolyticus* hemolysin (Vp-TRH) produced by environmental and clinical isolates. *FEMS Microbiol Lett* 71:157–161, 1992.

GLANDERS

ICD-10 A24.0

Synonyms: Farcy, cutaneous glanders, equine nasal phthisis, maliasmus.

Etiology: *Pseudomonas* (*Malleomyces, Actinobacillus*) *mallei*, a nonmotile, gram-negative bacillus that is not very resistant to environmental conditions; this is the only nonmotile species in the genus *Pseudomonas*.

Geographic Distribution: At one time, the disease was distributed worldwide. It was eradicated in Europe and the Americas, but foci reappeared in 1965 in Greece, Romania, and Brazil (FAO/WHO/OIE, 1972). The present distribution is not well known, but there are indications that it persists in some African and Asian countries; Mongolia is or was the area of greatest incidence. According to official country reports to the Food and Agriculture Organization of the United Nations (FAO), the International Office of Epizootics (OIE), and the World Health Organization (WHO), no government currently reports cases of glanders. Isolated suspected cases were noted in Mongolia and diagnostic tests were being conducted. No cases have been reported since 1991 in India and since 1987 in Iraq (FAO/WHO/OIE, 1992).

Occurrence in Man: At present, the disease in man is exceptional, if it occurs at all. Attenuated strains of *P. mallei* are found in Asia, where the infection is assumed to persist.

Occurrence in Animals: According to various sources, incidence in solipeds is now low or nonexistent in Myanmar (Burma), China, India, Indonesia, Vietnam, and Thailand, and the disease is seen only occasionally. Cases used to occur sporadically in Pakistan and rarely in Iran. In June 1982, 826 foci with 1,808 cases were reported in solipeds in Turkey and in 1984, 274 foci were reported (OIE, 1982, 1984). The incidence in Mongolia is believed to have been high. The present situation in Ethiopia and the Central African Republic is not known, but cases have occurred in these countries in recent years. The most recent information available is from the "Geographic Distribution" section of the *Animal Health Yearbook* (FAO/WHO/OIE, 1993). Based on the reports obtained, it would seem that the disease is becoming extinct.

In endemic areas, the incidence of infection was higher during the rainy season.

The Disease in Man: The incubation period is usually from 1 to 14 days. Cases of latent infection that became clinically evident after many years have been described. The disease course may be either acute or chronic. In addition, subclinical infections have been discovered during autopsy.

In man as well as in animals, *P. mallei* tends to localize in the lungs, nasal mucosa, larynx, and trachea. The infection is manifested clinically as pneumonia, bronchopneumonia, or lobar pneumonia, with or without bacteremia. Pulmonary abscesses, pleural effusion, and empyema may occur. In the acute forms, there is mucopurulent discharge from the nose, and in the chronic forms, granulomatous nodular lesions are found in the lungs.

Ulcers appear in the mucosa of the nostrils and may also be found in the pharynx. Cellulitis with vesiculation, ulceration, lymphangitis, and lymphadenopathy is seen on the skin at the etiologic agent's point of entry. Mortality in clinical cases is high.

The Disease in Animals: Glanders is primarily a disease of solipeds. The disease course is predominantly chronic in horses and is almost always acute in asses and mules. The acute form results in high fever, depression, dyspnea, diarrhea, and rapid weight loss. The animal dies in a few weeks. The chronic form may last years; some animals recover, others die.

Chronic glanders is characterized by three clinical forms, occurring alone or simultaneously: pulmonary glanders, upper respiratory tract disease, and cutaneous glanders.

Pulmonary glanders can remain inapparent for lengthy periods. When clinical symptoms do occur, they consist of intermittent fever, cough, depression, and weight loss. In more advanced stages, there is dyspnea with rales. Pulmonary lesions usually consist of nodules or pneumonic foci. The nodules are grayish white with red borders; in time, the center becomes caseous or soft, or undergoes calcification and becomes surrounded by grayish granulated or whitish fibrous tissue.

The upper respiratory disease is characterized by ulcerations of the mucosa (necrosis of the nodules is the initial lesion) of one or both nostrils and, frequently, of the larynx and trachea. The ulcers have a grayish center with thick, jagged borders. There is a mucous or mucopurulent discharge from one or both nostrils that forms dark scabs around them.

Figure 11. Glanders. Mode of transmission.

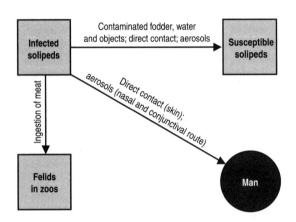

The cutaneous form (farcy) begins with superficial or deep nodules; these later become ulcers that have a gray center and excrete a thick, oily liquid that encrusts the hair. The lymph vessels form visible cords, and the lymph nodes are swollen.

Most authors consider upper respiratory glanders and cutaneous glanders to be secondary forms of pulmonary glanders.

In zoos and circuses, carnivores have contracted glanders as a consequence of eating meat from infected solipeds. The dog is another accidental host.

Source of Infection and Mode of Transmission (Figure 11): Man contracts the infection through contact with sick solipeds, especially those kept in crowded conditions, such as army stables. The portals of entry are the skin and the nasal and ocular mucosa. Nasal discharges, skin ulcer secretions, and contaminated objects constitute the source of infection.

Solipeds acquire the infection from conspecifics, mainly via the digestive route, but probably also through inhalation and wound infection.

Role of Animals in the Epidemiology of the Disease: The reservoir of *P. mallei* is solipeds. The great epizootics of glanders have occurred in metropolitan stables, especially during wartime. Horses with chronic or latent infection are responsible for maintaining the disease in an establishment or region, and their movement from one place to another contributes to its spread. Man and carnivores are accidental hosts.

Diagnosis: Diagnosis of glanders is based on: (a) bacteriologic examinations by means of culture or inoculation into hamsters of nasal or skin secretions or tissue from internal organs, especially the lungs; (b) allergenic tests with mallein (the intrapalpebral test is preferred); and (c) serologic tests, especially complement fixation. Although this last test is considered specific, false positives have occurred.

Control: Prevention in humans consists primarily of eradication of the infection in solipeds. Greatly improved diagnostic methods have made successful eradication campaigns possible, as have the disapperance of stables from cities and the almost complete substitution of automobiles for horses. Eradication procedures consist of identification of infected animals with allergenic or serologic tests, and sacrifice of reactors. Installations and equipment must then be disinfected.

Bibliography

Blood, D.C., J.A. Henderson. *Veterinary Medicine.* 4th ed. Baltimore: Williams & Wilkins; 1974.

Bruner, D.W., J.H. Gillespie. *Hagan's Infectious Diseases of Domestic Animals.* 6th ed. Ithaca: Comstock; 1973.

Cluff, L.E. Diseases caused by *Malleomyces. In:* Beeson, P., B.W. McDermott, J.B. Wyngaarden, eds. *Cecil Textbook of Medicine.* 15th ed. Philadelphia: Saunders; 1979.

Food and Agriculture Organization of the United Nations (FAO)/World Health Organization (WHO)/International Office of Epizootics (OIE). *Animal Health Yearbook, 1971.* Rome: FAO; 1972.

Food and Agriculture Organization of the United Nations (FAO)/World Health Organization (WHO)/International Office of Epizootics (OIE). *Animal Health Yearbook, 1984.* Rome: FAO; 1985.

Food and Agriculture Organization of the United Nations (FAO)/World Health Organization (WHO)/International Office of Epizootics (OIE). *Animal Health Yearbook, 1992.* Rome: FAO; 1993. (FAO Production and Animal Health Series 32).

Hagebock, J.M., L.K. Schlater, W.M. Frerichs, D.P. Olson. Serologic responses to the mallein test for glanders in solipeds. *J Vet Diagn Invest* 5:97–99, 1993.

Hipólito, O., M.L.G. Freitas, J.B. Figueiredo. *Doenças Infeto-Contagiosas dos Animais Domésticos.* 4th ed. São Paulo: Melhoramentos; 1965.

International Office of Epizootics (OIE). *Report on the Disease Status Worldwide in 1984. 53rd General Session.* Paris: IOE; 1985. (Document 53SG/2).

International Office of Epizootics (OIE). *Enfermedades animales señaladas a la OIE, estadísticas 1982.* Paris: OIE; 1982.

Langeneger, J., J. Dobereiner, A.C. Lima. Foco de mormo (Malleus) na região de Campos, Estado do Rio de Janeiro. *Arq Inst Biol Anim* 3:91–108, 1960.

Oudar, J., L. Dhennu, L. Joubert, A. Richard, J.C. Coutard, J.C. Proy, *et al.* A propos d'un récent foyer de morve du cheval en France. *Bull Soc Sci Vet Med Comp* 67:309–317, 1965.

Van der Schaaf, A. Malleus. *In:* Van der Hoeden, J., ed. *Zoonoses.* Amsterdam: Elsevier; 1964.

Van Goidsenhoven, C., F. Schoenaers. *Maladies Infectieuses des Animaux Domestiques.* Liège: Desoer; 1960.

INFECTION CAUSED BY *CAPNOCYTOPHAGA CANIMORSUS* AND *C. CYNODEGMI*

ICD-10 A28.8 other specified zoonotic bacterial diseases, not elsewhere classified; T14.1 open wound of unspecified body region

Synonyms: Infection caused by DF-2 and DF-2–like bacteria.

Etiology: Among the bacterial strains sent for identification to the US Centers for Disease Control and Prevention (CDC), there was a group that was named DF-2 (dysgonic fermenter-2). It consisted of small, gram-negative bacilli that grow slowly and with difficulty in common laboratory media. The first strain was received in 1961 and the first report on the human disease—a person bitten by two dogs—was published in 1976. Another group was named DF-2–like. These organisms were ultimately described according to the rules of nomenclature and bacterial classification.

There are two different species: *Capnocytophaga canimorsus* and *C. cynodegmi* (Brenner *et al.*, 1989). Both species consist of gram-negative bacilli 1 to 3 microns long that form filaments and are longer in blood agar. They do not have flagella, but do have gliding motility. They are microaerophilic and grow better in an atmosphere to which 5% to 10% carbon dioxide has been added. The best medium for their growth is heart infusion agar with 5% sheep or rabbit blood. They are oxidase- and catalase-positive, unlike CDC group DF-1 (*C. ochracea*, *C. gingivalis*, and *C. sputigena*), which is involved in dental processes and is not of zoonotic interest. *C. cynodegmi* differs from *C. canimorsus* in that it ferments raffinose, sucrose, and melibiose (Brenner *et al.*, 1989), and exhibits marked pathogenic differences.

Geographic Distribution: Worldwide, as are their reservoirs and sources of infection, cats and dogs. CDC received strains of *C. canimorsus* not only from the US, but also from Australia, Canada, Denmark, France, Great Britain, the Netherlands, New Zealand, South Africa, and Sweden.

Occurrence in Man: From 1961 to February of 1993, CDC received 200 cultures of *C. canimorsus* isolated from man (CDC, 1993). *C. canimorsus* occurs primarily in people who have had a splenectomy, alcoholics, and those with chronic pulmonary disease or a malignant blood disease. The disease may occur at any age, but people over age 50 predominated in a series of cases. In 77% of the cases, the disease was preceded by a dog bite or, less frequently, a cat bite, or some other exposure to these animals (a scratch, for example).

C. cynodegmi occurs in healthy individuals, without any preceding or concurrent disease.

Occurrence in Animals: *C. canimorsus* and *C. cynodegmi* have been isolated from the saliva of healthy dogs and cats, and thus are assumed to make up part of the normal flora in the mouths of these animals.

The Disease in Man: In infections caused by *C. canimorsus*, the spectrum of clinical manifestations varies from cellulitis that heals spontaneously to fatal septicemia. Serious cases are usually associated with people who have had a splenectomy or whose liver has been affected by alcoholism. This would indicate that *C. canimorsus* is opportunistic and not very virulent. However, a fatal case was described in Australia of a 66-year-old woman with septicemia who was hospitalized 48 hours after having been bitten by her dog. The patient presented with symptoms of septicemic shock, hemorrhagic eruption, and altered consciousness. She had no prior illness that could have predisposed her to this syndrome. She died 16 hours after being admitted, despite having received intravenous antibiotic treatment (Clarke *et al.*, 1992).

A similar case occurred in Belgium in a 47-year-old woman without any history of prior illness. She was admitted to the emergency room with septic shock five days after receiving a small lesion on the hand from her dog. *C. canimorsus* was isolated from her blood. Despite intensive treatment, she developed multiple organic deficiencies and died 27 days after being admitted (Hantson *et al.*, 1991).

The clinical picture includes meningitis, endocarditis, septic arthritis, gangrene, disseminated intravascular coagulation, and keratitis. The literature records a total of five cases of ophthalmic infections due to cat scratches or close exposure to this animal. There was also one case attributed to a dog (Paton *et al.*, 1988).

Capnocytophaga cynodegmi causes infection in wounds inflicted by dogs. It does not produce systemic infection.

C. canimorsus and *C. cynodegmi* are sensitive to various antibiotics, including penicillin, erythromycin, minocycline, and doxycycline. Penicillin G is usually preferred by doctors for wounds caused by dogs (Hicklin *et al.*, 1987). It should be kept in mind that 3% to 23% of the gram-negative bacteria isolated from the oropharynx of dogs may be resistant to penicillin (Hsu and Finberg, 1989).

The Disease in Animals: *C. canimorsus* and *C. cynodegmi* are normal components of the bacterial flora in the oropharynx of dogs, cats, sheep, and cattle. They are not pathogenic for these animal species.

Source of Infection and Mode of Transmission: The reservoir of the infection is dogs and cats. The source is the saliva of these animals and transmission is effected by a bite.

C. canimorsus was isolated from the nose and mouth of 4 out of 50 clinically normal dogs (8%). The agent was also isolated from dogs and cats whose bites caused infection in man (Bailie *et al.*, 1978; Chen and Fonseca, 1986; Martone *et al.*, 1980; Carpenter *et al.*, 1987). A broader study indicated that in a sample of 180 dogs, 24% were carriers of *C. canimorsus* and 11% were carriers of *C. cynodegmi*; in a sample of 249 cats, 17% carried *C. canimorsus* and 8% carried *C. cynodegmi* in their mouths. The agent was also isolated in a significant percentage of sheep and cattle (25% and 33%, respectively). In contrast, these agents could not be isolated from the normal flora of man (Westwell *et al.*, 1989).

C. canimorsus is primarily an opportunistic pathogen that infects individuals weakened by concurrent diseases. Those who have had a splenectomy comprise a high-risk group. Asplenic individuals suffer deficient IgM and IgG production and delayed macrophage mobilization. They also produce less tuftsin, a protein derived from IgG that stimulates phagocytosis (August, 1988). Liver disease caused by alcoholism is another predisposing factor for the infection. Predisposition is associated with susceptibility to bacteremia (Kanagasundaram and Levy, 1979).

Role of Animals in the Epidemiology of the Disease: This is a zoonosis in which dogs and, to a lesser extent, cats, play an essential role.

Diagnosis: *C. canimorsus* can be isolated from blood (see the culture medium and atmosphere indicated in the section on etiology). In asplenic patients, it is useful to make a gram-stained preparation of the leukocyte layer of the extracted blood sample. *C. cynodegmi* is isolated from wounds.

Prevention and Control: The treatment for any bite should first be thorough irrigation with water, then cleaning with soap and water. In the case of asplenic patients and alcoholics, it is advisable to administer antibiotics prophylactically. It is recommended that such people not own dogs or cats. However, not all authors agree with this recommendation.

Bibliography

August, J.R. Dysgonic fermenter-2 infections. *J Am Vet Med Assoc* 193:1506–1508, 1988.

Bailie, W.E., E.C. Stowe, A.M. Schmitt. Aerobic bacterial flora of oral and nasal fluids of canines with reference to bacteria associated with bites. *J Clin Microbiol* 7:223–231, 1978. Cited in: August, J.R. Dysgonic fermenter-2 infections. *J Am Vet Med Assoc* 193:1506–1508, 1988.

Brenner, D.J., D.G. Hollis, G.R. Fanning, R.E. Weaver. *Capnocytophaga canimorsus* sp. nov. (formerly CDC group DF-2), a cause of septicemia following dog bite, and *C. cynodegmi* sp. nov., a cause of localized wound infection following dog bite. *J Clin Microbiol* 27:231–235, 1989.

Carpenter, P.D., B.T. Heppner, J.W. Gnann. DF-2 bacteremia following cat bites. Report of two cases. *Am J Med* 82:621–623, 1987.

Chan, P.C., K. Fonseca. Septicemia and meningitis caused by dysgonic fermenter-2 (DF-2). *J Clin Pathol* 39:1021–1024, 1986.

Clarke, K., D. Devonshire, A. Veitch, *et al.* Dog-bite induced *Capnocytophaga canimorsus* septicemia. *Aust New Zealand J Med* 22:86–87, 1992.

Hantson, P., P.E. Gautier, M.C. Vekemans, *et al.* Fatal *Capnocytophaga canimorsus* septicemia in a previously healthy woman. *Ann Emerg Med* 20:93–94, 1991.

Hicklin, H., A. Verghese, S. Alvarez. Dysgonic fermenter 2 septicemia. *Rev Infect Dis* 9:884–890, 1987.

Hsu, H-W., R.W. Finberg. Infections associated with animal exposure in two infants. *Rev Infect Dis* 11:108–115, 1989.

Kanagasundaram, N., C.M. Levy. Immunologic aspects of liver disease. *Med Clin North Am* 63:631–642, 1979. Cited in: Hicklin, H., A. Verghese, S. Alvarez. Dysgonic fermenter 2 septicemia. *Rev Infect Dis* 9:884–890, 1987.

Martone, W.J., R.W. Zuehl, G.E. Minson, W.M. Scheld. Postsplenectomy sepsis with DF-2: Report of a case with isolation of the organism from the patient's dog. *Ann Intern Med* 93:457–458, 1980. Cited in: August, J.R. Dysgonic fermenter-2 infections. *J Am Vet Med Assoc* 193:1506–1508, 1988.

Paton, B.G., L.D. Ormerod, J. Peppe, K.R. Kenyon. Evidence for a feline reservoir of dysgonic fermenter 2 keratitis. *J Clin Microbiol* 26:2439–2440, 1988.

United States of America, Department of Health and Human Services, Centers for Disease Control and Prevention (CDC). *Capnocytophaga canimorsus* sepsis misdiagnosed as plague—New Mexico, 1992. *MMWR Morb Mortal Wkly Rep* 42:72–73, 1993.

Westwell, A.J., K. Kerr, M.B. Spencer, *et al.* DF-2 infection. *Br Med J* 298:116–117, 1989.

LEPROSY

ICD-10 A30.9 leprosy, unspecified

Synonyms: Hansen's disease, hanseniasis.

Etiology: *Mycobacterium leprae*, a polymorphic acid-alcohol-fast bacillus that up to now has been impossible to culture in artificial laboratory media or in tissue cultures. *M. leprae* is difficult to distinguish from other unculturable mycobacteria naturally affecting animals.

The failure of attempts to culture *M. leprae in vitro* constitutes a great barrier to better determining its biochemical characteristics for identification purposes as well as for therapeutic and immunologic studies. In part, this difficulty has been overcome, first by *in vivo* culture on mouse footpads and later in nine-banded armadillos (*Dasypus novemcinctus*). At present, the latter serve as a model for lepromatous leprosy and provide a large number of bacilli for research.

In identification of *M. leprae*, the dopa (3,4-dihydroxyphenylalanine) oxidation test and extraction with pyridine are of value. Homogenate of human leproma (granulomatous nodule rich in *M. leprae* and characteristic of lepromatous leprosy) oxidizes dopa to indole. Extraction with pyridine eliminates the acid-fast quality of *M. leprae*, but not that of other mycobacteria.

In recent years, more precise identification of *M. leprae* has been achieved by structural analysis of its mycolic acids, analysis by immunodiffusion of its antigens, and interaction of leprosy bacilli with bacteriophages specific for mycobacteria (Rastogi *et al.*, 1982).

Occurrence in Man: Leprosy is endemic in 93 countries. Eighty percent of all recorded cases are concentrated in five countries: India, Brazil, Nigeria, Myanmar (Burma), and Indonesia (WHO, 1988). The highest prevalence is found in the tropical and subtropical regions of Asia, Africa, Latin America, and Oceania. Leprosy is very prevalent in India, Southeast Asia, the Philippines, Korea, southern China, Papua New Guinea, and some Pacific islands. Ninety percent of the cases reported in Latin America come from five countries: Argentina, Brazil, Colombia, Mexico, and Venezuela (Brubaker, 1983). Chile is the only South American country free of the infection. In the United States, most cases occur among immigrants. Autochthonous cases arise in Hawaii, Puerto Rico, Texas, and Louisiana. The infection's prevalence is related to the population's socioeconomic level. The fact that the disease has practically disappeared in Europe is attributed to the improved standard of living there.

There are differences in the regional or racial prevalence of tuberculoid and lepromatous leprosy. Ninety percent of the cases in endemic areas of Africa and 80% of the cases in India are of the tuberculoid type. The lepromatous form represents 30% to 50% of cases among the white population or in some Asian countries such as Japan, China, and Korea (Bechelli *et al.*, 1972).

In countries with efficient control programs, it was expected that prevalence would fall by 60% to 80% by the year 2000. Of the cases reported worldwide, 49.1% were under multidrug treatment in 1990 (Noorden, 1990). The cumulative rate of coverage with polychemotherapy has reached 82%. Each year 1.4 million patients are freed from the disease (WHO, 1993).

Occurrence in Animals: Natural infection has been found in nine-banded armadillos (*Dasypus novemcinctus*) in Louisiana and Texas (USA) and in Mexico. By 1983, the infection had been observed in some 100 armadillos captured in Louisiana (Meyers *et al.*, 1983). Depending on their place of origin, between 4% and 29.6% of 1,033 armadillos examined were infected. On the Gulf Coast of Texas, leprosy lesions were found in 4.66% of 451 armadillos captured (Smith *et al.*, 1983). The disease form found in these animals was a lepromatous leprosy identical to the type produced by experimental inoculation with material from humans. On the other hand, the search for naturally infected armadillos carried out by other researchers in Louisiana, Texas, and Florida, as well as in Colombia and Paraguay, produced negative results (Kirchheimer, 1979).

At present, natural infection of nine-banded armadillos is a well-established fact. Its distribution is limited to some states in the US and Mexico. In Mexico, 1 of 96 armadillos was positive based on histopathology and mouse footpad inoculation (Amezcua *et al.*, 1984). In a study of armadillos found dead on the highways of Louisiana, 10 of 494 (2%) were positive based on histopathology and pyridine extraction (Job *et al.*, 1986a). The infection was also confirmed in an armadillo at the San Diego Zoo, California, and in another armadillo at the Centers for Disease Control and Prevention. The two armadillos originally came from Texas (Walsh *et al.*, 1981).

The ELISA method was adopted for serological study of leprosy in armadillos using phenolic glycolipid (PGL-1) antigen (Truman *et al.*, 1986), which is considered specific for *M. leprae* (Young and Buchanan, 1983). This test was conducted on armadillos captured in central Louisiana before being used in the laboratory (1960–1964). It was found that 17 of the 182 sera (9.3%) were serologically positive. This study was undertaken to refute the argument that free armadillos could have become infected by experimental armadillos through carelessness. The sera were collected at that time for a study on leptospirosis. Of 20 armadillos captured shortly before this study, four were positive.

Another study used ELISA and histopathological tests to examine 77 armadillos in an estimated population of 254 ± 60 animals in a defined area of Louisiana. Five of 67 (1.5%) sera tested with ELISA and 1 of 74 (1.3%) ears submitted for histopathological examination were positive (Stallknecht *et al.*, 1987).

On the Texas Gulf Coast, the presence of leprosy in armadillos was demonstrated (Smith *et al.*, 1983). More recently, 237 armadillo ears from 51 central Texas districts were examined; no positives were found upon histological examination (Clark *et al.*, 1987). A similar negative result was obtained for 853 ears from armadillos killed on the highways or captured for research purposes in five southeastern US states. The examination included microscopic and histopathological examination (Howerth *et al.*, 1990). An infected animal had previously been found in the state of Mississippi (Walsh *et al.*, 1986).

A spontaneous case of leprosy similar to the borderline or dimorphous form was described in a chimpanzee imported from Sierra Leone to the United States. Clinical and histopathologic characteristics (with invasion of dermal nerves by the agent) were identical to those of the human disease. Attempts to culture the bacteria were negative, and the chimpanzee did not respond to tuberculin or lepromin, just as humans infected with lepromatous or dimorphous leprosy give a negative reaction. As with *M. leprae* of human origin, experimental inoculation of rats with the isolated bacillus produced neither disease nor lesions. The only differences with *M. leprae* of human origin were negative results to the dopa oxidation and pyridine tests. However, the dopa oxidation test sometimes fails in animals (armadillos) inoculated experimentally with human *M. leprae* (Donham and Leininger, 1977). Results obtained by inoculating mouse foot pads were similar to those derived with *M. leprae* of human origin, i.e., reproduction of the bacterium in six months up to a quantity similar to that of *M. leprae* without dissemination from the inoculation point (Leininger *et al.*, 1978).

Another case of naturally acquired leprosy was discovered in a primate, *Cercocebus atys* or sooty mangabey monkey (identified in one publication as *Cercocebus torquatus atys*), captured in West Africa and imported to the United States in 1975 (Meyers *et al.*, 1980, 1981). The clinical picture and histopathology were similar to man's and the etiologic agent was identified as *M. leprae* based on the following criteria: invasion of the host's nerves, staining properties, electron microscopy findings, inability to grow in mycobacteriologic media, positive dopa oxidation reaction, reactivity to lepromin, patterns of infection in mice and armadillos, sensitivity to sulfones, and DNA homology (Meyers *et al.*, 1985). Simultaneous intravenous and intracutaneous inoculation succeeded in reproducing the infection and disease in other *Cercocebus* monkeys. The early appearance of signs (5 to 14 months), varying clinical disease forms, neuropathic deformities, bacillemia, and dissemination to various cool parts of the body make the mangabey monkey potentially the most complete model for the study of leprosy. It is the third animal species reported to be able to acquire leprosy by natural infection (Walsh *et al.*, 1981; Meyers *et al.*, 1983, 1985).

The Disease in Man: The incubation period is usually 3 to 5 years, but it can vary from 6 months to 10 years or more (Bullock, 1982). Clinical forms of leprosy cover a wide spectrum, ranking from mild self-healing lesions to a progressive and destructive chronic disease. Tuberculoid leprosy is found at one end of the spectrum and lepromatous leprosy at the other. Between them are found the intermediate forms.

Tuberculoid leprosy is characterized by often asymptomatic localized lesions of the skin and nerves. Basically, the lesion consists of a granulomatous, paucibacillary, inflammatory process. The bacilli are difficult to detect, and can be observed most frequently in the nerve endings of the skin. This form results from active destruction of the bacilli by the undeteriorated cellular immunity of the patient. On the other hand, the humoral response generally involves low titers. Nerve destruction causes lowered conduction; heat sensibility is the most affected, tactile sensibility less so. Trophic and autonomic changes are common, especially ulcers on the sole and mutilation of limbs (Toro-González *et al.*, 1983).

Lepromatous leprosy is characterized by numerous symmetrical skin lesions consisting of macules and diffuse infiltrations, plaques, and nodules of varying sizes (lepromas). There is involvement of the mucosa of the upper respiratory tract, of lymph nodes, liver, spleen, and testicles. Infiltrates are basically histiocytes with a few lymphocytes. Cellular immunity is absent (negative reaction to lepromin) and antibody titers are high. In this form of the disease, as in the dimorphous, erythema nodosum leprosum (ENL) often appears.

The indeterminate form of leprosy has still not been adequately defined from the clinical standpoint; it is considered to be the initial state of the disease. The first cutaneous lesions are flat, hypopigmented, and have ill-defined borders. If this initial form is not treated, it may develop into tuberculoid, dimorphous, or lepromatous leprosy. Bacilli are few and it is difficult to confirm their presence.

Finally, the dimorphous or borderline form occupies an intermediate position between the two polar forms (tuberculoid and lepromatous), and shares properties of both; it is unstable and may progress in either direction. Destruction of nerve trunks may be extensive. Bacilli are observed in scrapings taken from skin lesions.

A study group (WHO, 1985) has, primarily for practical treatment purposes, defined two types of the disease.

"a) *Paucibacillary*: This includes the categories described as indeterminate (I) and tuberculoid (T) leprosy in the Madrid classification, and the indeterminate (I), polar tuberculoid (TT) and borderline tuberculoid (BT) categories in the Ridley and Jopling classification, whether diagnosed clinically or histopathologically with a bacterial index of <2 according to the Ridley scale at all sites.

b) *Multibacillary*: This includes lepromatous (L) and borderline (B) leprosy in the Madrid classification and lepromatous (LL) and borderline lepromatous (BL) leprosy in the Ridley and Jopling classification, whether diagnosed clinically or histopathologically, with a bacterial index of ≥2 according to the Ridley scale at any site."

An estimated one-third of clinical cases become incapacitated, half of them completely. Nevertheless, these proportions are now changing, due to both prevention/control programs and early implementation of effective treatments.

There is evidence that inapparent infection may occur with a certain frequency among persons, especially family members, in contact with patients.

The Disease in Animals: The disease in armadillos (*Dasypus novemcinctus*) is similar to the lepromatous form in man. Infection in these animlas is characterized by macrophage infiltrates containing a large number of bacilli. Skin lesions range from mild to severe. The small dermal nerves are invaded by the etiologic agent. Many bacilli are seen in the macrophages of the lymph tissue, in the pulp of the spleen, and in Kupffer's cells in the liver.

M. leprae is known to prefer the coolest parts of the human or mouse body. For this reason, armadillos began to be used as experimental animals even before natural infection had been confirmed in these animals, since body temperature in nine-banded armadillos is between 30°C to 35°C. Experimental inoculation of armadillos with human leproma material reproduces the disease, characterized by broad dissemination of the agent, and involvement of the lymph glands, liver, spleen, lungs, bone marrow, meninges, and other tissues, in a more intense form than is usually observed in man (Kirchheimer *et al.*, 1972).

The disease in the chimpanzee appeared as a progressive, chronic dermatitis with nodular thickening of the skin on the ears, eyebrows, nose, and lips. Lesions of the nose, skin, and dermal nerves contained copious quantities of acid-fast bacteria (Donham and Leininger, 1977). The disease was histopathologically classified as dimorphous or borderline 12 months after the clinical symptoms were first observed, and as lepromatous in a subsequent biopsy (Leininger *et al.*, 1978).

In the case of the *Cercocebus* monkey, the initial lesion consisted of nodules on the face. Four months later, a massive infiltration and ulceration were seen on the face, and nodules on the ears and forearms. Sixteen months after cutaneous lesions were first observed, the animal began to suffer deformities and paralysis of the extremities. Histopathologic findings indicated the subpolar or intermediate lepromatous form, according to the Ridley and Jopling classification. The disease was progressive, with neuropathic deformation of the feet and hands. It seemed to regress when specific treatment was administered. The animal apparently acquired the disease from a patient with active leprosy. Experimental infections carried out to date have indicated that these animals may experience a spectrum of different forms similar to those seen in man (Meyers *et al.*, 1985).

Source of Infection and Mode of Transmission: Man is the principal reservoir of *M. leprae*. The method of transmission is still not well known due to the extended incubation period. Nevertheless, the principal source of infection is believed to be lepromatous patients, in whom the infection is multibacillary, skin lesions are often ulcerous, and a great number of bacilli are shed through the nose; similarly, bacilli are found in the mouth and pharynx. Consequently, transmission might be brought about by contact with infected skin, especially if there are abrasions or wounds. Currently, particular importance is attributed to aerosol transmission. Nasal secretions from lepromatous patients contain approximately 100 million bacilli per milliliter. In addition, *M. leprae* can survive for about seven days in dried secretions. Another possible route of transmission is mother's milk, which contains a large number of bacilli in lepromatous patients (Bullock, 1990). Oral transmission and transmission by hematophagous arthropods are not discounted, but they are assigned less epidemiological importance.

Until recently, leprosy was believed to be an exclusively human disease. However, research in recent years has demonstrated that the infection and the disease also occur naturally in wild animals. Although some researchers (Kirchheimer, 1979) have expressed doubt that the animal infection is identical to the human, the accumulated evidence indicates that the etiologic agent is the same. The criteria (Binford *et al.*, 1982) used to identify the bacillus in animals as *M. leprae* were as follows: (1) selective invasion of the peripheral nerves by bacilli, since the only *Mycobacterium* known to date to invade the nerves is *M. leprae*, (2) failure to grow on common laboratory media for mycobacteria, (3) positive pyridine test to eliminate acid-fastness, (4) positive dopa test, (5) characteristic multiplication in mouse foot pads and in armadillos, and (6) reactivity of lepromin prepared with animal bacilli compared to that of standard lepromin.

The origin of the infection in animals is unknown. Some authors believe that armadillos contracted the infection from a human source, perhaps from multibacillary patients before the era of sulfones. In this regard, it should be pointed out that leprosy bacilli may remain viable for a week in dried nasal secretions and that armadillos are in close contact with the soil. The high prevalence in some localities would also indicate that armadillos can transmit the disease to each other, either by inhalation or direct contact. Another possible transmission vehicle is maternal milk, in which the agent has been detected (Walsh *et al.*, 1981). It has also been suggested that transmission among armadillos may be brought about by thorns penetrating the ears, nose, or other body parts (Job *et al.*, 1986b), as apparently armadillos use places with spiny plants to hide from their predators. These authors have found thorns in the ears of 25.5% of 494 armadillos captured in Louisiana, and in the nose of 36.6% of them.

It is difficult to demonstrate that armadillos are a source of infection for man because of the long incubation period and the impossibility of excluding a human source in an endemic area. In Texas, a case of human leprosy was attributed to a patient's practice of capturing armadillos and eating their meat (Freiberger and Fudenberg, 1981). Subsequently, another five cases with hand lesions were detected in natives of the same state who habitually hunted and cleaned armadillos but had no known contact with leprosy patients (Lumpkin III et al., 1983). To determine if there was a significant association between contact with armadillos and human leprosy in Louisiana, a group of 19 patients was compared with another group of 19 healthy individuals from the same area. Of those with leprosy, four had had contact with armadillos, as opposed to five in the control group. Consequently, it was concluded that such an association did not exist (Filice et al., 1977). However, this conclusion was questioned, since the only valid comparison would be between persons who have handled armadillos and those who have had no contact with them (Lumpkin III et al., 1983).

The prevalence of leprosy in armadillos in Louisiana and Texas suggests that these animals could serve as a reservoir of *M. leprae*. However, nothing is known about the frequency of infection in nonhuman primates and the role they may play in transmission of the disease. The sources of the cases of leprosy in these animals were probably people with lepromatous leprosy.

Diagnosis: Clinically, an anesthetic or hypoesthetic cutaneous lesion raises suspicion of leprosy, even more so if the nerves are enlarged. Diagnosis is confirmed by biopsy of the skin lesion, which also permits classification of the form of the leprosy. For patients with lepromatous or borderline lepromatous leprosy, diagnosis can be made by using the Ziehl-Neelsen staining technique on a film of nasal mucosa scrapings or the interphase between erythrocytes and leukocytes from a centrifuged blood sample. Histopathologic preparations do not stain well using Ziehl-Neelsen and consequently a Fite-Faraco stain is recommended. Also used is the simplified staining method consisting of eliminating acid-fastness with pyridine in order to differentiate *M. leprae* (Convit and Pinardi, 1972). In tuberculoid and other paucibacillary forms of leprosy, it is difficult and at times impossible to confirm the presence of the etiologic agent; in any case, examination of many histologic sections is recommended in order to detect any bacteria present, especially in the nerve endings.

Skin tests have no diagnostic value, but they do serve as an aid to prognosis. Patients with tuberculoid leprosy or other paucibacillary forms react positively to the intradermal lepromin or Mitsuda test (with dead *M. leprae* bacilli and a reading after 28 days), since their cellular immunity is generally not affected. In contrast, lepromatous leprosy and other multibacillary forms give negative results to the Mitsuda test. The lepromin test has limited value for detecting infection in those in contact with patients or the general population in an endemic area (Jacobson, 1991). Serological tests are also of limited use.

The ELISA technique (Young and Buchanan, 1983) for measuring PGL-1 (phenolic glycolipid antigen) antibodies is a great step forward. The reactive titer depends on the patient's bacillary load and also serves to detect infection in those who are in contact with multibacillary patients, as well as in some people in endemic areas (Jacobson, 1991). In Malawi, Africa, where most cases are paucibacillary, the test was not sufficiently sensitive (unless its specificity were to be sacrificed), but it was used to detect a high percentage of multibacillary patients (Burgess *et al.*, 1988). A variation of this test is the use of the synthetic disaccharide epitope of PGL-1 as an antigen (Brett *et al.*, 1986).

Control: Control is based on early detection and chemotherapy. Given the multiple confirmed cases of resistance to dapsone, combination of this medication with rifampicin is presently recommended for paucibacillary leprosy, and the same two medications in combination with clofazimine are recommended for multibacillary leprosy. Rifampicin has a rapid bactericidal effect and eliminates contagion in patients in one to two weeks. To achieve the objective of eliminating leprosy, all patients should receive polychemotherapy. This treatment has been successful in reducing general prevalence from 5.4 million in 1986 to 3.7 million in 1990. Widespread testing began in 1992 on a new oral treatment that was developed over the preceding five years and combines two antibiotics, rifampicin and ofloxacin. Ofloxacin inhibits an enzyme that controls the way that DNA coils inside the bacterium. It is hoped that this combination will be able to cure leprosy in the course of one month. If testing is successful, all patients should have access to this medication (WHO, 1992). The isolation of patients in leprosariums is no longer necessary, since medication is effective in suppressing infectiousness and thus interrupts transmission of the disease.

Bibliography

Amezcua, M.E., A. Escobar-Gutierrez, E.E. Storrs, *et al.* Wild Mexican armadillo with leprosy-like infection [letter]. *Int J Lepr Other Mycobact Dis* 52:254–255, 1984.

Bechelli, L.M., V. Martínez Domínguez. Further information on the leprosy problem in the world. *Bull World Health Organ* 46:523–536, 1972. Cited in: Bullock, W.E. *Mycobacterium leprae* (Leprosy). *In*: Mandell, G.L., R.G. Douglas, Jr., J.E. Bennett, eds. *Principles and Practice of Infectious Diseases*. 3rd ed. New York: Churchill Livingstone, Inc.; 1990.

Binford, C.H., W.M. Meyers, G.P. Walsh. Leprosy. *JAMA* 247:2283–2292, 1982.

Binford, C.H., W.M. Meyers, G.P. Walsh, E.E. Storrs, H.L. Brown. Naturally acquired leprosy-like disease in the nine-banded armadillo (*Dasypus novemcinctus*): Histopathologic and microbiologic studies of tissues. *J Reticuloendothel Soc* 22:377–388, 1977.

Brett, S.J., S.N. Payne, J. Gigg, *et al.* Use of synthetic glycoconjugates containing the *Mycobacterium leprae* specific and immunodominant epitope of phenolic glycolipid I in the serology of leprosy. *Clin Experim Immunol* 64:476–483, 1986.

Brubaker, M. Leprosy Control in the Americas. Part I: General Considerations. *In*: Bolivar's Bicentennial Seminar on Leprosy Control: Report: Caracas 12–14 September 1983. Pan American Health Organization, 1983. (PNSP/84–05).

Bullock, W.E. Leprosy (Hansen's disease). *In*: Wyngaarden, J.B., L.H. Smith, Jr., eds. *Cecil Textbook of Medicine*. 16th ed. Philadelphia: W.B. Saunders; 1982.

Bullock, W.E. *Mycobacterium leprae* (Leprosy). *In*: Mandell, G.L., R.G. Douglas, Jr., J.E. Bennett, eds. *Principles and Practice of Infectious Diseases*. 3rd ed. New York: Churchill Livingstone, Inc.; 1990.

Burgess, P.J., P.E. Fine, J.M. Ponnighaus, C. Draper. Serological tests in leprosy. The sensitivity, specificity and predictive value of ELISA tests based on phenolic glycolipid antigens, and the implications for their use in epidemiological studies. *Epidemiol Infect* 101:159–171, 1988.

Clark, K.A., S.H. Kim, L.F. Boening, *et al.* Leprosy in armadillos (*Dasypus novemcinctus*) from Texas. *J Wildl Dis* 220–224, 1987.

Convit, J., M.E. Pinardi. A simple method for the differentiation of *Mycobacterium leprae* from other mycobacteria through routine staining technics. *Int J Lepr Other Mycobact Dis* 40:130–132, 1972.

Donham, K.J., J.R. Leininger. Spontaneous leprosy-like disease in a chimpanzee. *J Infect Dis* 136:132–136, 1977.

Filice, G.A., R.N. Greenberg, D.W. Fraser. Lack of observed association between armadillo contact and leprosy in humans. *Am J Trop Med Hyg* 26:137–139, 1977.

Fine, P.E. Leprosy: The epidemiology of a slow bacterium. *Epidemiol Rev* 4:161–188, 1982.

Freiberger, H.F., H.H. Fudenberg. An appetite for armadillo. *Hosp Practice* 16:137–144, 1981.

Howerth, E.W., D.E. Stallknecht, W.R. Davidson, E.J. Wentworth. Survey for leprosy in nine-banded armadillos (*Dasypus novemcinctus*) from the southeastern United States. *J Wildl Dis* 26:112–115, 1990.

Jacobson, R.R. Leprosy. *In*: Evans, A.S., P.S. Brachman, eds. *Bacterial Infections of Humans*. 2nd ed. New York: Plenum; 1991.

Job, C.K., E.B. Harris, J.L. Allen, R.C. Hastings. A random survey of leprosy in wild nine-banded armadillos in Louisiana. *Int J Lepr Other Mycobact Dis* 54:453–457, 1986a.

Job, C.K., E.B. Harris, J.L. Allen, R.C. Hastings. Thorns in armadillo ears and noses and their role in the transmission of leprosy. *Arch Pathol Lab Med* 110:1025–1028, 1986b.

Job, C.K., R.M. Sánchez, R.C. Hastings. Manifestations of experimental leprosy in the armadillo. *Am J Trop Med Hyg* 34:151–161, 1985.

Kirchheimer, W.F. Leprosy (Hansen's Disease). *In*: Stoenner, H., W. Kaplan, M. Torten, eds. Vol I, Section A: *CRC Handbook Series in Zoonoses*. Boca Raton: CRC Press; 1979.

Kirchheimer, W.F., E.E. Storrs, C.H. Binford. Attempts to establish the armadillo (*Dasypus novemcinctus Linn*) as model for the study of leprosy. II. Histopathologic and bacteriologic post-mortem findings in lepromatoid leprosy in the armadillo. *Int J Lepr Other Mycobact Dis* 40:229–242, 1972.

Leininger, J.R., K.J. Donham, W.M. Meyers. Leprosy in a chimpanzee. Postmortem lesions. *Int J Lepr Other Mycobact Dis* 48:414–421, 1980.

Leininger, J.R., K.J. Donham, M.J. Rubino. Leprosy in a chimpanzee. Morphology of the skin lesions and characterization of the organism. *Vet Pathol* 15:339–346, 1978.

Lumpkin III, L.R., G.F. Cox, J.E. Wolf, Jr. Leprosy in five armadillo handlers. *J Am Acad Dermatol* 9:899–903, 1983.

Martin, L.N., B.J. Gormus, R.H. Wolf, G.P. Walsh, W.M. Meyers, C.H. Binford, *et al.* Experimental leprosy in nonhuman primates. *Adv Vet Sci Comp Med* 28:201–236, 1984.

Meyers, W.M., G.P. Walsh, C.H. Binford, H.L. Brown, R.H. Wolf, B.J. Gormus, *et al.* Multibacillar leprosy in unaltered hosts, with emphasis on armadillos and monkeys [abstract]. *Int J Lepr Other Mycobact Dis* 50:584–585, 1982.

Meyers, W.M., G.P. Walsh, C.H. Binford, R.H. Wolf, B.J. Gormus, L.N. Martin, *et al.* Models of multibacillary leprosy in unaltered hosts: Current Status. *In*: Bolivar's Bicentennial Seminar on Leprosy Control: Report: Caracas 12–14 September 1983. Pan American Health Organization, 1983. (PNSP/84–05).

Meyers, W.M., G.P. Walsh, H.L. Brown, C.H. Binford, P.J. Gerone, R.H. Wolf, *et al.* Leprosy in a mangabey monkey (*Cercocebus torquatus atys* "sooty" mangabey) [abstract]. *Int J Lepr Other Mycobact Dis* 49:500–502, 1981.

Meyers, W.M., G.P. Walsh, H.L. Brown, C.H. Binford, G.D. Imes, Jr., T.L. Hadfield, *et al.* Leprosy in a mangabey monkey—naturally acquired infection. *Int J Lepr Other Mycobct Dis* 53:1–14, 1985.

Meyers, W.M., G.P. Walsh, H.L. Brown, Y. Fukunishi, C.H. Binford, P.J. Gerone, *et al.* Naturally-acquired leprosy in a mangabey monkey (*Cercocebus* spp.) [summary]. *Int J Lepr Other Mycobact Dis* 48:495–496, 1980.

Noorden, S.K. Multidrug therapy (MDT) and leprosy control. *Indian J Lepr* 62:448–458, 1990.

Rastogi, N., C. Frehel, A. Ryter, H.L. David. Comparative ultrastructure of *Mycobacterium leprae* and *M. avium* grown in experimental hosts. *Ann Microbiol* 133:109–128, 1982.

Smith, J.H., D.S. Folse, E.G. Long, J.D. Christie, D.T. Crouse, M.E. Tewes, *et al.* Leprosy in wild armadillos (*Dasypus novemcinctus*) of the Texas Gulf Coast: Epidemiology and mycobacteriology. *J Reticuloendothel Soc* 34:75–88, 1983.

Stallknecht, D.E., R.W. Truman, M.E. Hugh-Jones, C.K. Job. Surveillance for naturally acquired leprosy in a nine-banded armadillo population. *J Wildl Dis* 23:308–310, 1987.

Toro-González, G., G. Román-Campos, L. Navarro de Román. *Leprosy: neurología tropical.* Bogotá: Printer Colombiana; 1983.

Truman, R.W., E.J. Shannon, H.V. Hagstad, *et al.* Evaluation of the origin of *Mycobacterium leprae* infections in the wild armadillo, *Dasypus novemcinctus. Am J Trop Med Hyg* 35:588–593, 1986.

Walsh, G.P., W.M. Meyers, C.H. Binford. Naturally acquired leprosy in the nine-banded armadillo: A decade of experience 1975–1985. *J Leukoc Biol* 40:645–656, 1986. Cited in: Howerth, E.W., D.E. Stallknecht, W.R. Davidson, E.J. Wentworth. Survey for leprosy in nine-banded armadillos (*Dasypus novemcinctus*) from the southeastern United States. *J Wildl Dis* 26:112–115, 1990.

Walsh, G.P., W.M. Meyers, C.H. Binford, P.J. Gerone, R.H. Wolf, J.R. Leininger. Leprosy— a zoonosis. *Lepr Rev* 52(Suppl.1):77–83, 1981.

Walsh, G.P., E.E. Storrs, W.M. Meyers, C.H. Binford. Naturally acquired leprosy-like disease in the nine-banded armadillo (*Dasypus novemcinctus*): Recent epizootiologic findings. *J Reticuloendothel Soc* 22:363–367, 1977.

World Health Organization (WHO). *Epidemiology of leprosy in relation to control. Report of a WHO Study Group.* Geneva: WHO, 1985. (Technical Report Series 716).

World Health Organization (WHO). *WHO Expert Committee on Leprosy, Sixth Report.* Geneva: WHO; 1988. (Technical Report Series 768).

World Health Organization (WHO). Trials begin of new treatment for leprosy—disease could be conquered [press release]. Geneva: WHO; 3 February 1992. (Press Release WHO 5).

World Health Organization (WHO). Progress towards the elimination of leprosy as a public health problem. *Wkly Epidemiol Rec* 68(25):181–186, 1993.

Young, D.B., T.M. Buchanan. A serological test for leprosy with a glycolipid specific for *Mycobacterium leprae. Science* 221:1057–1059, 1983.

LEPTOSPIROSIS

ICD-10 A27.0 leptospirosis icterohaemorrhagica;
A27.8 other forms of leptospirosis

Synonyms: Weil's disease, swineherd's disease, rice-field fever, cane-cutter's fever, swamp fever, mud fever, and other local names; Stuttgart disease, canicola fever (dogs).

Etiology: Leptospires are spiral-shaped bacteria, with open, hooked ends; they are motile, aerobic, and culturable, and they measure some 6 to 20 microns long by 0.1 microns in diameter. They can be seen under a dark-field microscope and pass through filters that block other bacteria. Two species are recognized: *Leptospira interrogans* and *L. biflexa*. *L. interrogans* is pathogenic for man and animals; *L. biflexa*, a free-living saprophyte found in surface waters, is seldom associated with infection in mammals.

The species of interest as a zoonotic agent is *L. interrogans*. It has more than 200 serologic variants, or serovars, which constitutes the basic taxon. Serovars are grouped for convenience into 23 serogroups (which is not a recognized taxon) on the basis of the predominant agglutinogenic components they share (Faine, 1982; Alexander, 1991). Through the use of ribosomal RNA gene restriction patterns, an attempt is being made to characterize *L. interrogans* serovars in order to establish the bases for molecular typing (Perolat *et al.*, 1990).

Geographic Distribution: Worldwide. There are universal serovars, such as *L. interrogans* serovar *icterohaemorrhagiae* and serovar *canicola*, and serovars that occur only in certain regions. Each region has characteristic serotypes, determined by its ecology. Leptospirosis has a high prevalence in tropical countries with heavy rainfall and neutral or alkaline soils.

Occurrence in Man: Incidence varies in different parts of the world. The disease may occur sporadically or in epidemic outbreaks. In general, outbreaks are caused by exposure to water contaminated by the urine of infected animals. Several occupational groups are particularly at risk, such as workers in rice fields, sugarcane plantations, mines, sewer systems, and slaughterhouses, as well as animal caretakers, veterinarians, and members of the military.

Occurrence in Animals: The infection is common in rodents and other wild and domestic mammals. Worldwide, the infection occurs in approximately 160 mammalian species (Alexander, 1991). Each serovar has its preferred animal host or hosts, but each animal species may be host to one or more serovars. Thus, for example, the serovar *pomona* has pigs and cattle as its principal hosts, but it may transitorily infect other host animals. Dogs are the principal reservoir of *canicola*, but it may occasionally be found in foxes, swine, and cattle.

The Disease in Man: Man is susceptible to a large number of serovars. The incubation period lasts from one to two weeks, although cases with an incubation period of only two days or more than three weeks are known. The disease is characterized by two phases, the bacteremic phase, lasting 7 to 10 days, and the leptospiruric phase, lasting from a week to several months. Clinical manifestations vary and have differing degrees of severity. In addition, numerous cases of infection occur inapparently or subclinically. In general, two clinical types are distinguished: icteric and anicteric. The serious icteric, or hepatonephritic, type (Weil's disease) is much less frequent than the anicteric type. Some authors estimate that this form occurs in approximately 10% of cases. It is often associated with infection caused by *icterohaemorrhagiae*, but this is not the only serovar that can produce it. On the other hand, numerous infections caused by *icterohaemorrhagiae* occur in anicteric form. In the classical form of Weil's disease, the onset of symptoms is sudden, with fever, headache, myalgias, conjunctivitis, nausea, vomiting, and diarrhea or constipation. Prostration may be severe. Petechiae on the skin, hemorrhages in the gastrointestinal tract, and proteinuria are common. Hepatomegaly and jaundice, renal insufficiency with marked oliguria or anuria, azotemia, and electrolyte imbalance develop with the disappearance of leptospiremia and fever. If the patient's condition improves, diuresis is reestablished and jaundice decreases. Convalescence lasts one or two months, during which time fever, cephalalgia, myalgias, and general malaise may reappear for a few days.

In anicteric cases, the symptomatology is milder. The symptoms during leptospiremia, which occurs during the first week of the disease, are fever, myalgias (particularly in the calves), conjunctivitis, stiffness in the neck, nausea, and sometimes vomiting. Often, the disease resembles influenza. The anicteric form has a benign course and patients recover in about a month. Leptospiruria may continue for a week or several months after the disappearance of clinical symptoms.

Treatment should be started early in order to prevent tissue lesions. Penicillin G and amoxicillin were effective as late as one week after the onset of the disease (Benenson, 1990).

The Disease in Animals

CATTLE: At least 13 serovars have been isolated from cattle. In the Americas, the predominant serovars in cattle are *pomona, hardjo,* and *grippotyphosa*; at times, infections caused by *canicola* and *icterohaemorrhagiae*, as well as by other serovars, are found. The serovars *pomona* and *hardjo* are universal. As laboratory methods have improved, outbreaks caused by the latter have been confirmed with increasing frequency. In recent years, serovars belonging to the Hebdomadis group have been isolated more frequently. The importance of infection caused by some serovars is difficult to interpret. This is true of the serotype *paidjan* (Bataviae serogroup), isolated from the kidneys of cattle (obtained in an Argentine slaughterhouse), and the serotype *galtoni* (Canicola serogroup), isolated in Argentina and Colombia (Szyfres *et al.*, 1967; Tedesco *et al.*, 1969). To date, there are no known outbreaks caused by these serotypes in Argentina.

The infection may cause an acute or subacute disease or remain clinically inapparent. The disease manifests with a fever lasting four or five days, anorexia, conjunctivitis, and diarrhea. Leptospiremia begins to disappear when antibodies form, and the leptospires completely disappear from the bloodstream in approximately one week due to humoral immunity. The surviving leptospires are then harbored in the convoluted tubules of the kidneys and the infection enters a chronic phase. Leptospiruria sheds enormous quantities of leptospires to the outside environment, particularly during the first months of infection; later this decreases or ceases entirely. Leptospiruria caused by *hardjo* is much more prolonged than that caused by *pomona*. The *hardjo* serovar (Sejroe serogroup) in cattle is characterized by two syndromes: (a) agalactia, or a significant reduction in milk production, and (b) abortions or birthing of weak calves that die soon after birth. In infections caused by *hardjo*—but not by *pomona*— it was found that leptospires can reside in the genital tract (uterus and oviducts) in both pregnant and nonpregnant females (Ellis and Thiermann, 1986). Infection of the genital tract may indicate the possibility of sexual transmission (Prescott, 1991). *L. interrogans* is subdivided into two genotypes: *hardjo* hardjo-bovis and *hardjo* hardjo-prajitno. The first genotype is the most prevalent in the US.

Infertility may be a sequela of the infection. Serious cases include jaundice. However, the most notable symptoms in a certain proportion of the animals are abortion and hemoglobinuria. Abortions usually occur between one and three weeks after the onset of the disease. Up to 20% of aborting animals retain the placenta.

Cattle of all ages are susceptible. The course of the disease is more severe in calves, which experience stunted growth and variable mortality rates.

Quick-spreading epizootics are characterized by a high morbidity rate. It is possible that rapid passage of the leptospires from one animal to another intensifies their virulence. In slow-moving epizootics, the rate of inapparent infection varies from one herd to another.

Treatment with high doses of penicillin G or tetracycline is recommended for acute leptospirosis. Dihydrostreptomycin (12.5 mg/kg of bodyweight twice a day) may also be used, but due to its potential toxicity, treatment should be suspended after three days. Another suggested treatment is intramuscular sodium ampicillin (20 mg/kg of bodyweight twice a day). In the chronic disease caused by *pomona*, it has been repeatedly shown that a single intramuscular injection of dihydrostreptomycin (25 mg/kg of bodyweight) eliminates the infection from the kidneys of most animals treated. However, this treatment fails in the case of infection caused by *hardjo*, although the number of leptospires is apparently reduced (Ellis *et al.*, 1985).

SWINE: The serovars most often isolated from swine in the Americas and in the rest of the world are *pomona, tarassovi, grippotyphosa, canicola*, and *icterohaemorrhagiae*, as well as *bratislava* and *muenchen* of the Australis serogroup.

Swine are a very important reservoir of *pomona*, with abundant and prolonged leptospiruria. The clinical infection varies from one herd to another. In some cases, infection occurs subclinically, although the animals may exhibit a fever lasting a few days; in others, the infection produces such symptoms as abortion and birth of weak piglets. Stunted growth of piglets, jaundice, hemoglobinuria, convulsions, and gastrointestinal disorders have also been seen. At times, meningitis and nervous symptomatology are present. Abortion usually occurs between 15 and 30 days after infection. The principal serovars that cause abortions or stillborn piglets are *pomona, tarassovi*, and *canicola*. Infection that occurs during the last third of pregnancy is the most critical in interrupting gestation. Leptospires of the serovars *bratislava* and *muenchen* localize in the kidneys and in the genital tract of swine, as do *hardjo* leptospires in cattle.

As in cattle, a single intramuscular injection of dihydrostreptomycin (25 mg/kg of bodyweight) is recommended for chronic infections caused by *pomona*.

HORSES: Horses react serologically to many serotypes prevalent in the environment. *Pomona* has been isolated from these animals in the United States, and *hardjo* has been isolated in Argentina. In Europe, *icterohaemorrhagiae, sejroe*, and *canicola* have been isolated, as well as *pomona*. Most infections are inapparent. There may be photophobia, watery eyes, edema of the ocular conjunctiva, miosis, and iritis in the acute phase of the disease. In the chronic phase, there may be anterior and posterior adhesions, a turbid vitreous body, formation of cataracts, uveitis, and other ophthalmologic abnormalities (Sillerud *et al.*, 1987). Abortions may occasionally occur in infected mares (Bernard *et al.*, 1993).

Corneal opacity, which is frequently a sequela of the acute phase, can be reproduced through inoculation of inactivated leptospires from various serovars. An antigen relationship has also been demonstrated between *L. interrogans*, crystallin, and the cornea (Parma *et al.*, 1986). Often, the disease's sequela (periodic ophthalmia) is recognized instead of the acute, febrile phase. The onset of periodic ophthalmia occurs when the febrile phase has disappeared, after a latent phase that sometimes lasts several months. Leptospires have been detected in eye lesions of affected animals, and a high concentration of antibodies can be found in the aqueous humor. However, it should be borne in mind that leptospirosis is not the only cause of periodic ophthalmia. One hundred horses from the Minnesota River valley (USA) were examined ophthalmologically and serologically. A statistically significant association was found between uveitis and serology positive for *pomona*. Not all the seropositive horses were affected by uveitis, possibly due to different levels of exposure, strains of varying virulence, or different routes of infection (Sillerud *et al.*, 1987). Serious cases of leptospirosis with hepatonephritic and cardiovascular syndromes have been described in Europe.

SHEEP AND GOATS: Epizootics in these species are not very frequent. Various serovars that appear to have come from other animal species in the same environment have been isolated from sheep and goats in different countries (Faine, 1982), for example, *hardjo* in Australia and New Zealand, *pomona* in the United States and New Zealand, *grippotyphosa* in Israel, and *ballum* in Argentina. In Western Australia (Australia), a persistent leptospirosis caused by the serovar *hardjo* was found in sheep that had no contact with cattle infected by the same serovar (Cousins *et al.*, 1989). The authors conclude that, in addition to cattle, sheep could be a maintenance host for *hardjo*.

As in other ruminant species, the disease is characterized by fever, anorexia, and, in some animals, by jaundice, hemoglobinuria, anemia, abortion, birth of weak or stillborn animals, and infertility. The virulence of the infecting serovar and the condition of the animal determine the severity of the clinical picture.

DOGS AND CATS: The predominant serovars in dogs throughout the world are *canicola* and *icterohaemorrhagiae*. In addition to these serovars, *pyrogenes, paidjan*, and *tarassovi* have been isolated in Latin America and the Caribbean, and *ballum*, *grippotyphosa, pomona*, and *bratislava* have been isolated in the United States (Nielsen *et al.*, 1991). Similar serovars predominate in Europe. The infection may range from asymptomatic to severe. The most serious form is the hemorrhagic, which begins suddenly with a fever that lasts from three to four days, followed by stiffness and myalgia in the hind legs, and hemorrhages in the oral cavity with a tendency toward necrosis and pharyngitis. In a subsequent stage, there may be hemorrhagic gastroenteritis and acute nephritis. Jaundice may occur with infection by *canicola* or by *icterohaemorrhagiae*, particularly in infection caused by the latter serovar. Case fatality is estimated at 10%.

The disease rarely occurs in cats.

WILD ANIMALS: Many wild animals, including rodents, are perfectly adapted to leptospires and show no symptoms or lesions.

Source of Infection and Mode of Transmission (Figure 12): After a week of leptospiremia, animals shed leptospires in their urine, contaminating the environment. The best reservoirs of the infection are animals that have prolonged leptospiruria and generally do not suffer from the disease themselves. For example, this is true of rats, which harbor *icterohaemorrhagiae* and rarely have lesions. The infection in man and animals is contracted directly or indirectly, through skin abrasions and the nasal, oral, and conjunctival mucosa. Indirect exposure through water, soil, or foods contaminated by urine from infected animals is the most common route. An

Figure 12. Leptospirosis. Synanthropic transmission cycle.

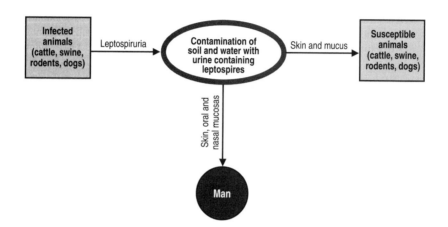

unusual case of transmission occurred in Great Britain, where an 11-year-old boy acquired the infection from a rat bite (Luzzi *et al.*, 1987).

People who work with livestock are often exposed to animal urine, directly or as an aerosol, which can contaminate the conjunctiva, nasal mucosa, or abrasions on exposed skin. They may also become infected indirectly by walking barefoot where animals have urinated. In many countries, domesticated animals, particularly swine and cattle, constitute important leptospire reservoirs and a frequent source of infection for man.

Rice-paddy workers are exposed to water contaminated by urine of rodents that infest the fields. Among agricultural workers, sugarcane harvesters are another high-risk group. Field mice nesting among crops are a source of infection for harvesters, particularly during the early morning hours, when workers' hands come into contact with dew mixed with urine.

Among pets, dogs are a common source of infection for man by serovars *canicola* and *icterohaemorrhagiae*.

Tropical regions are endemic areas of leptospirosis and the highest case rates correspond to areas with heavy rainfall. The highest number of cases occurs during the rainy season. Epidemic outbreaks erupt because of environmental changes, such as flooding, which cause rodents to move into cities. An example of this is the epidemics that occurred in the city of Recife (Pernambuco State, Brazil), in 1966 and 1970, with 181 and 102 cases, respectively. The predominant serovar was *icterohaemorrhagiae*. Humidity, high temperatures, and an abundance of rats were the principal factors that precipitated these outbreaks as well as others in tropical regions. Small epidemic outbreaks are also caused by recreational activities, such as swimming or diving in streams or ponds contaminated by the urine of infected animals. An outbreak occurred in a cattle- and swine-raising region of Cuba, where 21 cases were diagnosed in people who bathed in the Clavellina River and the Maniadero reservoir. The Pomona and Australis serogroups were predominant and two isolates of the latter were obtained from the river water (Suárez Hernández *et al.*, 1989). Epidemic outbreaks caused by several different serovars have occurred among soldiers wading in streams or camping by riverbanks during jungle maneuvers. Such epidemics have occurred in Panama and Malaysia; in these cases, the source of infection was the urine of infected wild animals.

Animals, either primary or secondary hosts, contract the infection in a similar way. The density of the host population and the environmental conditions in which it lives play important roles. On cattle ranches, the infection is usually introduced by a carrier animal with leptospiruria and, at times, by fields that flood with water contaminated at a neighboring establishment.

Pathogenic leptospires (*L. interrogans*) do not multiply outside the animal organism. Consequently, in addition to carrier animals, existence of a leptospirosis focus requires environmental conditions favorable to the survival of the agent in the exterior environment. Leptospires need high humidity, a neutral or slightly alkaline pH, and suitable temperatures. Low, inundated ground and artificial or natural freshwater receptacles (ponds, streams, reservoirs, etc.) are favorable to their survival, whereas salt water is deleterious. Soil composition, both its physiochemical and biological characteristics (microbe population), also acts to prolong or shorten life for leptospires in the environment. Temperatures in the tropics constitute a very favorable factor for survival of leptospires, but cases of leptospirosis may also occur in cold climates, although they are less frequent.

Role of Animals in the Epidemiology of the Disease: Wild and domesticated animals are essential for the maintenance of pathogenic leptospires in nature. Transmission of the infection from animals to man is effected directly or indirectly.

Human-to-human transmission is rare. Man is an accidental host and only in very special conditions can he contribute to the maintenance of an epidemic outbreak. Such was the case in an epidemic described in the forest northeast of Hanoi (Vietnam). The outbreak occurred among soldiers occupied in logging and transport of logs by buffalo through a swampy area. Leptospiruria was observed in 12% of 66 convalescent soldiers. In contrast, the rate of infection was insignificant among buffalo and rodents in the region. The pH of the surface water was neutral, the workers worked barefoot, and their urine had a pH that fluctuated around seven (their diet was vegetarian). Leptospiruria persisted in some of the soldiers for more than six months (Spinu *et al.*, 1963).

A case of transmission through mother's milk was described in the US (Songer and Thiermann, 1988). A female veterinarian continued nursing after being infected with the serovar *hardjo* while performing an autopsy on a cow. Twenty-one days after the appearance of clinical symptoms in the mother, the baby became ill with fever, anorexia, irritability, and lethargy. The serovar *hardjo* was isolated from the baby's urine and the baby recovered with antibiotic treatment.

Various cases of congenital infection have also been described (Faine, 1991).

Diagnosis: In man, the etiologic agent can be isolated from blood during the first week of the disease; afterwards, it can be isolated from the urine, either by direct culture or by inoculation into young hamsters. Repeated blood samples are necessary for serological examination. The patient has no antibodies during the first week; they appear in six to seven days and reach maximum levels in the third or fourth week. If the first sample is negative or low-titer and the second shows an appreciable increase in antibody titer (fourfold or more), leptospirosis is indicated.

The same diagnostic procedures are employed for animals as for man. Blood or urine may be used for the bacteriologic examination, depending on the stage of the illness. If a necropsy is performed on a sacrificed or dead animal, kidney cultures should be made. Examination of several tissue samples from the same individual is not always easily done in veterinary practice, but individual diagnosis of domestic animals is not as important as herd diagnosis. Discovery of high antibody titers in several members of a herd and a clinical picture compatible with leptospirosis indicate a recent infection.

Low titers may indicate residual antibodies from a past infection or recently formed antibodies that have not yet had time to reach a high level.

The serologic reference test that is used most for man as well as for animals is microscopic agglutination (MAT). This test should be carried out using representative serovars from different serogroups, especially those occurring in the region. It is necessary to bear in mind that cross-reactions are produced not only between different serovars of the same serogroup but, at the beginning of the infection (two to three weeks), also between serovars of different serogroups, and a heterologous serovar titer may predominate. Reaction to the homologous serovar becomes more pronounced with time. Cross-reactions are much more frequent in man than in animals.

The macroscopic plate test with inactivated antigens can be used as a preliminary or screening test for man and animals. It is fast and easy, and particularly useful for diagnosing disease in a herd.

Plate agglutination is a genus-specific test, which uses as an antigen the *patoc* strain of saprophytic leptospira (*L. biflexa*) to determine if the patient is suffering from leptospirosis (Mazzonelli *et al.*, 1974). Reaction to this test is marked during the acute phase of leptospirosis and then quickly becomes negative (Faine, 1982). Among more recent tests, those of interest are indirect immunofluorescence and enzyme-linked immunosorbent assay (ELISA). With both, the types of immunoglobulins (IgM or IgG) can be determined by using the corresponding antigens. IgM appears after the first week of the disease and IgG appears after several weeks. In some human cases, IgG antibodies cannot be detected for reasons as yet unknown.

The utility of ELISA for diagnosing infection due to *hardjo* was compared with MAT. It was found that a positive reaction can be obtained with MAT 10 days after the animal has been experimentally infected; ELISA does not give a positive reaction until 25 days after infection. In addition, there was a 90% concordance between both tests. Cross-reactions with sera from animals inoculated with other serotypes occurred in fewer than 1% (Bercovich *et al.*, 1990).

The serovar *hardjo* is subdivided into subserovars or genotypes: *hardjo* genotype hardjo-bovis and *hardjo* genotype prajitno. A DNA probe for genotype hardjo-bovis was developed by LeFebvre (1987). Three methods for detecting *hardjo* type hardjo-bovis were compared: with DNA hybridization, 60 of the 75 urine samples from cows experimentally exposed were positive; with immunofluorescence, 24 samples were positive; and with culturing, only 13 were positive. The DNA probe was shown to be much more sensitive than the other techniques in detecting the genotype hardjo-bovis (Bolin *et al.*, 1989a).

A very sensitive generic test is polymerase chain reaction (PCR), which can detect as few as 10 leptospires (Mérien *et al.*, 1992).

Control: In man, control measures include: (a) personal hygiene; (b) use of protective clothes during farm work; (c) drainage of lowlands whenever possible; (d) rodent-proof structures; (e) food protection and correct garbage disposal; (f) control of infection in domestic animals; (g) avoidance of swimming in streams and other fresh watercourses that may be contaminated, and (h) chemoprophylaxis of high-risk occupational groups (sugarcane harvesters, rice-paddy workers, or soldiers).

Human immunization has not been widely applied. It has been used with promising results in Italy, Poland, and the former Soviet Union. However, because of secondary, mainly allergic effects, its use did not spread. Tests of a vaccine made in a chemically defined, protein-free medium are under way (Shenberg and Torten, 1973). In China, a similar vaccine is being used on a wide scale.

The use of antibiotics in prophylaxis and treatment of human leptospirosis has yielded contradictory results. One study (Takafuji *et al.*, 1984) showed that doxycycline is effective in chemoprophylaxis; the same drug is probably also effective in treatment. Because leptospirosis caused many cases of disease among American soldiers training in Panama, a double-blind field test was undertaken to determine the efficacy of doxycycline in preventing the infection. Nine hundred forty soldier volunteers were randomly divided into two groups. One group was given an oral dose of 200 mg of doxycycline each week for three weeks, and the other group was given a placebo. After remaining in the jungle for three weeks, 20 cases of leptospirosis were diagnosed in the placebo group (attack rate of 4.2%) and only one case was diagnosed in the doxycycline group (attack rate of 0.2%), i.e., the drug was 95% effective (Takafuji *et al.*, 1984). It has been suggested (Sanford, 1984) that chemoprophylaxis would be justified in areas where incidence is 5% or higher. Mechanization of farm work has resulted in a decrease of outbreaks, for example, among rice-paddy workers.

Among domesticated animals, vaccination of pigs, cattle, and dogs is effective in preventing the disease, but it does not protect completely against infection. Vaccinated animals may become infected without showing clinical symptoms; they may have leptospiruria, although to a lesser degree and for a shorter time than unvaccinated animals. A few known human cases of leptospirosis were contracted from vaccinated dogs. There are bacterins to protect against the *pomona*, *hardjo*, and *grippotyphosa* serovars in cattle; against *pomona* in swine; and against *canicola* and *icterohaemorrhagiae* in dogs. Immunity is predominantly serovar-specific, and the serovar or serovars active in a focus must be known in order to correctly immunize the animals. Females should be vaccinated before the reproductive period to protect them during pregnancy. Young animals can be immunized after 3 or 4 months of age. Bacterins now in use require annual revaccination. For herds to which outside animals are being introduced, it is recommended that vaccination be repeated every six months. An effective measure is to combine vaccination with antibiotic treatment (Thiermann, 1984).

Vaccination against *hardjo* is not very satisfactory, not even if the prevalent genotype hardjo-bovis is used in combined vaccines (Bolin *et al.*, 1989b) or in monovalent vaccines (Bolin *et al.*, 1991).

It has been demonstrated that vaccination with bacterins initially stimulates the production of IgM antibodies, which disappear after a few months and are replaced by IgG antibodies. Vaccination generally does not interfere with diagnosis because of the quick disappearance of IgM antibodies, which are active in agglutination. IgG are the protective antibodies and can be detected with serum protection assays in hamsters or with the growth inhibition test in culture media.

A vaccine derived from the outer membrane of leptospires has been obtained and has yielded very promising results in laboratory tests by conferring resistance not only against the disease but also against the establishment of leptospiruria. Chemotherapy is promising. Experiments have shown that a single injection of dihydrostreptomycin at a dose of 25 mg/kg of bodyweight is effective against leptospiruria in cattle and swine. The infection has been eradicated in several herds with antibiotic treatment and proper environmental hygiene. The combination of vaccination and chemotherapy for the control of swine leptospirosis has been proposed.

Proper herd management is important for control. It has been repeatedly demonstrated that swine can transmit the *pomona* serovar to cattle. Therefore, separation of these two species is important for prophylaxis.

Bibliography

Alexander, A.D. Leptospira. *In*: Balows, A., W.J. Hausler, K.L. Hermann, H.D. Isenberg, H.J. Shadomy, eds. *Manual of Clinical Microbiology.* 5th ed. Washington, D.C.: American Society for Microbiology; 1991.

Alexander, A.D., W.E. Gochenour, Jr., K.R. Reinhard, M.K. Ward, R.H. Yagen. Leptospirosis. *In*: Bodily, H.L., ed. *Diagnostic Procedures for Bacterial, Mycotic and Parasitic Infections.* 5th ed. New York: American Public Health Association, 1970.

Alston, J.M., J.C. Broom. *Leptospirosis in Man and Animals.* Edinburgh, London: Livingstone; 1958.

Benenson, A.S., ed. *Control of Communicable Diseases in Man.* 15th ed. An official report of the American Public Health Association. Washington, D.C.: American Public Health Association; 1990.

Bercovich, Z., R. Taaijke, B.A. Bokhout. Evaluation of an ELISA for the diagnosis of experimentally induced and naturally occurring *Leptospira hardjo* infections in cattle. *Vet Microbiol* 21:255–262, 1990.

Bernard, W.V., C. Bolin, T. Riddle, *et al.* Leptospiral abortion and leptospiruria in horses from the same farm. *J Am Vet Med Assoc* 202:1285–1286, 1993.

Bolin, C.A., J.A. Cassells, R.L. Zuerner, G. Trueba. Effect of vaccination with a monovalent *Leptospira interrogans* serovar *hardjo* type hardjo-bovis vaccine on type hardjo-bovis infection of cattle. *Am J Vet Res* 52:1639–1643, 1991.

Bolin, C.A., R.L. Zuerner, G. Trueba. Comparison of three techniques to detect *Leptospira interrogans* serovar *hardjo* type hardjo-bovis in bovine urine. *Am J Vet Res* 50:1001–1003, 1989a.

Bolin, C.A., R.L. Zuerner, G. Trueba. Effect of vaccination with a pentavalent leptospiral vaccine containing *Leptospira interrogans* serovar *hardjo* type hardjo-bovis on type hardjo-bovis infection in cattle. *Am J Vet Res* 50:2004–2008, 1989b.

Cacchione, R.A. Enfoques de los estudios de la leptospirosis humana y animal en América Latina. *Rev Asoc Argent Microbiol* 5:36–53, 100–111, 143–154, 1973.

Cousins, D.V., T.M. Ellis, J. Parkinson, C.H. McGlashan. Evidence for sheep as a maintenance host for *Leptospira interrogans* serovar *hardjo*. *Vet Rec* 124:123–124, 1989.

Diesch, S.L., H.C. Ellinghausen. Leptospiroses. *In*: Hubbert, W.T., W.F. McCulloch, P.R. Schnurrenberger, eds. *Diseases Transmitted from Animals to Man.* 6th ed. Springfield: Thomas; 1975.

Ellis, W.A., J. Montgomery, J.A. Cassells. Dihydrostreptomycin treatment of bovine carriers of *Leptospira interrogans* serovar *hardjo*. *Res Vet Sci* 39:292–295, 1985.

Ellis, W.A., A.B. Thiermann. Isolation of leptospires from the genital tracts of Iowa cows. *Am J Vet Res* 47:1694–1696, 1986.

Everard, C.O., A.E. Green, J.W. Glosser. Leptospirosis in Trinidad and Grenada, with special reference to the mongoose. *Trans Roy Soc Trop Med Hyg* 70:57–61, 1976.

Faine, S., ed. Guidelines for the control of leptospirosis. Geneva: World Health Organization; 1982. (Offset Publication 67).

Faine, S. Leptospirosis. *In*: Evans, A.S., P.S. Brachman, eds. *Bacterial Infections of Humans*. 2nd ed. New York: Plenum Medical Book Co.; 1991.

Hanson, L.E., D.N. Tripathy, A.H. Killinger. Current status of leptospirosis immunization in swine and cattle. *J Am Vet Med Assoc* 161:1235–1243, 1972.

Hart, R.J., J. Gallagher, S. Waitkins. An outbreak of leptospirosis in cattle and man. *Brit Med J (Clin Res Ed)* 288(6435):1983–1984, 1984.

LeFebvre, R.B. DNA probe for detection of the *Leptospira interrogans* serovar *hardjo* genotype hardjo-bovis. *J Clin Microbiol* 25:2236–2238, 1987.

Leptospirosis in man, British Isles, 1983. *Br Med J (Clin Res Ed)* 288(6435):1984–1985, 1984.

Luzzi, G.A., L.M. Milne, S.A. Waitkins. Rat-bite acquired leptospirosis. *J Infect* 15:57–60, 1987.

Mazzonelli, J. Advances in bovine leptospirosis. *Bull Off Int Epizoot* 3:775–808, 1984.

Mazzonelli, J., G.T. Dorta de Mazzonelli, M. Mailloux. Possibilité de diagnostique sérologique des leptospires á l'aide d'un antigène unique. *Med Mal Infect* 4:253, 1974.

Mérien, F., P. Amouriaux, P. Perolat, *et al*. Polymerase chain reaction for detection of *Leptospira* spp. in clinical samples. *J Clin Microbiol* 30:2219–2224, 1992.

Myers, D.M. Serological studies and isolations of serotype *hardjo* and *Leptospira biflexa* strains from horses of Argentina. *J Clin Microbiol* 3:548–555, 1976.

Nielsen, J.N., G.K. Cochran, J.A. Cassells, L.E. Hanson. *Leptospira interrogans* serovar *bratislava* infection in two dogs. *J Am Vet Med Assoc* 199:351–352, 1991.

Parma, A.E., C.G. Santisteban, A.S. Fernández, *et al*. Relación antigénica entre *Leptospira interrogans*, cristalino y córnea equina, probada por enzimoinmunoensayo. *Rev Med Vet* 67:72–76, 1986.

Perolat, P., F. Grimont, F. Regnault, *et al*. rRNA gene restriction patterns of *Leptospira*: A molecular typing system. *Res Microbiol* 141:159–171, 1990.

Prescott, J. Treatment of leptospirosis [editorial]. *Cornell Vet* 81:7–12, 1991.

Sanford, J.P. Leptospirosis—time for a booster. *N Engl J Med* 310:524–525, 1984.

Shenberg, E., M. Torten. A new leptospiral vaccine for use in man. I. Development of a vaccine from *Leptospira* grown on a chemically defined medium. *J Infect Dis* 128:642–646, 1973.

Sillerud, C.L., R.F. Bey, M. Ball, S.I. Bistner. Serologic correlation of suspected *Leptospira interrogans* serovar *pomona*-induced uveitis in a group of horses. *J Am Vet Med Assoc* 191:1576–1578, 1987.

Songer, J.G., A.B. Thiermann. Leptospirosis. *J Am Vet Med Assoc* 193:1250–1254, 1988.

Spinu, I., V. Topcin, Trinh Thi Hang Quy, Vo Van Hung, Mguyen Sy Quoe, Chu Xnan Long, *et al*. L'homme comme réservoir de virus dans une épidémie de leptospirose survenue dans la jungle. *Arch Roum Path Exp* 22:1081–1100, 1963.

Stalheim, O.H. Vaccination against leptospirosis: Protection of hamsters and swine against renal leptospirosis by killed but intact gamma-irradiated or dihydrostreptomycin-exposed *Leptospira pomona*. *Am J Vet Res* 28:1671–1676, 1967.

Stalheim, O.H. Chemotherapy of renal leptospirosis in cattle. *Am J Vet Res* 30:1317–1323, 1969.

Stalheim, O.H. Duration of immunity in cattle in response to a viable, avirulent *Leptospira pomona* vaccine. *Am J Vet Res* 32:851–854, 1971.

Suárez Hernández, M., J. Bustelo Aguila, V. Gorgoy González, *et al*. Estudio epidemiológico de un brote de leptospirosis en bañistas en el poblado de Jicotea de la provincia Ciego de Ávila. *Rev Cubana Hig Epidemiol* 27:272–284, 1989.

Sulzer, C.R., W.L. Jones. *Leptospirosis Methods in Laboratory Diagnosis*. Atlanta: U.S. Centers for Disease Control and Prevention; 1974.

Szyfres, B. La leptospirosis como problema de salud humana y animal en América Latina y el área del Caribe. *In*: *VIII Reunión Interamericana sobre el Control de la Fiebre Aftosa y Otras Zoonosis*. Washington, D.C.: Organización Panamericana de la Salud; 1976. (Publicación Científica 316).

Szyfres, B., C.R. Sulzer, M.M. Galton. A new leptospiral serotype in the Bataviae serogroup from Argentina. *Trop Geogr Med* 19:344–346, 1967.

Takafuji, E.T., J.W. Kirkpatrick, R.N. Miller, *et al.* An efficacy trial of doxycycline chemoprophylaxis against leptospirosis. *N Engl J Med* 310:497–500, 1984.

Tedesco, L.F., G. Manrique, C.R. Sulzer. A new leptospiral serotype in the Canicola serogroup from Argentina. *Trop Geogr Med* 21:203–206, 1969.

Thiermann, A.B. Leptospirosis: Current developments and trends. *J Am Vet Med Assoc* 184:722–725, 1984.

Tripathy, D.N., A.R. Smith, L.E. Hanson. Immunoglobulins in cattle vaccinated with leptospiral bacterins. *Am J Vet Res* 36:1735–1736, 1975.

Van der Hoeden, J. Leptospirosis. *In*: Van der Hoeden, J., ed. *Zoonoses*. Amsterdam: Elsevier; 1964.

Waitkins, S.A. From the PHLS. Update on leptospirosis. *Brit Med J (Clin Res Ed)* 290(6480):1502–1503, 1985.

World Health Organization. Research needs in leptospirosis [memorandum]. *Bull World Health Organ* 47:113–122, 1972.

LISTERIOSIS

ICD-10 A32.1 listerial meningitis and meningoencephalitis; A32.7 listerial septicaemia; A32.8 other forms of listeriosis; P37.2 neonatal (disseminated) listeriosis

Synonyms: Leukocytosis, listerial infection, listeriasis, listerellosis, circling disease (in animals).

Etiology: The genus *Listeria* contains seven species, but only two are of interest in human and animal pathology: *L. monocytogenes* and *L. ivanovii* (formerly *L. bulgarica* or serovar 5 of *L. monocytogenes*). A notable difference between the two pathogenic species is their hemolytic ability.

The most important species for both man and animals is *L. monocytogenes*, a gram-positive, facultatively anaerobic bacillus 0.5 to 2 microns long and 0.5 microns in diameter that is motile at temperatures between 20°C and 25°C. It is beta-hemolytic in blood agar and forms a narrow band of hemolysis around the colonies (unlike *L. ivanovii,* which forms a wide band). A noteworthy characteristic of *L. monocytogenes* is its ability to grow at low temperatures; at a pH between 6 and 9, it can reproduce at temperatures from 3°C to 45°C. It is a facultative, intracellular parasite of the reticuloendothelial system. For purposes of epidemiological research, *L. monocytogenes* is subdivided into 11 serovars. Most human (92%) and animal cases are caused by serovars 4b, 1/2b, and 1/2a (Bortolussi *et al.*, 1985). Therefore, serotyping is of limited usefulness for identifying a source of infection (Gelin and Broome, 1989).

Of 161 isolates serotyped in the US, 33% belonged to serovar 4b; 31.5%, to serovar 1/2b; 30%, to serovar 1/2a; 4%, to serovar 3b; 1%, to serovar 3a; and 0.5%, to serovar 1/2c (Gelin *et al.*, 1987). When 71 isolates were serotyped in Brazil, seven different serovars were recognized; 50% were 4b and 29.6% were 1/2a (Hofer *et al.*, 1984).

Although serotyping has been useful as a preliminary approach, other schemes had to be devised in order to be able to specify the source of infection. Subtyping was done primarily with two methods: phage typing and electrophoretic enzyme typing. In Great Britain, 64% of the strains could be typed using 28 phages; in France, 78% could be typed using 20 phages. In both cases, a sizeable percentage of strains could not be typed. All strains of *L. monocytogenes* can be typed using the isoenzymatic subtyping method (Selander *et al.*, 1986). Recently, ribosomal RNA typing (ribotyping) has been used with success.

Geographic Distribution: Worldwide. *L. monocytogenes* is widely distributed in vegetation, soil, and human and animal intestines.

Occurrence in Man: Incidence is low, but it is an important disease because of its high mortality. In many developing countries, listeriosis is rare. There is greater concentration of cases in European countries and the United States, perhaps because medical personnel in these countries are more on the lookout for the disease and because better laboratory support is available. In the former Federal Republic of Germany (West Germany), there were 296 cases of listeriosis between 1969 and 1985, 60% of which occurred in urban areas. Fifty percent of the strains isolated were from newborns and the most common serovar was 4b (Schmidt-Wolf *et al.*, 1987). In Great Britain, information was obtained from 722 cases occurring from 1967 to 1985. In 246 cases (34%), the infection affected the mother, the fetus, or the newborn. Neonatal infection was diagnosed within the first two days postpartum in 133 (54%) cases; 56 cases (23%) were diagnosed later than two days postpartum. There were 47 (19%) cases of intrauterine death. There were also 10 cases (4%) of mothers with bacteremia that did not affect the fetus. Overall case fatality was 50% (McLauchlin, 1990a). The author estimates that these data must include less than 50% of the total number of cases that occurred in the country. In adults and youth, 474 cases were recorded; 275 (58%) were men and 199 (42%) were nonpregnant women. Case fatality was 44%. Seventy-six percent of these patients had an underlying illness. An increase in incidence was noted in autumn (McLauchlin, 1990b).

There were an estimated 800 cases per year in the US between 1980 and 1982, with an incidence of 3.6 per million inhabitants and at least 150 deaths (19% case fatality). The highest attack rates were seen in newborns (4.7 per 100,000 live births) and in persons 70 years of age or older (11 per million) (Gellin and Broome, 1989). There are few recognized cases in developing countries. Sporadic cases have been seen in several Latin American countries. In a Mexican hospital, hemocultures were carried out during a three-month period on all children whose mothers showed signs of amniotic infection; *L. monocytogenes* was isolated from 4 out of 33 newborns examined (Pérez-Mirabate and Giono, 1963). In Peru (Guevara *et al.*, 1979), serovars 4d and 4b of *L. monocytogenes* were isolated from three fatal cases of neonatal listeriosis and from five aborted fetuses. In Argentina, there are few data on the occurrence of human listeriosis. In Córdoba (Argentina), there are cases of neonatal listeriosis each year, and these constitute between 2% and 3% of bacteriologically confirmed sepsis (Paolasso, 1981). In a small town in the province of Buenos Aires, Manzullo (1981) isolated *L. monocytogenes* type 1a from a bovine fetus, the vaginal exudate of the woman who milked the cows, and from the household's female dog. In another town, Manzullo (1990) isolated the agent from a woman's vaginal exudate and from the woman's female cat. In a Buenos Aires medical center, nine cases of listeriosis were diagnosed in 15 years, two of them fatal. Only one patient was not immunocompromised (Roncoroni *et al.*, 1987).

Most cases occur sporadically, but epidemic outbreaks have occurred in several countries. In 1981, in a maternity hospital in Halifax (Canada), there were 34 perinatal cases and 7 cases in women without underlying illness or immunosuppression. Case fatality in the babies born live was 27%. There were five spontaneous abortions and four babies stillborn at term. The epidemic outbreak was attributed to coleslaw: *L. monocytogenes* serovar 4b was isolated from the cabbage as well as from the patients. On the farm where the cabbages were grown, two sheep had died from listeriosis the previous year; in addition, the farmer used sheep dung as fertilizer. It is also worth noting that the farmer kept the cabbage refrigerated at 4°C, which allowed the etiologic agent to multiply at the expense of other contaminant microorganisms (Schlech *et al.*, 1983).

An earlier outbreak occurred in 1979 in eight hospitals in Boston (USA); it affected 20 patients, 15 of whom acquired the infection in the hospital. Raw vegetables were assumed to be the source of infection.

In Massachusetts (USA), an epidemic outbreak caused by pasteurized milk was recorded in 1983. It affected 42 immunocompromised patients and seven immunocompetent patients; there were also perinatal cases. Case fatality was 29%. Of 40 isolates, 32 were type 4b. It is possible that the milk had been contaminated after pasteurization (Schuchat *et al.*, 1991).

The largest epidemic in the US was recorded in 1985 in Los Angeles, California (Linnan *et al.*, 1988). The epidemic affected pregnant women, their fetuses, and their newborns. Case fatality was 63% for the infected fetuses and newborns. The outbreak was due to a Mexican soft cheese; serovar 4b was isolated from the patients and the cheese. The incubation period was 11 to 70 days, with an average of 31 days (Schuchat *et al.*, 1991).

There have been epidemic outbreaks in Switzerland, Denmark, and France. In Switzerland, the 1987 outbreak that led to 64 perinatal cases and 58 nonperinatal cases was caused by a soft cheese. Case fatality was 28%. The strain of *L. monocytogenes* responsible was the same enzymatic type as the strain that caused the outbreak in California in 1985 (Gelin and Broome, 1989). One of the largest epidemics known to date occurred in France in 1992. It affected 691 persons and 40% of the cases were caused by serotype 4b. The epidemic strain was isolated from 91 pregnant women and their children. Of the remaining persons affected by the epidemic strain, 61% were immunodeficient. The phage type was the same as in California (1985), Switzerland (1983–1987), and Denmark (1985–1987). The epidemic strain was isolated from 163 samples of meat products, 35 cheese samples, and 12 other food samples. The epidemic lasted from 18 March to 23 December 1992 and caused

63 deaths and 22 abortions. The cause was attributed to pig's tongue in gelatin (WHO, 1993). In 1993 (January–August), 25 new cases occurred in France. This time the outbreak was again due to serogroup 4, but to a different lysotype than in the 1992 epidemic. Of the 25 cases, 21 were maternal-fetal, with 4 spontaneous abortions and 2 stillbirths at term. Most of the cases occurred in western France. The epidemiological investigation was able to attribute the infection to a pork product ("rillettes") distributed by a single commercial firm (*Bol Epidemiol Hebdom* No. 34, 1993).

There are various risk groups: pregnant women, fetuses, newborns, the elderly, and immunocompromised patients. However, there was some controversy regarding AIDS patients. Several authors maintained that AIDS patients were unlikely to contract listeriosis, even though their cellular immunity system was highly compromised. While it is true that listeriosis is not one of the principal conditions affecting AIDS patients, its incidence in those infected by HIV is 300 times higher than in the general population (Schuchat *et al.*, 1991).

Occurrence in Animals: Listeriosis has a wide variety of domestic and wild animal hosts. The infection has been confirmed in a large number of domestic and wild mammals, in birds, and even in poikilotherms. The most susceptible domestic species is sheep, followed by goats and cattle. The frequency of occurrence in these animals is not known.

Outbreaks in sheep have been described in several Latin American countries. The disease has been confirmed in alpacas in Peru, and in sheep, fowl, and cattle in Argentina and Uruguay.

The first epizootic outbreak (1924) was recognized in England in laboratory rabbits suffering from a disease characterized by mononucleosis, from whence the specific name of the agent, *monocytogenes*, comes. Mononucleosis rarely occurs in man or in animals other than rabbits and rodents.

Several outbreaks have been described in Great Britain and the US due to silage with a pH higher than 5, which favors multiplication of *L. monocytogenes*. As the use of silage increases, outbreaks, which occur when the quality of silage is poor and the pH high, increase as well.

The Disease in Man: The most affected group is newborns (50% of cases in France and 39% in the US), followed by those over age 50. The disease is very rare between 1 month and 18 years of age. According to data from two German obstetrical clinics, listerial infection caused 0.15% to 2% of perinatal mortality. Listerial abortion in women usually occurs in the second half of pregnancy, and is more frequent in the third trimester. Symptoms that precede miscarriage or birth by a few days or weeks may include chills, increased body temperature, cephalalgia, slight dizziness, and sometimes, gastrointestinal symptoms. These septicemic episodes may or may not recur before birth of a stillborn fetus or a seriously ill full-term baby. After delivery, the mother shows no disease symptoms, but *L. monocytogenes* can be isolated from the vagina, cervix, and urine for periods varying from a few days to several weeks. If the child is born alive but was infected *in utero*, it may show symptoms immediately after birth or within a few days. The symptomatology is that of sepsis or, less frequently, a disseminated granulomatosis (granulomatosis infantisepticum). There may also be symptoms of a respiratory tract disorder. Case fatality is high. The main lesion is a focal hepatic necrosis in the form of small, grayish-white nodules. Some children born apparently healthy fall ill with meningitis shortly thereafter (a few days to several weeks). In these cases, the infection was probably acquired *in utero* or during birth. In the US, neonatal meningitis is the most common clinical form, while in Europe, perinatal septicemia prevails. Hydrocephalus is a common sequela of neonatal meningitis.

Meningitis or meningoencephalitis is the most common clinical form in adults, especially in those over 50. Listerial meningitis often occurs as a complication in debilitated persons, alcoholics, diabetics, in patients with neoplasias, or in elderly patients with a declining immune system. Before the existence of antibiotics, case fatality was 70%. Listerial septicemia also occurs among weakened adults, especially patients undergoing long-term treatment with corticosteroids or antimetabolites. In addition, listeriosis may result in endocarditis, external and internal abscesses, and endophthalmitis. A cutaneous eruption has been described among veterinarians who handled infected fetuses.

The recommended treatment for maternal-fetal listeriosis is ampicillin. Various antibiotics, such as ampicillin (alone or in combination with aminoglycosides), tetracycline (not for those under 8 years of age), and chloramphenicol, may be used for the other forms of the disease (Benenson, 1990).

The Disease in Animals

SHEEP, GOATS, AND CATTLE: Listeriosis manifests itself in ruminants as encephalitis, neonatal mortality, and septicemia. The most common clinical form is encephalitis. In sheep and goats, the disease has a hyperacute course, and mortality may vary from 3% to more than 30%. In cattle, listerial encephalitis has a chronic course, with the animals surviving for 4 to 14 days. In general, only 8% to 10% of a herd is affected.

A ruminant with encephalitis isolates itself from the herd and shows symptoms of depression, fever, lack of coordination, torticollis, spasmodic contractions and paralysis of facial muscles and throat, profuse salivation, strabismus, and conjunctivitis. The animal tries to lean against some support while standing and, if able to walk, moves in circles. In the final phase of the disease, the animal lies down and makes characteristic chewing movements when attempting to eat.

Listerial encephalitis can affect animals of any age, but it is more common in the first three years of life. Nevertheless, it does not appear before the rumen becomes functional. Septicemia is much more common in young animals than adults. Abortion occurs mainly during the last months of gestation and is generally the only symptom of genital infection, the dam showing no other signs of disease. If uterine infection occurs in the cow before the seventh month of pregnancy, the dead fetus is usually retained in the uterus for several days and has a macerated appearance, with marked focal necrotic hepatitis. In addition, the placenta may be retained and metritus may develop. If infection occurs in the final months of pregnancy, the fetus is practically intact and shows minimal lesions.

L. monocytogenes can also cause mastitis in cows. There are few described cases, either because the presence of this agent in cows has not been studied or because its occurrence really is rare. Mastitis caused by *Listeria* varies in severity from subclinical to acute and chronic. Elimination of the agent in milk occurs over a long period of time and may have public health repercussions, especially since pasteurization does not guarantee complete safety if the viable bacteria count is high before heat treatment (Gitter, 1980).

A study carried out in 1970–1971 in Victoria (Australia) (Dennis, 1975) showed that listeriosis is an important cause of perinatal mortality in sheep. In 94 flocks, fetuses and lambs that died during the neonatal period were examined, and *L. monocytogenes* was found in 25%. The disease caused by this agent occurs mostly in winter. It has been estimated that the rate of abortion in flocks affected by listeriosis in Victoria varies from 2% to 20%.

L. ivanovii, which differs from *L. monocytogenes* on the basis of several phenotypic characteristics, was associated in several countries with abortions in sheep and, occasionally, in cows (Alexander *et al.*, 1992).

OTHER MAMMALS: Listeriosis is rare in swine; when it does occur in the first few weeks of life, it usually takes the septicemic form. Few cases are known in dogs, in which the disease may be confused with rabies. In other domestic and wild species, the disease generally appears as isolated cases and in the septicemic form. Outbreaks have been described in rabbit and guinea pig breeding colonies.

FOWL: Young birds are the most affected. Outbreaks are infrequent and mortality may range from the loss of a few birds on one farm to a high rate of losses on other farms. The septicemic form is the most common, with degenerative lesions of the myocardium, pericarditis, and focal hepatic necrosis. On rare occasions, the meningoencephalitic form is found, with marked torticollis. Since the generalized use of antibiotics in poultry feed began, few cases of listeriosis in this species have been reported.

Source of Infection and Mode of Transmission: The causal agent is widely distributed in animals and man, as well as in the environment. *L. monocytogenes* has been isolated from different mammalian and avian species and from the soil, plants, mud, pasture, wastewater, and streams. The presence of virulent and avirulent (for mice) strains in animals and in the environment complicates clarification of the epidemiology, but serotyping can be of considerable help. Cattle, sheep, and many other animal species eliminate the agent in their feces. *L. monocytogenes* has also been isolated from the feces of patients and their contacts, as well as from a small percentage of the general human population. However, it has been isolated from the stools of some 20% to 30% of pregnant women, and has also been found in the female genital tract. In addition to untypeable strains, potentially pathogenic serotype 1 and serovar 4b have been isolated (Kampelmacher and van Noorle Jansen, 1980). Consequently, the natural reservoir is wide and the number of hosts is large. Despite this, few people contract the disease. Many women from whose stools the agent has been isolated give birth to healthy children. Concurrent conditions, such as stress and other predisposing causes (particularly diseases or treatments that depress the immune system), come into play in initiating the disease. Another predisposing cause is the decline in the immune system that occurs with aging, as well as endocrine changes during pregnancy and deficiencies in immunoregulation at the placental level.

The source of infection for the fetus and newborn is evidently the infected mother herself. It is believed that the almost inapparent disease course manifested by the mother is caused by a mild bacteremia. Airborne infection might play a role, as suggested by the influenza-like symptoms exhibited by the mother. The mother's genital tract is probably infected via the fecal route, while the fetus is infected via the bloodstream or placenta. The discovery of the causal agent in the semen of a man whose wife's genitals were infected would indicate that, in some cases, the infection may be transmitted through sexual contact.

The oral route of transmission seems to be important, as indicated by the recent outbreaks occurring in the US, Switzerland, and France (see the section on occurrence in man), where some contaminated vegetables, milk and milk products, and meat were the vehicle of the infection. It is also interesting to note that the milk that led to one of the outbreaks came from establishments where listeriosis had been diagnosed in the animals. The disease affected two very susceptible groups: newborns and debilitated persons. Of 49 patients hospitalized with listerial septicemia or meningitis, 7 were newborns and 42 were adults. All the adults were suffering from other diseases or undergoing treatment with immunosuppressants.

A rise in listeriosis cases when animals feed on silage would indicate the digestive system as the portal of entry. The causal agent has been isolated from poorly prepared fodder that had a pH higher than 5. During an outbreak of encephalitis in sheep, the same serovar and phage type of *L. monocytogenes* was isolated from the silage and from the animals' brains. The silage contained 1 million listeriae per gram (Vázquez-Boland *et al.*, 1992).

L. monocytogenes is distributed in populations of healthy animals and the disease can be produced when stress lowers the host's resistance.

Although it has been demonstrated that food has been the source of infection in both human and animal outbreaks, the source of infection is not known with certainty in sporadic cases in man. However, it has been possible to confirm that a significant percentage of such cases were caused by the ingestion of a contaminated food (Schuchat *et al.*, 1992; Pinner *et al.*, 1992). Cases of listeriosis have been associated with ingestion of raw sausage and undercooked chicken (Schwartz *et al.*, 1988). It is likely that many cases with a food source cannot be detected because the extended incubation period makes it impossible for patients to associate a food with their infection (Gelin and Broome, 1989).

One case of listeriosis in a woman with cancer was associated with consumption of turkey franks. The investigation established that the franks in opened packages in her refrigerator were contaminated, but those in unopened packages were not. Cultures from other foods in the refrigerator also yielded positive results. The conclusion was that a cross-contamination was involved (CDC, 1989).

An interesting study was conducted in the US in 1992 (CDC, 1992). During the period 1988–1990, special epidemiological surveillance was conducted in four of the country's districts, with a population of 18 million inhabitants. There were 301 cases of listeriosis identified (7.4 per million inhabitants), 67 (23%) of whom died. The patients' food consumption histories indicated that the listeriosis patients ingested 2.6 times more soft cheeses than did the controls, or purchased 1.6 times more prepared foods. The patients' refrigerators were examined and it was found that 79 (64%) of 123 contained at least one food contaminated by *L. monocytogenes*; in 26 (33%) of the 79 refrigerators the same enzymatic strain as that found in the patients was isolated.

The wide distribution of *Listeria* spp. in nature and in animal feces explains why its presence in raw meats is almost inevitable. Prevalence in raw meats may vary from 0% to 68%. Pork is contaminated most often, but contamination is also frequent in uncooked chicken. There is little information regarding the virulence of *L. monocytogenes* strains isolated from meats (Johnson *et al.*, 1990).

There is no uniform criterion regarding when to reject foods according to the degree of contamination by *L. monocytogenes*. Several countries (France, US) require that there be no contamination at all, while others (Canada, Germany) have a certain tolerance. It is impossible to ensure the total absence of *Listeria* spp. in all foods (Dehaumont, 1992).

In California (USA), a six-month study was conducted on the prevalence of *Listeria* spp. in environmental samples from 156 milk-processing plants. *Listeria* spp. was isolated from 75 (12.6%) of the 597 environmental samples. Half of the isolates were identified as *L. monocytogenes*. Of the 156 plants, 46 gave positive samples for *Listeria* spp. and 19.9% of these isolates were identified as *L. monocytogenes* (Charlton et al., 1990).

Role of Animals in the Epidemiology of the Disease: The epidemiology of sporadic listeriosis is still not well known. Most researchers consider it a disease common to man and animals and not a zoonosis *per se*. It is likely that animals contribute to maintenance of listeria in general in nature and especially to its distribution.

Studies conducted in recent years suggest that man and animals can contract the infection from many sources. Most cases in man occur in urban areas, where there is little contact with animals. Nonetheless, animals may be the source of the infection. In one case, infection was confirmed in a woman who drank raw milk; the same serotype of *Listeria* was isolated from the raw milk and from the woman's premature twins. The etiologic agent was isolated from 16% of cows that had listerial abortions. The previously described outbreaks caused by milk, meat, or vegetables contaminated by manure from listeria-infected animals demonstrate that animals may be an important source of infection.

There are indisputable cases of direct transmission of the infection from animals to man. A cattleman assisted during the delivery of a cow, inserting his arms in the uterus. Within the next 24 hours, a rash appeared on his hands and one arm and developed into pustules. He later experienced fever, chills, and generalized pain. The same phage type was isolated from the cow's vagina and from the cattleman's pustules (Cain and McCann, 1986). The veterinary profession is particularly at risk of contracting cutaneous listeriosis. Many veterinarians have become ill after attending cows that aborted, fetuses, or newborns, or after conducting autopsies of septicemic animals. The most frequent lesion is a papular exanthema (Owen et al., 1960; Nieman and Lorber, 1980; Hird, 1987). Contact with sick birds may also cause human infection (Gray and Killinger, 1966).

Diagnosis: Diagnosis can be made only through isolation of the causal agent. If the sample is obtained from usually sterile sites, such as blood, cerebrospinal fluid, amniotic fluid, or biopsy material, seeding can be done directly in blood agar, with incubation at 35°C for a week and daily checks. Listeria can be isolated from any organ in septicemic fetuses.

In sheep, goats, or cattle with encephalitis, samples of the medulla oblongata should be cultured. In septicemic fowl, rodents, or neonatal ruminants, blood or internal organs should be cultured. The "cold enrichment" method is used especially in epidemiological investigations and is indicated for culturing highly contaminated specimens. However, this method has no diagnostic value for clinical cases because of the time it takes, since treatment with antibiotics (preferably ampicillin) should begin as soon as possible to be effective.

At present, contaminated samples as well as foods are cultured in an enrichment medium and then in a selective medium. One procedure is the US Department of Agriculture procedure; it uses nalidixic acid and acriflavin in broth to inhibit the growth of contaminating flora. The culture is incubated for 24 hours at 30°C and then a subculture is done in another broth of the same composition for another 24 hours at 30°C. Finally, a highly selective solid medium that contains lithium chloride and moxalactam is used (McClain and Lee, 1988).

A test has been developed to distinguish pathogenic from nonpathogenic strains of *L. monocytogenes*. This method is based on the potentiating and synergistic effect that the extrosubstance of *Rhodococcus equi* has for producing hemolysis in cultures of pathogenic strains of *L. monocytogenes* (Skalka *et al.*, 1982).

In general, serologic tests are confusing and not useful because of cross-reactions with enterococci and *Staphylococcus aureus,* especially by serogroups 1 and 3 of *Listeria.* DNA probes that specifically detect *L. monocytogenes* have been developed (Datta *et al.*, 1988).

Control: In regions where human neonatal listeriosis is common, a Gram stain can be made from the meconium of a newborn, and treatment with antibiotics can be rapidly initiated if bacteria suspected of being *Listeria* are found. Women who develop influenza-like symptoms in the final months of pregnancy should be carefully examined and treated, if necessary, with antibiotics. The limited arsenal of defense against the infection includes such measures as the pasteurization of milk, rodent control, and common practices of environmental and personal hygiene.

Special recommendations have been developed for food preparation (CDC, 1992): cook products of animal origin well, thoroughly wash vegetables that are eaten raw, keep raw meats separate from other foods, do not consume raw milk, wash utensils used in food preparation well, and reheat all food leftovers at a high temperature. Immunocompromised individuals must not eat soft cheeses and veterinarians must take precautions during delivery, and particularly during abortions and autopsies.

Animals with encephalitis or those that have aborted should be isolated and their placentas and fetuses destroyed. Recently acquired animals should only be added to a herd after undergoing a reasonable period of quarantine.

Bibliography

Alexander, A.V., R.L. Walker, B.J. Johnson, *et al.* Bovine abortions attributable to *Listeria ivanovii*: Four cases (1988–1990). *J Am Vet Med Assoc* 200:711–714, 1992.

Benenson, A.S., ed. *Control of Communicable Diseases in Man.* 15th ed. An official report of the American Public Health Association. Washington, D.C.: American Public Health Association; 1990.

Bojsen-Moller, J. Human listeriosis: Diagnostic, epidemiological and clinical studies. *Acta Pathol Microbiol Scand* (Suppl 229):1–157, 1972.

Bortolussi, R., W.F. Schlech III, W.L. Albritton. Listeria. *In*: Lennette, E.H., A. Balows, W.J. Hausler, Jr., H.J. Shadomy. *Manual of Clinical Microbiology.* 4th ed. Washington, D.C.: American Society for Microbiology; 1985.

Broadbent, D.W. Infections associated with ovine perinatal mortality in Victoria. *Aust Vet J* 51:71–74, 1975.

Cain, D.B., V.L. McCann. An unusual case of cutaneous listeriosis. *J Clin Microbiol* 23:976–977, 1986.

Charlton, B.R., H. Kinde, L.H. Jensen. Environmental survey for *Listeria* species in California milk processing plants. *J Food Protect* 53:198–201, 1990.

Datta, A.R., B.A. Wentz, D. Shook, M.W. Trucksess. Synthetic oligodeoxyribonucleotide probes for detection of *Listeria monocytogenes*. *Appl Environ Microbiol* 54:2933–2937, 1988.

Dehaumont, P. *Listeria monocytogenes* et produits alimentaires: "zérotolérance au moins." *Bull Epidemiol Hebdom* 24:109, 1992.

Dennis, S.M. Perinatal lamb mortality in Western Australia. 6. Listeric infection. *Aust Vet J* 51:75–79, 1975.

Fleming, D.W., S.L. Cochi, K.L. MacDonald, J. Brondum, P.S. Hayes, B.D. Plikaytis, *et al.* Pasteurized milk as a vehicle of infection in an outbreak of listeriosis. *N Engl J Med* 312(7):404–407, 1985.

Franck, M. Contribution a l'Étude de l'Épidémiologie des Listerioses Humaines et Animales [thesis]. École Nationale Vétérinaire de Lyon, France, 1974.

García, H., M.E. Pinto, L. Ross, G. Saavedra. Brote epidémico de listeriosis neonatal. *Rev Chil Pediatr* 54:330–335, 1983.

Gellin, B.G., C.V. Broome. Listeriosis. *JAMA* 261:1313–1320, 1989.

Gellin, B.G., C.V. Broome, A.W. Hightower. Geographic differences in listeriosis in the United States [abstract]. 27th Interscience Conference of Antimicrobial Agents and Chemotherapy. New York, Oct 5, 1987. Cited in: Gellin, B.G., C.V. Broome. Listeriosis. *JAMA* 261:1313–1320, 1989.

Gitter, M., R. Bradley, P.H. Blampied. *Listeria monocytogenes* infection in bovine mastitis. *Vet Rec* 107:390–393, 1980.

Gray, M.L., A.H. Killinger. *Listeria monocytogenes* and listeric infections. *Bact Rev* 30:309–382, 1966.

Green, H.T., M.B. Macaulay. Hospital outbreak of *Listeria monocytogenes* septicaemia: A problem of cross infection? *Lancet* 2:1039–1040, 1978.

Guevara, J.M., J. Pereda, S. Roel. Human listeriosis in Peru. *Tropenmed Parasitol* 30:59–61, 1979.

Hird, D.W. Review of evidence for zoonotic listeriosis. *J Food Protect* 50:429–433, 1987.

Hofer, E., G.V.A. Pessoa, C.E.A. Melles. Listeriose humana. Prevalência dos sorotipos de *Listeria monocytogenes* isolados no Brasil. *Rev Inst Adolfo Lutz* 44:125–131, 1984.

Johnson, J.L., M.P. Doyle, R.G. Cassens. *Listeria monocytogenes* and other *Listeria* spp. in meat and meat products. A review. *J Food Protect* 53:81–91, 1990.

Kampelmacher, E.H., L.M. van Noorle Jansen. Listeriosis in humans and animals in the Netherlands (1958–1977). *Zbl Bakt Hyg Orig A* 246:211–227, 1980.

Killinger, A.H. Listeriosis. *In*: Hubbert, W.T., W.F. McCulloch, P.R. Schnurrenberger, eds. *Diseases Transmitted from Animals to Man*. 6th ed. Springfield: Thomas; 1975.

Killinger, A.H., M.E. Mansfield. Epizootiology of listeric infection in sheep. *J Am Vet Med Assoc* 157:1318–1324, 1970.

Larsen, H.E. Epidemiology of listeriosis. The ubiquitous occurrence of *Listeria monocytogenes*. *In*: Proceedings, Third International Symposium on Listeriosis, Bilthoven, The Netherlands, 1966.

Linnan, M.J., L. Mascola, X.D. Lou, *et al.* Epidemic listeriosis associated with Mexican-style cheese. *N Engl J Med* 319:823–828, 1988.

Mair, N.S. Human listeriosis. *In*: Graham-Jones, O., ed. *Some Diseases of Animals Communicable to Man in Britain*. Oxford: Pergamon; 1968.

Manzullo, A. Epidemiología y epizootiología de la listeriosis. *Acta Bioq Clin Latinoam* 14:539–546, 1981.

Manzullo, A.C. Listeriosis [letter]. *An Acad Nacl Agr Vet* 44 (4):5–13, 1990.

McClain, D., W.H. Lee. Development of USDA-FSIS method for isolation of *Listeria monocytogenes* from raw meat and poultry. *J Assoc Off Anal Chem* 71:660–664, 1988.

McLauchlin, J. Human listeriosis in Britain, 1967–85, a summary of 722 cases. 1. Listeriosis during pregnancy and in the newborn. *Epidemiol Infect* 104:181–190, 1990a.

McLauchlin, J. Human listeriosis in Britain, 1967–85, a summary of 722 cases. 2. Listeriosis in non-pregnant individuals, a changing pattern of infection and seasonal incidence. *Epidemiol Infect* 104:191–201, 1990b.

Moro, M. Enfermedades infecciosas de las alpacas. 2. Listeriosis. *Rev Fac Med Vet* 16/17:154–159, 1961–1962.

Nieman, R.E., B. Lorber. Listeriosis in adults: A changing pattern. Report of eight cases and review of the literature, 1968–1978. *Rev Infect Dis* 2:207–227, 1980.

Owen, C.R., A. Neis, J.W. Jackson, H.G. Stoenner. A case of primary cutaneous listeriosis. *N Engl J Med* 362:1026–1028, 1960.

Paolasso, M.R. *Listeria* en Córdoba. *Acta Bioq Clin Latinoam* 14:581–584, 1981.

Pérez-Miravete, A., S. Giono. La infección perinatal listérica en México. II. Aislamiento de *Listeria monocytogenes* en septicemia del recién nacido. *Rev Inst Salubr Enferm Trop* 23:103–113, 1963.

Pinner, R.W., A. Schuchat, B. Swaminathan, *et al.* Role of foods in sporadic listeriosis. II. Microbiologic and epidemiologic investigation. The Listeria Study Group. *JAMA* 267:2046–2050, 1992.

Rocourt, J., J.M. Alonso, H.P. Seeliger. Virulence comparée des cinq groupes génomiques de *Listeria monocytogenes* (*sensu lato*). *Ann Microbiol* 134A:359–364, 1983.

Roncoroni, A.J., M. Michans, H.M. Bianchini, *et al.* Infecciones por *Listeria monocytogenes*. Experiencia de 15 años. *Medicina* 47:239–242, 1987.

Schlech, W.F., P.M. Lavigne, R.A. Bortolussi, *et al.* Epidemic listeriosis—evidence for transmission by food. *N Engl J Med* 308: 203–206, 1983.

Schmidt-Wolf, G., H.P.R. Seeliger, A. Schretten-Brunner. Menschliche Listeriose-Erkrankungen in der Bundesrepublik Deutschland, 1969–1985. *Zbl Bakt Hyg A* 265:472–486, 1987.

Schuchat, A., K.A. Deaver, J.D. Wenger, *et al.* Role of foods in sporadic listeriosis. I. Case-control study of dietary risk factors. *JAMA* 267:2041–2045, 1992.

Schuchat, A., B. Swaminathan, C.V. Broome. Epidemiology of human listeriosis. *Clin Microbiol Rev* 4:169–183, 1991.

Schwartz, B., C.A. Ciesielski, C.V. Broome, *et al.* Association of sporadic listeriosis with consumption of uncooked hot dogs and undercooked chicken. *Lancet* 2:779–782, 1988.

Seeliger, H.P.R. *Listeriosis*. New York: Hafner Publishing Co.; 1961.

Selander, R.K., D.A. Caugant, H. Ochman, *et al.* Methods of multilocus enzyme electrophoresis for bacterial population genetics and systematics. *Appl Environ Microbiol* 51:873–884, 1986.

Skalka, B., J. Smola, K. Elischerova. Routine test for *in vitro* differentiation of pathogenic and apathogenic *Listeria monocytogenes* strains. *J Clin Microbiol* 15:503–507, 1982.

Stamm, A.M., W.E. Dismukes, B.P. Simmons, C.G. Cobbs, A. Elliott, P. Budrich, *et al.* Listeriosis in renal transplant recipients: Report of an outbreak and review of 102 cases. *Rev Infect Dis* 4:665–682, 1982.

United States of America, Department of Health and Human Services, Centers for Disease Control and Prevention (CDC). Listeriosis associated with consumption of turkey franks. *MMWR Morb Mort Wkly Rep* 38(15):267–268, 1989.

United States of America, Department of Health and Human Services, Centers for Disease Control and Prevention (CDC). Update: Foodborne listeriosis—United States, 1988–1990. *MMWR Morb Mort Wkly Rep* 41:251, 257–258, 1992.

Vázquez-Boland, J.A., L. Domínguez, M. Blanco, *et al.* Epidemiologic investigation of a silage-associated epizootic of ovine listeric encephalitis, using a new *Listeria*-selective enumeration medium and phage typing. *Am J Vet Res* 53:368–371, 1992.

Weis, J., H.P.R. Seeliger. Incidence of *Listeria monocytogenes* in nature. *Appl Microbiol* 30:29–32, 1975.

World Health Organization (WHO). Outbreak of listeriosis in 1992. *Wkly Epidemiol Rec* 68(13):89–91, 1993.

Young, S. Listeriosis in cattle and sheep. *In*: Faulkner, L.C., ed. *Abortion Diseases of Livestock*. Springfield: Thomas; 1968.

LYME DISEASE

ICD-10 A69.2

Synonyms: Lyme borreliosis, Lyme arthritis, erythema migrans (formerly erythema chronicum migrans) with polyarthritis.

Etiology: The etiologic agent is a spirochete, transmitted by ticks of the *Ixodes ricinus* complex and named *Borrelia burgdorferi* in honor of the person who discovered it (Burgdorfer *et al.*, 1982; Steere *et al.*, 1983; Johnson *et al.*, 1984). The genus *Borrelia* belongs to the family *Spirochaetaceae* and is made up of spiral-shaped, actively motile bacteria. *B. burgdorferi* is 11 to 39 microns long and has 7 to 11 flagella. The strains of *B. burgdorferi* isolated in Europe have demonstrated some heterogeneity, particularly in the two principal plasmid-dependent surface proteins (Steere, 1990).

Geographical Distribution and Occurrence in Man: The human disease has been recognized in 46 states in the US. Areas with endemic foci in that country are the Atlantic coast (particularly in the Northeast), Wisconsin and Minnesota in the Midwest, and California and Oregon along the Pacific coast (Benenson, 1990). The natural foci of the infection are expanding. In New York State, the number of counties with recorded human cases increased from four to eight between 1985 and 1989 and the number of counties where the presence of the tick *Ixodes dammini*, the vector of the infection, was documented increased from 4 to 22 during the same period (White *et al.*, 1991).[1] In the US, more than 40,000 cases were recorded between 1982 and 1992, and it is currently the principal disease transmitted by ticks. The major vectors of the infection in the US are *Ixodes dammini* in the East and Midwest, and *I. pacificus* on the Pacific coast.

The etiological agent has also been isolated in Ontario (Canada). Many European countries record cases of Lyme borreliosis and the vector on that continent is *Ixodes ricinus*. The disease has also been recognized in Australia, China, Japan, and coun-

---

[1] A study indicates that *Ixodes dammini* and *I. scapularis* (a tick in the southern US) are geographic variants of the same species, which would correctly be named *I. scapularis* (Oliver *et al.*, 1993). Since there are differences in terms of ecology and the rate of infection (Kazmierczak and Sorhage, 1993), we feel it is advisable to retain the terminology commonly in use for both varieties in order to avoid confusion.

tries of the former Soviet Union. In the Asian countries, the tick that transmits the infection is *I. persulcatus*.

In the Northern Hemisphere, the disease has the highest incidence in summer during the months of June and July, but it may appear in other seasons depending on the tick life cycle in the region (Benenson, 1990).

Occurrence in Animals: In endemic areas and areas near to them, various species of domestic animals (dogs, horses, and cattle) are infected by *B. burgdorferi*.

In the natural foci of the infection, wild animals form the major part of the life cycle of the tick and of the agent it transmits. In these foci, high rates of reactors to the indirect immunofluorescence test, using antigens from the etiologic agent, have been found in several wild animal species. The prevalence of reactors among animals infested with *I. dammini* in eastern Connecticut from 1978 to 1982 was as follows (Magnarelli *et al.*, 1984): white-tailed deer (*Odocoileus virginianus*), 27%; white-footed mice (*Peromyscus leucopus*), 10%; eastern chipmunks (*Tamias striatus*), 17%; gray squirrels (*Sciurus carolinensis*), 50%; opossums (*Didelphis virginiana*), 17%; raccoons (*Procyon lotor*), 23%; and dogs, 24%. The spirochete was isolated from the bloodstream of 1 out of 20 white-footed mice examined (Anderson and Magnarelli, 1983; Bosler *et al.*, 1984).

Of 380 samples obtained from dogs from two locations selling animals in Wisconsin, 53% reacted positively to the immunofluorescence test and the pathogenic agent was isolated from the blood of 8 out of 111 dogs (Burgess, 1986). In Texas, the same test was used to examine 2,409 canine samples in 1988; of these, 132 (5.5%) yielded positive results. Many of the seropositive dogs were from the north-central part of the state, where most of the human cases are recorded (Cohen *et al.*, 1990).

It has been noted that horses are frequently bitten by *I. dammini*. In a serological study of 50 randomly selected horses in New England (USA), a known endemic area, 13 of the horses were reactive to the indirect immunofluorescence test.

In another serological survey using the enzyme-linked immunosorbent assay (ELISA) technique, 13 of 100 horses examined in the month of June tested positive and 6 of 91 (7%) tested positive in the month of October. The horses came from five eastern US states. The frequency of antibody responses was higher in horses from New Jersey than in horses from Pennsylvania (Bernard *et al.*, 1990). In contrast, no reactive horses were found in central Texas (Cohen *et al.*, 1992).

The Disease in Man: The characteristic cutaneous lesion, erythema migrans (EM), appears from 3 to 20 days after the tick bite. The lesion begins with a red macula or papule that widens. The borders are clearly delineated, the central lesion pales, and an annular erythema forms. The erythema may be recurrent, with secondary lesions appearing on other parts of the body. The cutaneous lesions may be accompanied for several weeks by malaise, fever, cephalalgia, stiff neck, myalgias, arthralgia, or lymphadenopathy. The EM constitutes the first stage or phase of the disease and lasts a few weeks, but may recur. In the second stage, after several weeks or months have passed and the agent has disseminated, some patients develop multiple EMs, meningoencephalitis, neuropathies, myocarditis, and atrioventricular tachycardia. Some suffer arthritic attacks in the large joints, which may recur for several years, at times taking a chronic course (Steere *et al.*, 1983). Months or years later, the third stage may occur in some patients; this stage sometimes includes acrodermatitis chronica atrophicans and neurological and articular changes.

It should be borne in mind that the connection between EM and arthritis might not be apparent, as several weeks or months transpire between the two episodes. Of 405 patients showing EM, 249 had later neurological, cardiac, and articular symptoms (Steere and Malawista, 1979). In Europe, cases with arthritis are rare, while neurological symptoms and acrodermatitis are more frequent.

Treatment for Lyme disease consists of giving the patient doxycycline for 10 to 30 days, or ceftriaxone, particularly if there is a neurological disorder (Benenson, 1990).

The Disease in Animals: The effect of the spirochete infection on wild animals is not known, but it may be asymptomatic. The predominant symptom in dogs is lameness due to arthritis in different joints, which may be migratory. Arthralgia is often accompanied by fever, anorexia, fatigue, and lymphadenitis. Arthritis is usually temporary, but may become chronic.

Different symptoms have been observed in horses, including arthritis, encephalitis, uveitis, dermatitis, edema of the limbs, and death of colts associated with natural infection in pregnant mares. However, the infection has not been confirmed in any of the cases described (Cohen *et al.*, 1992).

In cattle, infection caused by *B. burgdorferi* has also been associated with lameness. Serological analysis using Western blot, ELISA, and indirect immunofluorescence techniques on 27 milk cows from 17 herds in Minnesota and Wisconsin found that high serological titers were associated with arthritis (Wells *et al.*, 1993).

Source of Infection and Mode of Transmission: The etiologic agent is transmitted by a vector, which in the US is the tick *Ixodes dammini* on the Northeast Coast and northern states of the Midwest, but *I. pacificus* on the West Coast (Benenson, 1990). The vector is *I. ricinus* in Europe, possibly *I. holocyclus* in Australia (Stewart *et al.*, 1982), and *I. persulcatus* in Asia.

Isolation of the etiologic agent has made it possible to definitively establish the role of ticks as vectors. In fact, in the endemic area of Connecticut, a spirochete with the same antigenic and morphological characteristics as the one in Lyme disease patients was isolated from 21 (19%) of 110 nymphs and adult ticks (*I. dammini*). The high rate of infection of the vector was shown by direct immunofluorescence; in one locality, 30 (21%) of 143 *I. dammini* contained spirochetes, and in another, 17 (26%) of 66 contained spirochetes. These results were obtained only for nymphs and adults that had fed, while 148 larvae that had not fed were negative (Steere *et al.*, 1983). On Shelter Island, New York, more than 50% of ticks were infected (Bosler *et al.*, 1983). In contrast, only 2% of the *I. pacificus* ticks were infected.

The fact that the larvae were not infected prior to feeding on blood would indicate that the tick becomes infected from an animal reservoir. This reservoir would be small rodents and other wild mammals; among these the white-footed mouse (*Peromyscus leucopus*) is considered very important on the East Coast of the US. In Europe, the reservoir of the infection is also small, wild rodents, such as *Apodemus sylvaticus* and *Clethrionomys* spp. Tick larvae and nymphs feed on the blood of these small mammals and become infected with *B. burgdorferi*. The adult tick may transmit the etiologic agent to a very small percentage of the eggs, but there is a gradual loss of the agent when they go on to the larval and nymph stages until it disappears completely. The infection is renewed when larval and nymph ticks feed on rodents (Burgdorfer *et al.*, 1989). This fact is reflected in the high percentage of larvae and nymphs found on these small wild mammals, as well as their high rate of infection by *B. burgdorferi*. The adult tick has a predilection for deer (*Odocoileus virginianus*) in the foci along the eastern coast of the US. This cycle is repeated in other areas of the world, with different animal species whose blood feeds the stages of various tick species. The biotope where these cycles develop is wooded areas or areas of dense vegetation that retain the moisture that is favorable to ticks (Madigan and Tleitler, 1988).

Adult ticks are abundant in spring and fall; nymphs, in spring and early summer; and larvae, in late summer and early fall. All stages in the development of ticks are parasitic in humans, but the nymph stage is primarily responsible for the transmission of *B. burgdorferi* to man (Anderson, 1989; Steere, 1990).

Role of Animals in the Epidemiology of the Disease: On the basis of current information, it can be asserted that wild animals are primarily responsible for maintaining the infection in natural foci. Dogs and birds may spread ticks and increase endemic areas. Man is an accidental host.

Diagnosis: Until recently, diagnosis was based exclusively on the clinical picture, especially a history of EM, and on epidemiological information.

Although now possible, isolation of the infective agent by culture is still not very practical. In 1983, Steere *et al.* isolated the agent in only three patients, using a total of 142 clinical samples taken from 56 patients. Barbour, Stoener, Kelly (BSK) medium is used for isolation and is incubated at 33°C; it is easier to isolate the agent from cutaneous lesions than from blood. The indirect immunofluorescence test with conjugated IgM and IgG sera was widely used. Patients with EM had elevated IgM antibody titers only between the EM phase and convalescence two to three weeks later. Patients with late manifestations of the disease (arthritis, cardiac, or neurological anomalies) had elevated IgG antibody titers (Steere *et al.*, 1983). It was later shown that indirect ELISA was more sensitive and specific than immunofluorescence (Steere, 1990). In serological tests, there may be cross-reactions with other spirochetes. Given that all serological tests have limited specificity and sensibility, their use is not recommended for asymptomatic individuals.

Diagnosis in animals is similar to that in humans. Early treatment with antibiotics shortens the duration of EM and may prevent or lessen late manifestations of the disease; it may also have an effect on reducing the level of antibodies.

Control: The only methods of prevention consist of avoiding endemic areas and tick bites. Persons entering natural foci should use protective footwear and clothing, though this is not always possible. Insect repellents may provide some protection. It is advisable to check the body frequently and remove attached ticks by pulling gently with tweezers pressed as closely as possible to the skin. It is recommended that gloves be used during this operation.

Dogs should be checked frequently and ticks should be removed as carefully as with humans. The use of tickicides in powder form or collars is a good preventive measure. There is currently an inactivated commercial vaccine available for dogs. It is administered in two doses at three week intervals and annually thereafter (Chu *et al.*, 1992). Widespread and indiscriminate use of this vaccine is a matter of discussion, although it is recognized that the bacterin has no side effects (Kazmierczak and Sorhage, 1993).

Bibliography

Anderson, J.F. Epizootiology of *Borrelia* in *Ixodes* tick vectors and reservoir hosts. *Rev Infect Dis* 11(Suppl):1451–1459, 1989.

Anderson, J.F., L.A. Magnarelli. Spirochetes in *Ixodes dammini* and *Babesia microti* on Prudence Island, Rhode Island. *J Infect Dis* 148:1124, 1983.

Anderson, J.F., L.A. Magnarelli. Avian and mammalian hosts for spirochete-infected ticks and insects in a Lyme disease focus in Connecticut. *Yale J Biol Med* 57:627–641, 1984.

Barbour, A.G. Isolation and cultivation of Lyme disease spirochetes. *Yale J Biol Med* 57:521–525, 1984.

Benenson, A.S., ed. *Control of Communicable Diseases in Man.* 15th ed. An official report of the American Public Health Association. Washington, D.C.: American Public Health Association; 1990.

Bernard, W.V., D. Cohen, E.M. Bosler, D. Zamos. Serologic survey for *Borrelia burgdorferi* antibody in horses referred to a mid-Atlantic veterinary teaching hospital. *J Am Vet Med Assoc* 196:1255–1258, 1990.

Bosler, E.M., J.L. Coleman, J.L. Benach, *et al.* Natural distribution of the *Ixodes dammini* spirochete. *Science* 220:321–322, 1983.

Bosler, E.M., B.G. Ormiston, J.L. Coleman, *et al.* Prevalence of the Lyme disease spirochete in populations of white-tailed deer and white-footed mice. *Yale J Biol Med* 57:651–659, 1984.

Bruhn, F.W. Lyme disease. *Am J Dis Child* 138:467–470, 1984.

Burgdorfer, W., A.G. Barbour, S.F. Hayes, *et al.* Lyme disease—A tickborne spirochetosis? *Science* 216:1317–1319, 1982.

Burgdorfer, W., S.F. Hayes, D. Corwin. Pathophysiology of the Lyme disease spirochete, *Borrelia burgdorferi*, in ixodid ticks. *Rev Infect Dis* 11(Suppl 6):1442–1450, 1989.

Burgess, E.C. Natural exposure of Wisconsin dogs to the Lyme disease spirochete (*Borrelia burgdorferi*). *Lab Anim Sci* 36:288–290, 1986.

Chu, H.J., L.G. Chavez, B.M. Blumer, *et al.* Immunogenicity and efficacy study of a commercial *Borrelia burgdorferi* bacterin. *J Am Vet Med Assoc* 201:403–411, 1992.

Cohen, N.D., C.N. Carter, M.A. Thomas, Jr., *et al.* Clinical and epizootiologic characteristics of dogs seropositive for *Borrelia burgdorferi* in Texas: 110 cases (1988). *J Am Vet Med Assoc* 197:893–898, 1990.

Cohen, N.D., F.C. Heck, B. Heim, *et al.* Seroprevalence of antibodies to *Borrelia burgdorferi* in a population of horses in central Texas. *J Am Vet Med Assoc* 201:1030–1034, 1992.

Charmot, G., F. Rodhain, C. Perez. Un cas d'arthrite de Lyme observé en France. *Nouv Presse Med* 11:207–208, 1982.

Gerster, J.C., S. Guggi, H. Perroud, R. Bovet. Lyme arthritis appearing outside the United States: A case report from Switzerland. *Brit Med J* 283:951–952, 1981.

Hanrahan, J.P., J.L. Benach, J.L. Coleman, *et al.* Incidence and cumulative frequency of endemic Lyme disease in a community. *J Infect Dis* 150:489–496, 1984.

Hayes, S.F., W. Burgdorfer, A.G. Barbour. Bacteriophage in *Ixodes dammini* spirochete, etiological agent of Lyme disease. *J Bacteriol* 154:1436–1439, 1983.

Johnson, R.C., F.W. Hyde, C.M. Rumpel. Taxonomy of the Lyme disease spirochetes. *Yale J Biol Med* 57:529–537, 1984.

Johnson, R.C., F.W. Hyde, A.G. Steigerwalt, D.J. Brenner. *Borrelia burgdorferi* sp. nov.: Etiologic agent of Lyme disease. *Int J Syst Bacteriol* 34:496–497, 1984.

Kazmierczak, J.J., F.E. Sorhage. Current understanding of *Borrelia burgdorferi* infection, with emphasis on its prevention in dogs. *J Am Vet Med Assoc* 203:1524–1528, 1993.

Madigan, J.E., J. Teitler. *Borrelia burgdorferi* borreliosis. *J Am Vet Med Assoc* 192:892–896, 1988.

Magnarelli, L.A., J.F. Anderson, W. Burgdorfer, W.A. Chappel. Parasitism by *Ixodes dammini* (*Acari: Ixodidae*) and antibodies to spirochetes in mammals at Lyme disease foci in Connecticut, USA. *J Med Entomol* 21:52–57, 1984.

Oliver, J.N., M.R. Owsley, H.J. Hutcheson, *et al.* Conspecificity of the ticks *Ixodes scapularis* and *I. dammini* (*Acari: Ixodidae*). *J Med Entomol* 30:54–63, 1993.

Russell, H., J.S. Sampson, G.P. Schmid, *et al.* Enzyme-linked immunosorbent assay and indirect immunofluorescence assay for Lyme disease. *J Infect Dis* 149:465–470, 1984.

Schmid, G.P. The global distribution of Lyme disease. *Rev Infect Dis* 7:41–50, 1985.

Schulze, T., G.S. Bowen, E.M. Bosler, *et al.* *Amblyomma americanum*: A potential vector of Lyme disease in New Jersey. *Science* 224:601–603, 1984.

Stanek, G., G. Wewalka, V. Groh, *et al.* Differences between Lyme disease and European arthropod-borne *Borrelia* infections. *Lancet* 1(8425):401, 1985.

Steere, A.C. Borrelia burgdorferi (*Lyme disease, Lyme borreliosis*). *In*: Mandell, G.L., R.G. Douglas, Jr., J.E. Bennett, eds. *Principles and Practice of Infectious Diseases.* 3rd ed. New York: Churchill Livingstone, Inc.; 1990.

Steere, A.C., J. Green, R.T. Schoen. Successful parenteral penicillin therapy of established Lyme arthritis. *N Engl J Med* 312:869–874, 1985.

Steere, A.C., R.L. Grodzicki, A.N. Kornblatt, *et al.* The spirochetal etiology of Lyme disease. *N Engl J Med* 308:733–744, 1983.

Steere, A.C., S.E. Malawista. Cases of Lyme disease in the United States: Locations correlated with distribution of *Ixodes dammini*. *Ann Intern Med* 91:730–733, 1979.

Stevens, R., K. Hechemy, A. Rogers, J. Benach. Fluoroimmunoassay (FIAX) for Lyme disease antibody. Abstracts, Annual Meeting of the American Society for Microbiology, March 3–7, 1985.

Stewart, A., J. Glass, A. Patel, G. Watt, A. Cripps, R. Clancy. Lyme arthritis in the Hunter Valley. *Med J Aust* 1:139, 1982.

United States of America, Department of Health and Human Services, Centers for Disease Control and Prevention (CDC). Current Trends Update: Lyme disease and cases occurring during pregnancy—United States. *MMWR Morb Mortal Wkly Rep* 34:376–378, 383–384, 1985.

Wells, S.J., M. Trent, R.A. Robinson, *et al.* Association between clinical lameness and *Borrelia burgdorferi* antibody in dairy cows. *Am J Vet Res* 54:398–405, 1993.

White, D.J., H.G. Chang, J.L. Benach, *et al.* The geographic spread and temporal increase of the Lyme disease epidemic. *JAMA* 266:1230–1236, 1991.

Wilkinson, H.W. Immunodiagnostic tests for Lyme disease. *Yale J Biol Med* 57:567–572, 1984.

MELIOIDOSIS

ICD-10 A24.1 acute and fulminating melioidosis;
A24.2 subacute and chronic melioidosis; A24.3 other melioidosis

Synonyms: Whitmore's disease, rodent glanders.

Etiology: *Pseudomonas* (*Malleomyces*) *pseudomallei*, a small, aerobic, motile, gram-negative bacillus closely related to *P. mallei*, the agent of glanders. When stained with methylene blue or Wright stain, it shows bipolar coloration, in the shape of a safety pin. It is pleomorphic and sometimes forms chains. It is a saprophytic bacteria that lives in surface waters and in soil. *P. pseudomallei* can survive in moist, clayey soil; under laboratory conditions; at ambient temperature; and in shade for 30 months (Thomas and Forbes-Faulkner, 1981).

P. pseudomallei has several possible virulence factors, including an endotoxin, an exotoxin, and various digestive enzymes that can attack tissue. The role that each of these virulence factors plays in pathogenesis is still unknown. The exotoxin is the most toxic substance produced by the bacteria and can inhibit intracellular protein synthesis (Dance, 1991; Ismail *et al.*, 1991).

Geographic Distribution: Most human and animal cases have been recorded in Southeast Asia (Indonesia, Malaysia, Myanmar [Burma], and Thailand), which is considered the main endemic area. The disease has also been diagnosed in northeastern Australia, Guam, Iran, Korea, Madagascar, Papua New Guinea, Sri Lanka, and Turkey. Cases have also occurred in Bangladesh, India, and Pakistan. In the Americas, the infection has been confirmed in Aruba, the Bahamas, Ecuador, El Salvador, Mexico, Panama, and Puerto Rico. More recent investigations have revealed the agent's presence in other areas (Brazil, Burkina Faso, Côte d'Ivoire, Haiti, and Peru) by isolating it from people, animals, or soil and water samples. Sporadic cases have also occurred in human in Kenya and the Gambia, in swine in Burkina Faso and Niger, and in goats in Chad. The agent's distribution is predominantly tropical. The epizootic that occurred in the "Jardin des Plantes," in Paris, is the first reported outbreak in a temperate climate. In Europe, in addition to France, there have been cases in horses in Spain (Benenson, 1990; Galimard and Dodin, 1982; Dance, 1991a).

Occurrence in Man: Clinically apparent infection caused by *P. pseudomallei* is not very common. During the war in Indochina, several hundred French, American, and Vietnamese soldiers became ill with melioidosis. From 1965 to 1969, three cases per month occurred among US Army soldiers in Vietnam (Piggott, 1976). According to a serological survey, 9% of the 3 million US personnel participating in the Vietnam conflict were exposed to the agent. Cases confirmed in the US during the 1970s were almost all military personnel or travelers returning from Southeast Asia (CDC, 1977).

The numerous cases that occurred among military personnel during the Vietnam War provoked interest in the disease among medical professionals in Thailand. Prior to 1965, only three cases of melioidosis had been recorded in that country, while there were a total of about 1,000 cases between 1967 and 1988 (Kanai and Dejsirilert, 1988).

Melioidosis is currently recognized as the most common cause of pneumonia occurring in the Top End region in the Northern Territory of Australia (Currie, 1993).

Occurrence in Animals: In endemic zones, sporadic cases have been reported in different animal species. Occasional outbreaks have occurred among sheep (in Australia and Aruba), in swine (Vietnam), in goats, cattle, horses, dogs, dolphins, tropical fish, and zoo animals, as well as in monkeys imported for laboratories. A case occurred in macaques of the species *Macaca fascicularis* imported to Great Britain from the Philippines. There were a total of 13 confirmed or suspected cases in 50 imported animals. Most had splenic abscesses, but their general condition was not affected and infection was suspected on the basis of results from serological tests (Dance et al., 1992).

The Disease in Man: The incubation period may be a few days, but in some patients the agent lies dormant for months, or even years, before clinical signs are seen. The infection may occur subclinically, as was shown by a serologic survey of war veterans, or the disease may take an acute and fulminant, or subacute and chronic form. In the acute form, the patient dies in a few days, after suffering fever, pneumonia, and gastroenteritis. The disease generally appears as a respiratory illness that varies from mild bronchitis to severe and fatal pneumonia. Case mortality is approximately 30% (Kanai and Dejsirilert, 1988).

In septicemic cases of short duration, the principal lesion consists of small abscesses distributed throughout the body. When septicemia is prolonged, larger, confluent abscesses are found, often localized in one organ.

Lasting from a few months to many years, the subacute and chronic form is characterized by localization in some organ, such as the lungs, lymph glands, skin, or bones. The lesion consists of a combination of necrosis and granulomatous inflammation. The central zone of necrosis contains a purulent or caseous exudate that can be confused with a tubercular lesion.

In endemic areas, such as Southeast Asia, seroepidemiological surveys indicate that latent or subclinical forms are common. In latent cases, *P. pseudomallei* may remain inactive for years and become activated when there is some other disease or an individual's defenses are lowered due to the administration of steroids or other immunosuppressant therapy (Kanai and Dejsirilert, 1988).

In northern Australian aborigines, a form of the disease has been observed in which primary localization is in the lower urogenital system. This localization was observed in 6 of 16 aborigines with melioidosis (Webling, 1980).

Although the infection may occur in healthy individuals, *P. pseudomallei* is largely an opportunistic bacteria. In Thailand, 70% of patients have some concurrent disease, particularly diabetes or renal deficiency (Dance, 1991b). The ratio between men and women affected is 3:2. Most cases occur during or after tropical rains.

Various beta-lactamic agents are bactericides for *P. pseudomallei*. One of these compounds, ceftazidime, reduced mortality by 50% among individuals with acute and severe melioidosis (White et al., 1989).

The Disease in Animals: Many animal species are susceptible. Sporadic cases have been observed in sheep, goats, horses, swine, cattle, dogs, cats, nonhuman primates, wild and peridomestic rats, other wild animals, laboratory guinea pigs, and rabbits. The most susceptible species are sheep, swine, and goats, in which epidemic outbreaks have occurred.

As seen in Aruba, the disease in sheep consisted primarily of abscesses of the viscera, joints, and lymph nodes. In a few weeks, 25 of 90 sheep died from the disease and many survivors suffered weight loss and polyarthritis (Sutmöller et al., 1957). In cases in Australian sheep, cough and nervous symptoms were also observed (Laws and Hall, 1964).

In swine, the symptomatology consists of fever, prostration, dyspnea, cough, and arthritis. In suckling pigs, the disease is often fatal. In addition, the disease may be found through necropsy or when meat is seized in slaughterhouses. In northern Queensland (Australia), melioidosis occurs sporadically in swine bred in contact with the soil. In the southern part of the same state, which is not an enzootic area, veterinary inspection at a slaughterhouse uncovered cases in suckling pigs from eight intensive breeding facilities, during three successive years. These cases (159 out of 17,397 animals inspected) occurred after abundant rains and flooding. Abscesses were found in the bronchial ganglia of 40% and in the spleen of 34%. The outbreak was attributed to inhalation of aerosols from water (Ketterer *et al.*, 1986).

The disease is rare in cattle. The etiologic agent has been isolated from splenic abscesses, from the central nervous system, and from aborted fetuses.

In horses, the infection may become apparent due to the symptoms of septicemia, colic, diarrhea, and edemas in the legs.

The symptomatology is not very characteristic and the disease is difficult to diagnose in animal species in which it occurs sporadically. The lesions, which are similar to those in man, may suggest melioidosis and lead to its diagnosis.

Source of Infection and Mode of Transmission (Figure 13): Investigations have shown that the reservoirs of *P. pseudomallei* are surface waters and soil, as corroborated by sampling done in Southeast Asia. The highest isolation rates were obtained in rice fields and newly planted oil palm plantations (14.5%–33.3% of the isolations were from water samples). Seroepidemiologic studies also show that the highest reactor rates to the hemagglutination test came from workers or inhabitants of those areas. Human and animal infection occurs mainly during the rainy season. The etiologic agent can survive for many months in surface water and, with its low nutritional requirements, it can multiply in the hot, humid environment characteristic of endemic regions.

**Figure 13. Melioidosis (*Pseudomonas pseudomallei*).
Mode of transmission.**

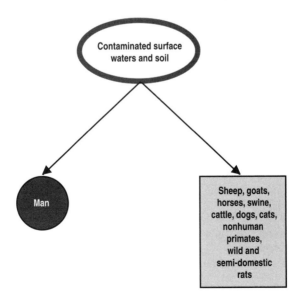

Transmission from animal to animal or from animal to man has not been proven, but it is thought that in some cases the infection may be passed from person to person. In addition to a case in Vietnam in which an American soldier with prostatitis seems to have transmitted the disease venereally to a woman, venereal transmission of the disease was also suspected among Australian aborigines with urogenital melioidosis. In accordance with tribal rituals, these aborigines smear their genitals with clay and coitus normally takes place in contact with the soil (Webling, 1980).

It is accepted that humans and animals acquire the infection through contact with contaminated water or soil, primarily through skin abrasions, but also through inhalation of dust and ingestion of contaminated water. During the war in Indochina, the number of recorded human cases climbed considerably due to contamination of war wounds with mud, traversal of flooded countryside, or prolonged stay in trenches.

The rat flea *Xenopsylla cheopis* and the mosquito *Aedes aegypti* are capable of transmitting the infection experimentally to laboratory animals. The etiologic agent multiplies in the digestive tract of these insects. The role of these possible vectors in natural transmission has not yet been evaluated, but it is thought to be of little importance.

Role of Animals in the Epidemiology of the Disease: Melioidosis seems to be a disease common to man and animals, with water and soil as reservoirs and sources of infection for both. Nevertheless, animals are believed to play a role as hosts in transporting the etiologic agent to new geographic areas.

Diagnosis: The only incontrovertible diagnostic method is isolation and identification of the etiologic agent, by either direct culture or inoculation of guinea pigs. *P. pseudomallei* can be isolated from abscesses, sputum, blood, urine, and various tissues.

The allergenic test using melioidin may be useful for diagnosis in animals, but gives many false negatives in swine and false positives in goats.

Of the serologic tests, indirect hemagglutination with melioidin-sensitized erythrocytes has proven to be sufficiently sensitive and specific in nonendemic areas. In endemic areas, titers of $\geq$ 1:160 would have to be considered significant reactions (Appassakij *et al.*, 1990). The indirect immunofluorescence and ELISA tests have proven to be more sensitive and specific (Dance, 1991). A latex agglutination test developed and evaluated by Smith *et al.* (1993) is considered highly sensitive and specific.

The ELISA test was used on Malaysian sheep to detect the anti-exotoxin. The antitoxin was confirmed in 49.3% of the sera taken from a sheep herd that had been naturally exposed to the infection. In sheep kept on a property without infection, the rate was 6% (Ismail *et al.*, 1991).

Control: Since it is an infrequent disease, specific preventive measures are not justified. In man, the use of boots during outdoor work can provide a certain amount of protection against the infection in endemic areas. Proper treatment of wounds and abrasions is important.

In animals, control of the infection is difficult, unless the environment is changed through such measures as drainage of low-lying, flooded fields.

Bibliography

Appassakij, H., K.R. Silpapojakul, R. Wansit, M. Pornpatkul. Diagnostic value of the indirect hemagglutination test for melioidosis in an endemic area. *Am J Trop Med Hyg* 42:248–253, 1990.

Benenson, A.S., ed. *Control of Communicable Diseases in Man*. 15th ed. An official report of the American Public Health Association. Washington, D.C.: American Public Health Association; 1990.

Biegeleisen, J.Z., Jr., M.R. Mosquera, W.B. Cherry. A case of human melioidosis. Clinical, epidemiological and laboratory findings. *Am J Trop Med Hyg* 13:89–99, 1966.

Currie, B. Medicine in tropical Australia. *Med J Aust* 158:609, 612–615, 1993.

Dance, D.A. *Pseudomonas pseudomallei*: Danger in the paddy fields. *Trans R Soc Trop Med Hyg* 85:1–3, 1991a.

Dance, D.A. Melioidosis: The tip of the iceberg? *Clin Microbiol Rev* 4:52–60, 1991b.

Dance, D.A., C. King, H. Aucken, *et al.* An outbreak of melioidosis in imported primates in Britain. *Vet Rec* 130:525–529, 1992.

Galimard, M., A. Dodin. Le point sur la melioidose dans le monde. *Bull Soc Pathol Exot* 75:375–383, 1982.

Hubbert, W.T. Melioidosis: Sources and potential. *Wildl Dis* 5(3):208–212, 1969.

Ismail, G., R. Mohamed, S. Rohana, *et al.* Antibody to *Pseudomonas pseudomallei* exotoxin in sheep exposed to natural infection. *Vet Microbiol* 27:277–282, 1991.

Kanai, K., S. Dejsirilert. *Pseudomonas pseudomallei* and melioidosis, with special reference to the status in Thailand. *Jpn J Med Sci Biol* 41:123–157, 1988.

Kaufman, A.E., A.D. Alexander, A.M. Allen, R.J. Cronkin, L.A. Dillingham, J.D. Douglas, *et al.* Melioidosis in imported nonhuman primates. *Wildl Dis* 6:211–219, 1970.

Ketterer, P.J., B. Donald, R.J. Rogers. Bovine melioidosis in south-eastern Queensland. *Aust Vet J* 51:395–398, 1975.

Ketterer, P.J., W.R. Webster, J. Shield, *et al.* Melioidosis in intensive piggeries in south-eastern Queensland. *Aust Vet J* 63:146–149, 1986.

Laws, L., W.T.K. Hall. Melioidosis in animals in north Queensland. IV. Epidemiology. *Aust Vet J* 40:309–314, 1964.

Piggott, J.A. Melioidosis. *In*: Binford, C.H., D.H. Connor, eds. *Pathology of Tropical and Extraordinary Diseases*. Washington, D.C.: Armed Forces Institute of Pathology; 1976.

Piggott, J.A., L. Hochholzer. Human melioidosis. A histopathologic study of acute and chronic melioidosis. *Arch Pathol* 90:101–111, 1970.

Redfearn, M.S., N.J. Palleroni. Glanders and melioidosis. *In*: Hubbert, W.T., W.F. McCulloch, P.R. Schnurrenberger, eds. *Diseases Transmitted from Animals to Man*. 6th ed. Springfield: Thomas; 1975.

Smith, M.D., V. Wuthiekanun, A.L. Walsh, T.L. Pitt. Latex agglutination test for identification of *Pseudomonas pseudomallei*. *J Clin Pathol* 46:374–375, 1993.

Strauss, J.M., M.G. Groves, M. Mariappan, D.W. Ellison. Melioidosis in Malaysia. II. Distribution of *Pseudomonas pseudomallei* in soil and surface water. *Am J Trop Med Hyg* 18:698–702, 1969.

Sutmöller, P., F.C. Kraneveld, A. Van der Schaaf. Melioidosis (*Pseudomalleus*) in sheep, goats, and pigs in Aruba (Netherlands Antilles). *J Am Vet Med Assoc* 130:415–417, 1957.

Thomas, A.D., J.C. Forbes-Faulkner. Persistence of *Pseudomonas pseudomallei* in soil. *Aust Vet J* 57:535–536, 1981.

United States of America, Department of Health and Human Services, Centers for Disease Control and Prevention (CDC). Melioidosis—Pennsylvania. *MMWR Morb Mortal Wkly Rep* 25:419–420, 1977.

Webling, D.D. Genito-urinary infections with *Pseudomonas pseudomallei* in Australian aboriginals. *Trans R Soc Trop Med Hyg* 74:138–139, 1980.

White, N.J., D.A. Dance, W. Chaowagul, *et al.* Halving of mortality of severe melioidosis by ceftazidime. *Lancet* 2:697–701, 1989.

NECROBACILLOSIS

ICD-10 A48.8 other specified bacterial diseases

Synonyms: Schmorl's disease, calf diphtheria, foot rot.

Etiology: *Fusobacterium necrophorum*, a nonsporulating, obligate anaerobe that is a pleomorphic, gram-negative bacillus of the family *Bacteroidaceae*. In broth cultures, *F. necrophorum* varies from coccoid shapes to filaments with granular inclusions. Rod shapes are more common in agar cultures. This bacteria is a component of the normal flora of the mouth, gastrointestinal tract, and urogenital tract of man and animals. Strains have varied virulence categories: pathogenic for mice; slightly pathogenic or not at all, but hemolytic, like the first category; and a third category (formerly called *Sphaerophorus pseudonecrophorus*) that is neither hemolytic nor pathogenic. There may be mutation from one category (or phase) to another. The validity of the identification of this bacteria in works prior to 1970 is questioned (Holdeman *et al.*, 1984).

Different species of *Bacteroides* play an important pathogenic role in necrobacillosis. They may appear alone or in conjunction with other species of the same genus, particularly in man, or with *F. necrophorus* in animals. *Bacteroides* spp. is also a nonsporulating, gram-negative, obligate anaerobe. *Bacteroides nodosus* is of particular interest in sheep pathology. These bacteria are nonmotile, and take the shape of straight or slightly curved rods sized 1 to 1.7 by 3 to 6 microns. They appear singly or in pairs and often have thickened ends (Holdeman *et al.*, 1984). They have numerous pili (fimbriae), an important virulence factor. The pili likely play an important role in colonization of the epidermal matrix of hooves. These appendices also make it possible to sub-classify the agent serologically into 9 serogroups containing 16 to 20 serovars or serotypes, according to their determination in different countries (Gradin *et al.*, 1991).

The polymicrobial nature of most anaerobic infections in man makes it difficult to distinguish the true pathogen or pathogens from those that merely accompany the infection (Kirby *et al.*, 1980). Singly or acting jointly with other nonsporulating, anaerobic bacteria, *F. necrophorum* causes different diseases and pathological conditions in man and animals. Different species of the genus *Bacteroides*, which belong to the same family as *F. necrophorum*, cause disease either by themselves (in man) or in combination and at times in synergistic action with *F. necrophorum* (in man and animals).

Geographic Distribution: Worldwide.

Occurrence in Man: Advances in laboratory technology for the isolation of anaerobes have led to greater recognition of their role in human pathology and, consequently, to an increase in the number of recorded cases in medical facilities.

Occurrence in Animals: Some diseases, such as foot rot in sheep, occur frequently in all countries where sheep are raised. Others, such as calf diphtheria (necrobacillary stomatitis), are less common. Bovine hepatic necrobacillosis causes appreciable economic losses in many countries due to confiscation of animals in slaughterhouses; it is more frequent in areas where cattle are fed grain in feedlots (Timoney *et al.*, 1988).

The Disease in Man: *F. necrophorum* causes a wide variety of necrotic lesions, empyema, pulmonary abscesses, arthritis, and ovariosalpingitic sepsis. *Bacteroides fragilis* and *F. necrophorum* are important agents of cerebral abscesses and, occasionally, of meningitis, almost always as a consequence of an otitis media (Islam and Shneerson, 1980). The formerly high incidence of septicemia caused by *F. necrophorum* in children and adolescents who had suffered from tonsillitis (Lemierre's syndrome) has now diminished notably and constitutes only 1% to 2% of all bacteremias caused by anaerobes. Patients with septicemia usually exhibit exudative pharyngitis or a peritonsillar abscess, but these symptoms may disappear by the time some patients obtain medical attention (Seidenfeld *et al.*, 1982). In most human clinical specimens, only the genera *Bacteroides*, *Prevotella*, *Porphyromonas*, and *Fusobacterium* should be considered among the anaerobic bacilli (Jousimies-Somer and Finegold, 1991). Infections in man come from the normal flora of adjacent cavities.

The most effective antibiotics for treating infections caused by gram-negative anaerobes are metronidazole, chloramphenicol, and imipenem (Jousimies-Somer and Finegold, 1991).

The Disease in Animals: *F. necrophorum* is more important in animal than in human pathology and is the cause of several common diseases.

SHEEP: Foot rot is the most common cause of lameness in sheep. The disease begins with interdigital dermatitis, progresses to the epidermal matrix of the hooves, and then causes destruction of the interdigital skin and detachment of the hoof. Environmental factors, such as wet soil and grass that soften the feet, are involved in producing the disease, along with two bacterial agents, *F. necrophorum* and *Bacteroides nodosus*. *F. necrophorum* establishes itself first and causes inflammation and destruction of the epidermis before penetrating to deeper layers. Hoof degeneration is due to the proteolytic properties of *B. nodosus*. The disease may appear in several forms: benign, usually caused by less virulent strains of *B. nodosus*; virulent, with deformation and detachment of the hoof; and chronic, which may last years, with or without producing lameness.

Other hoof diseases affecting sheep are interdigital dermatitis and infectious bulbar necrosis. The former, caused by *F. necrophorum*, is characterized by an edematous and erythematous inflammation of the interdigital skin, which may be covered by a layer of moist, gray, necrotic material. Infectious bulbar necrosis is caused by *F. necrophorum* and *Corynebacterium pyogenes* and is characterized by abscesses and suppuration of the bulbar area of the hoof, particularly on the hind feet. The disease results from the interaction of both bacteria. *C. pyogenes* produces a factor that stimulates proliferation of *F. necrophorum*, and the latter protects *C. pyogenes* from phagocytosis by producing a leukocidin (Cottral, 1978).

CATTLE: Calf diphtheria (necrobacillary stomatitis) is characterized by sialorrhea, anorexia, and necrotic areas in the oral cavity. Infection can spread to the larynx and, by inhalation, to the lungs, where it causes abscesses and pneumonia. The disease only occurs in animals under 2 years of age; mature animals seem immune. The disease is caused by *F. necrophorum* and is seen in dairy operations with deficient hygiene. The same disease also affects young goats.

Hepatic necrobacillosis is discovered by veterinary inspection in slaughterhouses and results in confiscation of carcasses. Lesions on the liver are characterized by well-delineated yellow areas with a firm consistency.

Foot rot in bovines is an acute or chronic necrotic infection of the interdigital skin and the coronary region. The chronic form frequently produces arthritis in the distal joint of the limb. *F. necrophorum* and *Bacteroides meleninogenicus* have been isolated from biopsy samples of foot rot lesions. A mixture of both bacteria administered by interdigital scarification or intradermal inoculation reproduced the typical lesions (Berg and Loan, 1975). Nevertheless, the etiology still has not been completely clarified, and it is possible that concurrent infection by *F. necrophorum* and other bacteria (*B. nodosus*, staphylococci) causes the disease (Timoney *et al.*, 1988). Mastitis caused by *Bacteroides fragilis* has also been described in cattle.

SWINE: Pathologies such as ulcerous stomatitis, necrotic enteritis, necrotic rhinitis, and abscesses have been described in this species.

OTHER ANIMAL SPECIES: Similarly to what happens in man, osteomyelitis in animals may be caused by anaerobes. Of a total of 39 anaerobic bacteria isolated from 19 marrow specimens, the most frequent genus was *Bacteroides* (18 isolates). *B. asaccharolyticus* was isolated from 26% of the specimens (Walker *et al.*, 1983).

Source of Infection and Mode of Transmission: *F. necrophorum* and *Bacteroides* spp. are part of the normal flora of several mucous membranes in humans and animals. The infection is endogenous, particularly in man. The relative infrequency of the disease in man indicates that predisposing factors are necessary for it to occur. These are usually traumas and debilitating illnesses. In sum, they are opportunistic agents. A lowered oxidation-reduction potential (E_h) resulting from insufficient blood supply, together with tissue necrosis and the presence of other facultative bacteria, creates a favorable environment for this and other anaerobic bacteria. Vascular disease, edema, surgery, and cold are some of the common factors favoring implantation and multiplication of anaerobes (Finegold, 1982). Most patients with anaerobic pulmonary infection (abscesses, necrotic pneumonia, pneumonitis, empyema) suffer from altered consciousness or dysphagia due to aspiration of the oropharyngeal content, which is rich in anaerobic flora. The underlying conditions are usually alcoholism, a cerebrovascular accident, general anesthesia, convulsions, and narcotics abuse, among others (Bartlett and Finegold, 1974).

An important predisposing factor in sheep and bovine foot rot is softening of the interdigital epidermis caused by moist ground, enabling *F. necrophorum* to implant itself and multiply. In addition, this bacteria abounds in humid environments (soil and grass contaminated by animal feces) and has been proved able to survive outside a host's body for several months. In contrast, *B. nodosus* is a parasite that can live for only a short time in the environment and is introduced in establishments by sick or carrier animals. *F. necrophorum* creates conditions necessary for the multiplication of *B. nodosus*. Thus, both bacteria are required to cause the disease.

As mentioned above, under different conditions other bacteria, such as *Corynebacterium pyogenes* (which causes infectious bulbar necrosis), interact synergistically with *F. necrophorum*.

Bovine hepatic necrobacillosis, the agent of which is *F. necrophorum*, has an endogenous origin. The agent possibly penetrates by way of the portal circulation from epithelial lesions in the rumen, which in turn may be caused by excessive acidity due to provision of concentrated foods.

Calf diphtheria, or necrobacillary stomatitis, is prevalent in environments where hygienic practices are markedly poor.

Role of Animals in the Epidemiology of the Disease: None. Necrobacillosis is a disease common to man and animals.

Diagnosis: When a nonsporulating, anaerobic bacterium is suspected as the cause of infection in a human patient, specimens collected from the lesions for bacteriologic diagnosis must be free of contaminants from the normal flora, of which these anaerobes are natural components. Thus, for example, when anaerobic origin is suspected for human pulmonary infection, transtracheal aspiration with a needle or direct penetration of the lung must be used. By contrast, the patient's sputum is not a suitable material for examination. In the case of empyema or abscesses, obtaining pus under aseptic conditions is not a problem (Finegold, 1982).

In veterinary practice, diagnosis of hoof diseases in sheep and cattle is based on clinical characteristics. Samples for laboratory diagnosis of hepatic necrobacillosis can be collected without difficulty. In calf diphtheria, ulcerous, necrotizing lesions with a strong, putrid odor point to the disease; if a bacteriologic examination is attempted, epithelial samples from the edges of the ulcer should be used (Guarino *et al.*, 1982).

Control: Prevention in man consists primarily of avoiding and properly treating predisposing conditions. Specific control measures are neither known nor justified.

Control of sheep foot rot is the subject of continuing research. An important preventive measure is avoiding introduction of animals from places where the disease exists, since *B. nodosus* is considered an obligate parasite. As with other contagious diseases, a period of isolation is recommended for recently acquired animals before introducing them into the flock. Once the disease is introduced, transmission may be reduced by chemoprophylaxis using a foot bath of 5% formalin, 10% zinc sulfate, or 10% copper sulfate. To control the disease, it is recommended that damaged hooves be cut during the dry season in order to expose the necrotic parts, and that the animals be given foot baths or topical treatment with the preparations indicated above, in addition to intramuscular administration of antibiotics. Studies are still under way to perfect a vaccine made with *B. nodosus*, but the existence of serogroups and serotypes within this bacterium complicates this task (Ribeiro, 1980). One study indicates that in addition to 9 serogroups (A to H), there are 16 or more serotypes. More than one serogroup of *B. nodosus* may exist in a single flock, and several serogroups are sometimes isolated from the hoof of a single sheep. Vaccines made from purified pili (which contain the principal protecting immunogen) of *B. nodosus* immunize satisfactorily against a homologous strain of the bacterium (Stewart *et al.*, 1983a). In addition to the pili, which only protect against homologous strains, there are two other immunogens that could give heterologous immunity. Vaccines made of whole cells tested against vaccines of purified pili (all having an equal pilus content) provided comparable protection. Although vaccines using whole cells are cheaper to produce and confer protection against heterologous strains, they are irritants and cause weight loss (Stewart, 1983b).

Control reduces but does not eliminate the problem. Some apparently healthy animals may harbor *B. nodosus* in their hooves and maintain the infection in the field.

Prevention of calf diphtheria is achieved principally by maintaining hygienic standards.

Chlortetracycline administered in feedlot foods helps to reduce the incidence of hepatic abscesses and allows the animals to gain weight normally (Timoney *et al.*, 1988). An important preventive measure is not allowing animals to change abruptly from their customary food to concentrated foods.

Bibliography

Bartlett, J.G., S.M. Finegold. Anaerobic infections of the lung and pleural space. *Am Rev Resp Dis* 110:56–77, 1974.

Berg, J.N., R.W. Loan. *Fusobacterium necrophorum* and *Bacteroides melaninogenicus* as etiologic agents of foot rot in cattle. *Am J Vet Res* 36:1115–1122, 1975.

Claxton, P.D., L.A. Ribeiro, J.R. Egerton. Classification of *Bacteroides nodosus* by agglutination tests. *Aust Vet J* 60:331–334, 1983.

Cottral, G.E., ed. *Manual of Standardized Methods for Veterinary Microbiology.* Ithaca: Comstock; 1978.

Finegold, S.M. Anaerobic bacteria. *In*: Wyngaarden, J.B., L.H. Smith, Jr., eds. *Cecil Textbook of Medicine.* 16th ed. Philadelphia: Saunders; 1982.

Gradin, J.L., J.A. Stephens, G.E. Pluhar, *et al.* Diversity of pilin of serologically distinct *Bacteroides nodosus. Am J Vet Res* 52:202–205, 1991.

Guarino, H., G. Uriarte, J.J. Berreta, J. Maissonnave. Estomatitis necrobacilar en terneros. Primera comunicación en Uruguay. *In*: Primer Congreso Nacional de Veterinaria, Montevideo, Sociedad de Medicina Veterinaria del Uruguay, 1982.

Holdeman, L.V., R.W. Kelley, W.E.C. Moore. Anaerobic gram-negative straight, curved and helical rods. *In*: Krieg, N.R., J.G. Holt. Vol I. *Bergey's Systematic Bacteriology.* Baltimore: Williams & Wilkins; 1984.

Islam, A.K.M.S., J.M. Shneerson. Primary meningitis caused by *Bacteroides fragilis* and *Fusobacterium necrophorum. Postgrad Med J* 56:351–353, 1980.

Jousimies-Somer, H.R., S. Finegold. Anaerobic gram-negative bacilli and cocci. *In*: Ballows, A., W.J. Hausler, Jr., K.L. Hermann, H.D. Isenberg, H.J. Shadomy, eds. *Manual of Clinical Microbiology.* 5th ed. Washington, D.C.: American Society for Microbiology; 1991.

Kirby, B.D., W.L. George, V.L. Sutter, *et al.* Gram-negative anaerobic bacilli: Their role in infection and patterns of susceptibility to antimicrobial agents. I. Little-known *Bacteroides* species. *Rev Infect Dis* 2:914–951, 1980.

Ribeiro, L.A.O. Foot-rot dos ovinos: etiología, patogenia e controle. *Bol Inst Pesq Vet Finamor* 7:41–45, 1980.

Seidenfeld, S.M., W.L. Sutker, J.P. Luby. *Fusobacterium necrophorum* septicemia following oropharyngeal infection. *JAMA* 248:1348–1350, 1982.

Stewart, D.J., B.L. Clark, D.L. Emery, J.E. Peterson, K.J. Fahey. A *Bacteroides nodosus* immunogen, distinct from the pilus, which induces cross-protective immunity in sheep vaccinated against footrot. *Aust Vet J* 60:83–85, 1983a.

Stewart, D.J., B.L. Clark, J.E. Peterson, D.A. Griffiths, E.F. Smith, I.J. O'Donnell. Effect of pilus dose and type of Freund's adjuvant on the antibody and protective responses of vaccinated sheep to *Bacteroides nodosus*. *Res Vet Sci* 35:130–137, 1983b.

Timoney, J.F., J.H. Gillespie, F.W. Scott, J.E. Barlough. *Hagan and Bruner's Infectious Diseases of Domestic Animals*. 8th ed. Ithaca: Comstock; 1988.

Walker, R.D., D.C. Richardson, M.J. Bryant, C.S. Draper. Anaerobic bacteria associated with osteomyelitis in domestic animals. *J Am Vet Med Assoc* 182:814–816, 1983.

NOCARDIOSIS

**ICD-10 A43.0 pulmonary nocardiosis; A43.1 cutaneous nocardiosis;
A43.8 other forms of nocardiosis**

Etiology: Three pathogenic species, *Nocardia asteroides*, *N. brasiliensis*, and *N. otitidiscaviarum* (*N. caviae*). The first was proposed as the type species.

Nocardia belong to the order *Actinomycetales* and are higher bacteria that resemble fungi in many characteristics. They are aerobic, gram-positive, weakly acid-fast, and form long, branched filaments that fragment into coccoid and bacillary forms. This fragmentation is the way the bacteria multiply.

Geographic Distribution: Worldwide. *Nocardia* are common members of the soil flora and act to decompose organic matter. They are not part of the normal flora of man or other animals. There seems to be a difference in the distribution of the species. *N. asteroides* has been identified all over the world, while *N. brasiliensis* is present mainly in tropical and subtropical climates in North, Central, and South America (Pier, 1979; Land *et al.*, 1991). *N. otitidiscaviarum* predominates in the soil in the US, India, Japan, Mexico, and Tunisia (Land *et al.*, 1991).

Occurrence in Man: Nocardiosis is not a reportable disease and there is no reliable information on its frequency. Cases are sporadic. In the US (Beaman *et al.*, 1976), an estimated 500 to 1,000 cases occur each year. Between 1972 and 1974, 81.2% of the cases were due to *N. asteroides*, 5.6% to *N. brasiliensis*, 3% to *N. otitidiscaviarum*, and 10.2% to unspecified *Nocardia*. The majority of cases occurred in people between 21 and 50 years of age, and the male to female ratio was 3 to 1.

Occurrence in Animals: The frequency of animal nocardiosis is not well known. Different diseases due to *Nocardia* spp. have been described in cattle, sheep, monkeys, dogs, cats, wild animals, marine mammals, and fish. In New Zealand, where little attention had been paid to this disease previously, 34 cases were reported between 1976 and 1978, and 26 of these were manifested as bovine mastitis (Orchard, 1979).

The Disease in Man: The principal agent is *N. asteroides*. Nocardiosis is a suppurative infection whose course varies from acute to chronic, with a tendency toward remission. The most common clinical form is pulmonary. Pulmonary nocardiosis may become chronic if not treated properly. Acute pneumonic forms occur primarily in immunodeficient patients (Lerner, 1991). The symptomatology is not specific: cough, respiratory difficulty, and hemoptysis when there is chronic cavitation. It usually begins with a primary pyogenous lesion in the lungs. Through hematogenous dissemination, the agent localizes in different organs and tissues. Cerebral abscesses are frequent. Between 20% and 38% of persons with nocardiosis show nervous symptoms. The case fatality rate in patients with cerebral abscesses is nearly 50%. A few cases of cerebral abscesses caused by *N. otitidiscaviarum* have been reported (Bradsher *et al.*, 1982). Other localizations include subcutaneous tissue, bones, and various organs.

Smego and Gallis (1984) analyzed 62 cases of infection caused by *N. brasiliensis* in the US, from their own files and from the literature. Of the 62 patients, 46 had both a cutaneous disease and a soft tissue disease. The cutaneous disease took the form of cellulitis, pustules, ulcers, pyoderma, subcutaneous abscesses, and mycetoma. Six patients had a pleuropulmonary disease and one of them also had a disease of the central nervous system. Dissemination of the disease, which is considered characteristic of *N. asteroides*, was seen in eight cases. Traumas were an important predisposing factor in cutaneous nocardiosis in 19 of 43 cases. All the patients with cutaneous or soft tissue disease recovered, as did 83% of the pulmonary patients. Case fatality was high in the cases of dissemination.

The recommended treatment is cotrimoxazole, sulfisoxazole, or sulfadiazine. It is important that treatment begin as soon as possible and continue for some time. In cases that are resistant to the sulfonamides, it is advisable to add amikacin or high doses of ampicillin (Benenson, 1990).

The incubation period is unknown. It most likely varies depending on the virulence and phase of multiplication of the *Nocardia* strain, as well as the host's resistance. Most (85%) cases of nocardiosis have occurred in immunologically compromised persons (Beaman *et al.*, 1976).

N. brasiliensis seldom causes pulmonary disease, but more frequently produces mycetomas.

The Disease in Animals: Cattle are the most affected species. *N. asteroides* and, more rarely, *N. otitidiscaviarum* are agents of bovine mastitis. The udder usually becomes infected one to two days after calving (Beaman and Sugar, 1983), but the disease may appear throughout lactation, frequently caused by unhygienic therapeutic infusions into the milk duct. The disease course varies from acute to chronic. The mammary gland becomes edematous and fibrotic. Fever is common and prolonged. Pus forms with small granules (microcolonies) as do fistulas to the surface. There may also be lymphatic or hematogenous dissemination to other organs. Among animals with acute infection, mortality is high.

Bovine nocardiosis may also manifest as pulmonary disease (especially in calves under 6 months of age), abortions, lymphadenitis of various lymph nodes, and lesions in different organs.

Canids are the second most affected group. The principal agent is *N. asteroides*, but infections caused by *N. brasiliensis* and *N. otitidiscaviarum* have also been described. The clinical picture is similar to that in man, and the most common clinical form is pulmonary. Dogs exhibit fever, anorexia, emaciation, and dyspnea.

Dissemination from the lungs to other organs is frequent and may affect the central nervous system, bones, and kidneys. The cutaneous form is also common in dogs, with purulent lesions usually located on the head or extremities. Nocardiosis is most frequent in male dogs under 1 year of age. The fatality rate is high (Beaman and Sugar, 1983).

Nocardiosis in cats is more unusual and is seen mostly in castrated males. Most cases are due to *N. asteroides*, but 30% have been attributed to *N. brasiliensis* or to other similar nocardias.

A disease with multiple pyogranulomatous foci in the liver, intestines, peritoneum, lungs, and brain was described in three macaque monkeys (*Macaca mulatta* and *M. menestrina*). *Nocardia* spp. was isolated in two cases. The assumption is that two monkeys were infected orally (Liebenberg and Giddens, 1985). Earlier references record five cases in monkeys, four of which had a localized infection. Pulmonary lesions were found in three of them. *N. otitidiscaviarum* was isolated from the hand of a baboon (*Papio* spp.) and a cynomolgus macaque (*M. fascicularis*) had lesions on the brain, jaws, lungs, heart, and liver (Liebenberg and Giddens, 1985).

The recommended treatment is prolonged administration of cotrimoxazole for some six weeks.

Source of Infection and Mode of Transmission: Nocardias are components of the normal soil flora. These potential pathogens are much more virulent during the logarithmic growth phase than during the stationary phase, and it is believed that actively growing soil populations are more virulent for man and animals (Orchard, 1979).

Man probably acquires the infection by inhaling contaminated dust. Predisposing causes are important in the pathogenesis of the disease, since most cases occur either in persons with deficient immune systems or those taking immunosuppressant drugs. An outbreak was confirmed among patients in a renal transplant unit and the strain of *N. asteroides* was isolated from the dust and air in the room (Lerner, 1991). Mycetomas caused by *N. brasiliensis* may be caused by a trauma to the skin. Wounds that come into contact with the soil may become infected by *Nocardia* spp. The most common route of infection by *N. brasiliensis* is through traumatic inoculation of the skin by thorns, nails, cat scratches, or burns (Smego and Gallis, 1984).

Animals probably contract pulmonary infections in the same way as man. Mastitis occurring later in the lactation period is produced by contaminated catheters. Mastitis at the beginning of lactation is more difficult to explain. It is possible that the focus of infection already exists in the nonlactating cow and that when the udder fills with milk, the infection spreads massively through the milk ducts and causes clinical symptoms (Beaman and Sugar, 1983). However, the origin of the initial infection remains an enigma, but it could also be due to the insertion of contaminated instruments. The multiple cases of nocardia-induced mastitis that are at times observed in a dairy herd are attributable to transmission of the infection from one cow to another by means of contaminated instruments or therapeutic infusions.

Role of Animals in the Epidemiology of the Disease: Nocardiosis is a disease common to man and animals; soil is the reservoir and source of infection. There are no known cases of transmission from animals to man or between humans.

Diagnosis: Microscopic examination of exudates can indicate nocardiosis, but only culture and identification of the agent provide a definitive diagnosis. In pulmonary nocardiosis, bronchoalveolar lavage and aspiration of abscesses or collection of fluids can be used, guided by radiology (Forbes *et al.*, 1990).

Various serological tests have been described. An enzyme immunoassay with an antigen (a 55-kilodalton protein) specific for *Nocardia asteroides* yielded good results in terms of both sensitivity and specificity (Angeles and Sugar, 1987). Serodiagnosis in immunodeficient patients—who currently suffer more frequently from nocardiosis—is very difficult. A more recent work (Boiron and Provost, 1990) suggests that the 54-kilodalton protein would be a good candidate as an antigen for a probe for detecting antibodies in nocardiosis.

Control: No specific control measures are available. Prevention consists of avoiding predisposing factors and exposure to dust (Pier, 1979). Environmental hygiene and sterilization of instruments are important.

For control of mastitis caused by *Nocardia* spp. in cows, it is recommended that udder hygiene practices be adopted as well as general hygiene rules for the dairy facility.

Bibliography

Angeles, A.M., A.M. Sugar. Rapid diagnosis of nocardiosis with an enzyme immunoassay. *J Infect Dis* 155:292–296, 1987.

Beaman, B.L., J. Burnside, B. Edwards, W. Causey. Nocardial infections in the United States, 1972–1974. *J Infect Dis* 134:286–289, 1976.

Beaman, B.L., A.M. Sugar. *Nocardia* in naturally acquired and experimental infections in animals. *J Hyg* 91:393–419, 1983.

Benenson, A.S., ed. *Control of Communicable Diseases in Man.* 15th ed. An official report of the American Public Health Association. Washington, D.C.: American Public Health Association; 1990.

Boiron, P., F. Provost. Use of partially purified 54-kilodalton antigen for diagnosis of nocardiosis by Western blot (immunoblot) assay. *J Clin Microbiol* 28:328–331, 1990.

Bradsher, R.W., T.P. Monson, R.W. Steele. Brain abscess due to *Nocardia caviae*: Report of a fatal outcome associated with abnormal phagoctye function. *Am J Clin Pathol* 78:124–127, 1982.

Forbes, G.M., F.A. Harvey, J.N. Philpott-Howard, *et al.* Nocardiosis in liver transplantation: Variation in presentation, diagnosis and therapy. *J Infect* 20:11–19, 1990.

Land, G., M.R. McGinnis, J. Staneck, A. Gatson. Aerobic pathogenic *Actinomycetales. In*: Balows, A., W.J. Hausler, K.L. Hermann, H.D. Isenberg, H.J. Shadomy, eds. *Manual of Clinical Microbiology.* 5th ed. Washington, D.C.: American Society for Microbiology; 1991.

Lerner, P.L. *Nocardia* species. *In*: Mandell, G.L., R.G. Douglas, Jr., J.E. Bennett, eds. *Principles and Practice of Infectious Diseases.* 3rd ed. New York: Churchill Livingstone, Inc.; 1990.

Liebenberg, S.P., W.E. Giddens. Disseminated nocardiosis in three macaque monkeys. *Lab Animal Sci* 35:162–166, 1985.

Orchard, V.A. Nocardial infections of animals in New Zealand, 1976–78. *N Z Vet J* 27:159–160, 165, 1979.

Pier, A.C. *Actinomycetes. In*: Stoenner, H., W. Kaplan, M. Torten, eds. Vol 1, Section A: *CRC Handbook Series in Zoonoses.* Boca Raton: CRC Press; 1979.

Smego, R.A., H.A. Gallis. The clinical spectrum of *Nocardia brasiliensis* infection in the United States. *Rev Infect Dis* 6:164–180, 1984.

PASTEURELLOSIS

ICD-10 A28.0

Synonyms: Shipping fever, bovine respiratory disease complex, fibrinous pneumonia (cattle); pasteurella pneumonia (lambs); hemorrhagic septicemia (cattle, lambs); fowl cholera; snuffles (rabbits).

Etiology: The genus *Pasteurella* was reclassified on the basis of DNA:DNA hybridization in order to determine the genetic relationship of the different accepted or proposed species (Mutters *et al.*, 1985). Based on the results of that study, the genus has been subdivided into 11 species. The species of interest here are: *Pasteurella multocida*, *P. dagmatis* sp. nov., *P. canis* sp. nov., and *P. stomatis* sp. nov. *P. caballi*, described more recently, should be added as well (Schater *et al.*, 1989). *P. haemolytica*, an important pathogen for animals and, occasionally, for man, is more related to the genus *Actinobacillus* and might receive its own generic name in the future (Mutters *et al.*, 1986). In addition, the DNA:DNA hybridization between strains of biotype A and biotype T ranges only from 3% to 13%, depending on the biotype used as the reference strain, and thus the two biotypes should be classified as separate species (Bingham *et al.*, 1990). The advantages of reclassification are not yet evident in epidemiological research, diagnosis, and treatment. Pasteurellae are small, pleomorphic, nonmotile, gram-negative, bipolar staining, nonsporulating bacilli, with little resistance to physical and chemical agents.

Subdivision of *P. multocida* and *P. haemolytica* into serotypes is important in the areas of epidemiology and control (vaccines). Subclassification of *P. multocida* into serotypes is based on its capsular (A, B1, D, and E) and somatic (1–16) antigens; the latter can occur in different combinations. *P. haemolytica* has been subdivided into two biotypes (A and T) and 15 serotypes.

Geographic Distribution: *P. multocida* and *P. haemolytica* are distributed worldwide. The distribution of the other species is less well-known, but based on their reservoirs they can be assumed to exist on all continents.

Occurrence in Man: Rare. It is not a reportable disease and its incidence is little known. According to laboratory records, 822 cases occurred in Great Britain from 1956 to 1965. A special survey in the US revealed 316 cases caused by *P. multocida* from 1965 to 1968. Data on the occurrence of human pasteurellosis in other countries are scarce. The disease caused by *P. haemolytica* is rare.

Occurrence in Animals: Common in domestic and wild species of mammals and birds.

The Disease in Man: The principal etiologic agent of human pasteurellosis is *P. multocida*. The other species make a lesser contribution to human disease. Fifty-six cultures from Göteborg University (Sweden), obtained from human cases of pasteurellosis, were reexamined. As a result, 26 strains were reclassified as *P. multocida* subspecies *multocida*; 11 as *P. multocida* ssp. *septica*; 12 as *P. canis*; 4 as *P. dagmatis*, and 1 as *P. stomatis*. Two strains were provisionally classified, one as *P. haemolytica* biogroup 2 (T) and another as belonging to the group that cannot be typed (Bisgaard and Falsen, 1986). The main clinical symptoms of the disease consist of infected bites or scratches inflicted by cats or dogs (or occasionally by other animals), diseases of the respiratory system, and localized infections in different organs and tissues. Cases of septicemia are rare. The English-language literature records 21 cases of meningitis (Kumar et al., 1990).

Various cases of pasteurellosis in pregnant women have been described. One primigravida who was carrying twins suffered from chorioamnionitis caused by P. multocida at 27 weeks, after her membranes had broken. The twin close to the cervix became infected and died shortly after birth, while the other twin did not become infected. It is believed that the infection rose upwards from the vagina, with asymptomatic colonization (Wong et al., 1992). Two pregnant women with no history of concurrent disease received phenoxymethylpenicillin in an early phase of pasteurellosis. Despite the treatment, one of them became ill with meningitis and the other suffered cellulitis with deep abscess formation. Both of them had animals (dog and cat), but had not been bitten (Rollof et al., 1992).

Most clinical cases arise from infected wounds. Most cats and dogs are normal carriers of Pasteurella and harbor the etiologic agent in the oral cavity. The microorganism is transmitted to the bite wound and a few hours later produces swelling, reddening, and intense pain in the region. The inflammatory process may penetrate into the deep tissue layers, reaching the periosteum and producing necrosis. Septic arthritis and osteomyelitis are complications that occur with some frequency. Septic arthritis often develops in patients suffering from rheumatoid arthritis. Cases have been described in which articular complications appeared several months and even years after the bite (Bjorkholm and Eilard, 1983). Of 20 cases of osteomyelitis with or without septic arthritis, 10 developed from cat bites, 5 from dog bites, 1 from dog and cat bites, and 4 had no known exposure (Ewing et al., 1980).

P. multocida may also aggravate certain respiratory tract diseases, such as bronchiectasis, bronchitis, and pneumonia. In terms of case numbers, chronic respiratory conditions from which the agent is isolated are second in importance to infection transmitted by animal bite or scratch. Septicemia and endocarditis are extremely rare.

The age group most affected is persons over 40 years old, despite the fact that bites are more frequent in children and younger people.

P. multocida is sensitive to penicillin, but some resistant animal and human strains have been found; thus, it is advisable to do an antibiogram. In vitro tests have also shown excellent sensitivity to ampicillin, third-generation cephalosporins, and tetracycline (Kumar et al., 1990).

The Disease in Animals: Pasteurellae have an extremely broad spectrum of animal hosts. Many apparently healthy mammals and birds can harbor pasteurellae in the upper respiratory tract and in the mouth. According to the most accepted hypothesis, pasteurellosis is a disease of weakened animals that are subjected to stress and poor hygienic conditions. In an animal with lowered resistance, pasteurellae harbored in the fauces or trachea may become pathogenic for their host. There is a marked difference in the level of virulence among different strains of P. multocida. In some diseases, P. multocida is the primary and only etiologic agent; in others, it is a secondary invader that aggravates the clinical picture.

A relationship exists between the serotype of Pasteurella, its animal host, and the disease it causes. Therefore, serologic typing is important for epizootiologic studies as well as for control (through vaccination).

Bovine hemorrhagic septicemia is caused by *P. multocida* serotype 6:B in Asia, and by 6:E and 6:B in Africa. In fibrinous pneumonia ("shipping fever") in cattle, serotype 1 of *P. haemolytica*, and serotype 2:A of *P. multocida* predominate.

CATTLE: Shipping fever, also called bovine respiratory disease complex, is a syndrome that causes large economic losses in the cattle industry of the Western Hemisphere. In the US, it causes annual losses estimated at more than US$ 25 million. Shipping fever is an acute respiratory disease that particularly affects beef calves and heifers as well as adult cows when they are subjected to the stress of prolonged transport. The symptomatology varies from a mild respiratory illness to a rapidly fatal pneumonia. Symptoms generally appear from 5 to 14 days after the cattle reach their destination, but some may be sick on arrival. The principal symptoms are fever, dyspnea, cough, nasal discharge, depression, and appreciable weight loss. The fatality rate is low.

The etiology of the disease has not been completely clarified, and it is noteworthy that the disease does not occur in Australia, even when animals are transported over long distances (Irwin *et al.*, 1979). Several concurrent factors are believed to cause the syndrome. Most prominent among these are such stress factors as fatigue, irregular feeding, exposure to cold or heat, and weaning. Viral infections, which occur constantly throughout a herd and are often inapparent, are exacerbated by factors such as overcrowding during transport. Moreover, susceptible animals suddenly added to a herd lead to increased virulence. The virus most often identified as the primary etiologic agent is parainfluenza virus 3 (PI3) of the genus *Paramyxovirus*. Infection by this virus alone usually causes a mild respiratory disease. However, the damage it causes to the respiratory tract mucosa aids such secondary invaders as *P. multocida* and *P. haemolytica*, which aggravate the clinical picture. On the other hand, virulent strains of *Pasteurella* can cause the disease by themselves. Pasteurellae frequently isolated in cases of shipping fever include *P. haemolytica* biotype A, serotype 1, and various serotypes of group A of *P. multocida*. The fact that treatment with sulfonamides and antibiotics gives good results also indicates that a large part of the symptomatology is due to pasteurellae. Another important viral agent that acts synergistically with pasteurellae is the herpesvirus of infectious bovine rhinotracheitis. Similarly, viral bovine diarrhea, chlamydiae, and mycoplasmas can play a part in the etiology of this respiratory disease.

An important disease among cattle and water buffalo in southern and southeastern Asia is hemorrhagic septicemia. In many countries, it is the disease responsible for the most losses once rinderpest has been eradicated. Hemorrhagic septicemia also occurs in several African countries, including Egypt and South Africa, and, less frequently, in southern Europe. The disease seems to be enzootic in American bison, and several outbreaks have occurred (the last one in 1967), without the disease spreading to domestic cattle (Carter, 1982). In tropical countries, hemorrhagic septicemia occurs during the rainy season. The main symptoms are fever, edema, sialorrhea, copious nasal secretion, and difficulty in breathing. Mortality is high. Surviving animals become carriers and perpetuate the disease. Cases of hemorrhagic septicemia have also been recorded in horses, camels, swine, yaks, and other species. It must be borne in mind that hemorrhagic septicemia is due to the specific *P. multocida* serotypes 6:B and 6:E. There is no evidence that the disease occurs in domestic cattle in the Americas.

P. multocida is also responsible for cases of mastitis.

SHEEP: *P. haemolytica* is the etiologic agent of two different clinical forms, pneumonia and septicemia. Biotype A serotype 2 is the most prevalent agent of pasteurella pneumonia among lambs in Great Britain (Fraser *et al.*, 1982). Pulmonary disease in sheep follows a viral infection (P13). Although *Pasteurella* is a secondary invader, it is the predominant pathogen. Occurrence of the disease is sporadic or enzootic. The main symptoms are a purulent nasal discharge, cough, diarrhea, and general malaise. Lesions consist of hemorrhagic areas in the lungs and petechiae in the pericardium. Pasteurella septicemia is caused by biotype T of *P. haemolytica* and appears in temperate climates in the fall, when the sheep's diet is changed (Gillespie and Timoney, 1981). In Mexico, 860 pneumonic lungs were examined, and 120 isolates of *P. haemolytica* type A were obtained from them. The most common serotypes were 1 (22%), 2 (16%), 5 (11%), and 9 (7%). Twenty-seven percent of the isolates could not be typed (Colin *et al.*, 1987). *P. haemolytica* is the only etiologic agent of sporadic sheep mastitis in the western US, Australia, and Europe (Blood *et al.*, 1979).

SWINE: Pasteurellosis also appears in the form of pneumonia and, more rarely, as septicemia. *Pasteurella* may be a primary or secondary agent of pneumonia, particularly as a complication of the mild form of classic swine plague (hog cholera) or mycoplasmal pneumonia. The anterior pulmonary lobes are the most affected, with hepatization and a sero-fibrinous exudate on the surface. Serotype 3:A of *P. multocida* is the most prevalent in chronic swine pneumonia (Pijoan *et al.*, 1983). Studies have revealed evidence of the etiologic role of toxigenic strains of *P. multocida* serotype D in atrophic rhinitis. *Bordetella bronchiseptica* acting synergistically with toxigenic strains of *P. multocida* probably causes this disease, the etiology of which has been the subject of much debate (Rutter, 1983).

Atrophic rhinitis is characterized by atrophy of the nasal turbinate bones, sometimes with distortion of the septum. Experiments have shown that the agents— *B. bronchiseptica* and toxigenic *P. multocida*—can cause the disease separately in 1-week-old gnotobiotic suckling pigs. However, turbinate atrophy is more severe and may become complete when the animals are inoculated with both agents (Rhodes *et al.*, 1987). Atrophic rhinitis could not be seen in some herds from which only *B. bronchiseptica* was isolated. The purified toxin of type D strains of *P. multocida*, inoculated intranasally, caused severe turbinate atrophy (Dominick and Rimler, 1986).

Various outbreaks of hemorrhagic septicemia caused by *P. multocida* 2:B have been reported in India. In one of these outbreaks, 40% of the herd died (Verma, 1988).

RABBITS: Pasteurellosis is common in rabbit hutches. The most frequent clinical manifestation is coryza. As in other animal species, the disease appears under stressful conditions. The principal symptoms are a serous or purulent exudate from the nose and sometimes from the eyes, sneezing, and coughing. The pathological process may spread to the lungs. Septicemia and death are not uncommon. Males that are kept together may show pasteurella-infected abscesses produced by bites. An atrophic rhinitis syndrome also occurs in rabbits. Autopsy of 52 adult rabbits revealed that 26 of them (50%) had turbinate atrophy. *P. multocida* and *B. bron-*

chiseptica were isolated from more than 70% of the rabbits. Six percent of those from which only *B. bronchiseptica* was isolated had the syndrome (DiGiacomo *et al.*, 1989).

WILD ANIMALS: Pasteurellosis occurs in many wild animal species, among which occasional epizootic outbreaks take place. The etiologic agent is *P. multocida; P. haemolytica* has not yet been isolated. Two disease forms are found: hemorrhagic septicemia, in which the whole animal body is invaded by pasteurellae, and the respiratory syndrome or pulmonary pasteurellosis.

FOWL: Fowl cholera is an acute septicemic disease with high morbidity and morality in all species of domestic fowl. Its incidence has diminished worldwide due to improved commercial poultry management practices. The disease usually appears on poultry farms where hygiene is deficient. Explosive outbreaks may occur two days after infected birds are introduced into a flock. Mortality is variable, at times reaching 60% of the poultry on a farm. Many of the survivors become carriers and give rise to new outbreaks. At the beginning of a hyperacute outbreak, fowl die without premonitory symptoms; mortality increases, but the only symptom seen is cyanosis of the wattle and comb. Later, the disease process slows down and respiratory symptoms appear. Cases of chronic or localized pasteurellosis may occur following an acute outbreak, or the disease may take this course from the outset of infection. The chronic disease is caused by attenuated strains of *P. multocida* and manifests itself mostly as "wattle disease" (edematization and later caseation of these appendages). Another localization can be the wing or foot joints. Fowl cholera is produced by *P. multocida* of serogroup A, predominantly serotypes 1 and 3 (Mushin, 1979); some strains of group D have also been isolated, but they seem to be less pathogenic. *P. multocida* causes outbreaks with high mortality among wild birds, especially waterfowl.

Source of Infection and Mode of Transmission: The reservoir includes cats, dogs, and other animals. The etiologic agent is harbored in the upper respiratory passages. Cats are the carriers of the agent 70% to 90% of the time, but dogs (20% to 50%), sheep, cattle, rabbits, and rats are also important carriers (Kumar *et al.*, 1990). The most common form of the disease (60% to 86% of cases) is a wound contaminated as the result of an animal bite. Cats are primarily responsible in 60% to 75% of the cases, followed by dogs. The mode of transmission for the pulmonary form is probably aerosolization of the saliva of cats or dogs. Some patients (7% to 13%) do not acknowledge having been bitten by or otherwise exposed to animals (Kumar *et al.*, 1990).

For human infections transmitted by animal bite or scratch, the source of the infection and the mode of transmission are obvious. Except in the case of bites, animal-to-man transmission is accomplished through the respiratory or digestive tract. An analysis of 100 cases of human pasteurella infections of the respiratory tract and other sites found that 69% of the patients had had contact with dogs or cats, or with cattle, fowl, or their products. Nevertheless, 31% of the patients denied all contact with animals; consequently, it is suspected that interhuman transmission may also occur.

Among fowl, where *P. multocida* is undoubtedly the primary agent of infection, the source of the outbreaks is carrier fowl, and transmission occurs predominantly by means of aerosols. Dogs and cats rarely suffer from pasteurellosis (with the exception of wounds infected with pasteurellae in fights) and are healthy carriers. Other mammals acquire the disease from members of their own species either through the respiratory or digestive tract, or by falling victim to the pasteurellae in their own respiratory tracts when stress lowers their defenses. There is much evidence that stress factors play an important enabling role in unleashing the respiratory syndrome of shipping fever, and that these factors permit multiplication of serotype 2 of *P. haemolytica* (Frank and Smith, 1983). Serotypes 6:B and 6:E, which cause hemorrhagic septicemia in cattle and water buffalo, are perpetuated by means of carriers and chronically ill animals that serve as a source of infection for their kind.

Role of Animals in the Epidemiology of the Disease: Pasteurellae survive only a very short time in the environment. It is certain that animals constitute the most important reservoir of the pasteurellae that are pathogenic for man.

Diagnosis: In the case of human infection, diagnosis is made by isolating and identifying the etiologic agent from wounds or other sites.

In hemorrhagic septicemia or fowl cholera, the etiologic agent can be cultivated from the animal's blood or viscera. In pneumonia of domestic animals, a pure culture of pasteurellae may indicate their role in the pathology, but does not reveal whether these bacteria are primary or secondary agents of the disease.

Control: Measures to reduce the likelihood of bites, such as elimination of stray dogs, can prevent some cases of human infection.

Control in animals lies mainly in adequate management of herds or poultry farms. Bacterins as well as live attenuated vaccines are in use, or are being tested, against *P. multocida* and *P. haemolytica*. Protection against homologous serotypes is satisfactory, but protection is only partial or irregular against heterologous serotypes. In general, attenuated live vaccines give better immunity than bacterins. In Asia, extensive experimentation proved that a bacterin with an oil adjuvant can offer solid immunity against hemorrhagic septicemia. A single dose of live vaccine with a streptomycin-dependent mutant strain conferred immunity against hemorrhagic septicemia in 66.6% to 83.3% of calves and in 100% of young buffalo (De Alwis and Carter, 1980).

The use of PI3 vaccine has been recommended for the control of shipping fever. It is better to vaccinate against the principal viral agents before weaning or transporting animals. The bacterins of *P. haemolytica* and *P. multocida* have been questioned. Attenuated live vaccines or vaccines from subunits, such as the cytotoxin (leukotoxin) of *P. haemolytica* (Confer *et al.*, 1988), are more reliable. Attenuated live vaccines of *P. haemolytica* are being tested. A bacterin containing multiple antigens of the prevalent serotypes, incorporated into a polyvalent anticlostridial biological with aluminum hydroxide adjuvant, has been tested against *P. haemolytica* pneumonia in lambs and has given satisfactory results (Wells *et al.*, 1984). Several live vaccines are available against avian cholera, some of which can be administered in the drinking water. Selection of *Pasteurella* strains within the serotypes that cause the disease is important in immunization.

Bovine hemorrhagic septicemia should be considered an exotic disease and appropriate measures should be taken to prevent its spread to disease-free areas.

Bibliography

Bingham, D.P., R. Moore, A.B. Richards. Comparison of DNA:DNA homology and enzymatic activity between *Pasteurella haemolytica* and related species. *Am J Vet Res* 51:1161–1166, 1990.

Bisgaard, M., E. Falsen. Reinvestigation and reclassification of a collection of 56 human isolates of *Pasteurellaceae*. *Acta Pathol Microbiol Immunol Scand [B]* 94:215–222, 1986.

Bisgaard, M., O. Heltberg, W. Fredriksen. Isolation of *Pasteurella caballi* from an infected wound on a veterinary surgeon. *Acta Pathol Microbiol Immunol Scand* 99(3):291–294, 1991.

Bjorkholm, B., T. Eilard. *Pasteurella multocida* osteomyelitis caused by cat bite. *J Infect* 6:175–177, 1983.

Blood, D.C., J.A. Henderson, O.M. Radostits. *Veterinary Medicine*. 5th ed. Philadelphia: Lea and Febiger; 1979.

Bruner, D.W., J.H. Gillespie. *Hagan's Infectious Diseases of Domestic Animals*. 6th ed. Ithaca: Comstock; 1973.

Burdge, D.R., D. Scheifele, D.P. Speert. Serious *Pasteurella multocida* infections from lion and tiger bites. *JAMA* 253:3296–3297, 1985.

Carter, G.R. Pasteurellosis: *Pasteurella multocida* and *Pasteurella haemolytica* [review]. *Adv Vet Sci* 11:321–379, 1967.

Carter, G.R. Pasteurella infections as sequelae to respiratory viral infections. *J Am Vet Med Assoc* 163:863–864, 1973.

Carter, G.R. Whatever happened to hemorrhagic septicemia? *J Am Vet Med Assoc* 180:1176–1177, 1982.

Colin, R., L. Jaramillo M., F. Aguilar R., *et al.* Serotipos de *Pasteurella haemolytica* en pulmones neumónicos ovinos en México. *Rev Latinoam Microbiol* 29:231–234, 1987.

Confer, A.W., R.J. Panciera, D.A. Mosier. Bovine pneumonic pasteurellosis: Immunity to *Pasteurella haemolytica* [review]. *J Am Vet Med Assoc* 193:1308–1316, 1988.

De Alwis, M.C., G.R. Carter. Preliminary field trials with a streptomycin-dependent vaccine against haemorrhagic septicaemia. *Vet Rev* 106:435–437, 1980.

DiGiacomo, R.F., B.J. Deeb, W.E. Giddens, *et al.* Atrophic rhinitis in New Zealand white rabbits infected with *Pasteurella multocida*. *Am J Vet Res* 50:1460–1465, 1989.

Dominick, M.A., R.B. Rimler. Turbinate atrophy in gnotobiotic pigs intranasally inoculated with protein toxin isolated from type D *Pasteurella multocida*. *Am J Vet Res* 47:1532–1536, 1986.

Ewing, R., V. Fainstein, D.M. Musher, M. Lidsky, J. Clarridge. Articular and skeletal infections caused by *Pasteurella multocida*. *South Med J* 73:1349–1352, 1980.

Frank, G.H, R.G. Marshall. Parainfluenza-3 virus infection of cattle. *J Am Vet Med Assoc* 163:858–859, 1973.

Frank, G.H., P.C. Smith. Prevalence of *Pasteurella haemolytica* in transported calves. *Am J Vet Res* 44:981–985, 1983.

Fraser, J., N.J. Gilmour, S. Laird, W. Donachie. Prevalence of *Pasteurella haemolytica* serotypes isolated from ovine pasteurellosis in Britain. *Vet Rec* 110:560–561, 1982.

Gillespie, J.H., J.F. Timoney. *Hagan's and Bruner's Infectious Diseases of Domestic Animals*. 7th ed. Ithaca: Comstock; 1981.

Harshfield, G.S. Fowl cholera. *In*: Biester, H.E., L.H. Schwarte, eds. *Diseases of Poultry*. 4th ed. Ames: Iowa State University Press; 1959.

Hoerlein, A.B. Shipping fever. *In*: Gibbons, W.J., ed. *Diseases of Cattle*. 2nd ed. Santa Barbara: American Veterinary Publications; 1963.

Hubbert, W.T., M.N. Rosen. *Pasteurella multocida* infection due to animal bite. *Am J Public Health* 60:1103–1108, 1970.

Hubbert, W.T., M.N. Rosen. *Pasteurella multocida* infections. II. *Pasteurella multocida* infection in man unrelated to animal bite. *Am J Public Health* 60:1109–1117, 1970.

Irwin, M.R., S. McConnell, J.D. Coleman, G.E. Wilcox. Bovine respiratory disease complex: A comparison of potential predisposing and etiologic factors in Australia and the United States. *J Am Vet Med Assoc* 175:1095–1099, 1979.

Kumar, A., H.R. Devlin, H. Vellend. *Pasteurella multocida* meningitis in an adult: Case report and review. *Rev Infect Dis* 12:440–448, 1990.

Mair, N.S. Some *Pasteurella* infections in man. *In*: Graham-Jones, O., ed. *Some Diseases of Animals Communicable to Man in Britain*. Oxford: Pergamon Press; 1968.

Mushin, R. Serotyping of *Pasteurella multocida* isolants from poultry. *Avian Dis* 23:608–615, 1979.

Mutters, R., M. Bisgaard, S. Pohl. Taxonomic relationship of selected biogroups of *Pasteurella haemolytica* as revealed by DNA:DNA hybridizations. *Acta Pathol Microbiol Immunol Scand* [B] 94:195–202, 1986.

Mutters, R., P. Ihm, S. Pohl, W. Frederiksen, W. Manuheim. Reclassification of the genus *Pasteurella* Trevisan 1887 on the basis of deoxyribonucleic acid homology with proposals for the new species *Pasteurella dagmatis*, *Pasteurella canis*, *Pasteurella stomatis*, *Pasteurella anatis*, and *Pasteurella langaa*. *Int J Syst Bacteriol* 35:309–322, 1985.

Namioka, S., M. Murata, R.V.S. Bain. Serological studies on *Pasteurella multocida*. V. Some epizootiological findings resulting from O antigenic analysis. *Cornell Vet* 54:520–534, 1964.

Pijoan, C., R.B. Morrison, H.D. Hilley. Serotyping of *Pasteurella multocida* isolated from swine lungs collected at slaughter. *J Clin Microbiol* 17:1074–1076, 1983.

Rhodes, M.B., C.W. New, P.K. Baker, *et al. Bordetella bronchiseptica* and toxigenic type D *Pasteurella multocida* as agents of severe atrophic rhinitis of swine. *Vet Microbiol* 13:179–187, 1987.

Rollof, J., P.J. Johansson, E. Holst. Severe *Pasteurella multocida* infection in pregnant women. *Scand J Infect Dis* 24:453–456, 1992.

Rosen, M.N. Pasteurellosis. *In*: Davis, J.W., L.H. Karstad, D.O. Trainer, eds. *Infectious Diseases of Wild Mammals*. Ames: Iowa State University Press; 1970.

Rutter, J.M. Virulence of *Pasteurella multocida* in atrophic rhinitis of gnotobiotic pigs infected with *Bordetella bronchiseptica*. *Res Vet Sci* 34:287–295, 1983.

Schlater, L.K., D.J. Brenner, A.G. Steigerwalt, *et al. Pasteurella caballi*, a new species from equine clinical specimens. *J Clin Microbiol* 27:2169–2174, 1989.

Verma, N.D. *Pasteurella multocida* B:2 in haemorrhagic septicaemia outbreak in pigs in India. *Vet Rec* 123:63, 1988.

Wells, P.W., J.T. Robinson, N.J. Gilmour, W. Donachie, J.M. Sharp. Development of a combined clostridial and *Pasteurella haemolytica* vaccine for sheep. *Vet Rec* 114:266–269, 1984.

Wong, G.P., N. Cimolai, J.E. Dimmick, T.R. Martin. *Pasteurella multocida* chorioamnionitis from vaginal transmission. *Acta Obstet Gynecol Scand* 71:384–387, 1992.

PLAGUE

ICD-10 A20.0 bubonic plague; A20.2 pneumonic plague; A20.7 septicaemic plague

Synonyms: Black death, pestilential fever, pest.

Etiology: The etiologic agent of plague is *Yersinia pestis*, a gram-negative, non-motile bacterium, coccobacillary to bacillary in form and showing bipolar staining that is not very resistant to physical and chemical agents. DNA hybridization studies demonstrated the close genetic relationship between *Yersinia pestis* and *Y. pseudotuberculosis* (Bercovier *et al.*, 1980). On the basis of this, the authors suggested calling the etiologic agent of plague *Y. pseudotuberculosis* subsp. *pestis* (International Committee on Systemic Bacteriology, List 7, 1981). However, the Committee's Judicial Commission (1985) decided to reject this nomenclature and retain the name *Y. pestis* in order, among other reasons, to avoid possible confusion. Three biological varieties are distinguished: *Orientalis* (oceanic), *Antiqua* (continental), and *Mediaevalis*. This distinction has a certain epidemiological significance, principally for nosography, but there is no difference in the biotypes' pathogenicity.

Some virulence factors of *Y. pestis* were defined in the 1980s. Apparently, the principal factor is a 45-megadalton plasmid. This plasmid encodes calcium dependency for growth at 37°C, but not at lower temperatures, as well as the virulence antigens V and W. The two proteins on the outer membranes that are assumed to be important in virulence (E and K) are also plasmid dependent. The precise role of each of these factors is not yet well defined (Butler, 1989).

Geographic Distribution: Natural foci of infection persist on nearly all continents; they do not exist in Australia, New Zealand, or New Guinea. In the Americas, sylvatic plague is maintained in rodents in the western third of the United States, the border region of Ecuador and Peru, southeastern Bolivia, and northeastern Brazil. Similarly, there are foci in north-central, eastern, and southern Africa, including Madagascar; the Near East; the border area between Yemen and Saudi Arabia; Kurdistan province (Iran); and central and Southeast Asia, in Myanmar (Burma) and Vietnam. There are also several natural foci in the former Soviet Union and in Indonesia (Benenson, 1990).

Occurrence in Man: Since the dawn of the Christian era, there have been three great pandemics: the first began in 542 (Justinian plague) and is estimated to have caused 100 million deaths; the second began in 1346, lasted three centuries, and claimed 25 million victims; and the last began in 1894 and continued until the 1930s. However, the data on incidence in the Middle Ages are very approximate and difficult to verify. As a result of the last pandemic, natural foci of infection were established in South America, West Africa, South Africa, Madagascar, and Indochina.

Urban plague has been brought under control in almost the entire world, and rural plague of murine origin is also on the decline. Nevertheless, epidemics have occurred in Indonesia, Nepal, and southern Vietnam. In this last country, there were 5,274 cases in 1967 due to contact with domestic rats and their fleas.

From 1958 to 1979, 46,937 cases of human plague were recorded in 30 countries; if Vietnam is excluded, the total number is reduced to 15,785. The large number of cases in Vietnam is attributed to military operations there and consequent ecologic changes. On the other hand, 16 of the 30 countries reporting plague cases were in Africa. However, incidence of the disease on that continent was very low, less than 6% of the world total (Akiev, 1982). Figure 14 shows the number of cases and deaths caused by human plague worldwide from 1971 to 1980.

The incidence of plague from 1977 to 1991 included 14,752 cases with 1,391 deaths distributed in 21 countries (WHO, 1993).

In 1991, there was a large increase of cases in Africa, with a total of 1,719 people affected, due primarily to an outbreak in Tanzania. In that country, there were 60 deaths among a total of 1,293 cases, 1,060 of which occurred in the Tanga region. There were also 137 cases reported in Madagascar and 289 in Zaire (WHO, 1993).

In Asia, there were 226 total cases, with 15 deaths. There were 100 cases in Myanmar, 94 in Vietnam, 29 in China (with 11 deaths), and the remainder in two other countries (WHO, 1993).

There are seven countries in the Americas with cases of plague: Bolivia, Brazil, Ecuador, Peru, the US, and occasionally, Colombia and Venezuela (Akiev, 1982). During the period 1971–1980, there were 2,312 cases in the Americas (Table 2), 1,551 of which occurred in Brazil, 316 in Peru, 247 in Bolivia, 123 in the US, and 75 in Ecuador (PAHO, 1981). In all the countries, the number of cases fluctuated greatly from year to year; at times, epidemic outbreaks have occurred. Plague continues to be a public health problem in the Americas because of the persistence of sylvatic plague and the link between domestic and wild rodents. In Ecuador, an outbreak of seven cases occurred in May 1976 in Nizac, Chimborazo Province, a settlement of 850 inhabitants. The outbreak was preceded by a large epizootic in rats and mortality among guinea pigs raised in homes for food. The worst outbreak since 1966 occurred in 1984 in northern Peru, with 289 cases reported in 40 localities. An association was presumed between this outbreak and a great abundance of rodents, possibly the result of ecologic changes due to flooding (Rust, 1985).

In the US, 35 cases were recorded from April to August 1983, the greatest number of cases since 1925. Almost all the cases occurred in five southwestern states.

Twenty-one cases of plague were reported in the Americas in 1991. Ten of these occurred in Brazil and 11 in the US, although there were no deaths (WHO, 1993). In 1992, there were 8 cases in Brazil (all in Bahia) and 13 in the US (4 in Arizona, 4 in New Mexico, and 1 each in five more states) (OPS, 1992). One of the cases in Arizona was primary pulmonary plague in a 31-year-old patient who died one day after being admitted to the hospital. Blood and urine cultures taken from the patient were negative. After the patient's death, *Y. pestis* was isolated from the sputum. The source of the infection was a sick cat. This is the third case in the US of primary pulmonary plague contracted from a cat. The incubation period is very short in these cases (two to three days) and the symptoms do not lead one to suspect plague (CDC, 1992). There have been no cases of direct human-to-human transmission in the US since 1924 (Benenson, 1990).

In October 1992, an outbreak of plague was reported in Cajamarca (Peru) which is still active. In nine localities affected, with an estimated at-risk population of 30,000, there were 547 cases and 19 deaths (up to mid-January 1994). The outbreaks were preceded by deaths among wild rodents and guinea pigs (*Cavia porcellus*) bred

Figure 14. Number of cases and deaths from human plague worldwide, 1971–1980.

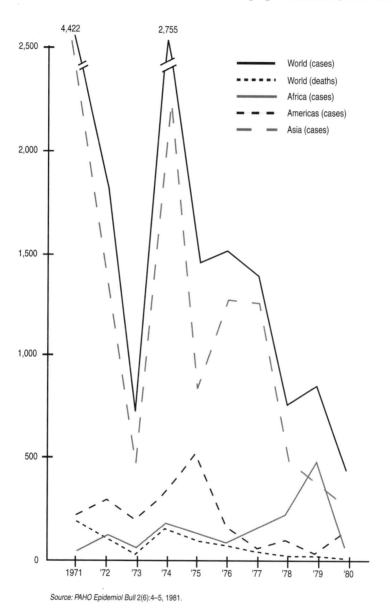

Source: PAHO Epidemiol Bull 2(6):4–5, 1981.

Table 2. Number of cases and deaths from human plague in the Americas, 1971–1980.

Country	1971 C	1971 D	1972 C	1972 D	1973 C	1973 D	1974 C	1974 D	1975 C	1975 D	1976 C	1976 D	1977 C	1977 D	1978 C	1978 D	1979 C	1979 D	1980 C	1980 D
Bolivia	19	3	0	0	0	0	14	5	2	0	24	5	29	9	68	2	10	0	26	2
Brazil	146	2	169	13	152	...	291	...	496	5	97	...	1	...	11	...	0	0	98	0
Ecuador	27	0	9	0	1	1	0	0	0	0	8	1	0	0	0	0	0	0	0	0
Peru	22	5	118	15	30	2	8	2	3	0	1	0	0	0	6	1			0	0
United States of America[a]	2	0	1	0	2	0	8	1	20	4	16	3	18	2	12	2	13	2	18	5
Total	216	10	297	28	185	3	321	8	521	9	146	9	48	11	97	5	23	2	142	7

C = Cases
D = Deaths
... Data unavailable
[a]Plague found in rodents.
Source: *PAHO Epidemiol Bull* 2(6):4–5, 1981.

at home by the peasants. One factor that helped to increase the number of cases was that rodenticides were used without simultaneous or prior use of flea pulicides (Report from Dr. Alfonso Ruiz to the Pan American Health Organization, February 8, 1994).

Occurrence in Animals: Natural infection by *Y. pestis* has been found in 230 species and subspecies of wild rodents. In natural foci, sylvatic plague is perpetuated through the continuous circulation of the etiologic agent, transmitted by fleas from one rodent to another. It is generally believed that the survival of the etiologic agent in a natural focus depends on the existence of rodent species, or individuals within a species, with differing levels of susceptibility. The most resistant individuals are host to and infect the fleas, which in turn infect susceptible animals in the area and can spread to domestic rodents. Susceptible animals generally die, but they increase the population of infected fleas by means of their bacteremia. When the number of susceptible individuals is large and climatic conditions favorable, an epizootic may develop in which many rodents die. As the epizootic diminishes, the infection continues in enzootic form in the surviving population until a new outbreak occurs. Infection may remain latent in enzootic foci for a long time, and the absence of human cases should not be interpreted as a sign that the natural focus is eliminated.

During the period 1966–1982, 861 isolates were taken of *Y. pestis* in foci in northeastern Brazil. Of these, 471 were from rodents or other small mammals, 236 were from batches of fleas, 2 from batches of *Ornithodorus*, and 152 from patients. In the rodents, the highest number of isolates were taken from *Zygodontomys lasiarus pixuna*, which also provided the highest number of fleas, primarily of the genus *Polygenis*; on only one occasion was the agent isolated from cat fleas (*Ctenocephalides felis*). The agent was isolated from human fleas (*Pulex irritans*) found on the floor of dwellings on 10 occasions. Human flea infection suggests the possibility of human-to-human transmission through flea bites, usually after a fatal case in the family (Almeida *et al.*, 1985).

House cats that come into contact with rodents and/or their fleas can become infected and fall ill, and can transmit the infection to man. In the US and South Africa, several cases of the disease in cats have been described (Kaufmann *et al.*, 1981; Rollag *et al.*, 1981). In New Mexico (USA), 119 cases of plague were reported in domestic cats from 1977 to 1988 (Eidson *et al.*, 1991). There is also evidence that camels and sheep in enzootic plague areas can contract the infection and that, in turn, man can become infected when sacrificing these animals. Such cases occurred in Libya (Christie *et al.*, 1980).

The Disease in Man: The incubation period lasts from two to six days, though it may be shorter. Three clinical forms of plague are recognized: bubonic, septicemic, and pneumonic. The symptoms shared by all three are fever, chills, cephalalgia, nausea, generalized pain, diarrhea, or constipation; toxemia, shock, arterial hypotension, rapid pulse, anxiety, staggering gait, slurred speech, mental confusion, and prostration are also frequent.

Bubonic plague—the most common form in interpandemic periods—is characterized by acute inflammation and swelling of peripheral lymph nodes (buboes), which can become suppurative. There may be a small vesicle at the site of the flea bite. The buboes are painful and the surrounding area is usually edematous.

Bacteremia is present at the beginning of the disease. The fatality rate in untreated cases is from 25% to 60%. At times, the disease may take the form of a mild, localized, and short-lived infection (pestis minor). Another, less frequent form is meningitis, which occurs primarily after ineffective treatment for bubonic plague (Butler, 1988). In septicemic plague, nervous and cerebral symptoms develop extremely rapidly. Epistaxis, cutaneous petechiae, hematuria, and involuntary bowel movements are seen. The course of the disease is very rapid, from one to three days, and case fatality may reach nearly 100%.

Pneumonic plague may be a secondary form derived from the bubonic or septicemic forms by hematogenous dissemination, or it may be primary, produced directly by inhalation during contact with a pneumonic plague patient (primary pneumonic plague). In addition to the symptoms common to all forms, dyspnea, cough, and expectoration are present. The sputum may vary from watery and foamy to patently hemorrhagic. This is the most serious form.

Primary pneumonic plague, the origin of which is human-to-human transmission by aerosol and which has caused outbreaks and sometimes devastating epidemics, is rare. The pneumonic form seen in present times is the secondary form, resulting from septicemic dissemination. Since 1925, the US has recorded very few cases of primary pneumonic plague, all of which have resulted from exposure to a cat with secondary pneumonia. The first case occurred in California in 1980 (CDC, 1982). A similar case occurred more recently in Arizona (CDC, 1992). In total, there have been three cases of primary pneumonia with the same characteristics. Secondary invasion of the lungs (secondary pneumonic plague) occurs in untreated patients and approximately 95% of them die without becoming transmitters of the agent by aerosol. If left untreated, the small number of patients who do not die may give rise to other cases of pneumonic plague by airborne transmission (Poland and Barnes, 1979). In countries that maintain epidemiologic surveillance and where physicians and the general population are alert to the disease, the high fatality rates caused by all forms of plague have been largely arrested by early diagnosis and prompt treatment with antibiotics, such as streptomycin, tetracycline, and chloramphenicol.

The Disease in Animals: *Y. pestis* primarily infects animals of the order *Rodentia*; if affects wild as well as domestic rodents and, to a lesser degree, rabbits and hares (lagomorphs). The infection may be acute, chronic, or inapparent. Different species of rodents and different populations of the same species show varying degrees of susceptibility. In this regard, it has been observed that a population in an enzootic area is more resistant than another in a plague-free area, a phenomenon attributed to natural selection. Domestic (commensal) rats are very susceptible; *Rattus rattus* die in large numbers during epizootics. By contrast, susceptibility varies greatly between different species in natural foci and must be determined for each situation. In the western United States, prairie dogs (*Cynomys* spp.) and the ground squirrel *Citellus beecheyi* are very susceptible, while certain species of *Microtus* or *Peromyscus* are resistant.

Lesions found in susceptible animals dead from plague vary with the course of the disease. In acute cases, hemorrhagic buboes and splenomegaly are present without other internal lesions; in subacute cases the buboes are caseous, and punctiform necrotic foci are found in the spleen, liver, and lungs.

Natural infection in cats has come under close scrutiny, as they have been a source of infection for man in several instances. Feline plague is characterized by formation of abscesses, lymphadenitis, lethargy, and fever (Rollag *et al.*, 1981). Secondary pneumonia may also be present, as in the case at Lake Tahoe, California, where a kitten transmitted the infection to a man by aerosol. Fatality is over 50% in cats infected experimentally. In contrast, dogs inoculated with the plague agent react only with fever. Other carnivores are not very susceptible, with the exception of individuals with greater than normal susceptibility, as might be expected in any animal population.

Natural infection has been recorded in camels and sheep in the former Soviet Union and Libya (Christie *et al.*, 1980) and, more recently, in camels from Saudi Arabia (A. Barnes, personal communication).

Source of Infection and Mode of Transmission (Figure 15): Wild rodents are the natural reservoir. The maintenance hosts vary in each natural focus, but they are almost always rodent species with low susceptibility, i.e., the animals become infected but do not die from the disease. Very susceptible species, in which many animals die during an epizootic, are important in amplification and diffusion of the infection as well as in its transmission to man, but they cannot be permanent hosts. The epizootics that afflict prairie dogs (*Cynomys* spp.) are devastating. In one epizootic, only some animals survived in two of seven colonies. Another explosive epizootic annihilated an entire colony of 1,000 to 1,500 animals in two months. A third epizootic reduced the population by 85% (Ubico *et al.*, 1988). *R. rattus* is very susceptible, but the infection usually dies out rapidly in this species. Only in some circumstances, as occurred in India, can it serve as a temporary host, but not for many years. Consequently, the persistence of a focus depends on rodent species that have a wide spectrum of partial resistance.

In a natural focus, the infection is transmitted from one individual to another by fleas. Different species of fleas vary greatly in their efficiency as vectors. Biological

Figure 15. Plague. Domestic and peridomestic transmission cycle.

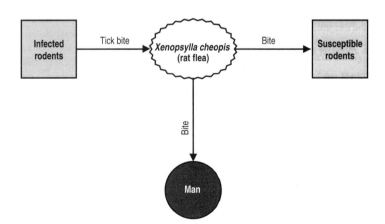

vectors are characterized by the blocking phenomenon. When *Y. pestis* is ingested with the septicemic host's blood, the agent multiplies in the flea's stomach and the proventriculum becomes blocked by the mass of bacteria. When a blocked flea tries to feed again, it regurgitates the bacteria into the bloodstream of the new host (this is the case with *Xenopsylla cheopis*, the domestic rat flea). Wild rodent fleas are generally less efficient and their capacity as biological vectors varies; it is believed that mechanical transmission may be important in natural foci. Also, these vectors are not very species-specific and can transmit the infection between different rodent species living in an enzootic area. The etiologic agent survives for a long time in fleas; some have remained infected for a period of 396 days. For this reason, fleas may be considered part of the natural reservoir, which would be an arthropod-vertebrate complex. More than 200 species of fleas have been implicated in the transmission of plague.

Infection from a natural focus may be passed to commensal rodents (domestic rats and mice) by members of the ubiquitous rodent species that approach human dwellings and can thus initiate an outbreak of plague within households. In the same way, peridomestic rodents may come into contact with wild rodents. Transmission is effected by means of fleas.

Other mammals (dogs, marsupials) may also serve as the link between the wild and domestic cycles by transporting fleas from one place to another. In northeastern Brazil, South American short-tailed gray opossums (*Monodelphis domestica*) naturally infected with the plague agent via *Polygenis bohlsi jordani* (a principal vector of sylvatic plague in this region) have been found to live near and enter houses. The natural plague foci can experience long periods of reduced activity, during which the proportion of infected rodents is small and no human cases occur. When these foci become active, epizootics among rodents and, at times, epidemic outbreaks can occur. Such could have been the case in the central Java (Indonesia) focus where no human plague had occurred since 1959, but where 100 cases were reported in 1968 and 40 in 1971.

When man enters a natural focus, he may contract the infection through bites of fleas of wild rodents or lagomorphs, or through skin abrasions or bites when handling these animals. Human cases are sporadic under these circumstances. When plague penetrates the domestic and peridomestic environment, man is infected via fleas of commensal rodents, and epidemic outbreaks may result. The domestic rat flea (*Xenopsylla cheopis*) is the biological vector *par excellence* of plague. The name zootic plague has been given to plague transmitted by insects. Indirect interhuman transmission via human ectoparasites (*Pulex irritans* and *Pediculus humanis*) is rare and has only been observed in heavily infected environments. In some areas of the Andes, this mode of transmission occurs with some frequency, especially during wakes for those who have died of plague. These outbreaks almost always occur within families.

Secondary pneumonia as a complication of bubonic or septicemic plague may give rise to a series of primary pneumonic plague cases through interhuman transmission via the respiratory route. This is so-called demic plague. At present, bubonic plague is eminently zoonotic and occurs primarily in semi-arid areas.

Cats have transmitted the infection in a small proportion of cases (in the US, 2.2% from 1930 to 1979). Because buboes in cats are located in the head and neck region, it is thought that cats contract the infection by consuming infected rodents. Transmission from cat to man has resulted from direct contact, bites, or scratches.

Role of Animals in the Epidemiology of the Disease: Perpetuation of plague depends on the *Y. pestis*-rodents-fleas complex in natural foci. Plague in commensal rats is usually a collateral phenomenon to sylvatic plague, and so, by extension, is demic plague.

Diagnosis: Early diagnosis is essential to protect the patient and the community. Diagnosis is confirmed in the laboratory by puncturing the bubo and collecting fluid from gelatinous edemas, cerebrospinal fluid, and sputum for preparation of a Gram- or Giemsa-stained smear, and culturing in appropriate media. The culture can be identified rapidly using specific phagocytolysis or the immunofluorescence and agglutination tests.

An index case (the first case in a community), which may be the precursor of an outbreak, can be provisionally diagnosed with the rapid immunofluorescence test, using material from a bubo, and confirmed later by culture or inoculation in laboratory animals (guinea pigs or mice).

Hemoculture can be used in the initial, septicemic period of bubonic plague.

The serological tests most often used for human patients are passive hemagglutination and the fluorescent antibody test. The enzyme-linked immunosorbent assay (ELISA) procedure for detecting the F1 antigen (Fraction 1) of *Y. pestis* with monoclonal antibodies yields apparently satisfactory results, but does not eliminate the need for bacteriological confirmation (Williams *et al.*, 1986).

Inoculation of laboratory animals has proven superior to culture on culture media for plague research in rodents or fleas. Passive hemagglutination is of great value for epizootic studies of the infection, both in native rodent populations and in sentinel animals in natural foci. Resistant animals, such as dogs, can fulfill the latter surveillance function. During a plague episode in which one man in southeastern Utah (USA) died, the only evidence of the infection's activity was the discovery of positive titers in two of the family dogs. In the same country, coyotes have proved useful as sentinels. Coyotes rarely die of plague, but produce antibodies against the disease agent; in addition, since they feed on sick and dead rodents, examining a coyote is equivalent to examining several hundred rodents. A rapid serological test (an enzymatic immunoassay) has been perfected for testing these animals (Willeberg *et al.*, 1979). The passive hemagglutination test, employing specific Fraction-1 antigen (pesticin), is also useful in retrospective studies of plague in human communities in enzootic areas. A DNA probe has been developed that could prove useful in epidemiological surveillance of plague (McDonough *et al.*, 1988).

Control: Prevention of human plague is based on control of rodents and vectors of infection. Eradication of natural foci is a long-term, costly, and difficult task that can be achieved by changing the ecology of the foci and dedicating the enzootic area to agriculture. In general, the objectives of prevention campaigns are more limited and consist mainly of emergency programs in situations with a high potential for human infection. In all areas where natural plague foci exist, continuous surveillance must be maintained (dogs have been used very successfully as sentinel animals) and emergency measures set in motion if cases of the disease develop. Essentially, these measures consist of the use of insecticides and rodenticides. Insecticides should be employed before or at the same time as rodenticides, but never after, as fleas abandon dead animal hosts and seek out new hosts, including man. During outbreaks, the main effort should be directed toward flea control, which is very effective and economical. If human plague cases occur, patients must be isolated (stringent isolation is required for pneumonic patients) and treated. All contacts should be disinfected and kept under surveillance; if deemed necessary, chemoprophylaxis (tetracycline and sulfonamides) should be given for six days; flea and rodent control should be continued. In such places as the Andes, where flea infestations on humans are prevalent, prophylactic measures are recommended for persons attending funerals of plague victims, along with strict control of these cases to prevent human-to-human transmission.

In the mountains of Tienshan (China), measures were taken to control the gray or Altai marmot (*Marmota baibacina*), a reservoir of plague. Between 1967 and 1987, the marmot population was reduced from 14.52 animals for every 10 hectares in 1967 to 0.91 in 1987. More recently, bacteriologic and serologic tests were performed on 5,000 marmots and 2,000 domestic dogs; with the exception of three dogs, the tests were negative. No more human cases were reported (Lu *et al.*, 1991).

The inactivated vaccine provides protection for no more than six months and vaccination is justified only for inhabitants of high-incidence areas, laboratory personnel who work with plague, and people who must enter a plague focus. It should be kept in mind that several doses are needed to obtain a satisfactory level of protection. The inactivated vaccine was used on US troops in Vietnam and is believed to have been very useful in protecting them.

Plague is subject to control measures established under the International Sanitary Code (World Health Organization).

Bibliography

Akiev, A.K. Epidemiology and incidence of plague in the world, 1958–79. *Bull World Health Organ* 60:165–169, 1982.

Almeida, A.M.P. de., D.P. Brasil, F.G. de Carvalho, C.R. de Almeida. Isolamento da *Yersinia pestis* nos focos pestosos do nordeste do Brasil no periodo de 1966 a 1982. *Rev Inst Med Trop Sao Paulo* 27:207–218, 1985.

Benenson, A.S., ed. *Control of Communicable Diseases in Man*. 15th ed. An official report of the American Public Health Association. Washington, D.C.: American Public Health Association; 1990.

Bercovier, H., H.H. Mollaret, J.M. Alonso, J. Brault, G.R. Fanning, A.G. Steigerwalt, *et al.* Intra- and interspecies relatedness of *Yersinia pestis* by DNA hybridization and its relationship to *Yersinia pseudotuberculosis*. *Curr Microbiol* 4:225–229, 1980.

Butler, T. Plague. *In*: Warren, K.S., A.A.F. Mahmoud, eds. *Tropical and Geographical Medicine*. New York: McGraw-Hill; 1984.

Butler, T. The black death past and present. 1. Plague in the 1980s. *Trans R Soc Trop Med Hyg* 83:458–460, 1989.

Christie, A.B., T.H. Chen, S.S. Elberg. Plague in camels and goats: Their role in human epidemics. *J Infect Dis* 141:724–726, 1980.

Davis, D.H.S., A.F. Hallett, M. Isaacson. Plague. *In*: Hubbert, W.T., W.F. McCulloch, P.R. Schnurrenberger, eds. *Diseases Transmitted from Animals to Man*. 6th ed. Springfield: Thomas; 1975.

Dinger, J.E. Plague. *In*: Van der Hoeden, J., ed. *Zoonoses*. Amsterdam: Elsevier; 1964.

Eidson, M., J.P. Thilsted, O.J. Rollag. Clinical, clinicopathologic, and pathologic features of plague in cats: 119 cases (1977–1988). *J Am Vet Med Assoc* 199:1191–1197, 1991.

Hudson, B.W., M.I. Goldenberg, J.D. McCluskie, H.E. Larson, C.D. McGuire, A.M.

Barnes, *et al.* Serological and bacteriological investigations of an outbreak of plague in an urban tree squirrel population. *Am J Trop Med Hyg* 20:225–263, 1971.

International Committee on Systemic Bacteriology, List 7. Validation of the publication of new names and new combinations previously effectively published outside USB. *Int J Syst Bacteriol* 31:382–383, 1981.

Judicial Commission of the International Commitee on Systemic Bacteriology. Opinion 60. Rejection of the name *Yersinia pseudotuberculosis* subsp. *Yersinia pestis* (Lehmann and Neumann) van Loghem 1944 for the plague bacillus. *Int J Syst Bacteriol* 35:540, 1985.

Kartman, L., M.I. Goldenberg, W.T. Hubbert. Recent observations on the epidemiology of plague in the United States. *Am J Public Health* 56:1554–1569, 1966.

Kaufmann, A.F., J.M. Mann, T.M. Gardiner, F. Heaton, J.D. Poland, A.M. Barnes, *et al.* Public health implications of plague in domestic cats. *J Am Vet Med Assoc* 179:875–878, 1981.

Lu, C.F. [Epidemiologic significance of the eradication of the gray marmot (*Marmota baibacina*) in natural foci in the mountains of Tienshan, in Hutubi District, Xinjang]. *Bull Endem Dis* 5:4–18, 1990–1991.

McDonough, K.A., T.G. Schwan, R.E. Thomas, S. Falkow. Identification of a *Yersinia pestis*-specific DNA probe with potential for use in plague surveillance. *J Clin Microbiol* 26:2515–2519, 1988.

Meyer, K.F. Pasteurella and Francisella. *In*: Dubos, R.J., J.G. Hirsch, eds. *Bacterial and Mycotic Infections of Man.* 4th ed. Philadelphia: Lippincott; 1965.

Olsen, P.F. Sylvatic (wild rodent) plague. *In*: Davis, J.W., L.H. Karstad, D.O. Trainer, eds. *Infectious Diseases of Wild Mammals.* Ames: Iowa State University Press; 1970.

Organización Panamericana de la Salud (OPS). Enfermedades sujetas al Reglamento Sanitario Internacional. *Bol Epidemiol* 13:16, 1992.

Pan American Health Organization (PAHO). *Health Conditions in the Americas, 1969–1972.* Washington, D.C.: PAHO; 1974. (Scientific Publication 287).

Pan American Health Organization (PAHO). Status of plague in the Americas, 1970–1980. *Epidemiol Bull* 2:5–8, 1981.

Pan American Health Organization (PAHO). *Plague in the Americas.* Washington, D.C.: PAHO; 1965. (Scientific Publication 115).

Pavlovsky, E.N. *Natural Nidality of Transmissible Diseases.* Urbana: University of Illinois Press; 1966.

Poland, J.D., A.M. Barnes. Plague. *In*: Stoenner, H., W. Kaplan, M. Torten, eds. Vol 1, Section A: *CRC Handbook Series in Zoonoses.* Boca Raton: CRC Press; 1979.

Pollitzer, R. A review of recent literature on plague. *Bull World Health Organ* 23:313–400, 1960.

Pollitzer, R., K.F. Meyer. The ecology of plague. *In*: May, J.M., ed. *Studies in Disease Ecology.* New York: Hafner Pub. Co.; 1961.

Rollag, O.J., M.R. Skeels, L.J. Nims, J.P. Thilsted, J.M. Mann. Feline plague in New Mexico: Report of five cases. *J Am Vet Med Assoc* 179:1381–1383, 1981.

Rust, J.H. Plague research in northern Peru. PAHO/WHO report, June 1985.

Stark, H.E., B.W. Hudson, B. Pittman. *Plague Epidemiology.* Atlanta: US Centers for Disease Control and Prevention; 1966.

Tirador, D.F., B.E. Miller, J.W. Stacy, A.R. Martin, L. Kartman, R.N. Collins, *et al.* Plague epidemic in New Mexico, 1965. An emergency program to control plague. *Public Health Rep* 82:1094–1099, 1967.

Ubico, S.R., G.O. Maupin, K.A. Fagerstone, R.G. McLean. A plague epizootic in the white-tailed prairie dogs (*Cynomys leucurus*) of Meeteetse, Wyoming. *J Wildl Dis* 24:399–406, 1988.

United States of America, Department of Health and Human Services, Centers for Disease Control and Prevention (CDC). Human plague—United States, 1981. *MMWR Morb Mortal Wkly Rep* 31:74–76, 1982.

United States of America, Department of Health and Human Services, Centers for Disease Control and Prevention (CDC). Pneumonic plague—Arizona, 1992. *MMWR Morb Mortal Wkly Rep* 41:737–739, 1992.

Willeberg, P.W., R. Ruppanner, D.E. Behymer, H.H. Higa, C.E. Franti, R.A. Thomson, *et al.* Epidemiologic survey of sylvatic plague by serotesting coyote sentinels with enzyme immunoassay. *Am J Epidemiol* 110:328–334, 1979.

Williams, J.E., L. Arntzen, G.L. Tyndal, M. Isaacson. Application of enzyme immunoassays for the confirmation of clinically suspect plague in Namibia, 1982. *Bull World Health Organ* 64:745–752, 1986.

World Health Organization (WHO). *WHO Expert Committee on Plague. Fourth Report.* Geneva: WHO; 1970. (Technical Report Series 447).

World Health Organization (WHO). Human plague in 1991. *Wkly Epidemiol Rec* 68(4):21–23, 1993.

PSEUDOTUBERCULOUS YERSINIOSIS

ICD-10 A28.2 extraintestinal yersiniosis

Etiology: *Yersinia pseudotuberculosis* is a coccobacillary, gram-negative bacteria that is motile at 25°C, nonmotile at 37°C, and can live a long time in soil and water. It belongs to the family *Enterobacteriaceae.* DNA hybridization studies have confirmed the close relationship between the agent of plague and that of pseudotuberculous yersiniosis.

Y. pseudotuberculosis is subdivided on the basis of its biochemical properties into five biotypes and on the basis of somatic (O) antigens into six serogroups (1–6), types 1, 2, 4, and 5 of which are divided into subgroups (Schiemann, 1989). More recently, Tsubokura *et al.* (1993) expanded the serogroups to 11 and also added a subgroup to O:1 (O:1C).

Virulent strains of *Y. pseudotuberculosis* have a plasmid that determines the virulence factors, including a kinase that determines the pathogenicity of the strains (Galyov *et al.*, 1993).

Geographic Distribution: The distribution of the etiologic agent is probably worldwide. The greatest concentration of animal and human cases is found in Europe, the Russian Far East, and Japan.

Occurrence in Man: For many years, pseudotuberculous yersiniosis was considered a disease that almost exclusively affected animals. However, since the 1950s, cases of lymphadenitis were described in children who had been operated on for appendicitis. In slightly more than three years, 117 cases of the disease were reported in Germany, most of which were diagnosed serologically. Hundreds of cases were diagnosed in Europe in later years (Schiemann, 1989).

Outbreaks occur as well as sporadic cases, which are possibly more numerous. An epidemic outbreak with 19 cases occurred in Finland (Tertti *et al.*, 1984). In the

Russian Far East, a scarlatiniform form of the disease has been described, with several thousand cases (Stovell, 1980). Three outbreaks occurred in the period 1982–1984 in Okayama Prefecture (Japan). In one outbreak, serogroup 5a was isolated from 16 patients and the infection was tied to contaminated foods. The other two outbreaks occurred in remote mountainous regions and affected a large number of preschool- and school-aged children, as well as adults. In these two outbreaks, a common source of infection could not be found, although it may have been well or stream water. Serotype 2c was detected in the feces of one patient and in well water. In another case, serotype 4b was detected in the feces of the patient and of a wild animal (Inoue et al., 1988).

Also in Japan, outbreaks occurred in 1991 in Aomori Prefecture in four primary schools and one secondary school. A total of 732 people became ill, including students, teachers, and administrative personnel; 134 were hospitalized. Y. pseudotuberculosis serotype 5a was isolated from 27 (81.8%) of the 33 samples examined. The strains isolated had the plasmid that determines various virulence factors, such as calcium dependence at 37°C and autoagglutination. The outbreak was attributed to food served in the schools, but no specific food could be pinpointed. The etiologic agent was also isolated from wastewater and the cooks' feces (Toyokawa et al., 1993). Serotypes 1, 2, and 3 have been isolated in Asia, Europe, Canada, and the US; serotypes 4 and 5 have been isolated in Europe and Japan; and serotype 6 has been isolated in a few cases in Japan (Quan et al., 1981).

Occurrence in Animals: Numerous species of domestic and wild mammals, birds, and reptiles are naturally susceptible to the infection. The disease occurs sporadically in domestic animals. In Europe, devastating epizootics have been described in hares. Epizootic outbreaks have occurred in guinea pigs, wild birds, turkeys, ducks, pigeons, and canaries. Serotype 1 predominates in animal disease.

The Disease in Man: The disease mainly affects children, adolescents, and young adults. In the past, the most recognized clinical form was mesenteric adenitis or pseudoappendicitis with acute abdominal pain in the right iliac fossa, fever, and vomiting. In the outbreaks in Okayama Prefecture, abdominal pains were accompanied by diarrhea. In another large outbreak in Japan, 86.4% of 478 patients had pyrexia, 73.8% had rashes, 66.7% had abdominal pain, and 63.4% experienced nausea and vomiting. Another frequent sign is strawberry tongue and painful pharyngeal redness. In the 19 patients studied in Finland (Tertti et al., 1984), the disease lasted from one week to six months. Twelve of the patients had complications: six had erythema nodosum, four had arthritis, one had iritis, and one had nephritis.

The incubation period is still unclear, but is estimated to last from one to three weeks.

Septicemia caused by Y. pseudotuberculosis is rare and usually appears in weakened individuals, particularly in the elderly or immunodeficient.

In the Russian Far East, a scarlatiniform type of the disease has been described. This syndrome is characterized by fever, a scarlatiniform rash, and acute polyarthritis. The disease can be reproduced in volunteers using cultures of the agent isolated from patients (Stovell, 1980).

Y. pseudotuberculosis is sensitive to tetracycline. Ofloxacin proved very effective in treatment tested on infected rats, but the beta-lactams were not effective (Lemaitre et al., 1991).

The Disease in Animals: Outbreaks of yersiniosis in guinea pig colonies have occurred in several parts of the world with some frequency. The course of the disease in these animals is usually subacute. The mesenteric lymph nodes become swollen and caseous, and sometimes there are nodular abscesses in the intestinal wall, spleen, liver, and other organs The animal rapidly loses weight and often has diarrhea. The disease lasts about a month. The septicemic form is rarer; the animal dies in a few days without showing significant symptoms. Mortality varies from 5% to 75%. Apparently healthy animals infected with *Y. pseudotuberculosis* that remain in the colony can perpetuate the infection and cause new outbreaks. Serotype 1 was isolated in an outbreak in a colony of guinea pigs in Argentina (Noseda *et al.*, 1987).

In cats, anorexia, gastroenteritis, jaundice, and often palpable mesenteric lymph nodes and hypertrophy of the spleen and liver are observed. Death can ensue two or three weeks after the onset of the disease.

Epizootics with abortions, suppurative epididymo-orchitis, and high mortality have been recorded in sheep in Australia and Europe. In Australian sheep, infection caused by serotype 3 of *Y. pseudotuberculosis* is common and occurs primarily in animals 1 to 2 years of age. The infection lasts up to 14 weeks during winter and spring (Slee and Skilbeck, 1992). Affected animals usually experience diarrhea and weight loss. Symptoms include characteristic microabscesses in the intestinal mucosa and increased thickness in the colonic and cecal mucosa (Slee and Button, 1990). Isolated cases with abortions and abscesses have been confirmed in sheep in several countries. Serotypes O:3 and O:1 have been isolated from goats in Australia. Diarrhea and loss of conditioning are the most notable symptoms (Slee and Button, 1990). Abortions and neonatal death were described in a herd of goats (Witte *et al.*, 1985).

The infection and disease in cattle have been recognized in several countries. In Australia, they are caused by serotype 3, which seems to prevail in the country's ruminants. In an episode of diarrhea in a dairy herd, 35 young animals died; in 20 of 26 examined histologically, the characteristic microabscesses were found in the intestinal mucosa. The disease occurred during the winter, spring, and early summer. In adult animals, there was a high rate of serologic reactors (Slee *et al.*, 1988). The disease has also been described in Australia in adult cattle in flooded fields, with diarrhea and death. Again, the serotype isolated was O:3 (Callinan *et al.*, 1988). More recently, the disease was described in two herds in Argentina. In one herd, 5.8% of the cattle became sick and 1.7% died. The symptoms consisted of cachexia, diarrhea, and lack of motor coordination. In the second herd, 0.6% of 700 animals died and deaths occurred suddenly without prior symptoms. The serotype responsible was also O:3 in Argentina (Noseda *et al.*, 1990). In Canada, there have also been cases in cattle, with abortions and pneumonia.

Cases of gastroenteritis have been observed in swine. *Y. pseudotuberculosis* has been isolated from the feces and particularly from the tonsils of apparently healthy animals.

Outbreaks in turkeys have been described in the US (Oregon and California) and England. An outbreak occurred on four farms in California (Wallner-Pendleton and Cooper, 1983). The main symptoms were anorexia; watery, yellowish-green diarrhea; depression; and acute locomotor impairment. The disease affected males 9 to 12 weeks old and had a morbidity rate of 2% to 15% and high mortality, principally due to cannibalism. Administration of high doses of tetracyclines in food seemed to arrest the disease, but the birds were condemned in the postmortem inspection because of septicemic lesions. The principal lesions were necrotic foci in the liver and spleen, catarrhal enteritis, and osteomyelitis.

The pseudotuberculosis agent is the most common cause of death in hares (*Lepus europaeus*) in France and Germany. Rabbits (*Oryctolagus cuniculus*) and the ringdove (*Columba palumbus*) are also frequent victims of the disease. Epizootics have been described among rats (*Rattus norvegicus*) in Japan.

In captive animals, disease caused by *Y. pseudotuberculosis* occurs with some frequency. Serotype O:1 was isolated in farm-bred nutrias (*Myocastor coypus*); it affected both young animals and adults with acute or chronic symptoms. The principal symptoms were diarrhea, swelling of the lymph nodes, formation of nodules in various organs, cachexia, and paralysis of the hindquarters (Cipolla *et al.*, 1987; Monteavaro *et al.*, 1990). In two London zoos, there were several deaths across a broad band of mammalian and avian species. Disease and death occurred sporadically, particularly in winter. The most affected species was the Patagonian mara (*Dolichotis patagonum*). Death in captive animals due to *Y. pseudotuberculosis* represents 0.66% to 0.79% of deaths each year. The serotypes isolated were 1a and 1b, which are the predominant types in many European countries. Some strains of 2a were also isolated (Parsons, 1991).

The disease also occurs in captive monkeys. In one colony, one green monkey (*Cercopithecus aethiops*) and nine squirrel monkeys (*Saimiri sciureus*) became sick. The digestive system was most affected during the acute phase and the lymphatic tissues, spleen, and liver suffered severe alteration in the chronic phase (Plesker and Claros, 1992). In another colony of New World monkeys, two different serotypes were isolated (O:1 and O:2), depending on the group of origin (Brack and Gatesman, 1991; Brack and Hosefelder, 1992).

Source of Infection and Mode of Transmission (Figure 16): Many facets of the epidemiology of pseudotuberculous yersiniosis still need to be clarified. The broad range of animal and bird species that are naturally susceptible to the infection and are carriers of *Y. pseudotuberculosis* suggests that animals are the reservoir of the etiologic agent. In this enormous reservoir, researchers emphasize the role of rodents and various bird species. In mountainous areas of Shimane Prefecture (Japan), a bacteriological study was conducted of 1,530 wild mice of the genera *Apodemus* and *Eothenomys*, and moles (*Urotrichus talpoides*). *Y. pseudotuberculosis* was isolated from the cecum of 72 animals and 10 of the strains had virulence plasmids. The etiologic agent was detected only in the mice, more frequently during the mating season and in newborns (Fukushima *et al.*, 1990). Another study in the same prefecture cultured feces from 610 wild mammals and 259 wild birds. Thirty-seven strains of *Y. pseudotuberculosis* were isolated from 34 mammals (5.6%) and from 2 anserine fowl (0.8%). The serotypes isolated were the same as those isolated from humans in that region of Japan, thus the inference of an epidemiological connection between the human infection and the infection in wild animals. The highest rate of infection (14%) was obtained in an omnivorous canine, the raccoon dog (*Nyctereutes procyonoides*), which is common in Japan, China, and Korea (Fukushima and Gomyoda, 1991).

In studies conducted in Germany and Holland, the agent was isolated from 5.8% and 4.3% of the tonsils of 480 and 163 clinically health swine, respectively, indi-

Figure 16. Pseudotuberculous yersiniosis (*Yersinia pseudotuberculosis*).
Probable mode of transmission.

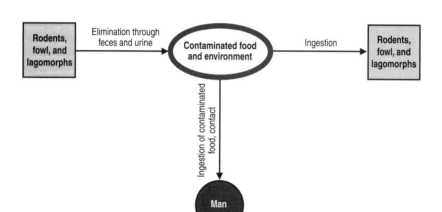

cating that this animal is a healthy carrier (Weber and Knapp, 1981a). In Japan, 2%
of pig tongues and 0.8% of chopped pork contained *Y. pseudotuberculosis*. When
samples taken from retail pork were examined, two of the four strains isolated (corresponding to serotype 4b) had the same pathogenic properties as the human strains
obtained from patients (Shiozawa *et al.*, 1988). One 4b strain was isolated previously from pork by Fukushima (1985). The agent was isolated in 0.58% of 1,206
samples of swine feces examined over 14 months. These isolations, as well as those
from tonsils, were done in the cold months, corresponding to the season in which
human cases occur (Weber and Knapp, 1981a). In New Zealand, the agent has frequently been isolated from deer. A study conducted in cattle in the same country isolated the agent from 134 (26.3%) of 509 fecal samples from 84% of 50 herds.
Serotype 3 was the most prevalent (93.2%), followed by 1 and 2. None of the herds
had prior history of disease due to *Y. pseudotuberculosis*, and thus were healthy carriers. The study was conducted in young animals during the winter (Hodges and
Carman, 1985). The authors note that diagnosis should not rely solely on examination of feces.

Several authors believe the soil is the reservoir of the agent, but isolations from
the soil in Europe have primarily yielded serotype 2, which is rarely found in the
human disease (Aldova *et al.*, 1979). However, in the focus of scarlatiniform
pseudotuberculosis in the Russian Far East, serotype 1 has been isolated from water
and soil possibly contaminated by animal feces, which would explain the large number of cases. In Khabarovsk Kray, in the Asiatic northeast of the Russian Federation,
the disease changed seasons in the period 1983–1989, going from winter to the middle of summer. This change could be explained by the early provision of vegetables
in stores, which could be contaminated by the feces of wild and synanthropic

Muridae (Dziubak *et al.*, 1991). In any case, animals and wild fowl undoubtedly contribute to environmental contamination. An epizootic or epornitic in one animal species often has repercussions in other species due to the excretion of the agent in feces and contamination of the environment.

The mode of transmission is fecal-oral. The localization of the infection in the mesenteric lymph nodes indicates that the digestive tract is the bacteria's principal route of entry.

In repeated outbreaks of yersiniosis in guinea pig colonies in Great Britain, the infection was transmitted by vegetables contaminated with feces of the ringdove (*Columba palumbus*). In the outbreak of pseudotuberculosis in turkeys in California (USA) (Wallner-Pendleton and Cooper, 1983), two dead squirrels were found near the feeders. The etiologic agent was isolated from necrotic lesions in the liver and spleen of one of the squirrels. The immediate source of infection for man is often difficult to ascertain. A common source of infection was not found for the epidemic outbreak in 19 patients in Finland (Tertti *et al.*, 1984).

The vehicles of infection are pork and possibly meat from other species; water from contaminated wells and streams; and vegetables contaminated by feces of wild animals, rodents, and other mammals and birds.

In both man and animals, the disease is prevalent in the cold months. Two reasons are suggested for this phenomenon. The agent survives better at low temperatures and many animals are healthy carriers that become ill when stressed by cold, moisture, and poor nutrition, and eliminate the agent in their feces (Carniel and Mollaret, 1990). Parturition is another stress factor. Young animals are more susceptible. The infection is transmitted from animal to animal in contaminated pastures.

Role of Animals in the Epidemiology of the Disease: Wild mammals, rodents, and others, as well as domestic mammals (swine) and wild birds, constitute the reservoir. The most common route of transmission to man is perhaps indirectly through contamination of the environment and foods by feces. The agent can survive for a relatively long time on vegetables and inanimate objects. A case of transmission by dog bite is also known.

Diagnosis: Definitive diagnosis can only be obtained through isolation and identification of the causal agent. The most suitable material is the mesenteric lymph nodes. The agent can be isolated from contaminated samples in culture media used for enterobacteria. A selective agar called cefsulodin-irgasan-novobiocin (CIN) can be used for epidemiological studies. Enrichment with diluted alkalis has been used successfully for isolations from meat samples (Fukushima, 1985). Serotyping of isolated strains is important from an epidemiological perspective. Serological tests commonly used to determine infection by *Y. pseudotuberculosis* are agglutination, hemagglutination, complement fixation, and more recently, enzyme-linked immunosorbent assay (ELISA) with the corresponding serotype, which is considered most sensitive and specific. Results should be carefully evaluated, since *Y. pseudotuberculosis* and *Y. enterocolitica* give cross-reactions and various serotypes have antigens in common with other enterobacteria.

Control: The principal preventive measure consists of protecting food and water against fecal contamination by rodents and fowl. Controlling peridomestic rodent populations and limiting the number of birds in public places are also recommended.

Meats and other animal products should be well cooked. Only chlorinated water should be consumed or, in its absence, water should be boiled for several minutes. Vegetables should be washed well with chlorinated water.

Bibliography

Aldova, E., A. Brezinova, J. Sobotkova. A finding of *Yersinia pseudotuberculosis* in well water. *Zbl Bakt Hyg [B]* 169:265–270, 1979.

Bercovier, H., H.H. Mollaret, J.M. Alonso, J. Brault, G.R. Fanning, A.G. Steigerwalt, *et al.* Intra and interspecies relatedness of *Yersinia pestis* by DNA hybridization and its relationship to *Yersinia pseudotuberculosis. Curr Microbiol* 4:225–229, 1980.

Brack, M., T.J. Gatesman [*Yersinia pseudotuberculosis* in New World monkeys]. *Berl Munch Tierarztl Wochenschr* 104:4–7, 1991.

Brack, M., F. Hosefelder. *In vitro* characteristics of *Yersinia pseudotuberculosis* of nonhuman primate origin. *Zentralbl Bakteriol* 277:280–287, 1992.

Callinan, R.B., R.W. Cook, J.G. Boulton, *et al.* Enterocolitis in cattle associated with *Yersinia pseudotuberculosis* infection. *Aust Vet J* 65:8–11, 1988.

Carniel, E., H.H. Mollaret. Yersiniosis [review]. *Comp Immunol Microbiol Infect Dis* 13:51–58, 1990.

Cipolla, A.L., P.E. Martino, J.A. Villar, M. Catena. Rodenciosis en nutrias (*Myocastor coypus*) de criadero: primeros hallazgos en Argentina. *Rev Argent Prod Animal* 7:481–486, 1987.

Dziubak, V.F., A.S. Maramovich, I.I. Lysanov, R.N. Liberova. [The epidemiological patterns of pseudotuberculosis in Khabarovsk Kray]. *Zh Mikrobiol Epidemiol Immunobiol.* October (10):25–28, 1991.

Fukushima, H. Direct isolation of *Yersinia enterocolitica* and *Yersinia pseudotuberculosis* from meat. *Appl Environ Microbiol* 50:710–712, 1985.

Fukushima, H., M. Gomyoda. Intestinal carriage of *Yersinia pseudotuberculosis* by wild birds and mammals in Japan. *Appl Environ Microbiol* 57:1152–1155, 1991.

Fukushima, H., M. Gomyoda, S. Kaneko. Mice and moles inhabiting mountainous areas of Shimane Peninsula as sources of infection with *Yersinia pseudotuberculosis. J Clin Microbiol* 28:2448–2455, 1990.

Galyov, E.E., S. Hakansson, A. Forsberg, H. Wolf-Watz. A secreted protein kinase of *Yersinia pseudotuberculosis* is an indispensable virulence determinant. *Nature* 361(6414): 730–732, 1993.

Hodges, R.T., M.G. Carman. Recovery of *Yersinia pseudotuberculosis* from faeces of healthy cattle. *N Z Vet J* 33:175–176, 1985.

Inoue, M., H. Nakashima, T. Ishida, M. Tsubokura. Three outbreaks of *Yersinia pseudotuberculosis* infection. *Zbl Bakt Hyg [B]* 186:504–511, 1988.

Joubert, L. La pseudo-tuberculose, zoonose d'avenir. *Rev Med Vet Lyon* 119:311–322, 1968.

Lemaitre, B.C., D.A. Mazigh, M.R. Scavizzi. Failure of beta-lactam antibiotics and marked efficacy of fluoroquinolones in treatment of murine *Yersinia pseudotuberculosis* infection. *Antimicrob Agents Chemother* 35:1785–1790, 1991.

Mair, N.S. Yersiniosis in wildlife and its public health implications. *J Wildl Dis* 9:64–71, 1973.

Mair, N.S. Yersiniosis (Infections due to *Yersiniosis pseudotuberculosis* and *Yersiniosis enterocolitica*). *In*: Hubbert, W.T., W.F. McCulloch, P.R. Schnurrenberger, eds. *Diseases Transmitted from Animals to Man.* 6th ed. Springfield: Thomas; 1975.

Monteavaro, C., A. Schettino, P. Soto, *et al.* Aislamiento de *Yersinia pseudotuberculosis* en nutrias de criadero. *Rev Med Vet* 71:220–224, 1990.

Noseda, R.P., J.C. Bardón, A.H. Martínez, J.M. Cordeviola. *Yersinia pseudotuberculosis*: epizootia en una colonia de *Cavia porcellus*. *Vet Argent* 4:134–136, 1987.

Noseda, R.P., A.H. Martínez, J.C. Bardón, *et al. Yersinia pseudotuberculosis* en bovinos de la Provincia de Buenos Aires. *Vet Argent* 7:385–388, 1990.

Parsons, R. Pseudotuberculosis at the zoological society of London (1981 to 1987). *Vet Rec* 128:130–132, 1991.

Plesker, R., M. Claros. A spontaneous *Yersinia pseudotuberculosis* infection in a monkey colony. *Zbl Vet Med [B]* 39:201–208, 1992.

Quan, T.J., A.M. Barnes, J.D. Poland. Yersinioses. *In*: A. Balows, W.J. Hausler, Jr., eds. *Diagnostic Procedures for Bacterial, Mycotic and Parasitic Infections*. Washington, D.C.: American Public Health Association; 1981.

Schiemann, D.A. *Yersinia enterocolitica* and *Yersinia pseudotuberculosis*. *In*: Doyle, M.P. *Foodborne Bacterial Pathogens*. New York: Marcel Dekker; 1989.

Shiozawa, K., M. Hayashi, M. Akiyama, *et al*. Virulence of *Yersinia pseudotuberculosis* isolated from pork and from the throats of swine. *Appl Environ Microbiol* 54:818–821, 1988.

Slee, K.J., P. Brightling, R.J. Seiler. Enteritis in cattle due to *Yersinia pseudotuberculosis* infection. *Aust Vet J* 65:271–275, 1988.

Slee, K.J., C. Button. Enteritis in sheep, goats and pigs due to *Yersinia pseudotuberculosis* infection. *Aust Vet J* 67:320–322, 1990.

Slee, K.J., N.W. Skilbeck. Epidemiology of *Yersinia pseudotuberculosis* and *Y. enterocolitica* infection in sheep in Australia. *J Clin Microbiol* 30:712–715, 1992.

Stovell, P.L. Pseudotubercular yersiniosis. *In*: Stoenner, H., W. Kaplan, M. Torten, eds. Vol 2, Section A: *CRC Handbook Series in Zoonoses*. Boca Raton: CRC Press; 1980.

Tertti, R., K. Granfors, O.P. Lehtonen, J. Mertsola, A.L. Makela, I. Valimaki, *et al*. An outbreak of *Yersinia pseudotuberculosis* infection. *J Infect Dis* 149:245–250, 1984.

Toyokawa, Y., Y. Ohtomo, T. Akiyama, *et al*. [Large scale outbreak of *Yersinia pseudotuberculosis* serotype 5a infection at Noheji-machi in Aomori Prefecture]. *Kansenshogaku Zasshi* 67:36–44, 1993.

Tsubokura, M., S. Aleksic, H. Fukushima, *et al*. Characterization of *Yersinia pseudotuberculosis* serogroups O9, O10 and O11; subdivision of O1 serogroup into O1a, O1b, and O1c subgroups. *Zentralbl Bakteriol* 278:500–509, 1993.

Wallner-Pendleton, E., G. Cooper. Several outbreaks of *Yersinia pseudotuberculosis* in California turkey flocks. *Avian Dis* 27:524–526, 1983.

Weber, A., W. Knapp. [Seasonal isolation of *Yersinia enterocolitica* and *Yersinia pseudotuberculosis* from tonsils of healthy slaughter pigs]. *Zbl Bakt Hyg A* 250:78–83, 1981a.

Weber, A., W. Knapp. [Demonstration of *Yersinia enterocolitica* and *Yersinia pseudotuberculosis* in fecal samples of healthy slaughter swine depending on the season]. *Zbl Vet Med B* 28:407–413, 1981b.

Wetzler, T.F. Pseudotuberculosis. *In*: Davis, J.W., L.H. Karstad, D.O. Trainer, eds. *Infectious Diseases of Wild Mammals*. Ames: Iowa State University Press; 1970.

Witte, S.T., D.P. Sponenberg, T.C. Collins. Abortion and early neonatal death of kids attributed to intrauterine *Yersinia pseudotuberculosis* infection. *J Am Vet Med Assoc* 187: 834, 1985.

RAT-BITE FEVER

ICD-10 A25.0 spirillosis; A25.1 streptobacillosis

Etiology: *Streptobacillus moniliformis* and *Spirillum minus* (*S. minor*).
Rat-bite fever is caused by two different bacteria: *Streptobacillus moniliformis* and *Spirillum minus*. Their geographic distribution and clinical picture are different and thus they will be treated separately.

1. Infection due to *Streptobacillus moniliformis*

Synonyms: Haverhill fever, epidemic arthritic erythema, streptobacillary fever.

Etiology: *Streptobacillus moniliformis* is a gram-negative, pleomorphous, nonmotile, nonsporogenic, microaerophilic bacillus 1 to 5 microns long and 0.1 to 0.7 in diameter. It occurs in isolated form or in chains 10 to 150 microns long, depending on the culture medium. Isolation of *S. moniliformis* requires media with a 20% supplement of serum, blood, or ascitic fluid (Savage, 1984).

Geographic Distribution: Worldwide.

Occurrence in Man: Very rare. It generally occurs in sporadic cases. Almost half of all cases are due to bites from laboratory rats. There have also been outbreaks in the US and Great Britain. The name Haverhill fever derives from an outbreak of "epidemic arthritic erythema" that occurred in 1926 in Haverhill, Massachusetts (USA). The largest outbreak to date occurred in Great Britain. It affected 304 people at a girls' school in a rural area, representing 43% of all the students and personnel at the school (McEvoy *et al.*, 1987).

Occurrence in Animals: The agent is isolated from the nasopharynx of a high percentage of healthy rats. Epizootics have been described in wild and laboratory mice. There have been some outbreaks in turkeys and isolated cases in other animals.

The Disease in Man: The incubation period lasts from 2 to 14 days after the bite from a rat or other rodent. The disease begins with symptomatology similar to that of influenza: fever, headache, chills, and myalgia. The bite wound heals spontaneously without complications. A maculopapular rash on the extremities as well as migratory arthralgia and myalgia are common. Polyarthritis is seen in the most severe cases. After a short time, body temperature returns to normal, but the fever may recur. Endocarditis is a possible complication. Mortality reaches 10% in untreated cases.

Haverhill fever has been attributed to the ingestion of milk contaminated by rat feces. Its characteristics were the severity of vomiting and the incidence of pharyngitis, as well as the usual symptoms of rat-bite fever (Washburn, 1990).

The outbreak that affected so many people at the school in Great Britain was attributed to water contaminated by rats. Many girls were hospitalized for weeks, with severe arthralgia and frequent relapses. There were also complications, such as endocarditis, pneumonia, metastatic abscesses, and anemia (McEvoy *et al.*, 1987).

The recommended treatment is intramuscular administration of penicillin for two weeks. McEvoy *et al.* (1987) recommend treatment with erythromycin to prevent the spontaneous development of L forms during the disease.

The Disease in Animals: Laboratory and wild rats are healthy carriers and harbor the etiologic agent in their nasopharynx. Purulent lesions have sometimes been observed in these animals. *S. moniliformis* is pathogenic for rats and has produced epizootics among rats in laboratories and in their natural habitat. In one epizootic among laboratory rats, high morbidity and mortality rates were recorded, with such symptoms as polyarthritis, gangrene, and spontaneous amputation of members. In guinea pigs, the agent can produce cervical lymphadenitis with large abscesses in the regional lymph nodes. Some outbreaks have been described among turkeys in which the most salient symptom was arthritis.

Source of Infection and Mode of Transmission: Rats are the reservoir of the infection. They harbor the etiologic agent in the nasopharynx and transmit it to humans by biting. In the Haverhill epidemic, the source was milk. According to the epidemiological investigation conducted on the school in Great Britain, the source of infection was drinking water contaminated by rat feces.

All outbreaks are due to a common source, whereas sporadic cases are due to a bite from a rat or other rodent. It would seem that man is not very susceptible, since there are very few recorded cases. Personnel working with laboratory rodents are exposed to infection. People who live in rat-infested houses can become infected without contact with rodents (Benenson, 1990). Infection among turkeys has been attributed to rat bites. It is suspected that infection in mice and other rodents in laboratories can be caused by aerosols when these rodents are kept in the same environment as rats.

Role of Animals in the Epidemiology of the Disease: Rats are the reservoir of the infection and play an essential epidemiological role.

Diagnosis: Diagnosis is accomplished by isolating *S. moniliformis* from the bloodstream or articular lesions in blood- or serum-enriched media. Inoculation of guinea pigs or rats from colonies that are demonstrably free of infection can also be used.

A few laboratories use serological tests, such as tube agglutination, complement fixation, or immunofluorescence (Wilkins *et al.*, 1988).

Control: The principal means of prevention is control of the rat population. Other important measures are pasteurization of milk and protection of food and water against rodents. Laboratory rats, mice, and guinea pigs should be kept in separate environments and personnel charged with their care should be instructed in proper handling techniques.

2. Infection due to *Spirillum minus*

Synonyms: Sodoku, spirillary fever.

Etiology: The etiologic agent is *Spirillum minus*. These bacteria are not well characterized and there are no reference strains because it is difficult to culture the spirillum. The genus name is still uncertain and the species name *minor* is considered incorrect. It is a spiral-shaped bacterium with two or three twists; it is motile, 3 to 5 microns long, and about 0.2 microns in diameter (Krieg, 1984).

Geographic Distribution: Worldwide, but more frequent in the Far East.

Occurrence in Man: Occasional.

Occurrence in Animals: The incidence of the infection in rats varies in different parts of the world. It affects 25% of rats in some regions.

The Disease in Man: It is similar to the disease caused by *S. moniliformis*. The most notable differences are that arthritic symptoms are rare and that four weeks after the bite there is a characteristic eruption with reddish or purple plaques. The incubation period is one to four weeks. Fever begins suddenly and lasts a few days, but it recurs several times over a period of one to three months. There is a generalized exanthematous eruption that may reappear with each attack of fever. Although the bite wound heals during the incubation period, it exhibits an edematous infiltration and often ulcerates. Similarly, the lymph nodes become hypertrophic.

Mortality is approximately 10% in untreated patients.

Treatment consists of intramuscular administration of procaine penicillin for two weeks.

The Disease in Animals: The infection is not apparent in rats.

Source of Infection and Mode of Transmission: The reservoir is rats and other rodents; their saliva is the source of infection for man. The infection is transmitted by bites.

Role of Animals in the Epidemiology of the Disease: Rats play the principal role. Human infections caused by bites from ferrets, dogs, cats, and other carnivores have also been described. It is presumed that these animals become contaminated while catching rodents and thus act as mechanical transmitters.

Diagnosis: Diagnosis is accomplished by dark-field microscopic examination of infiltrate from the wound, the lymph nodes, the erythematous plaques, and from the blood. The most reliable diagnosis is obtained by intraperitoneal inoculation of mice with blood or infiltrate from the wound, followed by microscopic examination of their blood and peritoneal fluid some two weeks after inoculation. The bacteria do not grow in laboratory culture media.

Control: Control is based on reduction of the rat population and on construction of rat-proof dwellings.

Bibliography

Anderson, L.C., S.L. Leary, P.J. Manning. Rat-bite fever in animal research laboratory personnel. *Lab Anim Sci* 33:292–294, 1983.

Benenson, A.S., ed. *Control of Communicable Diseases in Man.* 15th ed. An official report of the American Public Health Association. Washington, D.C.: American Public Health Association; 1990.

Bisseru, B. *Diseases of Man Acquired from His Pets.* London: Heinemann Medical; 1967.

Boyer, C.I., D.W. Bruner, J.A. Brown. A *Streptobacillus*, the cause of tendo-sheat infection in turkeys. *Avian Dis* 2:418–427, 1958.

Krieg, N.R. Aerobic/microaerophilic, motil, helical/vibroid gram-negative bacteria. *In*: Krieg, N.R., J.G. Holt, eds. Vol. 1: *Bergey's Manual of Systematic Bacteriology*. Baltimore: Williams & Wilkins; 1984.

McEvoy, M.B., N.D. Noah, R. Pilsworth. Outbreak of fever caused by *Streptobacillus moniliformis*. *Lancet* 2:1361–1363, 1987.

Ruys, A.C. Rat bite fevers. *In*: Van der Hoeden, J., ed. *Zoonoses*. Amsterdam: Elsevier; 1964.

Savage, N. Genus *Streptobacillus*. *In*: Krieg, N.R., J.G. Holt, eds. Vol. 1: *Bergey's Manual of Systematic Bacteriology*. Baltimore: Williams & Wilkins; 1984.

Washburn, R.G. *Streptobacillus moniliformis* (Rat-bite fever). *In*: Mandell, G.L., R.G. Douglas, Jr., J.E. Bennett, eds. *Principles and Practice of Infectious Diseases*. 3rd ed. New York: Churchill Livingstone, Inc.; 1990.

Wilkins, E.G.L., J.G.B. Millar, P.M. Cockroft, O.A. Okubadejo. Rat-bite fever in a gerbil breeder. *J Infect* 16:177–180, 1988.

Yamamoto, R., G.T. Clark. *Streptobacillus moniliformis* infection in turkeys. *Vet Rec* 79:95–100, 1966.

RHODOCOCCOSIS

ICD-10 J15.8 other bacterial pneumonia

Etiology: *Rhodococcus* (*Corynebacterium*) *equi* belongs to the order *Actinomycetales*; it has a coccoid or bacillary shape, is gram-positive, aerobic, non-motile, encapsulated, and nonsporogenic. Its normal habitat is the soil; it is a saprophytic bacteria that requires few nutrients and multiplies abundantly in fecal matter from herbivores.

Most strains of *R. equi* belong to 4 serogroups, which in turn contain 14 serotypes. Approximately 60% of the strains in North America belong to capsular serotype 1, and 26% belong to capsular serotype 2. In Japan, capsular serotype 3 predominates in cultures isolated from foals (Timoney *et al.*, 1988).

R. equi is an opportunistic pathogen and is harbored in the macrophages in the animal organism, causing a granulomatous inflammation (Prescott, 1991). A 15- to 17-kilodalton antigen has been identified that is probably associated with the virulence of *R. equi* (Takai *et al.*, 1991a) and could be used as a marker for it.

Geographic Distribution: Worldwide. Since 1923, when the first case of rhodococcosis was described in foals in Switzerland, the disease has been reported on all continents. *R. equi* is frequently and abundantly isolated from soil where there have been sick horses, but also from areas where there was no rhodococcosis, and even from soil where there have been no horses or other domestic animals recently (Barton and Hughes, 1980).

Occurrence in Man: Very rare. From the first human case described in 1977 up to 1983, the literature records no more than 13 human cases (Van Etta *et al.*, 1983).

Cases are more frequent due to the AIDS epidemic and at least 20 more cases were reported from 1983 to 1990 (Prescott, 1991). In many parts of the world, particularly in developing countries, physicians and hospital microbiologists know little about this disease. Consequently, underreporting is possible.

Occurrence in Animals: Infection due to *R. equi* is recognized worldwide as an important cause of bronchopneumonia, ulcerative enteritis, and lymphadenitis in foals, and less frequently in other animal species (Barton and Hughes, 1980).

The Disease in Man: As in other animals, in man the lungs are the organ most often affected. The disease appears with a fever lasting several days to several weeks, discomfort, dyspnea, unproductive cough, and, frequently, chest pain. Initially, x-rays show infiltration with nodular lesions, particularly in the superior lobes of the lungs. If the patient is not treated, the granulomatous lesion can develop into suppuration and cavitation. Extrapulmonary cases, such as osteomyelitis, hemorrhagic diarrhea and cachexia, pleurisy, abscesses, and lymphadenitis occur rarely (Prescott, 1991).

The infection and the disease appear in immunocompromised patients. *R. equi* is an intracellular parasite of the macrophages, which explains the pyogranulomatous nature of the disease and the predisposition of patients with cell-mediated immune system defects. Currently, AIDS patients represent 88% of cases. The remaining cases are patients undergoing immunosuppressive treatment due to neoplasias or an organ transplant. HIV-infected patients have a higher incidence of simultaneous secondary infections and higher mortality (54.5% as compared to 20% for patients not infected with HIV).

Given the intracellular nature of rhodococcosis, the efficacy of the antimicrobial agent depends on its ability to penetrate the phagocytes. *R. equi* is sensitive to erythromycin, vancomycin, amikacin, gentamicin, neomycin, and rifampicin. Surgical resection of the lesion or lesions is an important part of treatment (Prescott, 1991; Harvey and Sunstrum, 1991). The survival rate was 75% when antibiotic treatment was combined with surgical resection of the infected tissue. The survival rate for those who received only antibiotics was 61% (Harvey and Sunstrum, 1991).

The Disease in Animals: Rhodococcosis is a disease that occurs primarily in foals from 2 to 6 months of age, and particularly from 2 to 4 months of age. This susceptibility of young foals could be because at that age the passive immunity conferred by the mother is in decline and the animal's own immune system is still immature. Foals older than 6 months are resistant, unless they have a defect in cellular immunity or another concurrent disease with a debilitating effect (Yager, 1987).

Equine rhodococcosis appears as a subacute or chronic suppurative bronchopneumonia. Formation of abscesses is extensive, accompanied by a suppurative lymphadenitis. The lesions progress slowly. The degeneration of the macrophages coincides with the lysis of pulmonary parenchyma. Formation of abscesses continues with expansion of the purulent center. The infection is spread through the lymphatic system and affects the regional lymph nodes. Despite bacteremia no lesions are found in the liver or spleen, which would indicate that fixed macrophages could destroy *R. equi* in the circulatory system. It is estimated that approximately 50% of foals with bronchopneumonia develop concomitant ulcerative colitis and typhlitis. A small number of foals develop only intestinal lesions (Yager, 1987).

In infection caused by *R. equi*, we find both subclinical cases discovered upon autopsy and a disease with a fatal outcome in less than one week (26% of 89 foals who died from rhodococcosis).

The disease usually begins with a fever, rapid breathing, and cough and then becomes more intense. Mucopurulent nasal discharge and dyspnea are also common.

Most cases occur in summer, when there are more foals at a susceptible age and the temperature favors growth of the bacteria.

The recommended treatment is a combination of erythromycin and rifampicin, which have a synergistic effect, for 4 to 10 weeks. The two drugs are liposoluble and can penetrate the phagocytes. In the case of diarrhea, fluids and electrolytes should be replaced.

In swine, rhodococcosis appears as cervical and submaxillary lymphadenitis. *R. equi* has also been isolated from normal lymph nodes. Infection is rare in other species. Some sporadic cases have been reported in cattle, goats, sheep, reptiles, and cats. In cattle, the few cases reported were pyometra, chronic pneumonia, and lymphadenitis (Barton and Hughes, 1980).

Source of Infection and Mode of Transmission: *R. equi* is a saprophyte in soil. Its concentration depends on the presence of horses and ambient temperature. Feces of herbivores greatly favor their growth. It is believed that one of the feces' components, acetic acid, is the principal factor in the agent's multiplication (Fraser *et al.*, 1991). The prevalence of virulent *R. equi* (isolated from the soil and the feces of foals) on a horse-breeding farm where rhodococcosis is endemic is much higher than on a farm that has no history of the disease. Foals bred on an endemic farm are constantly exposed to virulent strains of *R. equi* (Takai *et al.*, 1991b). In New Zealand, samples of fecal matter from different animals and from the environment have been examined. The most frequent isolates came from the feces of foals (82%), mares (76%), deer (89%), sheep (97%), goats (83%), pigeons (64%), and soil samples (94%) (Carman and Hodges, 1987). However, *R. equi* could only be isolated from 2 of 521 human fecal samples (Mutimer *et al.*, 1979).

The route of infection for man is through inhalation. The gastroenteritis caused by *R. equi* that a few patients suffer from may be caused by swallowing sputum. A possible animal source of infection was assumed in 12 of 32 human patients (Prescott, 1991).

The airborne route is also preponderant in foals that inhale dust from the soil. In contrast, in swine the route of infection is probably oral, as indicated by their lesions (cervical and submaxillary lymphangitis). *R. equi* colonizes in the intestine of foals in the first 2 months of life. The formation of antibodies and the increased rate of formation would indicate a subclinical infection, acquired orally (Takai *et al.*, 1986; Hietala *et al.*, 1985; Yager, 1987).

Role of Animals in the Epidemiology of the Disease: Although many non–HIV-infected patients suffering from rhodococcosis acknowledged some exposure to animals, it is still unclear whether animals represent a source of infection for man. Herbivores contribute with their feces to the rapid multiplication of *R. equi* in the warm months and sick foals seem to be responsible for spreading virulent strains. The reservoir of *R. equi* is the soil.

Diagnosis: Positive diagnosis can be obtained by isolating the etiologic agent. *R. equi* grows in common laboratory media. Sputum can be used for isolation, but it is much more accurate to collect material from a bronchial sample obtained through percutaneous thoracic aspiration, or biopsy during a lobectomy. *R. equi* can sometimes be found in cultures with a variety of other bacteria and may be inadvertently discarded as "diphtheroid." The etiologic agent could be isolated from the blood of approximately one-third of human patients with pneumonia (Prescott, 1991).

Control: There are no practical measures for protecting humans or foals. It is more reasonable to prevent diseases that predispose humans to infection by *R. equi*, particularly AIDS. Another measure could be to reduce the dose of immunosuppressive medications whenever possible.

There are no preventive vaccines for equine rhodococcosis. On horse-breeding farms, the accumulation of feces and resulting multiplication of *R. equi* should not be permitted. Dusty conditions should be avoided in and around stables. On endemic farms, it is recommended that foals be examined frequently in the first months of life and that sick foals be treated (Fraser *et al.*, 1991).

Bibliography

Barton, M.D., K.L. Hughes. *Corynebacterium equi*: A review. *Vet Bull* 50:65–80, 1980.

Carman, M.G., R.T. Hodges. Distribution of *Rhodococcus equi* in animals, birds and from the environment. *N Z Vet J* 35:114–115, 1987.

Fraser, C.M., J.A. Bergeron, A. Mays, S.E. Aiello, eds. *The Merck Veterinary Manual*. 7th ed. Rahway: Merck; 1991.

Harvey, R.L., J.C. Sunstrum. *Rhodococcus equi* infection in patients with and without human immunodeficiency virus infection. *Rev Infect Dis* 13:139–145, 1991.

Hietala, S.K., A.A. Ardans, A. Sansome. Detection of *Corynebacterium equi*-specific antibody in horses by enzyme-linked immunosorbent assay. *Am J Vet Res* 46:13–15, 1985.

Mutimer, M.D., J.B. Woolcock, B.R. Sturgess. *Corynebacterium equi* in human faeces. *Med J Aust* 2:422, 1979. Cited in: Prescott, J.F. *Rhodococcus equi*: An animal and human pathogen. *Clin Microbiol Rev* 4:20–34, 1991.

Prescott, J.F. *Rhodococcus equi*: An animal and human pathogen. *Clin Microbiol Rev* 4:20–34, 1991.

Takai, S., K. Koike, S. Ohbushi, *et al.* Identification of 15- to 17-kilodalton antigens associated with virulent *Rhodococcus equi*. *J Clin Microbiol* 29:439–443, 1991a.

Takai, S., S. Ohbushi, K. Koike, *et al.* Prevalence of virulent *Rhodococcus equi* in isolates from soil and feces of horses from horse-breeding farms with and without endemic infections. *J Clin Microbiol* 29:2887–2889, 1991b.

Takai, S., H. Ohkura, Y. Watanabe, S. Tsubaki. Quantitative aspects of fecal *Rhodococcus* (*Corynebacterium*) *equi* in foals. *J Clin Microbiol* 23:794–796, 1986.

Timoney, J.F., J.H. Gillespie, F.W. Scott, J.E. Barlough. *Hagan and Bruner's Microbiology and Infectious Diseases of Domestic Animals*. 8th ed. Ithaca: Comstock; 1988.

Van Etta, L.L., G.A. Filice, R.M. Ferguson, D.N. Gerding. *Corynebacterium equi*: A review of 12 cases of human infection. *Rev Infect Dis* 5:1012–1018, 1983.

Yager, J.A. The pathogenesis of *Rhodococcus equi* pneumonia in foals. *Vet Microbiol* 14:225–232, 1987.

SALMONELLOSIS

ICD-10 A02.0 salmonella enteritis; A02.1 salmonella septicaemia; A02.8 other specified salmonella infections

Synonyms: Nontyphoid salmonellosis.

Etiology: The genus *Salmonella* belongs to the family *Enterobacteriaceae*. It is made up of gram-negative, motile (with a few exceptions), facultatively anaerobic bacteria. Salmonellae grow between 8°C and 45°C and at a pH of 4 to 8. They do not survive at temperatures higher than 70°C. Pasteurization at 71.1°C for 15 seconds is sufficient to destroy salmonellae in milk.

These bacteria can resist dehydration for a very long time, both in feces and in foods for human and animal consumption. In addition, they can survive for several months in brine with 20% salinity, particularly in products with a high protein or fat content, such as salted sausages; they also resist smoking. It has been indicated that they can survive for a long time in soil and water (WHO Expert Committee on Salmonellosis Control, 1988).

A study conducted in Great Britain showed that *S. typhimurium* can survive 4 to 14 months in the environment of facilities with infected calves, an important epidemiological factor (McLaren and Wray, 1991). It can survive in ripening cheddar cheese for 10 months at 7°C (el-Gazzar and Marth, 1992).

Le Minor and Popoff (1987) used DNA:DNA hybridization to show that they are genetically a single species. Various classification schemes have been proposed, leading to controversy and confusion. At present, the trend is to return to the scheme conceived by Kauffmann-White due to its simplicity and because it is clearer and more useful from a clinical and epidemiological standpoint. The nomenclature scheme of Edwards and Ewing that was frequently used, particularly in the Americas, is being abandoned (Farmer *et al.*, 1984). As a result, the serotype term is used directly as a species. Thus, *S. enterica* serotype *Typhimurium* according to one scheme or *Salmonella* subspecies I serotype *typhimurium* according to another scheme would currently be *S. typhimurium*.

The Kauffmann-White scheme divides salmonellae into serotypes. O somatic, H flagellar, and Vi capsular antigens are distinguished primarily on the basis of their antigenic structure. Currently, there are close to 2,200 serotypes.

Some serotypes have several different phenotypes, and their identification can be important in epidemiologic investigation. For example, biochemical tests were able to differentiate three biotypes of *S. typhimurium*, each of which was associated with a geographic and ecological region. *S. gallinarum* and *S. pullorum* are two non-motile salmonellae adapted to birds. Some authors consider them a single species or serotype because they are antigenically identical. However, each of these serotypes causes a different disease (fowl typhoid and pullorum disease). They can be distinguished because, unlike *S. gallinarum, S. pullorum* does not use dulcitol or d-tartrate (D'Aoust, 1989).

Phage typing is also useful for some serotypes. The Scottish Salmonella Reference Laboratory studied 2,010 cultures of *S. typhimurium* and differentiated 137 different groups of phage types/biotypes. Four major epidemic clones were recognized that accounted for 52% of the cultures, with a predominance of bovine and human strains. Epidemiological investigation shows that most salmonellosis outbreaks caused by *S. typhimurium* were caused by a lysotype/biotype that remained stable throughout the course of the epidemic (Barker *et al.*, 1980). Plasmid profiles and patterns of antibiotic resistance are also useful as epidemic markers.

Except for serotypes *S. typhi* and *S. paratyphi* A, and *S. paratyphi* C, which are strictly human and whose only reservoir is man, all serotypes can be considered zoonotic or potentially zoonotic.

Salmonellae have several virulence factors that contribute to causing diarrhea, bacteremia, and septicemia. These factors include the lipopolysaccharide of the outer wall, pili, flagella, cytotoxin, and enterotoxin (Murray, 1986).

Geographic Distribution: Worldwide. *S. enteritidis* is the most prevalent species, followed by *S. typhimurium*. Changes in the relative frequency of serotypes can be observed over short periods of time, sometimes within one or two years.

Only a limited number of serotypes is isolated from man or animals in a single region or country. The predominance of one or another can vary over time. Some serotypes, such as *S. enteritidis* and *S. typhimurium*, are found worldwide; in contrast, *S. weltevreden* seems to be confined to Asia.

Occurrence in Man: It is very common. Salmonellosis occurs both in sporadic cases and outbreaks affecting a family or several hundreds or thousands of people in a population. The true incidence is difficult to evaluate, since many countries do not have an epidemiological surveillance system in place, and even where a system does exist, mild and sporadic cases are not usually reported. In countries with a reporting system, the number of outbreaks has increased considerably in recent years; this increase is in part real and in part due to better reporting.

In 1980, *Salmonella* was isolated from slightly more than 30,000 people in the US (CDC, 1982). In 1986, 42,028 cases were isolated (Hargrett-Bean *et al.*, 1988). In the US and many other countries, the prevalent serotype was *S. typhimurium*. From 1976 to 1993, the rate of isolation of *S. enteritidis* increased (21% of all isolates) and overtook *S. typhimurium* as the most common serotype. During the period 1985–1991, 375 outbreaks caused by *S. enteritidis* were reported, with 12,784 cases, 1,508 hospitalized cases, and 49 deaths. Most of the cases were sporadic or small family outbreaks, and many of them were from the same phage type, indicating the possibility of a single source of infection (CDC, 1992a).

During a conference held in 1990 that was attended by 1,900 people from 30 states in the US, at least 23% became ill with gastroenteritis caused by *S. enteritidis*. The source of infection was a dessert prepared with eggs that were possibly undercooked (CDC, 1990).

In 1985, an outbreak occurred in Illinois (USA) that affected 20,000 people and was caused by pasteurized milk contaminated by *S. typhimurium* that was multiresistant to antibiotics (ampicillin and tetracycline).

Table 3 shows information on some outbreaks in the period 1981–1985 in various countries (WHO Expert Committee on Salmonellosis Control, 1988).

According to several authors' estimates, the number of human cases occurring each year in the US ranges from 740,000 to 5,300,000. In Canada, the data were similar (Bryan, 1981). Rates for reported cases are about 10 per 100,000 inhabitants in Denmark, 44 per 100,000 in Finland, and 43 per 100,000 in Sweden, one-third to two-thirds of which were probably contracted by international travelers (Silliker,

Table 3. Outbreaks of foodborne salmonellosis in selected countries, 1981–1985.

Year	Country	Food	Serotype	Approx. number of cases
1981	England	Chicken	montevideo	500
1981	The Netherlands	Cold buffet	indiana	700
1981	Scotland	Raw milk	typhimurium	654
1982	England	Chocolate	napoli	245
1982	Norway	Black pepper	oranienburg	126
1984	England	Cooked meat	virchow	274
1984	England	Cold roast beef	typhimurium	450
1984	Canada	Cheddar cheese	typhimurium	2,000
1984	Worldwide[a]	Meat gelatin	enteritidis	766
1985	England	Cooked meats	infantis	150
1985	England	Powdered milk for infants	ealing	60
1985	United States of America	Pasteurized milk	typhimurium	20,000

[a]Meals prepared in London for airlines.
Source: World Health Organization, 1988.

1982). In the former West Germany, 33,215 cases were reported in 1978, 40,717 in 1979, and 48,607 in 1980 (Poehn, 1982). In Australia, from 1980 to 1983, annual incidence was 32.2 per 100,000 inhabitants and in 1985 it was 27.0 per 100,000 (D'Aoust, 1989).

Seven of the 23 outbreaks of gastroenteritis that occurred on transatlantic flights to the US between 1947 and 1984 were due to salmonellosis (Tauxe *et al.*, 1987).

It is difficult to evaluate the situation of this disease in developing countries because of the lack of epidemiological surveillance data, but epidemic outbreaks are known to occur. In 1977, an extensive outbreak took place in Trujillo (Peru) among university students who lunched in the university dining hall. Of 640 students who ate regularly in the hall, 598 (93%) became ill and 545 were hospitalized, resulting in temporary overcrowding of community medical services. Serotype *S. thompson* was isolated from the patients' stools, and epidemiologic evidence pointed to eggs used in the food as the source of the infection (Gunn and Bullón, 1979). In the period 1969–1974, 3,429 cases of acute diarrhea in children in Buenos Aires (Argentina) and its environs were studied. Isolations of 932 strains of *Salmonella* were obtained from 3,429 stool samples. Between 1969 and 1972, isolation of *S. typhimurium* predominated, revealing the existence of an epidemic. The clinical picture was serious and the mortality rate reached 14% of the 246 children studied. After 1972, isolations of serotype *S. oranienburg* increased, and those of *S. typhimurium* decreased. Seventy-three percent of the children acquired the infection at home; 27% first showed symptoms in the hospital after being admitted for causes other than gastrointestinal disorders (Binsztein *et al.*, 1982). Starting in 1986, there was a notable increase in *S. enteritidis* in Europe, the US, South America, and some African countries. From 1986 to 1988, 39 outbreaks occurred in Argentina, affecting more than 2,500 people, with a serious clinical picture (Eiguer *et al.*, 1990; Rodrigue *et al.*, 1990).

Occurrence in Animals: It is very common. The rate of infection in domestic animals has been estimated at from 1% to 3%. In 1980, 16,274 strains of 183 serotypes of *Salmonella* were isolated in the former West Germany from animals, foods of animal origin, water, and other sources (Pietzsch, 1982). In 1985, *Salmonella* was isolated from 1.25% of 222,160 samples of meat obtained during veterinary inspection in slaughterhouses. In other examinations of animals and animal organs, *Salmonella* was isolated from 4.81% of 81,851 examined. Positive cultures were obtained from 4.59% of 141,827 bovine fecal samples. In the US, 2,515 cultures of nonhuman origin were obtained in 1980 (CDC, 1982). Several surveys have found the incidence of avian salmonellosis to be lower than 1% in Sweden, approximately 5% in Denmark, and approximately 7% in Finland. Its incidence in other countries is higher. In Great Britain, there were 3,626 isolations in 1980 and 2,992 in 1981. Epidemiologic surveillance of animals, including birds, is of the utmost importance, since the source of the large majority of nontyphoid salmonellosis cases is food of animal origin. There are no data from developing countries in this regard.

Some reports on pets indicate that salmonellosis occurs frequently. In the former West Germany between 1967 and 1983, different researchers isolated salmonellae from 8.4% to 12.8% of the dogs examined and from 9.8% to 11.2% of 908 cats. In the US, 0.04% of 124,774 dogs examined during the same time period gave positive cultures, as did 0.1% of 29,613 cats. In Iran, 7.7% of 672 dogs and 13.6% of 301 cats were positive (D'Aoust, 1989).

Infection caused by *Salmonella* is also spread among wild mammals, birds, amphibians, reptiles, and invertebrates.

The Disease in Man: With the exception of *S. typhi* and the paratyphoid serotypes (particularly A and C), which are species-specific for man, all other infections caused by *Salmonella* may be considered zoonoses. Salmonellosis is perhaps the most widespread zoonosis in the world.

Salmonellae of animal origin cause an intestinal infection in man characterized by a 6- to 72-hour incubation period after ingestion of the implicated food, and sudden onset of fever, myalgias, cephalalgia, and malaise. The main symptoms consist of abdominal pain, nausea, vomiting, and diarrhea. Salmonellosis normally has a benign course and clinical recovery ensues in two to four days. The convalescent carrier may shed salmonellae for several weeks and, more rarely, for a few months. Conversely, the carrier state is persistent in infections due to *S. typhi* or paratyphoid salmonellae. Although salmonellosis may occur in persons of all ages, incidence is much higher among children and the elderly. Dehydration can be serious.

Extraintestinal infections caused by zoonotic salmonellae are relatively infrequent. Of the 6,564 strains of *Salmonella* spp. isolated from 1969 to 1983 in a hospital in Liverpool (England), 3% were extraintestinal infections. Of the 194 extraintestinal cultures, 34% were from blood, 32% from urine, 23% from pus and inflamed tissues, 5% from bones, 5% from cerebrospinal fluid, and 3% from sputum (Wilkins and Roberts, 1988).

Serotypes adapted to a particular animal species are usually less pathogenic for man (*pullorum, gallinarum, abortus equi, abortus ovis*). An exception is *S. choleraesuis*, which produces a serious disease with a septicemic syndrome, splenomegaly, and high fever a few days to a few weeks after the onset of gastroenteritis. Bacteremia is present in more than 50% of patients with *S. choleraesuis* infections and the fatality rate may reach 20%. Serotypes *sendai* and *dublin* can also cause septicemia ("enteric fever") and often metastatic abscesses.

Zoonotic salmonellae usually heal without complications and the only treatment recommended is rehydration and electrolyte replacement. A small proportion of patients, particularly those weakened by other diseases (AIDS, neoplasias, diabetes, etc.), can suffer from bacteremia. There may also be different localizations, such as the lungs, pleura, joints, and, more rarely, the endocardium. Children under the age of 5 and the elderly are more susceptible to complications. Children younger than 2 months, the elderly, and patients with concurrent diseases should be given antibiotics (ampicillin, amoxycillin, cotrimoxazole, and chloramphenicol). Antibiotics should also be given to patients with a prolonged fever with extraintestinal complications (Benenson, 1990).

A high proportion of *Salmonella* strains with multiple antibiotic resistance has been seen in many countries. The main cause of this in industrialized countries has been the overuse of antibiotics in animal feed as a growth enhancer, as well as the indiscriminate prescription-drug treatment of people and animals. In Great Britain, the prophylactic use of antibiotics against bovine salmonellosis has resulted in the emergence of multiresistant strains of *S. typhimurium*, which have caused epizootics with high mortality. Outbreaks and epidemics of multiresistant strains of several serotypes have occurred in nurseries and pediatric clinics, with complications of septicemia or meningitis and high mortality. An epidemic caused by multiresistant strains of serotype *wien* originated in Algeria in 1969 and spread to several European and Asian countries; the source in the food chain was not discovered. Other epidemics spreading to several countries have been caused by *S. typhimurium* phage type 208 (WHO Scientific Working Group, 1980) and, in more recent years, by *S. enteritidis*. In developing countries, the principal cause of the emergence of multiresistant *Salmonella* strains may be self-medication, made possible by the public's easy access to antibiotics without a prescription.

The Disease in Animals: Salmonellae have a wide variety of domestic and wild animal hosts. The infection may or may not be clinically apparent. In the subclinical form, the animal may have a latent infection and harbor the pathogen in its lymph nodes, or it may be a carrier and eliminate the agent in its fecal material briefly, intermittently, or persistently. In domestic animals, there are several well-known clinical entities due to species-adapted serotypes, such as *S. pullorum* or *S. abortus equi*. Other clinically apparent or inapparent infections are caused by serotypes with multiple hosts.

CATTLE: The principal causes of clinical salmonellosis in cattle are serotype *dublin* and *S. typhimurium*. Other serotypes can sometimes be isolated from sick animals.

Salmonellosis in adult cattle occurs sporadically, but in calves it usually acquires epizootic proportions. The disease generally occurs when stress factors are involved. Serotype *dublin*, adapted to cattle, has a focal geographic distribution. In the Americas, outbreaks have been confirmed in the western United States, Venezuela, Brazil, and Argentina. It also occurs in Europe and South Africa.

In adult cattle, the disease begins with high fever and the appearance of blood clots in the feces, followed by profuse diarrhea, and then a drop in body temperature to normal. Signs of abdominal pain are very pronounced. Abortion is common. The disease may be fatal within a few days or the animal may recover, in which case it often becomes a carrier and new cases appear. Calves are more susceptible than adults, and in them the infection gives rise to true epidemic outbreaks, often with high mortality. Septicemia and death are frequent in newborns. The carrier state is less frequent among young animals and occurs primarily in adult cattle. The infection is almost always spread by the feces of a cow that is shedding the agent, but it may also originate from milk.

SWINE: Swine are host to numerous *Salmonella* serotypes and are the principal reservoir of *S. choleraesuis*. Serotypes that attack swine include *S. enteritidis*, *S. typhimurium*, and *S. dublin*. These serotypes are generally isolated from the intestine and from the mesenteric lymph nodes. *S. choleraesuis* is very invasive and causes septicemia; it may be isolated from the blood or from any organ. Swine are particularly susceptible and experience epidemic outbreaks between 2 and 4 months of age, but the infection also appears in mature animals, almost always as isolated cases.

Swine paratyphoid (*S. choleraesuis*) or necrotic enteritis occurs mostly in poorly managed herds living in poor hygienic conditions. It is frequently associated with classic swine plague (cholera) or with such stress factors as weaning and vaccination. The most frequent symptoms are fever and diarrhea. The infection usually originates from a carrier pig or contaminated food.

Infection by other serotypes may sometimes give rise to serious outbreaks of salmonellosis with high mortality.

Because of the frequency with which swine are infected with different types of salmonellae, pork products have often been a source of human infection.

SHEEP AND GOATS: Cases of clinical salmonellosis in these species are infrequent. The most common serotype found in gastroenteritis cases is *S. typhimurium*, but many other serotypes have also been isolated. Serotype *S. abortus ovis*, which causes abortions in the last two months of pregnancy and gastroenteritis in sheep and goats, seems to be restricted to Europe and the Middle East (Timoney *et al.*, 1988).

HORSES: The most important pathogen among horses is *S. abortus equi*, which causes abortions in mares and arthritis in colts. It is distributed worldwide. As in other types of salmonellosis, predisposing factors influence whether the infection manifests itself clinically. Pregnant mares are especially susceptible, particularly if other debilitating conditions are present. Abortion occurs in the last months of pregnancy, and the fetus and placenta contain large numbers of bacteria. This serotype is adapted to horses and is rarely found in other animal species.

Horses are also susceptible to other types of salmonellae, particularly *S. typhimurium*. Salmonella enteritis occurs in these animals, sometimes causing high mortality. Calves suffer from acute enteritis with diarrhea and fever; dehydration may be rapid. Nosocomial transmission has been seen in hospitalized horses. From April 1990 to January 1991, in an outbreak among hospitalized horses, 97.8% of the animals contracted the infection due to *S. typhimurium* var. *copenhagen* with the same plasmid profile. Other strains of *S. typhimurium* var. *copenhagen* with a different plasmid profile and *S. enteritidis* began to appear in February 1991 (Bauerfeind *et al.*, 1992).

DOGS AND CATS: In recent years, a high prevalence of infection caused by numerous serotypes has been confirmed in cats and dogs. These animals may be asymptomatic carriers or may suffer from gastroenteritic salmonellosis with varying degrees of severity.

Dogs can contract the infection by eating the feces of other dogs, other domestic or peridomestic animals, or man. Dogs and cats can also be infected by contaminated food. In addition, dogs can transmit the disease to man.

Treatment for these animals consists mainly of fluid and electrolyte replacement. Antibiotic treatment is reserved for septicemic cases and is effective if begun early in the course of the disease. The antibiotics indicated for invasive salmonellosis are ampicillin, chloramphenicol, and sulfamethoxazole with trimethoprim (Timoney *et al.*, 1988).

Multiresistant animal strains that can be transmitted to man are another problem. The indiscriminate use of antibiotics in animals often results in changes in flora in the colon, allowing rapid multiplication of resistant bacteria. In addition, the number of carrier animals in the group that shed the etiologic agent can increase (Timoney *et al.*, 1988).

FOWL: Two serotypes, *S. pullorum* and *S. gallinarum*, are adapted to domestic fowl. They are not very pathogenic for man, although cases of salmonellosis caused by these serotypes have been described in children. Many other serotypes are frequently isolated from domestic poultry; for that reason, these animals are considered one of the principal reservoirs of salmonellae.

Pullorum disease, caused by serotype *S. pullorum*, and fowl typhoid, caused by *S. gallinarum*, produce serious economic losses on poultry farms if not adequately controlled. Both diseases are distributed worldwide and give rise to outbreaks with high morbidity and mortality. Pullorum disease appears during the first 2 weeks of life and causes high mortality. The agent is transmitted vertically as well as horizontally. Carrier birds lay infected eggs that contaminate incubators and hatcheries. Fowl typhoid occurs mainly in adult birds and is transmitted by the fecal matter of carrier fowl. On an affected poultry farm, recuperating birds and apparently healthy birds are reservoirs of infection.

Salmonellae unadapted to fowl also infect them frequently. In the US, more than 200 serotypes of *Salmonella* spp. have been isolated from chickens and/or turkeys (Nagaraja *et al.*, 1991). Nearly all the serotypes that attack man infect fowl as well. Some of these serotypes are isolated from healthy birds. The infection in adult birds is generally asymptomatic, but during the first few weeks of life, its clinical picture is similar to pullorum disease (loss of appetite, nervous symptoms, and blockage of the cloaca with diarrheal fecal matter). The highest mortality occurs during the first 2 weeks of life. Most losses occur between six and ten days after hatching. Mortality practically ceases after a month. The clinically apparent form of the disease is rare after three weeks of life, but many birds survive as carriers (Nagaraja *et al.*, 1991).

The most common agent in ducks and geese is *S. typhimurium*. The infection may be transmitted from the infected ovary to the egg yolk, as in pullorum disease, or by contamination of the shell when it passes through the cloaca.

The most common agent of salmonellosis in pigeons is *S. typhimurium* var. *copenhagen.*

Salmonellosis is frequent in wild birds. In one species of seagull (*Larus argenta-tus*), it was found that 8.4% of 227 birds examined were carriers of salmonellae and that the serotypes were similar to those in man. Wild birds have also been implicated as vectors of outbreaks of serotype *S. montevideo* in sheep and cattle in Scotland (Butterfield *et al.*, 1983; Coulson *et al.*, 1983).

OTHER ANIMALS: Rodents become infected with the serotypes prevalent in the environment in which they live. The rate of wild animal carriers is not high. Rodents found in and around food processing plants can be an important source of human infection.

Of 974 free-living wild animals examined in Panama, 3.4% were found to be infected, principally by serotype *S. enteritidis* and, less frequently, by *S. arizonae* (*Arizona hinshawii*) and *Edwardsiella*. The highest rate of infection (11.8%) was found among the 195 marsupials examined. *Salmonella* was isolated from only 8 of 704 spiny rats (*Proechimys semispinosus*).

Outbreaks of salmonellosis among wild animals held in captivity in zoos or on pelt farms are not unusual.

Salmonella infection in cold-blooded animals has merited special attention. Because of the high rate of infection among small turtles kept as house pets in the US, their import was prohibited and a certificate stating them to be infection-free was required for interstate commerce.

An infection rate of 37% was found in 311 reptiles examined live or necropsied at the National Zoo in Washington, D.C. The highest rate of infection was observed in snakes (55%) and the lowest in turtles (3%). The salmonellae isolated were 24 different serotypes formerly classified under the common name of *S. enteritidis*, 1 strain of *S. choleraesuis*, and 39 of *S. arizonae*. No disease in their hosts was attributed to these bacteria, but they may act together with other agents to cause opportunistic infections (Cambre *et al.*, 1980).

Source of Infection and Mode of Transmission (Figure 17): Animals are the reservoir of zoonotic salmonellae. Practically any food of animal origin can be a source of infection for man. The most common vehicles are contaminated poultry, pork, beef, eggs, milk, and milk and egg products. Foods of vegetable origin contaminated by animal products, human excreta, or dirty utensils, in both commercial processing plants and household kitchens, have occasionally been implicated as vehicles of human salmonellosis. An outbreak of enteritis occurred in June and July of 1991 in the US and Canada. It affected 400 people who ate melons contaminated by *S. poona*, a relatively rare serotype. It is assumed that the salmonellae penetrated the soft portion of the fruit from the rind when contaminated knives were used and the melons were left at ambient temperature in the summer (Publ Hlth News. Abst Hyg Comm Dis 60 (9): 210, 1991). Contaminated public or private water supplies are important sources of infection in typhoid fever (*S. typhi*) and, less frequently, in other salmonella infections. An outbreak caused by *S. typhimurium* occurred in 1965 in Riverside, California due to contaminated water. The causal agent was isolated from 100 patients examined, though it probably affected 16,000 people (Aserkoff *et al.*, 1970).

Fowl (chickens, turkeys, and ducks) represent the most important reservoir of salmonellae entering the human food chain (D'Aoust, 1989). In England and Wales from 1981 to 1983, 51.3% of 347 vehicles of human salmonellosis were associated with fowl; in 1984–1985, 32.2% of 177 vehicles were of avian origin (Humphrey *et*

**Figure 17. Salmonellosis. Mode of transmission
(except *Salmonella typhi* and the paratyphoid serotypes).**

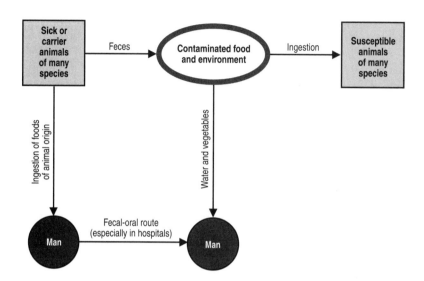

al., 1988). Another important source of salmonellae is raw or poorly cooked eggs, whether alone or as a component of various foods. An outbreak of *S. enteritidis* during a wedding celebration in a London hotel affected 173 people. The agent, phage type 4, was isolated from 118 of those affected and another 17 asymptomatic people. The source of infection was a sauce made from eggs imported from the continent. An unusual aspect of this outbreak was that some people fell ill only three hours after consuming the food. The percentage of eggs infected with *S. enteritidis* is low (an estimated 0.001%) but the risk increases when a large number of eggs is used to prepare a dish (Stevens *et al.*, 1989). Pork, beef, milk, and milk products (ice cream, cheeses) are other sources of human infection. Important contributing factors are inadequate cooking, slow cooling of the food, lack of refrigeration for many hours, and inadequate reheating before serving. Large outbreaks are invariably due to improper handling of food in restaurants and institutional dining facilities. Man can also contract the infection directly from domestic animals or house pets, such as dogs, turtles, monkeys, hamsters, and others. Young children are especially susceptible to salmonellae in reptiles, even without direct contact. In Indiana (USA), two cases were described in children; one child was less than 2 weeks old and the other less than 3 months. They were infected indirectly by *S. marina*. The source of the infection was iguanas kept in the house. These animals harbor a wide variety of serotypes and their rate of infection varies from 36% to 77% (CDC, 1992b). There are numerous reports from Asia, Canada, the US, and Europe on transmission from small turtles to humans, particularly children. This led several countries to prohibit their import. The serotypes isolated most frequently are *S. poona* and *S. arizonae* (D'Aoust *et al.*, 1990). The long period of survival (many months) of salmonellae in fecal matter can explain why direct contact is not always necessary, as in the case of some reptiles kept in or near a house (Morse and Duncan, 1974). Interhuman transmission is particularly important in hospitals; children and the elderly are the principal victims. In Baden-Würtenberg (Germany), an outbreak of *S. enteritidis*, phage type 4, occurred in a home for elderly disabled persons. The same serotype and phage type was isolated from 95 residents and 14 employees. The source of infection was a dessert made of orange cream prepared with eggs with contaminated shells (WHO Surveillance Programme for Control of Foodborne Infections and Intoxications in Europe, 1991).

Institutional and nosocomial outbreaks are usually due to food that is undercooked and kept at the wrong temperature, or to a kitchen employee who is an asymptomatic carrier. Nosocomial cases require prompt epidemiological investigation because they can involve patients who, given their age or illness, can experience severe cases of salmonellosis (CDC, 1991).

Insects, particularly flies, may have some role as mechanical vectors in very contaminated environments.

Carrier animals perpetuate the animal-to-animal cycle by means of their excreta or, in the case of fowl, infected eggs. Feed contaminated by such ingredients as bone, meat, or fish meal plays an important role as a vehicle of infection.

Intensive cattle-raising in developed countries is a very important contributing factor in the epidemiology of salmonellosis. Close contact between animals and the use of concentrated feed or ingredients that may be contaminated create conditions favorable to outbreaks. In developing countries, the source of infection is mainly the contaminated environment and water sources where animals crowd together.

Animal-to-animal transmission occurs not only at the home establishment, but also during shipping, at auctions and fairs, and even at slaughterhouses prior to sacrifice. Meat can become contaminated in abattoirs by means of contaminated equipment and utensils during skinning and butchering. Contaminated water can be a source of infection for man and animals.

The cycle of infection in fowl begins with contaminated eggshells or yolks. Contaminated eggs spread the infection in the incubator. When the eggs hatch, the newborn chicks become infected and many of those that do not die become carriers. This is the most important mechanism at work when fowl in poultry yards become infected. Another vehicle of infection may be contaminated feed. Cannibalism and the ingestion of contaminated eggs also contribute to transmission of the infection.

Non–species-specific serotypes spread easily from one animal species to another and also to humans.

Role of Animals in the Epidemiology of the Disease: Since animals constitute the reservoir of salmonellae (except *S. typhi* and the paratyphoid serotypes), they play an essential role in its epidemiology.

Diagnosis: In humans, clinical diagnosis of gastroenteritis due to *Salmonella* is confirmed by isolation of the etiologic agent from the patient's stool, serologic typing, and, when necessary, phage typing and plasmid profiling. In the few cases of septicemia, the agent may be isolated from the blood during the first week of the disease, and from feces in the second and third weeks.

Diagnosis of animal salmonellosis is also made by culturing fecal material. For infections caused by *S. pullorum* and *S. gallinarum* in fowl, serologic diagnosis is important to identify and eliminate individual carriers. Infection by *S. dublin* can be diagnosed serologically in a herd, but not in individual cattle. As a screening test, the *S. pullorum* antigen can also be used in detecting antibodies for the lipopolysaccharide of *S. enteritidis* in chickens. Seroagglutination with the *S. abortus equi* antigen can be used as a preliminary test prior to culture in mares that have aborted. Postmortem examinations of animals primarily use cultures from the mesenteric lymph nodes.

Surveillance of food processing requires that cultures be made from product samples at different stages of preparation, and from utensils and surfaces that come into contact with the food. Special sampling methods have been developed for different kinds of foods.

Control: Given current conditions under which cattle and poultry are raised, transported, marketed, and slaughtered, as well as existing food processing practices, it is impossible to obtain salmonellae-free foods of animal origin. Control is currently based on protecting man from infection and reducing its prevalence in animals. Veterinary meat and poultry inspection and supervision of milk pasteurization and egg production are important for consumer protection.

Another important control measure is the education of food handlers, both in commercial establishments and in the home, about correct cooking and refrigeration practices for foods of animal origin, and about personal and environmental hygiene.

Epidemiological surveillance by health authorities is necessary to evaluate the magnitude of the problem in each country, locate the origins of outbreaks, and adopt methods designed to reduce risks.

In animals, salmonellosis control consists of: (a) elimination of carriers, which is currently possible for pullorum disease and fowl typhoid by means of serologic tests; (b) bacteriologic control of foods, mainly of such ingredients as fish, meat, and bone meal; (c) immunization; and (d) proper management of herds and poultry farms.

Immunization may be an important method for preventing animal salmonellosis. Two types of vaccines are being used: bacterins and live attenuated vaccines. Bacterins are administered parenterally, usually in two doses two to four weeks apart. Commercially available bacterins act against *S. dublin, S. typhimurium,* and *S. abortus equi.* Live salmonellae vaccines are administered orally; they are usually genetically defective mutants. In the US, strains of *S. dublin* and *S. typhimurium* that are unable to synthesize aromatic amino acids are used. Vaccines that are unable to synthesize purines are used against these serotypes and *S. choleraesuis* in Germany. These vaccines are avirulent and do not revert to the virulent state.

In the US, a vaccine has been developed against *S. choleraesuis,* with a strain attenuated through repeated selection of a virulent strain with passes of neutrophils from salmonellosis-free swine. In this way, the vaccine strain lost the 50-kilobase plasmid, which is a virulence factor (Kramer *et al.,* 1992). Live vaccines stimulate a greater cell-mediated immune response than bacterins, which primarily promote a humoral response with little or no association with protection. Oral administration (whether of bacterins or live vaccines) has the advantage of producing local immunity in the intestine and reducing elimination of salmonellae in feces. Parenteral administration of live vaccines can sometimes cause adverse reactions due to endotoxins (WHO Expert Committee on Salmonellosis Control, 1988).

The results of many tests conducted to date indicate that immunization with vaccines and some bacterins can prevent the disease (particularly in its severe form), but not the infection or carrier status.

A control measure known as Nurmi's method originated in Finland. Salmonella-free cultures of fecal organisms from the cecum of adult birds are administered orally to newly hatched chickens and turkey chicks. The cecal flora (some 60 species of bacteria) from the adult birds compete with the salmonellae and thus protect the chicks against salmonellosis at their most susceptible age. Treated chicks resist high doses of salmonellae. It is believed to work by competitive exclusion.

Various countries have had success combating pullorum disease (*S. pullorum*) and fowl typhoid (*S. gallinarum*), reducing the rate of infection to a minimum. Several countries have undertaken control programs for *S. enteritidis* in fowl. Control is important to reduce both public health risk and economic losses. In general terms, the first step is to ensure that establishments that provide eggs for incubation and 1-day-old chicks are free of infection. Each group of egg layers must be examined serologically and bacteriologically to certify those that are disease-free and destroy those that are infected. After the surroundings and the installations are disinfected, they should be repopulated from a safe source. Once a reliable source of eggs and chicks is assured, clean-up of commercial farms should begin.

Some countries limit the control program to *S. enteritidis*, others to all invasive serotypes, including *S. typhimurium* and *S. hadar*. In Sweden, during the first year of control (1991–1992), infection was found in 6% of the layer establishments. This fell to 2% in the second year. An organization of broiler breeders in Northern Ireland had a successful program that eradicated infection by *S. enteritidis* in the establishments of their associates (McIlroy *et al.*, 1989).

Bibliography

Ager, E.A., F.H. Top, Sr. Salmonellosis. *In*: Top, F.H., Sr., P.F. Wehrle, eds. *Communicable and Infectious Diseases*. 7th ed. Saint Louis: Mosby; 1972.

Aserkoff, B., S.A. Schroeder, P.S. Brachman. Salmonellosis in the United States—a five-year review. *Am J Epidemiol* 92:13–24, 1970.

Barker, R., D.C. Old, J.C. Sharp. Phage type/biotype groups of *Salmonella typhimurium* in Scotland 1974–6: Variation during spread of epidemic clones. *J Hyg* 84:115–125, 1980.

Bauerfeind, R., L.H. Wieler, R. Weiss, G. Baljer. [Comparative plasmid profile analysis of *Salmonella typhimurium* var. *Copenhagen* strains from a *Salmonella* outbreak in hospitalized horses.] *Berl Münch Tierärztl Wochenschr* 105:38–42, 1992.

Benenson, A.S., ed. *Control of Communicable Diseases in Man*. 15th ed. An official report of the American Public Health Association. Washington, D.C.: American Public Health Association; 1990.

Binsztein, N., T. Eiguer, M. D'Empaire. [An epidemic of salmonellosis in Buenos Aires and its suburbs.] *Medicina* 42:161–167, 1982.

Bryan, F.L. Current trends in food-borne salmonellosis in the United States and Canada. *J Food Protect* 44:394–402, 1981.

Butterfield, J., J.C. Coulson, S.V. Kearsey, P. Monaghan, J.H. McCoy, G.E. Spain. The herring gull *Larus argentatus* as a carrier of *Salmonella*. *J Hyg* 91:429–436, 1983.

Buxton, A., H.I. Field. Salmonellosis. *In*: Stableforth, A.W., I.A. Galloway, eds. *Infectious Diseases of Animals*. London: Butterworth; 1959.

Cambre, R.C., D.E. Green, E.E. Smith, R.J. Montali, M. Bush. Salmonellosis and arizonosis in the reptile collection at the National Zoological Park. *J Am Vet Med Assoc* 177:800–803, 1980.

Clarenburg, A. Salmonellosis. *In*: Van der Hoeden, J., ed. *Zoonoses*. Amsterdam: Elsevier; 1964.

Coulson, J.C., J. Butterfield, C. Thomas. The herring gull *Larus argentatus* as a likely transmitting agent of *Salmonella montevideo* to sheep and cattle. *J Hyg* 91:437–443, 1983.

D'Aoust, J.Y. *Salmonella. In*: M.P. Doyle, ed. *Foodborne Bacterial Pathogens*. New York: Marcel Dekker; 1989.

D'Aoust, J.Y., E. Daley, M. Crozier, A.M. Sewell. Pet turtles: A continuing international threat to public health. *Am J Epidemiol* 132:233–238, 1990.

Edwards, P.R., W.H. Ewing. *Identification of* Enterobacteriaceae. 3rd ed. Minneapolis: Burgess; 1972.

Edwards, P.R., M.M. Galton. Salmonellosis. *Adv Vet Sci* 11:1–63, 1967.

Eiguer, T., M.I. Caffar, G.B. Fronchkowsky. [Significance of Salmonella enteritidis in outbreaks of diseases transmitted by foods in Argentina, 1986–1988]. *Rev Argent Microbiol* 22:31–36, 1990.

Farmer, J.J., III, A.C. McWhorter, D.J. Brenner, *et al.* The *Salmonella-Arizona* group of *Enterobacteriaceae*: Nomenclature, classification and reporting. *Clin Microbiol Newsletter* 6:63–66, 1984.

el-Gazzar, F.E., E.H. Marth. Salmonellae, salmonellosis, and dairy foods: A review. *J Dairy Sci* 75:2327–2343, 1992.

Gunn, R.A., Bullón, F. Salmonella enterocolitis: Report of a large foodborne outbreak in Trujillo, Peru. *Bull Pan Am Health Organ* 13(2):162–168, 1979.

Hargrett-Bean, N.T., A.T. Pavia, R.V. Tauxe. *Salmonella* isolates from humans in the United States, 1984–1986. *MMWR Morb Mortal Wkly Rep* 37 (Suppl 2):25–31, 1988.

Humphrey, T.J., G.C. Mead, B. Rowe. Poultry meat as a source of human salmonellosis in England and Wales. Epidemiological Overview. *Epidemiol Infect* 100:175–184, 1988.

Kourany, M., L. Bowdre, A. Herrer. Panamanian forest mammals as carriers of *Salmonella*. *Am J Trop Med Hyg* 25:449–455, 1976.

Kramer, T.T., M.B. Roof, R.R. Matheson. Safety and efficacy of an attenuated strain of *Salmonella choleraesuis* for vaccination of swine. *Am J Vet Res* 53:444–448, 1992.

Le Minor, L., M.Y. Popoff. Request for an opinion. Designation of *Salmonella enterica* sp. nov., nom. rev., as the type and only species of the genus *Salmonella*. *Int J Syst Bacteriol* 37:465–468, 1987.

McIlroy, S.G., R.M. McCracken, S.D. Neill, J.J. O'Brien. Control, prevention and eradication of *Salmonella enteritidis* infection in broiler and broiler breeder flocks. *Vet Rec* 125(22):545–548, 1989.

McLaren, I.M., C. Wray. Epidemiology of *Salmonella typhimurium* infection in calves: Persistence of salmonellae on calf units. *Vet Rec* 129:461–462, 1991.

Morse, E.V., M.A. Duncan. Salmonellosis—an environmental health problem. *J Am Vet Med Assoc* 165:1015–1019, 1974.

Murray, M.J. *Salmonella*: Virulence factors and enteric salmonellosis. *J Am Vet Med Assoc* 189:145–147, 1986.

Nagaraja, K.V., B.S. Pomeroy, J.E. Williams. Paratyphoid infections. *In*: Calnek, B.W., H.J. Barnes, C.W. Beard, W.M. Reid, H.W. Yoder, Jr., eds. *Diseases of Poultry*. 9th ed. Ames: Iowa State University Press; 1991.

Peluffo, C.A. Salmonellosis in South America. *In*: Van Ove, E., ed. *The World Problem of Salmonellosis*. The Hague: Junk; 1964.

Pietzsch, O. Salmonellose-Überwachung in der Bundesrepublik Deutschland einschl. Berlin (West). *Bundesgesundhbl* 25:325–327, 1982.

Pietzsch, O. Salmonellose-Überwachung bei Tieren, Lebens-und Futtermitteln in der Bundesrepublik Deutschland einschl. Berlin (West), 1984/85. *Bundesgesundhbl* 29:427–429, 1986.

Poehn, H.P. Salmonellose-Überwachtung beim Menschen in der Bundesrepublik Deutschland einschl. Berlin (West). *Bundesgesundhbl* 25:320–324, 1982.

Rodrigue, D.C., R.V. Tauxe, B. Rowe. International increase in *Salmonella enteritidis*: A new pandemic? *Epidemiol Infect* 105:21–27, 1990.

Silliker, J.H. The *Salmonella* problem: Current status and future direction. *J Food Protect* 45:661–666, 1982.

Skerman, V.B.D., V. McGowan, P.H.A. Sneath. Approved list of bacterial names. *Int J Syst Bacteriol* 30:225–420, 1980.

Smith, B.P., M. Reina-Guerra, S.K. Hoiseth, B.A. Stocker, F. Habasche, E. Johnson, *et al.* Aromatic-dependent *Salmonella typhimurium* as modified live vaccines for calves. *Am J Vet Res* 45:59–66, 1984.

Stevens, A., C. Joseph, J. Bruce, *et al.* A large outbreak of *Salmonella enteritidis* phage type 4 associated with eggs from overseas. *Epidemiol Infect* 103:425–433, 1989.

Tauxe, R.V., M.P. Tormey, L. Mascola, *et al.* Salmonellosis outbreak on transatlantic flights; foodborne illness on aircraft: 1947–1984. *Am J Epidemiol* 125:150–157, 1987.

Taylor, J., J.H. McCoy. *Salmonella* and *Arizona* infections. *In*: Riemann, H., ed. *Food-Borne Infections and Intoxications*. New York: Academic Press; 1969.

Timoney, J.F., J.H. Gillespie, F.W. Scott, J.E. Barlough. *Hagan and Bruner's Microbiology and Infectious Diseases of Domestic Animals*. 8th ed. Ithaca, New York: Comstock; 1988.

United States of America, Department of Health and Human Services, Centers for Disease Control and Prevention (CDC). *Salmonella Surveillance. Annual Summary 1980*. Atlanta: CDC; 1982.

United States of America, Department of Health and Human Services, Centers for Disease Control and Prevention (CDC). Update: *Salmonella enteritidis* infections and shell eggs— United States, 1990. *MMWR Morb Mortal Wkly Rep* 39:909–912, 1990.

United States of America, Department of Health and Human Services, Centers for Disease Control and Prevention (CDC). Foodborne nosocomial outbreak of *Salmonella reading*— Connecticut. *MMWR Morb Mortal Wkly Rep* 40 (46):804–806, 1991.

United States of America, Department of Health and Human Services, Centers for Disease Control and Prevention (CDC). Outbreak of *Salmonella enteritidis* infection associated with consumption of raw shell eggs, 1991. *MMWR Morb Mortal Wkly Rep* 41:369–372, 1992a.

United States of America, Department of Health and Human Services, Centers for Disease Control and Prevention (CDC). Iguana-associated salmonellosis—Indiana, 1990. *MMWR Morb Mortal Wkly Rep* 41 (3):38–39, 1992b.

United States of America, National Academy of Sciences, National Research Council. An evaluation of the *Salmonella* problem. Washington, D.C.: National Academy of Sciences; 1969.

WHO Expert Committee on Microbiological Aspects of Food Hygiene. *Microbiological aspects of food hygiene. Report of a WHO expert committee with the participation of FAO*. Geneva: WHO; 1968. (Technical Report Series 399).

WHO Expert Committee on Salmonellosis Control. *Salmonellosis Control: The Role of Animal and Product Hygiene. Report of a WHO Expert Committee*. Geneva: WHO, 1988. (Technical Report Series 774).

WHO Scientific Working Group. Enteric infections due to *Campylobacter, Yersinia, Salmonella*, and *Shigella*. *Bull World Health Organ* 58:519–537, 1980.

WHO Surveillance Programme for Control of Foodborne Infections and Intoxications in Europe N° 28:4–5, 1991.

Wilkins, E.G., C. Roberts. Extraintestinal salmonellosis. *Epidemiol Infect* 100:361–368, 1988.

Williams, L.P., B.C. Hobbs. *Enterobacteriaceae* infections. *In*: Hubbert, W.T., W.P. McCulloch, P.R. Schnurrenberger, eds. *Diseases Transmitted from Animals to Man*. 6th ed. Springfield: Thomas; 1975.

SHIGELLOSIS

ICD-10 A03.0 shigellosis due to *Shigella dysenteriae*;
A03.1 shigellosis due to *Shigella flexneri*;
A03.2 shigellosis due to *Shigella boydii*;
A03.3 shigellosis due to *Shigella sonnei*; A03.8 other shigellosis

Synonyms: Bacillary dysentery.

Etiology: The genus *Shigella* belongs to the family *Enterobacteriaceae*. Shigellae are small gram-negative, nonmotile, unencapsulated bacilli; they are anaerogenic (with a few exceptions) and non-lactose fermenting (or slow fermenters).

The genus *Shigella* may be considered genetically as a single species, closely related in DNA analyses to *E. coli*. However, it is divided into four species based on phenotype traits. Each species is a distinct serogroup: *Shigella dysenteriae* (serogroup A), *S. flexneri* (serogroup B), *S. boydii* (serogroup C), and *S. sonnei* (serogroup D). The four serogroups contain a total of 38 serotypes. Serotyping is important in epidemiological investigation. Diagnostic laboratories are generally limited to identifying the serogroup and sending cultures to a reference laboratory for identification of the serotype.

The primary virulence factor of a *Shigella* strain is its ability to invade cells of the intestinal mucosa. The invasive capacity depends on factors controlled by both chromosomic and plasmidic genes (Keusch and Bennish, 1991).

The invasive capacity of a strain can be demonstrated with the Sereny test, which consists of inoculating a culture in a guinea pig's conjunctival sac. Invasive strains produce keratoconjunctivitis in 24 to 48 hours. Cultures obtained from clinical cases always yield a positive Sereny test result. Shigellae also produce cytotoxins, particularly in the case of *S. dysenteriae* serotype 1 (Shiga toxin).

Geographic Distribution: Worldwide.

Occurrence in Man: Shigellosis can be either epidemic or endemic. Epidemic or pandemic shigellosis is usually caused by *S. dysenteriae* serotype 1 (Shiga bacillus), the most virulent and toxigenic strain. In 1969–1970, a widespread epidemic caused by *S. dysenteriae* serotype 1 occurred in Central America and Mexico, with high morbidity and mortality rates, particularly in children. More than 13,000 patients died as a result. The infection was introduced in the US, where 140 cases occurred from 1970 to 1972. The epidemic spread to Central Africa and Asia (India, Bangladesh, and Sri Lanka). Plasmid analysis demonstrated that the pandemic was not produced by a single bacterial clone. Thus, it is difficult to explain the appearance of the disease in such distant areas. The strains isolated in all areas proved to be multiresistant to antibiotics (WHO, 1987). In Guatemala, there were 112,000 cases with 10,000 deaths from 1969 to 1972. A new outbreak appeared in Guatemala in 1991 caused by *S. dysenteriae* serotype 1; it affected 540 people in the course of one month, both in Guatemala City and in Verapaz, a city of 10,000 inhabitants (CDC, 1991).

Endemic shigellosis is usually caused by *S. flexneri* and *S. sonnei*. The first occurs primarily in developing countries, the second, in economically advanced countries. Morbidity and mortality rates are high in developing countries, particularly in children aged 1 to 5 years (WHO, 1987). Of 16,567 isolations done in the US during 1987, 67.7% were *S. sonnei*, 22.2% were *S. flexneri*, 2.1% were *S. boydii*, 1.4% were *S. dysenteriae*, and 6.6% were unidentified species (Keusch and Bennish, 1991).

It is very difficult to calculate the number of cases worldwide, but they are estimated at more than 200 million each year, 650,000 of whom die (WHO, 1991). In the US, there are an estimated 300,000 clinical cases (Bennett, cited in Wachsmuth and Morris, 1989).

An outbreak affecting large numbers of people occurred in 1987 during a mass "Rainbow Family" gathering in a forest in North Carolina (USA). It is estimated that more than 50% of the 12,700 participants were affected. The location's sanitary infrastructure was insufficient for so many people. The outbreak was caused by *S. sonnei*, which is resistant to many antibiotics (ampicillin, tetracycline, and trimethoprim with sulfamethoxazole), and which contained a 90-kilobase plasmid not found in strains not related to this epidemic. When the participants dispersed, they became the source of infection for outbreaks in three US states (Wharton *et al.*, 1990).

Those who suffer most from the disease are those who cannot follow personal hygiene rules, such as patients or residents confined in different institutions. Children are the principal victims of the disease in endemic areas. Resistance in adults is due to acquired immunity to the prevalent serotype. Adult travelers visiting endemic areas contract the disease because they have had no previous exposure. Similarly, when a new serotype is introduced into a susceptible population, the disease affects all age groups (Levine and Lanata, 1983).

Occurrence in Animals: It is common in captive nonhuman primates and rare in other animal species. All species of *Shigella*, including *S. dysenteriae* type 1 (Shiga bacillus), which is considered the most pathogenic form for man, have been isolated from nonhuman primates (L'Hote, 1980). In 1984, an epizootic caused by *S. flexneri* occurred at the National Zoo in Washington, DC (USA), and since then, shigellosis has become endemic. The infected species were gibbons (*Hylobates concolor* and *H. syndactylies*), macaques (*Macaca silenus, M. nigra,* and *M. sylvanus*), colobus monkeys (*Colobus guerzea*), and gorillas (*Gorilla gorilla*). From 1984 to 1988, the two species of gibbons (species in danger of extinction) had a high rate of infection and disease (Banish *et al.*, 1993a). *S. sonnei* was isolated from mangabey monkeys (*Cercocebus albigena*) and spider monkeys (*Ateles susciceps*) in the same zoological collection (Banish *et al.*, 1993a).

The Disease in Man: It is seen most often in preschool-aged children. When a new serotype is introduced in tropical areas in which the population is undernourished, the disease affects all age groups, particularly children, the elderly, and debilitated individuals. The incubation period is one to seven days, but usually four days.

The clinical picture may vary from an asymptomatic infection to a serious and fatal disease. The disease begins with fever and abdominal pains, as well as diarrhea that may be watery at first and later dysenteric with blood and mucus. The rectum and colon are the parts of the intestine most affected. In the final stages, there is an intense tenesmus with frequent elimination of small amounts of feces consisting almost entirely of blood and mucus. The disease is self-limiting in well-nourished individuals, but may last for weeks or months in undernourished persons (Keusch and Bennish, 1991). Convulsions are frequent in hospitalized children.

Shigellae rapidly acquire resistance to antimicrobials. The choice of an antimicrobial will depend on the antibiogram of the strain isolated or local patterns of susceptibility. Fluids and electrolytes must be replaced if dehydration occurs. Antiperistaltics are contraindicated, both for intestinal infections caused by shigellae and for other intestinal infections.

In many countries, strains of *Shigella* resistant to sulfonamides and to several antibiotics have been observed.

The Disease in Animals: It occurs in monkeys, with a clinical picture similar to that in man. In nonhuman primate colonies, strains resistant to many antibiotics are frequently found. As in man, an antibiogram must be done to identify the most appropriate antimicrobial. Enrofloxacine was used with good results at the National Zoo in Washington, DC (Banish *et al.*, 1993a).

Source of Infection and Mode of Transmission: The principal reservoir of the infection for man is other humans who are sick or carriers. The sources of infection are feces and contaminated objects. The most common mode of transmission is the fecal-oral route. Outbreaks with numerous cases have had their origin in a common source of infection, such as foods contaminated by hands or feces of carrier individuals. Insects, particularly flies, can also play a role as mechanical vectors.

There is a direct relationship between the frequency of shigellosis and a country's degree of economic development, as well as between poor and well-off classes within a country. Lack of health education, health infrastructure (potable water and sewer system), environmental hygiene, and personal hygiene habits are all factors that contribute to the spread of infection. Shigellosis is a disease of poverty.

Bacillary dysentery is a serious disease with high mortality in nonhuman primates in captivity, but there is doubt that monkeys can harbor the etiologic agent in their natural habitat. Monkeys probably contract the infection though contact with infected humans. The infection spreads rapidly in nonhuman primate colonies because the monkeys defecate on the cage floor and often throw their food there.

Role of Animals in the Epidemiology of the Disease: Of little significance. Cases of human bacillary dysentery contracted from nonhuman primates are known. The victims are mainly children. In highly endemic areas, dogs may shed *Shigella*, at least temporarily.

The etiologic agent has been isolated rarely from bats and rattlesnakes. Nevertheless, animals other than nonhuman primates play an insignificant role.

Diagnosis: Definitive diagnosis depends on isolation of the etiologic agent by culture of fecal material on selective media. There are several selective media, which are based on the suppression of lactose fermenters. One of these is MacConkey agar with bile salts, xylose, lysine, and deoxycholate (XLD). Serologic identification and typing, at least of the serogroup, are important for diagnosis and for epidemiological research.

Control: In man, control measures include: (a) environmental hygiene, especially disposal of human waste and provision of potable water; (b) personal hygiene; (c) education of the public and of food handlers about the sources of infection and modes of transmission; (d) sanitary supervision of the production, preparation, and preservation of foods; (e) control of flies; (f) reporting and isolation of cases and sanitary disposal of feces; and (g) search for contacts and the source of infection.

A live streptomycin-dependent vaccine, administered orally in three or four doses, provided good protection against the clinical disease for 6 to 12 months. However, it is currently not in use due to side effects such as vomiting in a small number of those who have been given the vaccine. Another undesirable and more serious effect of this vaccine is the instability of the strain and reversion to its original virulence (WHO, 1991). Different types of vaccines have been developed, including hybrids of *Shigella* and *E. coli*, and of *Shigella* and *Salmonella*; vaccines obtained through deletions and mutations; and oral vaccines of dead shigellae. All these vaccines are awaiting evaluation (WHO, 1991).

In two military camps in Israel, intensive measures (primarily bait and strategically located traps) were taken in the early summer of 1988 to control flies for 11 weeks. The test was repeated in the summer of 1989. The number of flies was reduced by 64% and clinic visits for diarrhea caused by shigellosis fell by 42% in the first year and 85% in the second. These results indicate that flies, acting as mechanical vectors, are an important factor in the transmission of shigellosis (Cohen *et al.*, 1991).

Indiscriminate use of antibiotics must be avoided in order to prevent the emergence of multiresistant strains and to ensure that these medications remain available for use in severe cases.

In animals, control consists of: (a) isolation and treatment of sick or carrier monkeys; (b) careful cleaning and sterilization of cages; (c) prevention of crowding in cages; and (d) prompt disposal of wastes and control of insects.

At the National Zoo in Washington, DC, carrier status for multiresistant *S. flexneri* was eliminated through intramuscular administration of enrofloxacine (5 mg/kg of bodyweight every 24 hours for 10 days). The large primates received the same medicine orally. In this way, it was possible to eradicate *S. flexneri* from a colony of 85 primates, although after 10 to 12 months *S. sonnei* was isolated from the feces of three animals (Banish *et al.*, 1993b).

Bibliography

Banish, L.D., R. Sims, D. Sack, *et al.* Prevalence of shigellosis and other enteric pathogens in a zoologic collection of primates. *J Am Vet Med Assoc* 203:126–132, 1993a.

Banish, L.D., R. Sims, M. Bush, *et al.* Clearance of *Shigella flexneri* carriers in a zoologic collection of primates. *J Am Vet Med Assoc* 203:133–136, 1993b.

Benenson, A.S., ed. *Control of Communicable Diseases in Man.* 15th ed. An official report of the American Public Health Association. Washington, D.C.: American Public Health Association; 1990.

Bennett, J.V. Cited in: Wachsmuth, K., G.K. Morris. *Shigella. In*: Doyle, M.P. *Foodborne Bacterial Pathogens.* New York: Marcel Dekker; 1989.

Cohen, D., M. Green, M. Block, *et al.* Reduction of transmission of shigellosis by control of houseflies (*Musca domestica*). *Lancet* 337:993–997, 1991.

Edwards, P.R., W.H. Ewing. *Identification of* Enterobacteriaceae. 3rd ed. Minneapolis: Burgess; 1972.

Fiennes, R. *Zoonoses of Primates.* Ithaca: Cornell University Press; 1967.

Keusch, G.T., M.L. Bennish. Shigellosis. *In*: Evans, A.S., P.S. Brachman, eds. *Bacterial Infections of Humans.* 2nd ed. New York: Plenum Medical Book Co.; 1991.

Keusch, G.T., S.B. Formal. Shigellosis. *In*: Warren, K.S., A.A.F. Mahmoud, eds. *Tropical and Geographical Medicine.* New Jersey: McGraw-Hill; 1984.

Levine, M.M., C. Lanata. Progresos en vacunas contra diarrea bacteriana. *Adel Microbiol Enf Inf* 2:67–118, 1983.

Lewis, J.N., E.J. Gangarosa. Shigellosis. *In*: Top, F.H., Sr., P.F. Wehrle, eds. *Communicable and Infectious Diseases*. 7th ed. Saint Louis: Mosby; 1972.

L'Hote, J.L. Contribution à l'étude des salmonelloses et des shigelloses des primates. Zoonoses [thesis]. École Nationale Vétérinaire de Lyon, 1980.

Ruch, T.C. *Diseases of Laboratory Primates*. Philadelphia: Saunders; 1959.

United States of America, Department of Health and Human Services, Centers for Disease Control and Prevention (CDC). *Shigella dysenteriae* type 1—Guatemala, 1991. *MMWR Morb Mortal Wkly Rep* 40(25):421, 427–428, 1991.

Wachsmuth, K., G.K. Morris. *Shigella. In*: Doyle, M.P. *Foodborne Bacterial Pathogens*. New York: Marcel Dekker; 1989.

Wharton, M., R.A. Spiegel, J.M. Horan, *et al.* A large outbreak of antibiotic-resistant shigellosis at a mass gathering. *J Infect Dis* 162:1324–1328, 1990.

WHO Scientific Working Group. Enteric infections due to *Campylobacter, Yersinia, Salmonella*, and *Shigella. Bull World Health Organ* 58:519–537, 1980.

Williams, L.P., B.C. Hobbs. *Enterobacteriaceae* infections. *In*: Hubbert, W.T., W.F. McCulloch, P.R. Schnurrenberger, eds. *Diseases Transmitted from Animals to Man*. 6th ed. Springfield: Thomas; 1975.

World Health Organization (WHO). Development of vaccines against shigellosis: Memorandum from a WHO meeting. *Bull World Health Organ* 65:17–25, 1987.

World Health Organization (WHO). Research priorities for diarrhoeal disease vaccines: Memorandum from a WHO meeting. *Bull World Health Organ* 69(6):667–676, 1991.

STAPHYLOCOCCAL FOOD POISONING

ICD-10 A05.0 foodborne staphylococcal intoxication

Synonyms: Staphylococcal alimentary toxicosis, staphylococcal gastroenteritis.

Etiology: It is caused by an enterotoxin preformed in food by *Staphylococcus aureus*. The overwhelming majority of outbreaks are due to coagulase-positive strains of *S. aureus*. Very few coagulase-negative strains are capable of producing enterotoxins. Some outbreaks may be due to *S. intermedius* and *S. hyicus*.

The genus *Staphylococcus* consists of gram-positive bacteria in the form of cocci grouped in clusters. The bacteria is not very heat-resistant, but the enterotoxin is. There are five known types of enterotoxins (A, B, C, D, and E), but enterotoxin A is most prevalent in outbreaks. Some strains of *S. aureus* can produce both the enterotoxins and toxic shock syndrome toxin-1.

Geographical Distribution: Worldwide.

Occurrence in Man: In some countries, the disease is an important cause of food poisoning. Most sporadic cases are not recorded. Outbreaks affecting several or many people are those that are primarily known and recorded.

In the US during the period 1977–1981, 131 outbreaks were reported, affecting 7,126 people. In the last three years of that five-year period, only enterotoxin A was incriminated. Milk (the most common source of toxins C and D) and commercially packaged foods are the least common causes of the disease in the United States (Holmberg and Blake, 1984). In Japan, the annual average of food poisoning outbreaks from 1976 to 1980 was 827. Of a total of 8,742 cases, 28.2% were caused by staphylococcal poisoning (Genigeorgis, 1989).

It has been suggested that a proportion of the intestinal disorders frequently observed in developing countries are caused by staphylococcal food poisoning. Evidence of this is the fact that titers of antibodies to enterotoxins are higher in residents of these countries than in travelers (Bergdoll, 1979).

Occurrence in Animals: Spontaneous cases of staphylococcal poisoning in domestic animals are not known. The rhesus monkey (*Macaca mulatta*) is susceptible to the enterotoxin through the digestive tract and is used as an experimental animal to show the presence of the toxin in implicated foods. Intravenous or peritoneal inoculation with the enterotoxin in cats and kittens has also been used for the same purpose. Dogs possibly suffer from gastroenteritis similar to that in man.

Mastitis in cattle caused by staphylococci is of interest from a public health perspective. In modern milking systems, *S. aureus* is a common pathogen in cows' udders. The agent is transmitted by means of milking machines or the milker's hands, and enters through the milk duct or superficial lesions on the teat. Mastitis caused by *S. aureus* in cattle may vary from the prevalent subclinical form of infection to a severe gangrenous form. Both forms are economically important because of the losses they cause in milk production (Gillespie and Timoney, 1981). Studies conducted in five northern European countries and in Japan have shown that a large proportion of the staphylococci isolated from cases of bovine mastitis are toxigenic. In Europe, 41.4% of 174 strains isolated produced enterotoxins, and of these, 48.6% produced A; 5.6%, B; 29.2%, C; and 33.3%, D; either singly or in combination. In Japan, 34.4% of 1,056 strains isolated from cows with subclinical mastitis were toxigenic, and of these 31.1% produced enterotoxin A; 54.3%, C; 27% D; and 10.7%, B; either singly or in combination. Enterotoxins A, C, or D are the predominant types in staphylococcal poisoning in many countries (Kato and Kume, 1980). Nevertheless, the types of enterotoxins produced by strains isolated from milk seem to vary in prevalence in different countries; this may often be because an unrepresentative number of strains has been studied.

S. intermedius and *S. aureus* are the most common agents in canine skin infections and cause pyoderma, impetigo, folliculitis, and furunculosis. *S. aureus* is frequently a complicating agent of demodectic mange, producing cellulitis in the deep layers of the skin. Enterotoxigenic staphylococci were isolated from 13% of 115 domestic dogs in Japan. The strains isolated were producers of enterotoxins A, C, and D that can cause food poisoning in man (Kaji and Kato, 1980). A study conducted in Brazil in dogs with pyodermatitis confirmed that 13 of 52 isolates of *S. intermedius* and 6 of 21 of *S. aureus* produced enterotoxins. There were six isolates of enterotoxin C, seven of D, and six of E. Four strains produced toxic shock syndrome toxin-1 (Hirooka *et al.*, 1988).

In fowl, staphylococcal infection can cause diseases ranging from pyoderma to septicemia with different localizations (salpingitis, arthritis, and other disorders).

Purulent staphylococcal synovitis is a disease that causes appreciable losses in chickens and turkeys. In the former Czechoslovakia, one of the principal sources of staphylococcal food poisoning is thought to be infected poultry (Raska *et al.*, 1980). Staphylococcal strains isolated from poultry farms in that country and others produce enterotoxin D. Many researchers have isolated *S. aureus* from the nasal passages and skin of 100% of the birds examined, as well as from the nose and skin of 72% of swine (Genigeorgis, 1989). These data indicate that meat- and milk-producing animals may make a significant contribution to contamination of the food chain.

The Disease in Man: The incubation period is short, generally three hours after ingestion of the food involved. The interval between ingestion and the first symptoms may vary from 30 minutes to 8 hours depending on the amount of toxin ingested and the susceptibility of the individual.

The major symptoms are nausea, vomiting, abdominal pain, and diarrhea. Some patients may show low fever (up to 38°C). More serious cases may also show prostration, cephalalgia, abnormal temperature, and lowered blood pressure as well as blood and mucus in the stool and vomit. The course of the disease is usually benign and the patient recovers without medication in 24 to 72 hours.

There are patients who require hospitalization due to the severity of the symptoms. It is assumed that these are people who have ingested foods with high doses of the enterotoxin, who were not exposed to the enterotoxin in the past, or who may be debilitated due to other causes.

Source of Infection and Mode of Transmission: The principal reservoir of *S. aureus* is the human carrier. A high proportion of healthy people (30% to 35%) have staphylococci in the nasopharynx and on the skin. A carrier with a respiratory disease can contaminate foods by sneezing, coughing, or expectorating. Similarly, he may contaminate food he handles if he has a staphylococcal skin lesion. However, even if not sick himself, the carrier may contaminate food by handling different food ingredients, equipment, utensils, or the finished product. According to various authors, the proportion of enterotoxin-producing *S. aureus* strains of human origin varies from 18% to 75% (Pulverer, 1983). The proportion of toxigenic strains isolated from various sources (humans, animals, and food) is very high.

Strains of human origin predominate in epidemics, but animals are also reservoirs of the infection. Milk from cow udders infected with staphylococci can contaminate numerous milk products. Many outbreaks of staphylococcal poisoning have been caused by the consumption of inadequately refrigerated raw milk or cheeses from cows whose udders harbored staphylococci. The largest outbreak affected at least 500 students in California (USA) between 1977 and 1981 and was traced to chocolate milk (Holmberg and Blake, 1984). Another outbreak occurred in the US in which 850 students became ill after drinking chocolate milk. The average amount of enterotoxin A in the milk was 144 ng per half-pint carton (Evenson *et al.*, 1988).

Goat milk is implicated more rarely. A small outbreak occurred in Israel among Bedouin children who drank *semna*, goat milk that is skimmed, sweetened, and heated. The milk came from a goat with mastitis caused by *S. aureus* enterotoxin B (Gross *et al.*, 1988).

Small outbreaks and sporadic cases occurred in a town in Scotland between December 1984 and January 1985, in which cheeses made from sheep milk were implicated. Bacteriological examination of the various samples of the cheese was unsuccessful in isolating *Staphylococcus*, but the presence of enterotoxin A was confirmed (Bone *et al.*, 1989). In various Mediterranean countries, *Staphylococcus* is one of the most important agents in ovine mastitis. Not only can ovine staphylococcus cause economic losses, it could also be a public health problem. Food poisoning is probably the most important foodborne disease in Spain and other countries of the region. The vehicle of poisoning could be cheese made from sheep's milk. In Spain, 46 of 59 isolates of *S. aureus* produced enterotoxin C; 2, enterotoxin A; 1, enterotoxin D; and 2, enterotoxins A and C (Gutiérrez *et al.*, 1982). In developing countries, where the refrigeration of milk after milking leaves much to be desired, it is possible that milk and milk products are an important source of staphylococcal intoxication.

According to recent studies, a high proportion of strains isolated from staphylococcal mastitis produce enterotoxin A, which causes many human outbreaks.

Several studies were successful in isolating the *S. aureus* phage type 80/81 from skin lesions and cow's milk, which is related to epidemic infections in man. One of the studies proved that phage type 80/81 produced interstitial mastitis in cows. The same phage type was found among animal caretakers, which indicates that the bacterium can be transmitted between man and animals and that the latter may reinfect man.

Infected fowl and dogs (see the section on occurrence in animals) may also give rise to and be a source of staphylococcal poisoning in man.

One subject that deserves special attention is the appearance of antibiotic-resistant strains in animals whose food contains antibiotics. There is concern regarding the possible transmission of these strains to man. On several occasions, resistant strains have been found both in animals (cows, swine, and fowl) and in their caretakers, with the same antibiotic resistance. Moreover, "human" strains (phage typed) have occasionally been isolated from the nostrils and lesions of other species of domestic animals.

A variety of foods and dishes may be vehicles of the toxin. If environmental conditions are favorable, *S. aureus* multiplies in the food and produces enterotoxins. Once made, the toxin is not destroyed even if the food is subjected to boiling for the usual cooking time. Consequently, the toxin may be found in food while staphylococci are not.

Poisoning is usually caused by primarily protein-based cooked foods that are contaminated during handling and left at room temperature. Red meat and fowl were responsible for 47.3% of the outbreaks in the US (ham was the most common source in that country) and 77.2% in England. In Spain, primarily mayonnaise and foods containing mayonnaise were implicated; in Germany, four outbreaks were due to meat and three to eggs and milk products (Genigeorgis, 1989). During a Caribbean cruise, 215 of 715 passengers were poisoned by cream-filled pastries served at two different meals on board. The remaining pastries were thrown out and could not be studied, but enterotoxigenic strains of *S. aureus* phage type 85/+ were isolated from the feces of 5 of 13 patients and from none of the controls. Isolates of the same phage were obtained from a perirectal sample and from a forearm lesion from two of seven members of the ship's crew who were in charge of pastry preparation (Waterman *et al.*, 1987).

An important causal factor in poisoning is keeping food at room temperature or inadequate refrigeration, practices which allow staphylococci to multiply. Lack of hygiene in food handling is another notable factor. Outbreaks of food poisoning may often be traced to a single dish.

Role of Animals in the Epidemiology of the Disease: Most outbreaks are caused by human strains and, to a lesser degree, by strains from cattle or other animals.

Animal products, such as meat, milk, cheese, cream, and ice cream, usually constitute a good substrate for staphylococcal multiplication. Pasteurization of milk does not guarantee safety if toxins were produced prior to heat treatment, as the toxins are heat-resistant. Outbreaks have also been caused by reconstituted powdered milk, even when the dried powder contained few or no staphylococci.

Diagnosis: The short incubation period between ingestion of the food involved and the appearance of symptoms is the most important clinical criterion. Laboratory confirmation, when possible, is based mainly on demonstration of the presence of enterotoxin in the food. Biological methods (inoculation of cats with cultures of the suspect food, or of rhesus monkeys with the food or cultures) are expensive and not always reliable. As substitutes, serological methods, such as immunodiffusion, immunofluorescence, hemagglutination inhibition, enzyme-linked immunosorbent assay (ELISA), and reverse passive latex agglutination are used (Windemann and Baumgartner, 1985; Shinagawa *et al.*, 1990). These tests are useful in epidemiological research but not in daily practice (Benenson, 1990).

The isolation of enterotoxigenic staphylococcal strains from foods and typing by phage or immunofluorescence have epidemiological value. Quantitative examination of staphylococci in processed or cooked foods serves as an indicator of hygiene conditions in the processing plant and of personnel supervision.

Control: Control measures include the following: (a) education of those who prepare food at home and other food handlers, so that they will take proper personal hygiene measures; (b) prohibiting individuals with abscesses or other skin lesions from handling food; (c) refrigeration at 4°C or lower of all foods in order to prevent bacterial multiplication and the formation of toxins. Foods must be kept at room temperature for as little time as possible.

The veterinary milk inspection service should supervise dairy installations, the correct operation of refrigeration units and their use immediately after milking, and refrigerated transport of the milk to pasteurization plants.

The veterinary meat inspection service should be responsible for enforcing hygiene regulations before and after slaughter as well as during handling and processing of meat products. Control of hygiene conditions in meat retail establishments is also important.

Bibliography

Benenson, A.S., ed. *Control of Communicable Diseases in Man.* 15th ed. An official report of the American Public Health Association. Washington, D.C.: American Public Health Association; 1990.

Bergdoll, M.S. The enterotoxins. *In*: Cohen, J.O., ed. *The Staphylococci.* New York: Wiley; 1972.

Bergdoll, M.S. Staphylococcal intoxications. *In*: Riemann, H., F.L. Bryan, eds. *Food-Borne Infections and Intoxications.* 2nd ed. New York: Academic Press; 1979.

Bergdoll, M.S., C.R. Borja, R.N. Robbins, K.F. Weiss. Identification of enterotoxin E. *Infect Immun* 4:593–595, 1971.

Bergdoll, M.S., B.A. Crass, R.F. Reiser, R.N. Robbins, J.P. Davis. A new staphylococcal enterotoxin, enterotoxin F, associated with toxic-shock-syndrome *Staphylococcus aureus* isolates. *Lancet* 1:1017–1021, 1981.

Bergdoll, M.S., R. Reiser, J. Spitz. Staphylococcal enterotoxin detection in food. *Food Techn* 30:80–83, 1976.

Bone, F.J., D. Bogie, S.C. Morgan-Jones. Staphylococcal food poisoning from sheep milk cheese. *Epidemiol Infect* 103:449–458, 1989.

Casman, E.P., R.W. Bennett. Detection of staphylococcal enterotoxin in food. *Appl Microbiol* 13:181–189, 1965.

Cohen, J.O., P. Oeding. Serological typing of staphylococci by means of fluorescent antibodies. *J Bact* 84:735–741, 1962.

De Nooij, M.P., W.J. Van Leeuwen, S. Notermans. Enterotoxin production by strains of *Staphylococcus aureus* isolated from clinical and non-clinical specimens with special reference to enterotoxin F and toxic shock syndrome. *J Hyg* 89:499–505, 1982.

Evenson, M.L., M.W. Hinds, R.S. Bernstein, M.S. Bergdoll. Estimation of human dose of staphylococcal enterotoxin A from a large outbreak of staphylococcal food poisoning involving chocolate milk. *Int J Food Microbiol* 7:311–316, 1988.

Fluharty, D.N. Staphylococcocis. *In*: Hubbert, W.T., W.F. McCulloch, P.R. Schnurrenberger, eds. *Diseases Transmitted from Animals to Man.* 6th ed. Springfield: Thomas; 1975.

Genigeorgis, C.A. Present state of knowledge on staphylococcal intoxication. *Int J Food Microbiol* 9:327–360, 1989.

Gillespie, J.H., J.F. Timoney. *Hagan and Bruner's Infectious Diseases of Domestic Animals.* 7th ed. Ithaca: Comstock; 1981.

Gross, E.M., Z. Weizman, E. Picard, *et al.* Milkborne gastroenteritis due to *Staphylococcus aureus* enterotoxin B from a goat with mastitis. *Am J Trop Med Hyg* 39:103–104, 1988.

Gutiérrez, L.M., I. Menes, M.L. García, *et al.* Characterization and enterotoxigenicity of staphylococci isolated from mastitic ovine milk in Spain. *J Food Protect* 45:1282–1285, 1982.

Hirooka, E.Y., E.E. Müller, J.C. Freitas, *et al.* Enterotoxigenicity of *Staphylococcus intermedius* of canine origin. *Int J Food Microbiol* 7:185–191, 1988.

Holmberg, S.D., P.A. Blake. Staphylococcal food poisoning in the United States. New facts and old misconceptions. *JAMA* 251:487–489, 1984.

Kaji, Y., E. Kato. Occurrence of enterotoxigenic staphylococci in household and laboratory dogs. *Jpn J Vet Res* 28:86–94, 1980.

Kato, E., T. Kume. Enterotoxigenicity of bovine staphylococci isolated from California mastitis test-positive milk in Japan. *Jpn J Vet Res* 28:75–85, 1980.

Live, I. Staphylococci in animals: Differentiation and relationship to human staphylococcosis. *In*: Cohen, J.O., ed. *The Staphylococci.* New York: Wiley; 1972.

Merchant, I.A., R.A. Packer. *Veterinary Bacteriology and Virology.* 7th ed. Ames: Iowa State University Press; 1967.

Mossel, D.A.A., F. Quevedo. *Control microbiológico de los alimentos.* Lima: Universidad Nacional Mayor de San Marcos; 1967.

Pulverer, G. Lebensmittelvergiftugen durch Staphylokokken. *Bundesgesundhbl* 26:377–381, 1983.

Raska, K., V. Matejosvska, L. Polak. To the origin of contamination of foodstuff by enterotoxigenic staphylococci. Proceedings of the World Congress of Foodborne Infections and Intoxications. Berlin: Institute of Veterinary Medicine; 1980.

Shinagawa, K., K. Watanabe, N. Matsusaka, *et al.* Enzyme-linked immunosorbent assay for the detection of staphylococcal enterotoxins in incriminated foods and clinical specimens from outbreaks of food poisoning. *Jpn J Vet Sci* 52:847–850, 1990.

Thatcher, F.S., D.S. Clark. *Análisis microbiológico de los alimentos.* Zaragoza: Acribia; 1972.

Waterman, S.H., T.A. Demarcus, J.G. Wells, P.A. Blake. Staphylococcal food poisoning on a cruise ship. *Epidemiol Infect* 99:349–353, 1987.

Windemann, H., E. Baumgartner. Bestimmung von Staphylokokken-Enterotoxinen A, B, C und D in Lebensmitteln mittels Sandwich-ELISA mit markierten Antikörper. *Zbl Bak Hyg I Abt Orig B* 181:345–363, 1985.

STREPTOCOCCOSIS

(*S. suis* and other species of interest)

ICD-10 A38 scarlet fever; G00.2 streptococcal meningitis; J02.0 streptococcal pharyngitis

Synonyms: Streptococcal infection, streptococcal sore throat, scarlatina.

Etiology: The genus *Streptococcus* includes many species that display notable differences in their biological properties and their pathogenicity for man and animals. Streptococci are round, nonmotile, gram-positive bacteria that occur in pairs or long chains, particularly in fluid cultures. *Streptococcus* does not form spores and certain species, such as *S. suis*, have capsules that can be seen when cultured in serum media.

Lancefield's serological classification is very useful for identifying these bacteria. This scheme currently distinguishes 20 serogroups and identifies them with the letters A to V, excluding I and J. Many components of the serogroups have not been given specific names. Lancefield's classification is based on a precipitation test with antisera for the different dominant polysaccharide antigens located on the bacterium wall. Capsular species can in turn be divided into serotypes. This is true of *S. suis,* which is currently subdivided into 29 capsular serotypes (Higgins *et al.*, 1992). Several serogroups produce additional antigens that serve to identify serotypes. Serotyping is useful in epidemiology.

A single serogroup may include strains that are physiologically and biochemically different, thus classification cannot be based solely on serology (Timoney *et al.*, 1988). Moreover, some strains cannot be typed serologically in a serogroup and can only be identified on the basis of biochemical and physiological properties or by the combination of these characteristics plus serology (Kunz and Moellering, 1981).

A common technique for preliminary identification consists of dividing the streptococci into three categories according to their hemolytic reactivity: alpha (incomplete hemolysis and greenish discoloration on blood agar), beta (complete lysis of erythrocytes), and gamma (nonhemolytic). β-hemolytic streptococci are usually the cause of acute diseases and suppurative lesions, while α-hemolytic and Γ-streptococci cause subacute disease, with some exceptions.

S. suis serotype 2 is of particular interest in terms of zoonoses because transmission from swine to man has been confirmed. This agent belongs to Lancefield's group D. There are other *Streptococcus* species that are common to both man and animals, but which may or may not have specific reservoirs for different animal species.

Geographic Distribution: Streptococci are distributed worldwide. *S. suis* is probably prevalent in all areas where swine are bred.

Occurrence in Man: Disease caused by *S. suis* in man is rare. Between 1968 and 1984, it was isolated from 30 cases of meningitis in the Netherlands; another 30 cases caused by this agent occurred outside that country from 1968 to 1985 (Arends and Zanen, 1988).

Infections caused by group A (*S. pyogenes*) are common in man, with an apparently higher prevalence in temperate climates. For a long time, streptococci belonging to serogroup B (*S. agalactiae*) were considered mainly pathogenic for animals. They are now recognized as one of the major causes of septicemia, pneumonia, and meningitis in human newborns. In addition, streptococci belonging to serogroup D (*S. bovis*) are a frequent cause of endocarditis and bacteremia in man. There are sporadic cases of disease caused by streptococci belonging to groups C, G, F, H, and others. In man, there have been rare cases due to *S. acidominimus*, which is found in milk and in the genital and intestinal tracts of cattle; to *S. uberis*, which causes mastitis in cows and is found in milk, the oropharynx, skin, and intestinal tract; to *S. lactis* and *S. cremoris*, which cause mastitis in cows and are found in cow milk; and to *S. equi* and its subspecies, *S. zooepidemicus*, which produce various diseases in animals. Finally, there is *S. canis*, groups G, L, and M (Gallis, 1990).

Occurrence in Animals: Some diseases are very common and economically important. These include mastitis in cows caused by *S. agalactiae* (group B) and strangles caused by *S. equi* (group C) in horses and *S. suis* in swine.

The Disease in Man: In the 60 cases recorded up to 1988, the clinically predominant form of infection caused by *S. suis* was meningitis. Most patients showed classic symptoms of meningitis: severe headache, high fever, confusion, and stiff neck. More than 50% experienced a loss of auditory acuity. Other complications were arthritis and endophthalmitis. Mortality was 7%. Most patients were employed in occupations involving the handling of swine or their products (swine breeders, slaughterhouse workers, butchers, swine transporters). Of the 30 patients in the Netherlands, 28 cases were caused by *S. suis* type 2, 1 by type 4, and 1 by a strain that could not be typed (Arends and Zanen, 1988). The same authors estimate that in that country the risks for slaughterhouse workers and swine breeders would be 3 per 100,000 inhabitants.

S. pyogenes is the principal pathogen among hemolytic streptococci. This agent frequently causes epidemics of septic sore throat and scarlet fever (streptococcal tonsillitis and pharyngitis), various suppurative processes, septicemias, puerperal sepsis, erysipelas, ulcerative endocarditis, and other localized infections. Streptococcal sore throat and scarlet fever are epidemiologically similar. The latter is differentiated clinically by the exanthema caused by strains producing an erythrogenic toxin. The disease is mild or inapparent in a high percentage of those infected. Rheumatic fever is a sequela of streptococcal sore throat or scarlet fever and may be caused by any strain of group A. Glomerulonephritis is another complication, produced only by certain nephritogenic strains of the same group.

Group B streptococci are important causal agents of neonatal disease. Group A streptococci and *Staphylococcus aureus* were replaced by *Escherichia coli* and serogroup B streptococci as the principal agents of neonatal infection. In infections caused by group B streptococci (*S. agalactiae*), two clinical syndromes are distinguished, depending on the age of the infant at the onset of disease. The acute or early-onset syndrome appears between the first and fifth day of life and is characterized by sepsis and respiratory difficulty. The delayed-onset syndrome generally appears after the tenth day and is characterized by meningitis, with or without sepsis. Affected children show lethargy, convulsions, and anorexia. Mortality is high in both forms, but higher in the early-onset syndrome.

In older children and adults, group B streptococci cause a variety of clinical syndromes: urinary tract infections, bacteremia, gangrene, postpartum infection, pneumonia, endocarditis, empyema, meningitis, and other pathological conditions (Patterson and el Batool Hafeez, 1976).

Disease caused by group C streptococci (*S. equi*) is sporadic and rare in man. However, in 1983, an epidemic outbreak occurred in New Mexico (USA), with 16 cases caused by the consumption of white cheese made at home with unpasteurized milk. The agent was identified as *S. zooepidemicus*, one of the four species that make up group C. The disease in these patients consisted of fever, chills, and vague constitutional symptoms, but five of them had a localized infection, which manifested in such varied symptoms as pneumonia, endocarditis, meningitis, pericarditis, and abdominal pains (CDC, 1983).

In England and Wales between 1983 and 1984, there were eight deaths during 32 outbreaks associated with milk and milk products contaminated by *S. zooepidemicus* (Barrett, 1986). There were 11 cases in Hong Kong between 1982 and 1990 in patients suffering from septicemia associated with a cardiovascular illness. Mortality was 22%. Five of the 11 patients had a predisposing disease. The source of infection was undercooked or raw pork (Yuen *et al.*, 1990).

In sporadic cases caused by streptococcus group C, the most common clinical manifestation is exudative pharyngitis or tonsillitis. With some exceptions, group C streptococci isolated from these cases belong to *S. equisimilis*, which produces septicemia in suckling pigs. An outbreak of pharyngitis caused by group C streptococci, due to the consumption of raw milk, was followed by a high incidence of glomerulonephritis (Duca *et al.*, 1969).

Both enterococcal and nonenterococcal group D streptococci cause serious diseases in man. *S. bovis* causes bacteremia and endocarditis, and enterococci cause urinary tract infections, abdominal abscesses, and a significant percentage of cases of bacterial endocarditis. *S. suis*, already described, belongs to group D.

Streptococci belonging to other serogroups, as well as those not serologically grouped, cause a wide variety of clinical manifestations, including dental caries and abscesses, meningitis, puerperal sepsis, wound infections, endocarditis, and other pathological conditions (Kunz and Moellering, 1981).

Nonhemolytic streptococci and "viridans" type (a-hemolytic) streptococci can cause subacute endocarditis.

The preferred antimicrobial for treatment is penicillin (Benenson, 1990).

The Disease in Animals: *S. suis* belongs to group D and can be β- or α-hemolytic (Timoney *et al.*, 1988). This agent frequently causes septicemia, meningitis, pneumonia, and arthritis. Less frequently, it causes endocarditis, polyserositis, encephalitis, and abscesses. Although the rate of infection in a herd can be high, it does not usually affect more than 5% (Clifton-Hadley, 1984). Of 663 strains isolated from sick swine in Canada, 21% belonged to type 2 (the most frequently occurring type in all countries), followed by types 1/2 (which has capsular antigens from 1 and 2) and 3, with 12% each. Types 20 and 26 were the only types not found (Higgins and Gottschalk, 1992). In Denmark, types 2 and 7 represented 75% of the isolates. Type 7 was isolated more frequently than in other countries, usually in suckling pigs younger than 3 weeks. Experimental inoculation with *S. suis* type 7 in suckling pigs under 7 days old caused severe disease (Boetner *et al.*, 1987). In Australia, type 1 has caused septicemia, meningitis, and polyarthritis in suckling pigs (Cook *et al.*, 1988). In weaned piglets from various regions of Australia, type 2 is predominant (Ossowicz *et al.*, 1989), although types 3, 4, and 9 have also been isolated and there are indications that they can produce the same disease picture. In another study in New South Wales and Victoria (Australia), type 9 was predominant (Gogolewski *et al.*, 1990).

In cattle, sheep, and goats, strains of types 5 and 2 were isolated from purulent lesions in the lungs and from other extramammary sites (Hommez *et al.*, 1988).

Most isolates of *S. suis* type 2 are sensitive to penicillin.

S. agalactiae (*S. mastitidis*), in Lancefield's group B, is the principal agent of chronic catarrhal mastitis in dairy cows. *S. dysgalactiae* (group C) and *S. uberis* (group E) cause sporadic cases of acute mastitis in bovines. *S. pyogenes*, a human pathogen, can infect the cow's udder, producing mastitis and leading to epidemic outbreaks in man.

Horse strangles, caused by *S. equi* (group C), is an acute disease of horses characterized by inflammation of the pharyngeal and nasal mucosa, with a mucopurulent secretion and abscesses of the regional lymph nodes.

S. equisimilis (group C) infects different tissues in several animal species. Group C streptococci that are adapted to animals and classified as *S. zooepidemicus* produce cervicitis and metritis in mares and often cause abortions. They also cause septicemia in colts. They are pathogenic for bovines, swine, and other animals, in which they produce various septicemic processes.

S. zooepidemicus (group C) is an opportunistic pathogen in many animal species. It is a commensal on the skin, the mucosa of the upper respiratory tract, and in the tonsils of many animal species. In horses, it is the common agent of wound infections and is a secondary disease agent after a viral infection in the upper respiratory tract of colts and young animals. It is also the agent of other infections in horses (Timoney *et al.*, 1988). In cows, *S. zooepidemicus* can cause acute mastitis when it enters a wound in the teat. A fatal case of septicemia was described in a chicken (Timoney *et al.*, 1988).

Streptococci belonging to other groups cause abscesses and different disease processes in several animal species. The many diseases caused by streptococci are clinically differentiated by the agent's portal of entry and the tissue it affects.

Source of Infection and Mode of Transmission: The reservoir of *S. pyogenes* is man. Transmission of this respiratory disease agent (septic sore throat, scarlet fever) results from direct contact between an infected person, whether patient or carrier, and another susceptible person. The disease is most frequent among children from 5 to 15 years old, but also occurs at other ages.

In Germany, Denmark, the US, Great Britain, and Iceland, important epidemics have had their origin in the consumption of raw milk or ice cream made with milk from cows with udders infected by *S. pyogenes*. These epidemics were due to infection in the cows' udders contracted from infected milkers. Between 1920 and 1944, 103 such epidemics of septic sore throat and 105 of scarlet fever were recorded in the US due to consumption of raw milk from cows with infected udders. In other instances, the milk was contaminated directly (without the udders' being infected by people with septic sore throat or localized infections). In several epidemic outbreaks, the milk became contaminated after pasteurization.

According to the WHO Expert Committee on Streptococcal and Staphylococcal Infections (1968), contamination of milk products has caused small outbreaks of streptococcal respiratory disease, but these are increasingly less frequent.

Pasteurization has been the most important factor in the reduction of streptococcal outbreaks resulting from milk. In Third World countries, much milk is still consumed raw, and even in developed countries, outbreaks are produced by products made with raw milk.

Special attention has been given to neonatal sepsis caused by group B streptococci (*S. agalactiae*). Research has shown that *S. agalactiae* colonizes a high percentage of women (7% to 30% or more) in different locations, such as the intestinal tract, the cervicovaginal region, and the upper respiratory tract. The agent is possibly transferred from the rectal region to the vaginal canal, since most of the bacteria are intestinal. Infants can become contaminated *in utero* or during childbirth. Only a small percentage of neonates (approximately 1%) become infected and fall ill; in most, the agent colonizes the skin and the mucosa without affecting their health. The principal victims of the infection, especially in the case of the early-onset syndrome, are premature infants, low birthweight babies, and those born after a difficult labor. The principal reservoir of group B streptococci causing neonatal disease is clearly the mother. The *S. agalactiae* serotypes isolated from mothers and sick newborns are always the same. Although *S. agalactiae* is an agent of bovine mastitis and has also been isolated from other animal species, there is no evidence that the infection is transmitted from animals to man. In general, human and animal strains differ in some biochemical, metabolic, and serologic properties. It has been experimentally shown that human strains of *S. agalactiae* can produce mastitis in bovines (Patterson and el Batool Hafeez, 1976). However, some studies have suggested that a percentage of human infections may have derived from a bovine source (Van den Heever and Erasmus, 1980; Berglez, 1981) or that there is reciprocal transmission between humans and bovines. Nonetheless, research findings seem to indicate that if such transmission occurs, its importance is probably limited.

The outbreak of disease caused by *S. zooepidemicus* (group C) in New Mexico (USA) (see the section on the disease in man) clearly indicates that raw milk and unpasteurized milk products can be the source of infection for man. The epidemiological investigation of this outbreak sampled milk from cows on the establishment where the cheese was made as well as samples of the cheese itself. *S. zooepidemicus* was isolated from many of the samples. In Europe, there have also been cases of *S. zooepidemicus* infection caused by ingestion of raw milk. A case of pneumonia caused by *S. zooepidemicus* in a woman who cared for a sick horse has been described (Rose *et al.*, 1980). The cases of disease caused by *S. zooepidemicus* that occurred in Hong Kong were attributed to the consumption of cooked or raw pork (Yuen *et al.*, 1990).

Infection caused by *S. suis* type 2 is a true zoonosis. It is a highly occupational disease among those who breed pigs or participate in slaughtering, processing, or marketing them. Man contracts the infection primarily through skin lesions.

The infection in swine is widespread in areas where these animals are bred. In an endemic herd, both sick and healthy pigs carry the agent in their nasal cavities and tonsils. The percentage of carrier animals can reach 50% or more of the herd during outbreaks and fall to only 3% when there are no clinical cases. Carrier status can last for at least 45 days and may persist in animals treated with penicillin (Clifton-Hadley and Alexander, 1980). Among swine, the infection is transmitted through the air and possibly through the digestive route as well. Pigs can also be carriers of *S. suis* in the vaginal canal and piglets can become infected during delivery (Robertson *et al.*, 1991).

Animals can also transmit groups G, L, and M to man, but the epidemiology of these cross-infections has not yet been elucidated.

Role of Animals in the Epidemiology of the Disease: Swine are the reservoir and source of *S. suis* infection in man. Animals do not act as maintenance hosts for *S. pyogenes*, but can sometimes cause important epidemic outbreaks by contracting the infection from man and retransmitting it by means of contaminated milk. There is no firm evidence that animals play any significant role in the transmission of group B streptococci causing neonatal sepsis. Raw cow milk can be a source of group C streptococcal infection in humans.

Diagnosis: If milk is suspected as the source of an epidemic outbreak in man, an attempt should be made to isolate the etiologic agent. Obviously, a correct identification of the agent is required. From either a human or animal source, it is advisable to identify the serogroup of streptococci involved, and to establish the species whenever possible. However, few laboratories have the human and material resources necessary for this task.

A method has been described for identifying pregnant women with heavy colonization of the genital tract by group B streptococci (Jones *et al.*, 1983). The goal of this procedure is to start treating the newborn with drugs immediately after birth to reduce morbidity and mortality due to neonatal sepsis caused by group B streptococci.

Infection by *S. suis* should be suspected if the patient presents the clinical manifestations described and his or her occupation involves contact with swine or their by-products. Culture, isolation, and typing can confirm the diagnosis.

In swine, definitive diagnosis also depends on isolation and identification of the agent. In endemic herds, the symptomatology may be sufficiently clear to make a clinical diagnosis during new outbreaks. In a study conducted in Quebec (Canada) with 1,716 weaned pigs belonging to 49 herds and 23 control herds, nasal and tonsil samples were taken with swabs. The samples were cultured in a brain-heart infusion broth, strengthened with a supplement selective for *Streptococcus* and 5% anti-*S. suis* type 2 serum developed in goats. After the diameter of the precipitation zone was measured in 539 isolates, serum plate agglutination was used to identify isolates of *S. suis* serotype 2. This method successfully identified 93.1% of the cultures isolated using the diameter of the precipitation zone as the sole criterion. Specificity was 94.5% and relative sensitivity was 88.7% (Moreau *et al.*, 1989).

Control: Those who work with swine or their by-products should pay attention to cuts or abrasions and treat them properly to prevent infection by *S. suis* type 2.

As for preventing the disease in swine, there are doubts regarding the efficacy of the bacterins used against *S. suis*. However, many veterinarians and breeders maintain that they prevent outbreaks of acute illness. Adding penicillin to feed when piglets are being weaned early can also control acute disease. The disadvantage is that penicillin becomes inactive in feed (Fraser *et al.*, 1991). Experimental tests showed that tiamulin administered in water was effective in reducing the effects of *S. suis* type 2 (Chengappa *et al.*, 1990).

Prevention of human infection transmitted through milk is achieved primarily by pasteurization. Infected persons should not participate in milking or handling milk or other foods.

The prevention of neonatal sepsis has been attempted by active immunization of pregnant women with capsular polysaccharides of group B streptococci, as well as by passive immunization with immunoglobulin preparations given intravenously. Both immunization methods are in the experimental stage. Promising results have been obtained with prophylactic intravenous administration of ampicillin to women in labor. In this way, a significant level of the antibiotic is obtained in the amniotic fluid and in samples of the umbilical cord. Among the newborns of obstetric patients receiving this treatment, only 2.8% were colonized by group B streptococci and none became ill, while in the control group, 35.9% of the newborns were colonized and four developed the early-onset syndrome (Fischer *et al.*, 1983).

To reduce the prevalence of mastitis caused by *S. agalactiae* in dairy herds, cows testing positive to the California Mastitis Test (CMT) are treated with penicillin by extramammary infusion. However, this procedure does not eradicate the infection, probably because of reinfection. Application of antiseptic creams to teat lesions can help to prevent mastitis caused by *S. dysgalactiae* and *S. zooepidemicus*. Bacterins have been tried for preventing equine strangles caused by *S. equi*. Although they confer satisfactory immunity, they produce a local and systemic reaction (Timoney *et al.*, 1988).

Bibliography

Arends, J.P., H.C. Zanen. Meningitis caused by *Streptococcus suis* in humans. *Rev Infect Dis* 10:131–137, 1988.

Barrett, N.J. Communicable disease associated with milk and dairy products in England and Wales: 1983–1984. *J Infect* 12:265–272, 1986.

Benenson, A.S., ed. *Control of Communicable Diseases in Man*. 15th ed. An official report of the American Public Health Association. Washington, D.C.: American Public Health Association; 1990.

Berglez, I. Comparative studies of some biochemical properties of human and bovine *Streptococcus agalactiae* strains. *Zbl Bakt Hyg I Abst Orig* 173:457–463, 1981.

Boetner, A.G., M. Binder, V. Bille-Hansen. *Streptococcus suis* infections in Danish pigs and experimental infection with *Streptococcus suis* serotype 7. *Acta Pathol Microbiol Scand [B]* 95:233–239, 1987.

Chengappa, M.M., L.W. Pace, J.A. Williams, *et al*. Efficacy of tiamulin against experimentally induced *Streptococcus suis* type 2-infection in swine. *J Am Vet Med Assoc* 197:1467–1470, 1990.

Clifton-Hadley, F.A. Studies of *Streptococcus suis* type 2 infection in pigs. *Vet Res Commun* 8:217–227, 1984.

Clifton-Hadley, F.A., T.J. Alexander. The carrier site and carrier rate of *Streptococcus suis* type II in pigs. *Vet Rec* 107:40–41, 1980.

Cook, R.W., A.R. Jackson, A.D. Ross. *Streptococcus suis* type 1 infection of suckling pigs. *Aust Vet J* 65:64–65, 1988.

Davies, A.M. Diseases of man transmissible through animals. *In*: Van der Hoeden, J., ed. *Zoonoses*. Amsterdam: Elsevier; 1964.

Duca, E., G. Teodorovici, C. Radu, A. Vita, P. Talasman-Niculescu, E. Bernescu, *et al.* A new nephritogenic streptococcus. *J Hyg* 67:691–698, 1969.

Eickhoff, T.C. Group B streptococci in human infection. *In*: Wannamaker, L.W., J.M. Matsen, eds. *Streptococci and Streptococcal Diseases: Recognition, Understanding, and Management*. New York: Academic Press; 1972.

Fischer, G., R.E. Horton, R. Edelman. From the National Institute of Allergy and Infectious Diseases. Summary of the National Institutes of Health workshop on group B streptococcal infection. *J Infect Dis* 148:163–166, 1983.

Fluharty, D.M. Streptococcosis. *In*: Hubbert, W.T., W.F. McCulloch, P.R. Schnurrenberger, eds. *Diseases Transmitted from Animals to Man*. 6th ed. Springfield: Thomas; 1975.

Fraser, C.M., J.A. Bergeron, A. Mays, S.E. Aiello, eds. *The Merck Veterinary Manual*. 7th ed. Rahway: Merck; 1991.

Gallis, H.A. Viridans and β-hemolytic (Non-Group A, B, and D) streptococci. *In*: Mandell, G.L., R.G. Douglas, Jr., J.E. Bennett, eds. *Principles and Practice of Infectious Diseases*. 3rd ed. New York: Churchill Livingstone, Inc.; 1990.

Gogolewski, R.P., R.W. Cook, C.J. O'Connell. *Streptococcus suis* serotypes associated with disease in weaned pigs. *Aust Vet J* 67:202–204, 1990.

Higgins, R., M. Gottschalk. Distribution of *Streptococcus suis* capsular types in Canada in 1991. *Can Vet J* 33:406, 1992.

Hommez, J., J. Wullepit, P. Cassimon, *et al. Streptococcus suis* and other streptococcal species as a cause of extramammary infection in ruminants. *Vet Rec* 123:626–627, 1988.

Jones, D.E., E.M. Friedl, K.S. Kanarek, J.K. Williams, D.V. Lim. Rapid identification of pregnant women heavily colonized with group B streptococci. *J Clin Microbiol* 18:558–560, 1983.

Kunz, L.J., R.C. Moellering. Streptococcal infection. *In*: Balows, A., W.J. Hausler, Jr., eds. *Diagnostic Procedures for Bacterial, Mycotic, and Parasitic Infections*. 6th ed. Washington, D.C.: American Public Health Association; 1981.

MacKnight, J.F., P.J. Ellis, K.A. Jensen, B. Franz. Group B streptococci in neonatal deaths. *Appl Microbiol* 17:926, 1969.

Merchant, I.A., R.A. Packer. *Veterinary Bacteriology and Virology*. 7th ed. Ames: Iowa State University Press; 1967.

Moreau, A., R. Higgins, M. Bigras-Poulin, M. Nadeau. Rapid detection of *Streptococcus suis* serotype 2 in weaned pigs. *Am J Vet Res* 50:1667–1671, 1989.

Ossowicz, C.J., A.M. Pointon, P.R. Davies. *Streptococcus suis* isolated from pigs in South Australia. *Aust Vet J* 66:377–378, 1989.

Patterson, M.J., A. el Batool Hafeez. Group B streptococci in human disease. *Bacteriol Rev* 40:774–792, 1976.

Robertson, I.D., D.K. Blackmore, D.J. Hampson, Z.F. Fu. A longitudinal study of natural infection of piglets with *Streptococcus suis* types 1 and 2. *Epidemiol Infect* 107:119–126, 1991.

Rose, H.D., J.R. Allen, G. Witte. *Streptococcus zooepidemicus* (group C) pneumonia in a human. *J Clin Microbiol* 11:76–78, 1980.

Stollerman, G.H. Streptococcal disease. *In*: Beeson, P.B., W. McDermott, eds. *Cecil-Loeb Textbook of Medicine*. 12th ed. Philadelphia: Saunders; 1967.

Timoney, J.F., J.H. Gillespie, F.W. Scott, J.E. Barlough. *Hagan and Bruner's Microbiology and Infectious Diseases of Domestic Animals.* 8th ed. Ithaca: Comstock; 1988.

United States of America, Department of Health and Human Services, Centers for Disease Control and Prevention (CDC). Group C streptococcal infections associated with eating home-made cheese—New Mexico. *MMWR Morb Mortal Wkly Rep* 32(39):510, 515–516, 1983.

Van den Heever, L.W., M. Erasmus. Group B *Streptococcus*—comparison of *Streptococcus agalactiae* isolated from humans and cows in the Republic of South Africa. *J S Afr Vet Assoc* 51:93–100, 1980.

WHO Expert Committee on Streptococcal and Staphylococcal Infections. *Streptococcal and Staphylococcal Infections. Report of a WHO Expert Committee.* Geneva: WHO; 1968. (Technical Report Series 394).

Yuen, K.Y., W.H. Seto, C.H. Choi, *et al. Streptococcus zooepidemicus* (Lancefield group C) septicaemia in Hong Kong. *J Infect* 21:241–250, 1990.

TETANUS

ICD-10 A33 tetanus neonatorum; A34 obstetrical tetanus; A35 other tetanus

Synonyms: Trismus, lockjaw.

Etiology: *Clostridium tetani*; the pathology is produced by the neurotoxin of the infectious agent, since the bacterium does not invade the animal body. *C. tetani*, like all clostridia, is a gram-positive, anaerobic, motile bacillus, 2–2.5 microns long by 0.3–0.5 microns in diameter. It forms terminal ovoid spores, giving it the appearance of a tennis racket. While multiplying logarithmically, *C. tetani* amasses an intracellular neurotoxin called tetanospasmin, which is released when the cell lyses. Tetanospasmin is a very potent toxin. It is estimated that less than 2.5 ng/kg of body-weight would be fatal for man and that 0.3 ng/kg of bodyweight would be fatal for a guinea pig (Orenstein and Wassilak, 1991). Production of the neurotoxin is determined by a plasmid gene (Finn *et al.*, 1984).

C. tetani spores are very resistant to environmental factors and can survive in the soil for many years.

Geographic Distribution: Worldwide. The etiologic agent is a soil microorganism that can also be found in the feces of animals and man. The spores of *C. tetani* are found primarily in cultivated land rich in organic matter, or in pastures. The disease occurs more frequently in the tropics than in temperate or cold climates.

Occurrence in Man: The incidence of the disease is low in industrialized countries; in developing countries, it still represents an important public health problem. In the decade 1951–1960, the mortality rate from tetanus was 0.16 per 100,000 inhabitants in the US and Canada and 8.50 per 100,000 in Latin America, excluding

Argentina and Brazil. In 1987, it was estimated that 1,680,000 cases and 1,030,000 deaths occurred worldwide. In 1973, 60% to 90% of cases occurred in newborns during the first month of life (Orenstein and Wassilak, 1991). Currently, the distribution of the disease by age group is completely different in the US. In the period 1989–1990, there were 117 cases of tetanus in 34 states, with an annual incidence of 0.02 per 100,000 inhabitants. In marked contrast to developing countries, 58% of the patients were 60 years of age or older and only one case occurred in a newborn. Case fatality bore a direct relationship to age: 17% in patients aged 40 to 49, and 50% in those aged 80 or older (CDC, 1993).

Inhabitants of rural areas are more exposed than those in urban areas. Case fatality is high despite improved treatment.

A study conducted in Paraguay demonstrated that tetanus is more frequent in men than in women, and more common in newborns and children than in adults (Vera Martínez *et al.*, 1976).

In Argentina, the annual rates of incidence for the period 1965–1977 were 1.2 to 1.7 per 100,000 inhabitants (except in 1967, when the rate was 3.1 per 100,000 inhabitants). The disease was more frequent in subtropical or temperate provinces than in the cold Patagonian provinces. Average hospital admissions for tetanus in Buenos Aires between 1968 and 1973 were higher during the hot months. Tetanus mortality in these municipal hospitals reached 35.8% and was eight times higher in children younger than 15 days than in other age groups (Mazzáfero *et al.*, 1981). Table 4 shows the morbidity distribution by climate for tetanus in Argentina during the period 1967–1977. In 1990, 49 cases were reported; in 1991, there were 38 cases of all ages; and in 1992, there were 7 neonatal cases. Underreporting is evident, since the number of deaths exceeds the number of patients, as indicated by the authorities in charge of the National Disease Surveillance System (Argentina, Ministerio de Salud y Acción Social, 1990, 1991, and 1992).

Occurrence in Animals: The disease is infrequent in animals. There are enzootic areas, particularly in the tropics. Horses are the most susceptible species. Cases also occur in sheep and cattle.

The Disease in Man: It is characterized by painful spasms of the masseter muscles (trismus) and neck muscles (rictus), but it frequently affects other muscles in the body. Although the average incubation period is 14 days, it may vary from less than two days to several months. If the disease is not complicated by other infections, temperature may be normal or only slightly elevated. Reflexes are exaggerated, and rigidity of the abdominal muscles, urine retention, and constipation are common. The case fatality rate is high, but varies from one country to another. In the US, fatality fell from 90% in 1947 to 60% in 1969. In 1989–1990, it was 17% in patients aged 40 to 49 and 50% in those aged 80 or older. The disease is much more severe when the incubation period is short and convulsions appear early. The longer, more frequent, and more intense the convulsions become, the worse the prognosis.

The symptomatology of neonatal tetanus is the same as that of the disease in adults; only the infection's portal of entry differs. In newborns, the infection usually enters through the umbilical stump. At other ages, the route of entry is a wound. Puncture wounds produced by contaminated objects or trauma wounds are especially dangerous. Surgical interventions and induced abortions performed without adequate asepsis have given rise to tetanus.

Table 4. Distribution of tetanus morbidity according to political division and climate, Argentina, 1967–1977.

Political division and climate	Average number of notified cases per year	Population at middle of reporting period (in thousands)	Rate per 100,000 inhabitants
Subtropical	168.8	4,221	3.9
Catamarca	3.4	175	1.9
Corrientes	19.2	587	3.3
Chaco	38.5	572	6.7
Formosa	14.2	248	5.6
Jujuy	6.7	323	2.1
Misiones	15.3	470	3.3
Salta	20.4	533	3.8
Santiago del Estero	15.7	519	3.0
Tucumán	32.6	794	4.1
Temperate	217.6	19,409	1.1
Federal District	18.5	2,974	0.6
Buenos Aires	111.9	9,289	1.2
Córdoba	20.9	2,177	0.9
Entre Ríos	16.5	838	1.9
La Pampa	3.4	177	2.2
La Rioja	0.6	139	0.4
Mendoza	4.5	1,025	0.4
San Juan	3.1	403	0.7
San Luis	1.5	187	0.8
Santa Fe	36.2	2,200	1.6
Cold	3.7	762	0.5
Chubut	0.6	202	0.3
Río Negro	1.3	281	0.4
Neuquén	1.6	170	0.9
Santa Cruz	0.2	94	0.2
Tierra del Fuego	—	15	0.0

Source: Bull Pan Am Health Organ 15:328, 1981.

C. tetani is not an invasive bacteria. The spores enter through a wound that may be an anaerobic medium, especially if there is tissular necrosis. Under such conditions, *C. tetani* enters a vegetative state, multiplies, and releases the neurotoxin as it lyses. The disease is due to tetanospasmin, a very potent neurotoxin (see the section on etiology). It enters the nervous system through the neuromuscular junctions of alpha motor neurons. Tetanospasmin inhibits the release of various neurotransmitters, allowing the lower motor neurons to increase muscle tone and produce convulsions simultaneously in the agonist and antagonist muscles (Cate, 1990).

The patient must be kept in an intensive care unit and treated with benzodiazepines to reduce anxiety, and to obtain a central anticonvulsive effect and muscular relaxation. It is often necessary to continue with tracheal intubation or a tracheostomy. Simultaneously with these measures, human antitetanus immunoglobulin must be administered (intramuscular administration of 500 IU). Administration of penicillin or other antibiotics is recommended to reduce the toxin load (Cate, 1990).

The Disease in Animals: Horses are very susceptible to tetanus and usually acquire it from shoeing nails. They may also contract it from any other wound contaminated with *C. tetani* if anaerobic conditions favor its multiplication. Their symptoms are similar to those of human tetanus. Localized rigidity appears first, due to tonic convulsions of the masseter muscles, the neck muscles, and the hind legs, followed by generalized rigidity. Reflexes are increased and the animals are easily startled by noise, which causes general convulsions.

Postpartum cases are seen in cows, especially if the placenta is retained. Cattle have a high rate of neutralizing antibodies against the neurotoxin (tetanospasmin) of *C. tetani*, but the antibody level drops markedly after parturition, leaving the animal very susceptible to the disease. In calves and lambs, tetanus often follows castration, especially when rubber bands are used, since the necrotic tissue left by this operation favors anaerobiosis.

Dehorning, tail docking, and shearing may also give rise to the disease.

Iatrogenic tetanus sometimes occurs after surgical operations and vaccinations.

The incubation period lasts 2 to 14 days. The symptomatology is similar to that in man. Death occurs in 4 to 10 days.

Treatment consists of tranquilizers, curariform agents, and 300,000 IU of tetanus antitoxin every 12 hours. Good results can be obtained in horses if they are treated at the onset of the disease. The wound must also be cleaned and drained, and broad spectrum antibiotics administered (Fraser *et al.*, 1991).

Source of Infection and Mode of Transmission: The reservoir and source of infection is soil containing *C. tetani*. The etiologic agent is found in many soils, particularly cultivated soil rich in organic matter. Areas where the exposure risk is high are referred to as "telluric foci" of *C. tetani*.

The agent is commonly found in horse feces. It has also been found in other species, such as cattle, sheep, dogs, rats, and chickens; similarly, man may harbor *C. tetani* in the intestinal tract.

Transmission is effected through wounds. Scabs or crusts promote multiplication of the etiologic agent. Some cases are due to dog bites. Tetanospasmin is produced after the spores have germinated, i.e., by the vegetative form of the bacteria.

In Paraguay, of 2,337 cases studied from 1946 to 1972, the portal of entry was the umbilical stump in 31.7%, small wounds in 38.7%, wounds caused by removal of the chigoe flea *Tunga penetrans* in 7.7%, and the remainder followed induced abortions, surgical interventions, burns, and injections without proper asepsis (Vera Martínez *et al.*, 1976).

Role of Animals in the Epidemiology of the Disease: Tetanus is a disease common to man and animals, not a zoonosis. Some authors ascribe the role of reservoir to animals (McComb, 1980; Benenson, 1990), but it is more likely that the disease agent derives from the soil, and that it is present in the digestive tract of herbivores and omnivores only transitorily and does not multiply there (Wilson and Miles, 1975; Smith, 1975). Nevertheless, domesticated animals can disseminate toxigenic strains of *C. tetani* by means of their feces, in cultivated as well as uncultivated areas.

Diagnosis: Prior existence of a wound and accompanying symptoms are the bases for diagnosis. Direct microscopic examination of wound material is useful. Given the urgency of diagnosis, the value of culturing *C. tetani* is doubtful. It is not always possible to isolate the etiologic agent from a wound.

Control: In man, given the soil origin of the infection, the only rational means of control is active immunization with toxoid. Children 2 to 3 months of age should receive three doses of the toxoid in the triple DPT vaccine (diphtheria, pertussis, tetanus) at intervals of one month to six weeks. They should then receive a booster, preferably administered 18 months after the last dose. An initial series of three doses induces protective titers of antitoxin for 5 to 13 years in 90% or more of those vaccinated. Booster shots ensure higher titers of the antitoxin and probably confer immunity throughout a woman's childbearing years (Halsey and de Quadros, 1983). Periodic boosters of tetanus toxoid every 10 years are recommended, particularly for population groups most at risk. The effectiveness of the toxoid was confirmed during World War II. US soldiers who were vaccinated with three doses of tetanus toxoid experienced one case of tetanus among 455,803 wounded, while in the unvaccinated Japanese army, the incidence was 10 cases per 100,000 wounded soldiers.

In developing countries, immunization is recommended for pregnant mothers to prevent tetanus mortality in newborns. The effectiveness of prenatal immunization with tetanus toxoid (anatoxin) has been demonstrated. Primary immunization consists of administering two doses, one at the start of pregnancy and another one month later, but not beyond three weeks before birth. If a pregnant woman has already been immunized, she only needs a booster and probably has enough antibodies to protect the children she bears over the next five years (Stanfield and Galazka, 1984).

Passive immunization with antitoxin should be reserved for persons with no previous active immunization who must undergo surgical operations, as well as for women after abortion or birth and for their newborn children in high-risk areas. The use of human antitoxin serum is preferable, but if unavailable, horse or bovine hyperimmune serum can be used after the patient is tested for a possible allergic reaction to the serum.

Wounds should be cleaned and debrided. Persons who have previously received basic toxoid treatment should be given a booster if the wound is small and more than 10 years have passed since the last dose. If the patient has a large, contaminated wound, a booster toxoid should be given if he was not vaccinated in the last five years. Persons who did not receive a full primary series of tetanus toxoid should receive a dose of toxoid and may require an injection of human tetanus immunoglobulin, if it is a major wound and/or is contaminated (Benenson, 1990).

Control procedures in animals are similar. Horses in particular should be vaccinated with toxoid; two doses given one to two months apart are sufficient. If the horse suffers from a potentially dangerous wound, another toxoid injection should be given. If the animal has not received toxoid previously, 2,000 to 3,000 IU of antitoxin should be given. At the same time, one dose of toxoid should be given and repeated one month later. The antitoxin confers passive immunity for approximately two weeks. Colts are given toxoid at 2 months of age and mares are given toxoid in the last six weeks of pregnancy (Fraser *et al.*, 1991). Operations such as dehorning, castration, and tail docking should be done in the most aseptic conditions possible and antiseptics should be applied to surgical wounds.

Lambs in the first month of life can become passively immunized when the ewe is vaccinated with two doses of aluminum phosphate-adsorbed toxoid. The first injection should be administered eight weeks and the second, three or four weeks before the birth (Cameron, 1983).

Bibliography

Argentina, Ministerio de Salud y Acción Social. Boletines Epidemiológicos Nacionales, 1990, 1991, and 1992.

Benenson, A.S., ed. *Control of Communicable Diseases in Man*. 15th ed. An official report of the American Public Health Association. Washington, D.C.: American Public Health Association; 1990.

Bytchenko, B. Geographical distribution of tetanus in the world, 1951–60. *Bull World Health Organ* 34:71–104, 1966.

Cameron, C.M., B.J. Van Biljon, W.J. Botha, P.C. Knoetze. Comparison of oil adjuvant and aluminium phosphate-adsorbed toxoid for the passive immunization of lambs against tetanus. *Onderstepoort J Vet Res* 50:229–231, 1983.

Cate, T.R. *Clostridium tetani* (Tetanus). *In*: Mandell, G.L., R.G. Douglas, Jr., J.E. Bennett, eds. *Principles and Practice of Infectious Diseases*. 3rd ed. New York: Churchill Livingstone, Inc.; 1990.

Cvjetanovic, B. Epidemiología del tétanos considerada desde un punto de vista práctico de salud pública. *Bol Oficina Sanit Panam* 75:315–324, 1973.

Finn, C.W., Jr., R.P. Silver, W.H. Habig, M.C. Hardegree, *et al.* The structural gene for tetanus neurotoxin is on a plasmid. *Science* 224:881–884, 1984.

Fraser, C.M., J.A. Bergeron, A. Mays, S.E. Aiello, eds. *The Merck Veterinary Manual*. 7th ed. Rahway: Merck; 1991.

Halsey, N.A., C.A. de Quadros. *Recent Advances in Immunization*. Washington, D.C.: Pan American Health Organization; 1983. (Scientific Publication 451).

Mazzáfero, V.E., M. Boyer, A. Moncayo-Medina. The distribution of tetanus in Argentina. *Bull Pan Am Health Organ* 15(4):327–332, 1981.

McComb, J.A. Tetanus (Lockjaw). *In*: H. Stoenner, W. Kaplan, M. Torten, eds. Vol 2, Section A: *CRC Handbook Series in Zoonoses*. Boca Raton: CRC Press; 1980.

Orenstein, W.A., S.G.F. Wassilak. Tetanus. *In*: Evans, A.S., P.S. Brachman, eds. *Bacterial Infection of Humans*. 2nd ed. New York: Plenum Medical Book Co.; 1991.

Rosen, H.M. Diseases caused by clostridia. *In*: Beeson, P.B., W. McDermott, J.B. Wyngaarden, eds. *Cecil Textbook of Medicine*. 15th ed. Philadelphia: Saunders; 1979.

Rosen, M.N. Clostridial infections and intoxications. *In*: Hubbert, W.T., W.F. McCulloch, P.R. Schnurrenberger, eds. *Diseases Transmitted from Animals to Man*. 6th ed. Springfield: Thomas; 1975.

Smith, J.W.G. Diphtheria and tetanus toxoids. *Br Med Bull* 25(2):177–182, 1969.

Smith, L.D. Clostridial diseases of animals. *Adv Vet Sci* 3:465–524, 1957.

Smith, L.D. *The Pathogenic Anaerobic Bacteria*. 2nd ed. Springfield: Thomas; 1975.

Spaeth, R. Tetanus. *In*: Top, F.H., Sr., P.F. Wehrle, eds. *Communicable and Infectious Diseases*. 7th ed. St. Louis: Mosby; 1972.

Stanfield, J.P., A. Galazka. Neonatal tetanus in the world today. *Bull World Health Organ* 62:647–669, 1984.

Tavares, W. Profilaxis do tetano. Fundamentos e critica de sua realização. *Rev Assoc Med Bras* 28:10–14, 1982.

United States of America, Department of Health and Human Services, Centers for Disease Control and Prevention (CDC). Tetanus surveillance—United States, 1989–1990. *MMWR Morb Mortal Wkly Rep* 42:233, 1993.

Vera Martínez, A., C.M. Ramírez Boettner, V.M. Salinas, R. Zárate. Tétanos: estudio clínico y epidemiológico de 2.337 casos. *Bol Oficina Sanit Panam* 80:323–332, 1976.

Wilson, G.S., A. Miles. Vol. 2. *Topley and Wilson's Principles of Bacteriology, Virology, and Immunity*. 6th ed. Baltimore: Williams & Wilkins; 1975.

World Health Organization (WHO). Guidelines for the prevention of tetanus. *WHO Chron* 30:201–203, 1976.

TICK-BORNE RELAPSING FEVER

ICD-10 A68.1

Synonyms: Endemic relapsing fever, spirochetosis, spirochetal fever, recurrent typhus, borreliosis.

Etiology: Spirochetes of the genus *Borrelia* (syn. *Spirillum, Spirochaeta, Spironema*). Given the close relationship of specificity between the tick species and the *Borrelia* strains it harbors, classification of the etiologic agent according to its vector has been proposed. Thus, the agent transmitted by *Ornithodoros hermsii* would be named *Borrelia hermsii*, the one found in *O. brasiliensis* would be *B. brasiliensis*, etc. Other borreliae derive their species name from their geographical region of origin. These include *B. hispanica*, transmitted by *O. erraticus*; *B. venezuelensi*, transmitted by *O. rudis*; and *B. caucasica,* transmitted by *O. verrucosus*.

However, not all researchers agree with this taxonomy. Some maintain that all the strains adapted to different *Ornithodoros* species are merely variants of a single species, *Borrelia recurrentis*, the agent of epidemic relapsing fever, transmitted by lice.

Borreliae are helical bacteria 3–20 microns long by 0.2–0.5 microns in diameter. They are gram-negative, have flagella between the external and internal membranes, are actively motile, and change direction frequently. Some species (*B. duttoni, B. parkeri, B. turicata*) grow in laboratory culture media (Kelly, 1984).

Geographic Distribution: Natural foci of *Borrelia* transmissible to man are found worldwide, with the exception of Australia, New Zealand, and Oceania.

Occurrence in Man: The incidence is low. Man contracts the infection only upon entering the natural foci where infected *Ornithodoros* are found. In some regions of Africa, the vector *O. moubata* has become established in dwellings, where it lives in dirt floors. In Latin America, *O. rudis* (*O. venezuelensis*) and *O. turicata* also have an affinity for dwellings.

In 1969, the number of cases in South America was 278, with one death. In 1976, 15 cases were reported in the US. Sporadic cases occur in the western US states, in

Canada (British Columbia), Mexico, Guatemala, Panama, Colombia, Venezuela, Ecuador, and Argentina.

Although endemic relapsing fever is usually sporadic, at times group outbreaks occur. In 1973, there was an outbreak with 62 cases (16 confirmed and 46 clinically diagnosed) among tourists at Grand Canyon National Park in Arizona (USA) who were lodged in rustic wooden cabins infested by rodents and their ticks. In 1976, an outbreak occurred under similar circumstances in California, with 6 cases among 11 tourists (Harwood and James, 1979).

A telephone and mail survey was conducted of 10,000 people who visited the Grand Canyon. The results showed that there were 14 cases of relapsing fever among the tourists, and that 7 of these had to be hospitalized. There was laboratory confirmation of 4 cases and clinical diagnosis of 10 cases. Rodent nests were found beneath the ceilings and underneath the floors of the cabins where the tourists were lodged. These nests may have sheltered the vectors of the infection, as frequently happens with *Ornithodoros* (CDC, 1991).

Occurrence in Animals: In natural foci, many wild animal species are infected, among them rodents, armadillos, opossums, weasels, tree squirrels, and bats.

The Disease in Man: Epidemic relapsing fever (transmitted by lice) and endemic relapsing fever (transmitted by ticks) have similar clinical pictures. The average incubation period is 7 days after the tick bite, but may vary from 4 to 18 days. The disease is characterized by an initial pyrexia that lasts three to four days and begins and disappears suddenly. The fever, which may reach 41°C, is accompanied by chills, profuse sweating, vertigo, cephalalgia, myalgia, and vomiting. At times, erythemas, petechiae, epistaxis, and jaundice of varying degrees of severity may be observed. After several days without fever, the attacks of fever recur several times, lasting longer than in the first episode. The primary characteristic of the disease is the syndrome of periodic fevers. There are generally three to seven relapses of fever, with intervals of four to seven days (Barbour, 1990). Periodic recurrences are attributed to antigenic changes or mutations in the borreliae, against which the patient cannot develop immunity. Borreliae in the first attack are antigenically different from those isolated in relapses and there is no protective immunity among these serotypes. The variable antigens are proteins on the outer membrane and their variation is the result of a new DNA arrangement (Barbour, 1990).

Treatment is based on tetracyclines. Complications consist of meningitis and some other neurological disorders, but these occur in a small percentage of patients. Endemic fever is fatal in 2% to 5% of cases.

The Disease in Animals: Little is known about the natural course of the infection and its possible clinical manifestations in wild animals. As with many other reservoirs of infectious agents in natural foci, the hosts and borreliae are probably well adapted to each other, and the latter likely have little or no pathogenic effect on their hosts.

Borreliosis (spirochetosis) of fowl is a serious disease in geese, ducks, and chickens. It is caused by *B. anserina* and transmitted by *Argus persicus* and *A. miniatus*. The bovine infection in South Africa produced by *B. theileri* and transmitted by *Margaropus decoloratus* and *Rhipicephalus evertsi* causes a benign disease. These borrelioses affect only animals and are not transmitted to man.

**Figure 18. Tick-borne relapsing fever (*Ornithodoros* spp.).
Mode of transmission.**

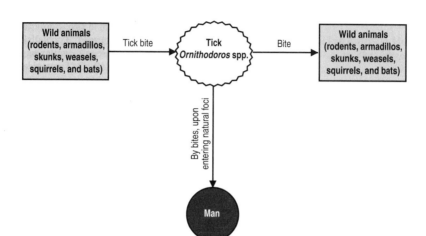

Source of Infection and Mode of Transmission (Figure 18): The borreliae that cause endemic relapsing fever have as their reservoir wild animals and ticks of the genus *Ornithodoros*; in addition, the latter are vectors of the infection. These ticks are xerophilic argasids that are long-lived and very resistant to dessication and long periods of fasting in environments with low humidity and high temperatures. Borreliae survive in the ticks for a long time. Depending on the species of *Ornithodoros*, transovarial transmission may vary from less than 1% to 100%. In the Western Hemisphere, the most important vectors of *Borrelia* are *O. hermsii*, *O. turicata*, *O. rudis*, and possibly *O. talaje*. The continuous circulation of borreliae in nature is ensured by the ticks' characteristics and their feeding on infected wild animals. *O. hermsii* lives at altitudes of over 1,000 meters, feeds on the blood of squirrels, and can be found in rodent burrows and wooden huts. *O. turicata* attacks sheep and goats, as well as other animals, and infests hides, rodent and snake burrows, and pigsties.

Transmission to humans is caused by a bite from an infected tick.

Role of Animals in the Epidemiology of the Disease: Several species of wild animals constitute the reservoir of the etiologic agent. The relative importance of ticks and wild animals as reservoirs is the subject of debate, but both undoubtedly play important roles in maintaining the infection in nature. An exception is infection by *B. duttoni* in Africa, which has not been found in animals and is transmitted directly to man by the tick *O. moubata*.

Diagnosis: Diagnosis is based on demonstrating the presence of the etiologic agent in the patient's blood during the febrile phase by dark-field microscopy using fresh smears or films stained by Giemsa or Wright techniques, or by inoculation in mice. The number of borreliae diminishes or disappears at the end of a fever attack;

thus, intraperitoneal inoculation of young mice and examination of their blood 24 to 72 hours after inoculation is advisable.

Control: Control measures are difficult to apply and are impractical, since cases in the Western Hemisphere are rare and usually widely dispersed. The principal recommendation is to avoid being bitten by ticks living in caves, burrows of rodents and other animals, or primitive huts.

Human dwellings should be built to keep out the hosts (rodents or others) of *Ornithodoros*. In addition, the storage of wood inside or near buildings should be avoided. People entering natural foci should examine themselves for ticks periodically, in addition to using protective footwear and clothing. Repellents provide partial protection; dimethyl phthalate is the most highly recommended.

Bibliography

Barbour, A.G. Antigenic variation of a relapsing fever *Borrelia* species. *Ann Rev Microbiol* 44:155–171, 1990.

Bruner, D.W., J.H. Gillespie. *Hagan's Infectious Diseases of Domestic Animals*. 6th ed. Ithaca: Comstock; 1973.

Coates, J.B., B.C. Hoff, P.M. Hoff, eds. *Preventive Medicine in World War II*. Vol. VII: *Communicable Diseases: Arthropod-borne Diseases other than Malaria*. Washington, D.C.: Department of the Army; 1964.

Felsenfeld, O. *Borreliae*, human relapsing fever, and parasite-vector-host relationships. *Bact Rev* 29:46–74, 1965.

Francis, B.J., R.S. Thompson. Relapsing fever. *In*: Hoeprich, P.D., ed. *Infectious Diseases*. Hagerstown: Harper & Row; 1972.

Geigy, R. Relapsing fevers. *In*: Weinmann, D., M. Ristic, eds. Vol 2: *Infectious Blood Diseases of Man and Animals*. New York: Academic Press; 1968.

Harwood, K.F., M.T. James. *Entomology in Human and Animal Health*. 7th ed. New York: Macmillan; 1979.

Jellison, W.J. The endemic relapsing fevers. *In*: Hubbert, W.T., W.F. McCulloch, P.R. Schnurrenberger, eds. *Diseases Transmitted from Animals to Man*. 6th ed. Springfield: Thomas; 1975.

Kelly, R.T. Genus IV *Borrelia*. *In*: Krieg, N.R., J.G. Holt, eds. Vol 1: *Bergey's Manual of Systematic Bacteriology*. Baltimore: Williams & Wilkins; 1984.

Pan American Health Organization. *Reported Cases of Notifiable Diseases in the Americas, 1969*. Washington, D.C.: PAHO; 1972. (Scientific Publication 247).

United States of America, Department of Health and Human Services, Centers for Disease Control and Prevention (CDC). Outbreak of relapsing fever—Grand Canyon National Park, Arizona, 1990. *MMWR Morb Mortal Wkly Rep* 40(18):296–297, 303, 1991.

TULAREMIA

ICD-10 A21.0 ulceroglandular tularaemia; A21.1 oculoglandular tularaemia; A21.2 pulmonary tularaemia; A21.7 generalized tularaemia; A21.8 other forms of tularaemia

Synonyms: Francis' disease, deer-fly fever, rabbit fever, Ohara's disease.

Etiology: *Francisella tularensis*, a highly pleomorphic, gram-positive, nonmotile bacillus; it has a fine capsule and can survive for several months in water, mud, and decomposing cadavers.

Two biovars are recognized: *F. tularensis* biovar *tularensis* (Jellison type A) and *F. tularensis* biovar *palaearctica* (Jellison type B). Names have also been suggested for some local biovars, such as *mediaasiatica* (Olsufjev and Meshcheryakova, 1982) and *japonica*. Classification into biovars is not based on antigenic differences, but on the agent's biochemical, virulence, and ecologic characteristics, and its nosography.

Geographic Distribution: Natural foci of infection are found in the Northern Hemisphere. In the Americas, the disease has been confirmed in Canada, the US, and Mexico. It is found in most European countries, Tunisia, Turkey, Israel, Iran, China, and Japan. In the former Soviet Union, there are extensive areas with natural foci.

F. tularensis biovar *tularensis* predominates in North America and causes 70% to 90% of human cases in that part of the world. The principal sources of infection by this biovar are lagomorphs (mainly those of the genus *Sylvilagus)* and ticks. Biovar *palaearctica* (syn. *holarctica*) causes 10% to 30% of human cases; its principal hosts are rodents. Biovar *tularensis* is more virulent than biovar *palaearctica* (Bell and Reilly, 1981).

Biovar *palaearctica* is found in western and northern Europe, Siberia, the Far East, in some parts of central Europe, and less frequently, in North America. Biovar *palaearctica* is distributed in natural foci among *Rodentia* spp. and *Lagomorpha* spp. In the Asian part of the former Soviet Union, where there are natural foci among *Lepus* and *Gerbilinae*, the name *F. tularensis* var. *mediaasiatica* has been suggested for the etiologic agent. This biovar, like *palaearctica*, is moderately virulent. Genetic studies have shown that the *mediaasiatica* and *japonica* varieties hybridize with *F. tularensis* var. *tularensis*, indicating the possibility of genetically related strains outside of North America. The strains of Central Asia differ from the two main biovars in their glucose fermentation properties (Sandström *et al.*, 1992).

Occurrence in Man: It is not an internationally reportable disease and its global incidence is hard to establish. The countries with the best data are the US and the former Soviet Union. In both, the number of human cases has apparently declined sharply. In the former Soviet Union, where in the 1940s some 100,000 cases were reported annually, the incidence has diminished to a few hundred cases per year. In the US, the average number of annual cases fell from 1,184 in the 1940s to some 274 cases between 1960 and 1969 and has continued to fall.

In the period 1977–1986, the average number of cases per year was 225. Many mild cases are not reported (Rohrbach, 1988). Current incidence is approximately

0.6 to 1.3 per million inhabitants (Boyce, 1990). The reduced incidence is attributed to, among other factors, limited demand for beaver (*Castor canadensis*) and muskrat (*Ondatra zibethicus*) skins and the resulting decline in hunting for these animals. In the US, 50% or more of the cases appear in a few states, such as Arkansas, Missouri, Oklahoma, Tennessee, and Texas. Although sporadic cases have occurred in all states except Hawaii, their numbers have fallen.

In areas where transmission is effected primarily by arthropods, incidence peaks in spring and summer. In contrast, in areas where cases of infection transmitted by wild rabbits predominate, the peaks occur in winter (Boyce, 1990), during the hunting season.

Epidemiological data on 1,026 human cases in the midwestern US states indicated that 63% involved an attached tick and 23% exposure to wild rabbits or other animals, such as squirrels, cats, and raccoons (Taylor *et al.*, 1991). In Canada, there were 31 cases between 1975 and 1979 (Akerman and Embil, 1982).

Occurrence in Animals: The disease affects a large number of vertebrates (more than 100 species of wild and domestic animals) and invertebrates (more than 100 species). Natural infection has been found in ticks, mosquitoes, horseflies, fleas, and lice that parasitize lagomorphs and rodents.

Epizootic outbreaks have been described in sheep, commercially bred furbearers (mink, beaver, and fox), and wild rodents and lagomorphs.

In Sweden, epizootics occur in hares (*Lepus timidus*), the principal source of human infection caused by *F. tularensis* biovar *palaearctica*. Between 1973 and 1985, 1,500 samples were submitted to the National Veterinary Institute in Uppsala, divided nearly equally into *Lepus europeus* and *L. timidus*. Tularemia was diagnosed by immunofluorescence in 109 samples of *L. timidus*, but in none of the *L. europeus* samples. The rate of animals infected varied by year; the highest rates occurred in autumn (Mörner *et al.*, 1988).

Few serological surveys have been conducted in domestic animals (Rohrbach, 1988). In endemic areas of Georgia and Florida, titers of ≥ 1/80 were found in 2 (6.2%) of 32 stray cats. As a result of an outbreak of 12 human cases of tularemia on the Crow Indian reservation in southern Montana (USA), 90 dogs were tested serologically. Of these, 56 had agglutination titers of ≥ 1/40, whereas in a nearby town, only 6 of 34 yielded similar titers (Schmid *et al.*, 1983).

A study conducted in western Georgia and northwestern Florida (USA) used the serum agglutination test on 2,004 mammals of 13 species; 344 animals of 10 species were positive with titers of ≥ 1/80 (McKeever *et al.*, 1958).

The Disease in Man: It is seen most commonly as sporadic cases, but epidemic outbreaks have occurred in the US and the former Soviet Union.

The incubation period usually lasts from three to five days, but may range from one to ten days. Several clinical forms of the disease are known; they are determined principally by the agent's route of entry. In all its forms, the disease is of sudden onset, with rising and falling fever, chills, asthenia, joint and muscle pain, cephalalgia, and vomiting. The most common clinical form is ulceroglandular, which represents 85% of all cases in the Western Hemisphere. A local lesion is seen at the site of entry (an arthropod bite, or a scratch or cut inflicted by contaminated nails or knife), which progresses to a necrotic ulceration accompanied by swelling of the nearby lymph node. The node frequently suppurates, ulcerates, and becomes sclerotic. In untreated cases, the disease course lasts three to five weeks and convalescence takes several weeks or months, with intermittent bouts of fever. A variety of this form is the glandular, in which there is no primary lesion; this is the most prevalent type in Japan. The oculoglandular form develops when contaminated material comes into contact with the conjunctiva. The primary lesion localizes on the lower eyelid and consists of an ulcerated papule; at the same time, the regional lymph nodes swell. The primary pulmonary form, caused by aerosols, affects rural and laboratory workers, and produces pneumonia in one or both lungs. The typhoidal form is rare; it is caused by ingestion of contaminated foods (usually infected wild rabbit meat) or water. It is a systemic disease that has very varied symptoms and is difficult to diagnose. It is sometimes expressed as gastroenteritis, fever, and toxemia. Pneumonia is frequent in typhoidal tularemia. If not treated early, the course of this clinical form may be short and fatal. Mortality in the pulmonary forms is high. Prior to the existence of antibiotics, mortality for all cases of tularemia in the US was close to 7%. Mortality outside of the Americas has rarely exceeded 1%. This difference is attributed to the greater virulence of the tick-transmitted strains of *F. tularensis* (biovar *tularensis*) in the US. In the former Soviet Union, untreated cutaneous infections (ulceroglandular form) are fatal for less than 0.5% of patients (biovar *palaearctica*).

The results of serologic and skin sensitivity tests carried out among exposed groups show that inapparent infections are common.

Streptomycin is the preferred antibiotic for all forms of tularemia. Recommended treatment is 15 to 20 mg/kg/day of streptomycin via intramuscular administration, divided into various doses over 7 to 14 days (Boyce, 1990). Laboratory tests with Scandinavian strains of *F. tularensis* biovar *palaearctica* obtained the lowest minimal inhibitory concentration with quinolones, as compared to other antibiotics. This result should be taken into account in clinical assays. In the Scandinavian countries, where most tularemia patients are ambulatory, quinolones have the additional advantage that they can be administered orally (Scheel *et al.*, 1993).

The Disease in Animals: In has been demonstrated experimentally that susceptibility to *F. tularensis* varies in different species of wild animals. Three groups have been established based on the infecting dose and the lethal dose. Group 1, the most susceptible, contains most species of rodents and lagomorphs, which generally suffer a fatal septicemic disease. Group 2 is composed of other species of rodents and birds, which though highly susceptible to the infection, rarely die from it. Group 3 consists of carnivores, which require high doses to become infected, rarely develop bacteremia, and only occasionally manifest overt disease.

Group 1 animals are an important source of infection for arthropods, other animals, man, and the environment. The clinical picture of the natural disease in these animals is not well known, since they are usually found dead or dying. Experimentally inoculated hares show weakness, fever, ulcers, abscesses at the inoculation site, and swelling of the regional lymph nodes. Death ensues in 8 to 14 days. The lesions resemble those of plague and pseudotuberculosis, with caseous lymph nodes and grayish white foci in the spleen.

High-mortality outbreaks have occurred in sheep in enzootic areas in Canada, the US, and the former Soviet Union. In addition to causing economic losses, tularemia in sheep is a source of infection for man. In the US, the infection is transmitted by the tick *Dermacentor andersoni*, which during outbreaks is found in great numbers at the base of the sheep's ears and on the neck. Sick animals separate themselves from the flock and manifest fever, rigid gait, diarrhea, frequent urination, and respiratory difficulty. Most deaths occur among young animals. Pregnant ewes may abort. Reactions to serologic tests indicate that many animals have an inapparent infection. Sheep can be classified in group 2 based on their susceptibility to the infection. Autopsy reveals infarcts of the regional lymph nodes, mainly those of the head and neck, as well as pneumonic foci. In this species, tularemia is a seasonal disease, coinciding with tick infestations.

The disease has been confirmed on occasion in horses, with symptoms that include lack of coordination, fever, and depression. The animals were parasitized by a large number of ticks. Infected young swine can manifest fever, dyspnea, and depression. Cattle seem to be resistant (Rohrbach, 1988).

Cats can become infected and fall ill when hunting rodents in endemic areas or by consuming dead lagomorphs. Cats can, in turn, transmit the infection to man. In a case that occurred in Georgia (USA), a young man who contracted ulceroglandular tularemia had three Siamese cats that had fallen ill two weeks earlier. The cats had fever, anorexia, and apathy; the veterinarian prescribed streptomycin and penicillin. The animals were cared for by their owner, who developed a necrotic ulcerous lesion that started with a wound on his finger, although he did not recall having been scratched or bitten. The three cats died despite treatment. On autopsy, necrotic foci were found in the liver and spleen that contained coccobacilli positive for *F. tularensis* with immunofluorescence.

Another case was described in New Mexico (USA). The patient found his cat under the bed eating a dead wild rabbit. He tried to remove the cat and was bitten; four days later he fell ill with tularemia. The cat fell ill one day earlier, with apathy, anorexia, and fever, but no other symptoms. The veterinarian did not prescribe any treatment and the animal was found to be healthy when examined a week later. Serum agglutination yielded a titer of 1/160. The owner also recovered, after being treated with streptomycin (CDC, 1982). In Oklahoma (USA), a state considered endemic, a case of acute tularemia in three cats was diagnosed clinically and then confirmed by culture and immunofluorescence. The three animals showed signs of depression, lethargy, ulcerated tongue and palate, moderate lymphadenomegaly, hepatosplenomegaly, and panleukopenia, with a severe toxic change in the neutrophils. Upon necropsy, multiple necrotic foci were found in the lymph nodes, liver, and spleen, as well as severe enterocolitis. The diagnosis was confirmed by immunofluorescence and culture (Baldwin *et al.*, 1991). Although tularemia is rare in cats, it should be kept in mind in enzootic areas. Since 1928, only 51 human cases have been described that involve exposure to infected cats (Capellan and Fong, 1993).

Source of Infection and Mode of Transmission (Figure 19): In natural foci, the infection circulates among wild vertebrates, independently of man and domestic animals. Ticks are biological vectors of *F. tularensis*; not only do they transmit the etiologic agent from donor animals to other animals, they also constitute an important interepizootic reservoir. They are also responsible for transtadial and transovarial transmission of the bacteria. Each enzootic region has one or more species of vertebrate animals and of ticks that play the primary roles of transmitting and maintain-

Figure 19. Tularemia. Mode of transmission in the Americas.

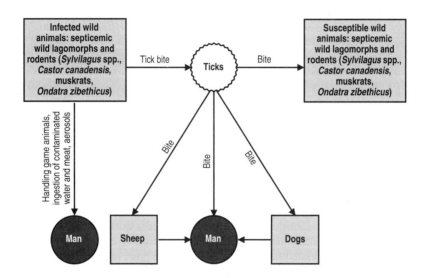

ing the infection in nature. It is a matter of debate whether very susceptible lago-morphs and rodents (group 1) are true reservoirs or only amplifiers and the main source of infection for man. Less susceptible animals (group 2), together with ticks, are thought to be important reservoirs.

Domestic animals, such as sheep and cats, are accidental hosts, but they may also constitute sources of infection for man.

Humans contract the infection upon entering the natural foci of tularemia. The sources of infection and modes of transmission of the causal agent are many. In North America, the animals that most frequently serve as the source of infection for man are wild rabbits (*Sylvilagus* spp.), hares (*Lepus californicus*), beavers (*Castor canadensis*), muskrats (*Ondatra zibethicus*), meadow voles (*Microtus* spp.), and sheep. The biovar *tularensis* is generally transmitted by wild rabbits or by their ticks (*Dermacentor variabilis*, *D. andersoni*, *Amblyomma americanum*). The biovar *palaearctica* is more common among rodents, particularly aquatic rodents, but also in some species of lagomorphs, such as *Lepus europaeus* and *L. variabilis*. Tularemia in Sweden is transmitted from *L. variabilis* by means of mosquitoes. The European hare plays no role in Sweden, but it does in other European countries. Rodents such as beavers and muskrats are important in aquatic cycles. In different ecological areas, other ticks (e.g., *Ixodes* spp., *Haemophysalis* spp.) and arthropods are also involved. In many enzootic areas, the principal route of penetration is through the skin (by means of hematophagous arthropods, scratches, or knife cuts). Another portal of entry is the conjunctiva, which can be contaminated by materials splashed into the eyes or, in the case of hunters or sheep shearers, by hands soiled from handling sick animals. Infection via the oral route occurs as a result of ingest-ing water contaminated by dead animals or the urine and feces of infected animals, or by eating undercooked meat of lagomorphs or other infected animals. In addition, the disease can be contracted through the respiratory system by inhaling aerosols contaminated in the laboratory or dust from fodder, grain, or wool contaminated with rodent excreta.

Some cases of human infection by cat scratches or bites have been described. It is assumed that these animals had recently hunted and captured sick rodents or had eaten dead lagomorphs. Another case occurred in a person exposed to a cat with an ulcer (CDC, 1982). The disease was also contracted by a Canadian zoo veterinarian who was bitten on the finger when treating a sick primate (*Sanguinus nigricollis*). In this zoo, four primates in adjacent cages died from tularemia, possibly transmitted by fleas from squirrels that often came near the cages. *F. tularensis* was isolated from one of the squirrels. The primate responsible for infecting the veterinarian had sialorrhea, ocular and nasal discharges, and ulcers on the tongue (Nayar *et al.*, 1979).

The highest incidence of cases occurs in the summer, when ticks are most active. Hunters are an especially vulnerable group, and the number of human cases increases in hunting season.

Role of Animals in the Epidemiology of the Disease: Human-to-human transmission has not been confirmed. Tularemia is a zoonosis that is transmitted to man (an accidental host) through contact with wild or domestic animals (of the latter, usually sheep), by a contaminated environment, or by such vectors as ticks, horseflies, and mosquitoes.

Diagnosis: In man, clinical diagnosis is based on the symptomatology and prior contact with a likely source of infection. Laboratory confirmation is based on: (a) isolation of the etiologic agent from the patient's local lesion, lymph nodes, and sputum by means of direct culture or inoculation into laboratory animals; (b) the immunofluorescence test on exudates, sputum, and other contaminated materials; (c) the skin test with bacterial allergen, which gives delayed hypersensitivity reactions (these reagents can give a diagnosis during the first week of illness); and (d) serologic tests, such as tube agglutination or microagglutination (Snyder, 1980; Sato *et al.*, 1990). An enzyme-linked immunosorbent assay with sonicated antigen has been perfected (Viljanen *et al.*, 1983). This test has the advantage of permitting an early diagnosis, which is important for treatment; it can also detect IgM, IgA, or IgG antibodies. However, the microagglutination test is used more often due to its simplicity and reliability; other tests are used only in case of doubt (Syrjälä *et al.*, 1986). In the agglutination test, a four-fold increase in titer is significant. Antibodies appear in the second week of illness and may persist for years. Cross agglutination with *Brucella* antigen can occur, but at a lower level than with the homologous antigen. Absorption of the patient's serum with *Brucella* antigen removes all doubt.

In sheep, laboratory confirmation is obtained by isolating the causal agent or by serologic tests.

Due to the risk to laboratory personnel, methods to isolate the causal agent should only be used at reference laboratories that have the required safety measures.

Control: To prevent the disease in man, general and individual protective measures may be taken. General measures include reducing the source of infection, controlling vectors, changing the environment, and educating the public. Except for the last one, these control measures are costly and difficult to apply. In the former Soviet

Union, where tularemia was an important health problem, anti-tularemia institutes have been established in epizootic regions to carry out these control activities.

An important protective measure consists of immunizing at-risk individuals, populations, or occupational groups with attenuated live vaccines. In the former Soviet Union, the drastic reduction achieved in human morbidity is attributed to this single activity. In the US, there is an attenuated vaccine for high-risk groups (Burke, 1977) that has proven effective in reducing the incidence of the typhoidal form and attenuating the ulceroglandular form (Rohrbach, 1988). Other protective measures consist of using insect repellents and protective clothing to avoid tick infestation and bites of other arthropods, promptly removing ticks from the body, using gloves to handle and skin wild animals, avoiding consumption of untreated water in areas where contamination by *F. tularensis* is suspected, and thoroughly cooking wild animal meat in enzootic areas.

Controlling the infection in sheep involves applying tickicides by spray or dip, and administering antibiotics (streptomycin, tetracyclines) in case of an outbreak.

Bibliography

Akerman, M.B., J.A. Embil. Antibodies to *Francisella tularensis* in the snowshoe hare (*Lepus americanus struthopus*) populations of Nova Scotia and Prince Edward Island and in the moose (*Alces alces americana* Clinton) population of Nova Scotia. *Can J Microbiol* 28:403–405, 1982.

Arata, A., H. Chamsa, A. Farhang-Azad, O. Mescerjakova, V. Neronov, S. Saidi. First detection of tularaemia in domestic and wild mammals in Iran. *Bull World Health Organ* 49:597–603, 1973.

Baldwin, C.J., R.J. Panciera, R.J. Morton, *et al.* Acute tularemia in three domestic cats. *J Am Vet Med Assoc* 199:1602–1605, 1991.

Bell, J.F, J.R. Reilly. Tularemia. *In*: Davis, J.W., L.H. Karstad, D.O. Trainer, eds. *Infectious Diseases of Wild Mammals*. 2nd ed. Ames: Iowa State University Press; 1981.

Benenson, A.S., ed. *Control of Communicable Diseases in Man*. 15th ed. An official report of the American Public Health Association. Washington, D.C.: American Public Health Association; 1990.

Boyce, J.M. *Francisella tularensis* (Tularemia). *In*: Mandell, G.L., R.G. Douglas, Jr., J.E. Bennett, eds. *Principles and Practice of Infectious Diseases*. 3rd ed. New York: Churchill Livingstone, Inc.; 1990.

Burke, D.S. Immunization against tularemia: Analysis of the effectiveness of live *Francisella tularensis* vaccine in prevention of laboratory-acquired tularemia. *J Infect Dis* 135:55–60, 1977.

Capellan, J., I.W. Fong. Tularemia from a cat bite: Case report and review of feline-associated tularemia. *Clin Infect Dis* 16:472–475, 1993.

Frank, F.W., W.A. Meinershagen. Tularemia epizootic in sheep. *Vet Med* 56:374–378, 1961.

Gelman, A.C. Tularemia. *In*: May, J.M., ed. *Studies in Disease Ecology*. New York: Hafner; 1961.

Hornick, R.B. Tularemia. *In*: Hoeprich, P.D., ed. *Infectious Diseases*. Hagerstown: Harper & Row; 1972.

Marsh, H. *Newsom's Sheep Diseases*. 2nd ed. Baltimore: Williams & Wilkins; 1958.

McKeever, S., J.H. Schubert, M.D. Moody, *et al.* Natural ocurrence of tularemia in marsupials, carnivores, lagomorphs, and large rodents in southwestern Georgia and northwestern Florida. *J Infect Dis* 103:120–126, 1958.

Meyer, K.F. *Pasteurella* and *Francisella*. *In*: Dubos, R.J., J.G. Hirsch, eds. *Bacterial and Mycotic Infections of Man*. 4th ed. Philadelphia: Lippincott; 1965.

Mörner, T., G. Sandström, R. Mattsson, P.O. Nilsson. Infections with *Francisella tularensis* biovar *palaearctica* in hares (*Lepus timidus, Lepus europaeus*) from Sweden. *J Wildl Dis* 24:422–433, 1988.

Nayar, G.P., G.J. Crawshaw, J.L. Neufeld. Tularemia in a group of nonhuman primates. *J Am Vet Med Assoc* 175:962–963, 1979.

Olsen, P.F. Tularemia. *In*: Hubbert, W.T., W.F. McCulloch, P.R. Schnurrenberger, eds. *Diseases Transmitted from Animals to Man*. 6th ed. Springfield: Thomas; 1975.

Olsufjev, N.G., I.S. Meshcheryakova. Subspecific taxonomy of *Francisella tularensis*, McCoy and Chapin, 1912. *Int J Syst Bacteriol* 33:872–874, 1983.

Pavlosky, E.N. *Natural Nidality of Transmissible Diseases*. Urbana: University of Illinois Press; 1966.

Reilly, J.R. Tularemia. *In*: Davis, J.W., L. Karstad, D.O. Trainer, eds. *Infectious Diseases of Wild Mammals*. Ames: Iowa State University Press; 1970.

Rohrbach, B.W. Tularemia. *J Am Vet Med Assoc* 193:428–432, 1988.

Sandström, G., A. Sjöstedt, M. Forsman, *et al*. Characterization and classification of strains of *Francisella tularensis* isolated in the central Asian focus of the Soviet Union and in Japan. *J Clin Microbiol* 30:172–175, 1992.

Sato, T., H. Fujita, Y. Ohara, M. Homma. Microagglutination test for early and specific serodiagnosis of tularemia. *J Clin Microbiol* 28:2372–2374, 1990.

Scheel, O., T. Hoel, T. Sandvik, B.P. Berdal. Susceptibility pattern of Scandinavian *Francisella tularensis* isolates with regard to oral and parenteral antimicrobial agents. *APMIS* 101:33–36, 1993.

Schmid, G.P., A.N. Kornblatt, C.A. Connors, *et al*. Clinically mild tularemia associated with tick-borne *Francisella tularensis*. *J Infect Dis* 148:63–67, 1983.

Snyder, M.J. Immune response to *Francisella*. *In*: Rose, H.R., H. Friedman, eds. *Manual of Clinical Immunology*. 2nd ed. Washington, D.C.: American Society for Microbiology; 1980.

Syrjälä, H., P. Koskela, T. Ripatti, *et al*. Agglutination and ELISA methods in the diagnosis of tularemia in different clinical forms and severities of the disease. *J Infect Dis* 153:142–145, 1986.

Taylor, J.P., G.R. Istre, T.C. McChesney, *et al*. Epidemiologic characteristics of human tularemia in the southwest-central states, 1981–1987. *Am J Epidemiol* 133:1032–1038, 1991.

Thorpe, B.D., R.W. Sidwell, D.E. Johnson, K.L. Smart, D.D. Parker. Tularemia in the wildlife and livestock of the Great Salt Lake Desert Region, 1951 through 1964. *Am J Trop Med Hyg* 14:622–637, 1965.

Tiggert, W.D. Soviet viable *Pasteurella tularensis* vaccines. A review of selected articles. *Bacteriol Rev* 26:354–373, 1962.

United States of America, Department of Health and Human Services, Centers for Disease Control and Prevention (CDC). Tularemia associated with domestic cats—Georgia, New Mexico. *MMWR Morb Mortal Wkly Rep* 31:39–41, 1982.

Viljanen, M.K., T. Nurmi, A. Salminen. Enzyme-linked immunosorbent assay (ELISA) with bacterial sonicate antigen for IgM, IgA, and IgG antibodies to *Francisella tularensis*: Comparison with bacterial agglutination test and ELISA with lipopolysaccharide antigen. *J Infect Dis* 148:715–720, 1983.

Woodward, T.E. Tularemia. *In*: Beeson, P.B., W. McDermott, eds. *Cecil Textbook of Medicine*. 15th ed. Philadelphia: Saunders; 1979.

Zidon, J. Tularemia. *In*: Van der Hoeden, J., ed. *Zoonoses*. Amsterdam: Elsevier; 1964.

ZOONOTIC TUBERCULOSIS

**ICD-10 A16 respiratory tuberculosis, not confirmed
bacteriologically or histologically; A18 tuberculosis of other organs**

Etiology: The etiologic agents of mammalian tuberculosis are *Mycobacterium tuberculosis*, the main cause of human tuberculosis; *M. bovis*, the agent of bovine tuberculosis; and *M. africanum*, which causes human tuberculosis in tropical Africa. This last species has characteristics halfway between those of *M. tuberculosis* and *M. bovis*. *M. microti*, which causes tuberculosis in rodents, should be added to these agents, although it is not of zoonotic interest (nontuberculous mycobacteria are presented in the chapter, "Diseases Caused by Nontuberculous Mycobacteria").

The principal agent of zoonotic tuberculosis is *M. bovis*; the agent in man and other primates is *M. tuberculosis*, which is the type species of the genus.

Tuberculous mycobacteria are alcohol- and acid-resistant, nonsporogenic, grampositive bacilli. These mycobacteria are resistant to many disinfectants, desiccation, and other adverse environmental factors because the cell wall has a high lipid content.

Phage typing is being used in epidemiological research on *M. tuberculosis*, and the API ZIM system divides the genus into seven biovars (Casal and Linares, 1985; Humble *et al.*, 1977). The use of phage typing was not widespread and the method practically fell into disuse. It has been replaced by DNA hybridization.

Analysis of DNA fragments obtained through the digestive action of one or more restriction endonucleases is useful for identifying strains of both *M. tuberculosis* and *M. bovis* (Collins and De Lisle, 1985; Shoemaker *et al.*, 1986).

Many authors prefer to refer to a single species (*M. tuberculosis*) and human and bovine types.

Geographic Distribution: The distribution of *M. bovis* and *M. tuberculosis* is worldwide. *M. africanum* is prevalent in Africa, but it has also been isolated in Germany and England. *M. africanum* strains phenotypically related to *M. tuberculosis* are nitrase positive and are found in western Africa; those that are similar to *M. bovis* are nitrase negative and are isolated more frequently in eastern Africa (Grange and Yates, 1989).

Occurrence in Man: The prevalence of human tuberculosis of animal origin has diminished greatly in countries where mandatory pasteurization of milk has been implemented and where successful campaigns to control and eradicate the bovine infection have been carried out. The British Isles, where the incidence of human infection due to *M. bovis* is currently low and is limited to the elderly, were once the most affected area due to the consumption of raw milk. However, despite the great reduction in rates of human infection by bovine strains in Great Britain, tuberculosis originated by these strains continues to occur. From 1977 to 1979 in southeast England, isolations from 5,021 tuberculosis patients revealed 63 patients (1.25%) infected with "classic bovine strains" (*M. bovis*), 53 of which were Europeans and 10, immigrants. Of these cases, 27 (42.85%) had pulmonary tuberculosis and 36 (57.14%) had extrapulmonary tuberculosis. There was a marked difference in the frequency of renal tuberculosis caused by *M. bovis* (23.8%) and *M. tuberculosis*

(8.2%). Commenting on these results, Collins *et al.* (1981) suggested the possibility of human-to-human transmission, given that bovine tuberculosis had practically disappeared from Great Britain, that milk is pasteurized, and that some cases occurred in young people. Also in southeast England, human cases caused by *M. bovis* continued to occur nearly 30 years after the program to eradicate bovine tuberculosis ended in 1960. From 1977 to 1987, there were 201 new confirmed human cases caused by *M. bovis*, or 1.20% of all isolations of tuberculous mycobacteria (Yates and Grange, 1988). Most cases occurred in the elderly, who may have acquired the infection when it was still prevalent in cattle (in 1935, before the start of the eradication program, 40% of cattle were positive to tuberculin). The pulmonary and genitourinary forms are currently the most common forms in humans infected by *M. bovis* (Yates and Grange, 1988). In Slovakia, 52 human cases caused by the bovine bacillus were recorded during the period 1979–1983, 10 to 15 years after the eradication of bovine tuberculosis. The average age of the patients was 61. Of these, 88% suffered from pulmonary tuberculosis; 17% of these were relapses and 71% were new cases (Burjanova and Nagyova, 1985). In the Czech Republic, 47 patients infected by *M. bovis* were reported during the period 1981–1983 (Kubin *et al.*, 1985). In Germany during the period 1953–1957, when the prevalence of tuberculosis in cattle was still high, 45% of tuberculous adenitis cases in children were caused by *M. bovis*. Later, as prevalence declined in cattle, this form of tuberculosis as well as cutaneous tuberculosis declined notably. In the US at the beginning of the 20th century, up to 20% of human tuberculosis was attributed to *M. bovis*; in 1980, barely 0.1% of human tuberculosis was so attributed (Good and Snider, 1980). In the Netherlands, where bovine tuberculosis had been eradicated, 125 people were infected by *M. bovis* from 1972 to 1975 (Schonfeld, 1982). More than 80% of these patients were born when transmission of *M. bovis* via milk was still possible. The five patients younger than 20 years, who were born after the bovine infection was eradicated, were presumed to have contracted the infection outside the Netherlands. Interhuman transmission is still a matter of controversy, but it is undeniable that eradication campaigns against bovine tuberculosis have drastically reduced the incidence of human cases of this origin. For example, in Great Britain in 1945, 5% of all fatal tuberculosis cases and 30% of cases of the disease in children under 5 years old were due to bovine strains (Collins and Grange, 1983).

In countries where milk is routinely boiled, as in Latin America, the incidence of infection by *M. bovis* has always been low. Nevertheless, pulmonary and extrapulmonary forms of human tuberculosis of animal origin continue to be a problem in areas where the prevalence of infection in cattle is high, because not all milk consumed is boiled, many products are prepared from unpasteurized milk, and cases of infection are contracted via aerosols. In Peru, a study of 853 strains of pulmonary tuberculosis identified 38 (4.45%) as *M. bovis* (Fernández Salazar *et al.*, 1983). Several laboratories in Argentina studied a total of 7,195 strains, primarily between 1978 and 1981. Most of the strains were isolated from adult pulmonary tuberculosis patients, and 82 (1.1%) were classified as *M. bovis* (Argentina, Comisión Nacional de Zoonosis, 1982).

Occurrence in Animals: In industrialized countries, bovine tuberculosis has been eradicated or is in an advanced stage of control, while in several developing countries the situation has not improved or prevalence is increasing. Almost all Western

European countries report a prevalence of bovine infection lower than 0.1%. In the Western Hemisphere, Canada and the US have reduced the infection rate to very low levels. In the US in 1969, 0.06% of 4.5 million cattle examined reacted to tuberculin (most of the reactors showed no evident lesions when slaughtered). In 1989, 33.5 million cattle were slaughtered in the US (excluding reactors to tuberculin), of which only 143 had tuberculous lesions (0.0004%). In Latin America, Costa Rica, Cuba, Jamaica, Panama, Uruguay, and Venezuela have national control programs. Cuba is already in the post-eradication surveillance phase. The rate of infection is very low in several Central American and Caribbean countries. The highest infection rates are found in the milk-producing regions near large cities in South America. In South American countries in which hogs are fed unpasteurized milk products, the infection rate in swine is similar to or higher than in cattle, judging by records of confiscations at slaughterhouses. However, it should be kept in mind that these figures include a large percentage of lesions caused by nontuberculous mycobacteria (see the chapter, "Diseases Caused by Nontuberculous Mycobacteria").

Bovine tuberculosis is important not only because it is a source of human infection, but also because of the economic losses it causes.

Mycobacterium africanum, isolated for the first time from a human patient in Senegal and described in 1969 (Castets *et al.*, 1969), is capable of infecting nonhuman primates and causing pulmonary, lymph node, and renal lesions. Thorel (1980) isolated these strains from chimpanzees and from a *Cercopithexus* monkey of African origin that were found in experimental stations in Europe. These animals had probably contracted the infection from man. There is a potential danger of retransmission to those who work with them. There is also a report on bovine infection in Malawi caused by *M. africanum* (Berggren, 1981), but it fails to provide details on typing (Pritchard, 1988).

Man can transmit *M. tuberculosis* to monkeys, dogs, cats, and psittacine birds (see the section on the disease in animals).

The Disease in Man: *M. bovis* can cause the same clinical forms and pathologic lesions as *M. tuberculosis* (the agent of human tuberculosis). Historically, the most prevalent forms caused by *M. bovis* were extrapulmonary, and children were among those most affected. The reason for extrapulmonary localization of the bovine bacillus is not that it has an affinity for other tissues, but that it is most commonly transmitted by consumption of raw milk or raw milk products. Thus, in those countries where the prevalence of bovine tuberculosis was high and raw milk was consumed, many cases of extrapulmonary tuberculosis, such as cervical adenitis, genitourinary infections, tuberculosis of the bones and joints, and meningitis, were caused by *M. bovis*. According to data on typing of tuberculosis bacilli in the British Isles prior to control of bovine infection, 50% or more of cervical adenitis cases were caused by *M. bovis*. Pulmonary tuberculosis caused by the bovine bacillus occurs less frequently, but its incidence is significant in occupational groups in contact with infected cattle or their carcasses, particularly in countries where animals are stabled. This form cannot be distinguished clinically or radiologically from the disease caused by *M. tuberculosis*. Transmission occurs by aerosol droplets micromillimeters in diameter. In countries where the incidence of the human infection caused by *M. tuberculosis* has declined and the bovine infection has not been controlled, it is believed that *M. bovis* could assume a principal role in human pulmonary tuberculosis. Although Denmark was declared free of bovine tuberculosis in 1952, 127 cases of human infection caused by *M. bovis*, 58% of which were pulmonary tuberculosis, were detected between 1959 and 1963 in middle-aged and elderly persons.

In countries where the control of bovine tuberculosis is advanced, human cases caused by *M. bovis* are observed mainly in the elderly, who were exposed to the pathogenic agent in their youth or childhood.

Reduction or elimination of *M. bovis* in cattle and compulsory pasteurization of milk have helped reduce the incidence of infection in man. At the same time, the clinical picture of human infection caused by the bovine agent has changed. Currently, pulmonary tuberculosis predominates, followed by urogenital tuberculosis.

Interhuman transmission of *M. bovis* is possible, but few cases have been satisfactorily confirmed. As is the case with most zoonoses, man is generally an accidental host of *M. bovis* and human infection depends on the animal source. Since *M. tuberculosis* and *M. bovis* are very similar in their pathogenic effect on man, it is not understood why large-scale interhuman transmission of the bovine infection does not occur. A possible explanation is that pulmonary patients infected by *M. bovis* shed fewer bacteria in their sputum than do those infected by *M. tuberculosis* (Griffith, 1937).

Inhabitants of Latin America have been assumed to be protected from infection by the bovine bacillus because of the widespread custom of boiling milk. Undoubtedly, if this practice were not followed, the rate of human infection by *M. bovis* would be much higher there, considering the infection's wide distribution and the rate of infection in dairy cattle in many Latin American countries. However, some people in rural areas do drink raw milk and frequently consume products (cream, butter, soft cheese) made at home from raw milk. In Latin America and other parts of the world, children are the main victims, as indicated by typing data from Brazil, Peru, and Mexico. These data also confirm that some children are fed milk or milk products that are not heat-treated.

Although it is not customary to stable cattle in Latin America, cases of pulmonary tuberculosis caused by *M. bovis* have been recorded, with rural laborers and employees of abattoirs and locker plants being the most exposed groups. In Argentina, the bovine bacillus was isolated from 8% of 85 pulmonary patients from rural areas, while only 1 case due to *M. bovis* was found among 55 patients in the capital.

People suffering from pulmonary tuberculosis of bovine origin can, in turn, retransmit the infection to cattle. This occurrence is particularly evident in herds from which tuberculosis has been eradicated and which later become reinfected, the source of exposure often being a ranch hand with *M. bovis* tuberculosis. Such episodes have occurred in the US and in several European countries. Between 1943 and 1952, 128 herds containing more than 1,000 head of cattle were reinfected in Denmark by 107 individuals with tuberculosis. Similar occurrences continued in Denmark until 1960, despite advances made in the eradication of bovine tuberculosis. Huitema (1969) reports on 50 herds that were infected by people with tuberculosis caused by *M. bovis*; 24 of the patients suffered from renal tuberculosis. It is possible that this phenomenon (retransmission of the infection from man to cattle) also occurs in the Southern Hemisphere, but goes unnoticed due to high rates of tuberculosis in cattle.

In regions where bovine tuberculosis has been eradicated, cattle cease to be a source for human infection, but man may continue to be a potential source of infection for cattle for years.

Persons with pulmonary or genitourinary tuberculosis due to the human type species (*M. tuberculosis*) can temporarily infect and sensitize cattle. Cattle are very resistant to *M. tuberculosis*; the agent does not cause a progressive tuberculosis in these animals, but the bacillus can survive for some time in their tissues, especially the lymph nodes, sensitizing the animal to mammalian tuberculin and confusing the diagnosis. Sensitization can persist for some six to eight months after the human source of infection is removed. Elimination of *M. tuberculosis* in milk has occasionally been confirmed, but tuberculous lesions of the udder were not present. Man can transmit the human bacillus to several other animals, principally monkeys and dogs, in which it produces a progressive tuberculosis.

In many countries, direct or indirect exposure of man to bovine tuberculosis is an important source of sensitization to tuberculin. In Denmark, a relationship was found between the prevalence of bovine tuberculosis and the rate of reactors to tuberculin in the human population. In the same country, statistical data indicate that a third of the population between the ages of 30 and 35 owes its tuberculin sensitization to infection by *M. bovis*. The same study suggests that the risk of developing pulmonary tuberculosis later is much smaller among those sensitized by the bovine bacillus than by the human bacillus, perhaps because *M. bovis* infection is contracted mainly through the digestive tract and not via aerosols. Another interesting conclusion is that less calcification occurs in pulmonary tuberculosis resulting from *M. bovis* than from *M. tuberculosis*.

The treatment for humans infected by *M. bovis* is the same as for those infected by *M. tuberculosis* (isoniazid, rifampicin, ethambutol), except that pyrazinamide should be excluded, as it is not active against the bovine bacillus.

The Disease in Animals: Many mammalian species are susceptible to the agents of tuberculosis. Bovine tuberculosis is the most important form in economic terms and as a zoonosis. Tuberculosis in swine also causes substantial economic losses.

CATTLE: The principal etiologic agent for cattle is *M. bovis*. As in man, the bacillus enters the body mainly by inhalation. The intestinal tract is an important route of infection in calves nursed on contaminated milk. The most common clinical and pathological form is pulmonary tuberculosis. The causal agent enters the lungs and multiplies there, forming the primary focus; this is accompanied by tuberculous lesions in the bronchial lymph nodes of the same side, thus producing the primary complex. These lesions can remain latent or develop further, depending on the interaction between the agent and the host's body. If the animal's resistance to tuberculosis bacilli breaks down, the infection will spread to other organs via the lymph or blood vessels, giving rise to early generalization of the infection. If the immune system is unable to destroy the bacilli, they will cause tubercles to form in organs and tissues where they lodge. New foci are produced, mainly in the lungs, kidneys, liver, spleen, and their associated lymph nodes. Dissemination may also give rise to acute miliary tuberculosis.

In most cases, tuberculosis has a chronic course, with effects limited to the lungs. The disease process is slow and may remain clinically inapparent for a long time. In fact, some animals spend their entire useful lives without any evident symptomatology, although they constitute a potential threat for the rest of the herd. Other animals develop chronic bronchopneumonia, accompanied by coughing and reduced milk production. In advanced cases, when the lungs are largely destroyed, there is pronounced dyspnea.

Pearl disease, a tuberculous peritonitis or pleurisy, is another form sometimes observed in infected herds in countries with no tuberculosis control program.

It is estimated that about 5% of tuberculous cows, especially in advanced cases, have tuberculous uterine lesions or tuberculous metritus, and that 1% to 2% have tuberculous mastitis. This clinical form not only has public health repercussions, but also serves as a source of infection for calves nursed naturally or artificially. One of the main signs of tuberculosis acquired by the oral route is swelling of the retropharyngeal lymph nodes. In calves, the primary lesion is usually located in the mesenteric lymph nodes and the intestinal mucosa is not affected.

The disease appears more frequently in older animals because the disease is chronic and because older animals have had more time to be exposed to the infection. The infection is more prevalent among dairy cattle than among beef cattle, not only because their useful economic life is longer, but because dairy cattle are in closer contact with one another when gathered for milking or when housed in dairy sheds.

Cattle are resistant to the *M. avium* complex (MAC) and rarely suffer progressive tuberculosis due to these agents. Nevertheless, they are very important in control programs because cattle can become paraspecifically sensitized to mammalian tuberculin, leading to difficulties in diagnosis. *M. avium* infects cattle through the digestive tract. When lesions are present, they are generally limited to the intestine and mesenteric lymph nodes. However, lesions can occasionally be found in the lungs and regional lymph nodes but not in other tissues, indicating that the entry route may sometimes be the respiratory tract. Lesions tend to heal spontaneously. Bovine-to-bovine transmission of *M. avium* infection does not occur (see the chapter, "Diseases Caused by Nontuberculous Mycobacteria").

Cattle are very resistant to *M. tuberculosis*, and rarely develop anatomicopathologic lesions. In several countries, *M. tuberculosis* has been isolated from the lymph nodes of some positive reactors to tuberculin that showed no lesions in postmortem examination. Again in this instance, the infection's importance lies in sensitizing these animals to tuberculin.

An experiment comparing the pathogenicity of *M. africanum*, *M. bovis*, and *M. tuberculosis* for calves inoculated intravenously showed that *M. africanum* (at least the strain used in this experiment) was as pathogenic for calves as *M. bovis* (de Kantor *et al.*, 1979).

SWINE: This species is susceptible to the following agents: *M. bovis*, *M. avium* complex, and *M. tuberculosis*. *M. bovis* is the most pathogenic and invasive for swine and is the cause of most cases of generalized tuberculosis.

The principal route of infection is the digestive tract through consumption of contaminated milk or milk products, kitchen and abattoir scraps, and excreta from tuberculous fowl and cattle. The primary infection complex is found in the oropharynx and the submaxillary lymph nodes, or in the intestines and the mesenteric lymph nodes. The lesions are usually confined in the primary complex. Chronic lesions are not found in single organs, as they often are in cattle. Prevalence is lower in young animals than in adults, but the former show a greater tendency toward generalization of the infection. Eradication programs for bovine tuberculosis directly help to reduce the infection rate among swine. In the US in 1924, tuberculous lesions were found in 15.2% of hogs butchered, while in 1989, they were found in only 0.67%.

Most cases of swine tuberculosis are due to the *M. avium* complex. Thus, the reduction of avian tuberculosis has also helped lower the rate of infection in swine. In Great Britain, as tuberculosis of bovine origin declined, infections caused by MAC increased proportionally (Lesslie *et al.*, 1968). The total number of confiscations due to generalized tuberculosis was reduced even more drastically. In some Latin American countries, *M. bovis* is the cause of 80% to 90% of tuberculous lesions in swine. The relative proportions of *M. bovis* and MAC as the cause of swine tuberculosis are reversed when *M. bovis* infection is controlled in cattle, as it has been in several European countries and in the US.

MAC usually causes adenitis of the digestive tract and, more rarely, a generalized disease (see the chapter, "Diseases Caused by Nontuberculous Mycobacteria").

Swine are also susceptible to the human bacillus (*M. tuberculosis*), which produces an infection of the lymph nodes that drain the digestive system and, more rarely, generalized tuberculosis. The main sources of infection are kitchen scraps and leftovers from tuberculosis sanatoriums. This infection has been confirmed in several countries in the Americas, Europe, and Africa.

Swine-to-swine transmission of the infection is insignificant. Intestinal lesions are hyperplastic, and ulcers that would cause the agent to be shed are not observed. However, swine may transmit the infection to other swine when they have pulmonary, uterine, or mammary lesions (Thoen, 1992).

If there is generalization of the infection caused by MAC, the lesions appear in diffuse form and there is little tendency toward encapsulation. The cutaway view of a lesion generally shows a smooth surface and there may be foci of caseation, but calcification is minimal. Lesions caused by *M. bovis* or *M. tuberculosis*, in contrast, are caseous and well-circumscribed by fibrosis with pronounced calcification (Thoen, 1992). Other bacteria, for example *Rodococcus equi*, can produce lesions similar to tuberculous lesions.

SHEEP AND GOATS: Tuberculosis in sheep is generally rare and sporadic. In the few cases described, the most important agent was *M. avium*, followed by *M. bovis*. Only two cases involved *M. tuberculosis*. In research in New Zealand stemming from a program to eradicate bovine tuberculosis, multiples cases of infection by *M. bovis* were confirmed among sheep sharing the same pasture with infected cattle. In one area, 597 sheep were given the tuberculin test on the inner thigh and 108 (18%) reactors were discovered. Lesions, mostly in the lymph nodes, were found in 43 (61%) out of 70 necropsies. The lungs were affected in eight sheep (Davidson *et al.*, 1981). A similar result was observed in another region of New Zealand, on land where the prevalence of tuberculosis in cattle and opossums (*Trichosurus vulpecula*) was high. The tuberculin test yielded positive results in 11% of the sheep, and was judged to have a sensitivity of 81.6% and a specificity of 99.6% (Cordes *et al.*, 1981).

Prevalence in goats seems to be low. In countries with advanced programs to eradicate bovine tuberculosis, the infection in goats is monitored, since this species is susceptible to *M. bovis*, frequently suffers from pulmonary tuberculosis, and can reinfect cattle. Nannies also suffer from tuberculous mastitis and their milk may constitute a danger to the consumer. In addition, goats are susceptible to *M. avium* and *M. tuberculosis*, and the latter agent sometimes causes generalized processes. Little is known about the disease's occurrence in goats in developing countries, since these animals are generally slaughtered without veterinary inspection.

HORSES: Tuberculosis is infrequent in horses. In countries where the incidence of bovine infection is high, the principal agent of the disease in horses is *M. bovis*. The infection's predominant route of entry is the digestive system. Lesions are generally confined to the lymph nodes of the digestive tract, where they produce a tissue reaction that resembles tumors. Some cases of generalized infection, caused by both *M. bovis* and *M. avium*, have been described. Often, no lesions are found in infections produced by *M. avium*. In Germany, the avian bacillus was isolated from 30% of 208 horses with no apparent lesions.

M. tuberculosis is seldom isolated from horses. In a study carried out some time ago, only 13 of 241 typed strains corresponded to the human bacillus (Francis, 1958).

The disease is very rare in asses and mules.

It is interesting to note that horses are hypersensitive to tuberculin, and thus the allergenic test does not give reliable results.

DOGS AND CATS: Dogs are resistant to experimental tuberculosis infection. Recorded cases in dogs are probably due to massive and repeated exposure brought about by living with humans with tuberculosis or frequently eating contaminated food. Infection may be produced by aerosols, or by ingestion of sputa, milk, and viscera. Almost 75% of the cases are due to the human bacillus and the rest to the bovine. The clinical picture is not characteristic. The only symptoms found in eight tuberculous dogs in New York City were anorexia, weight loss, lethargy, vomiting, and leukocytosis. Radiology revealed pleural and pericardial effusion, ascites, and hepatomegaly. Granulomatous lesions in soft tissues were similar to those observed in neoplasias (Liu *et al.*, 1980). Infection mainly localizes in the lungs or mesenteric lymph nodes; intestinal ulcers and renal lesions are sometimes found as well. Consequently, dogs can shed bacilli by coughing and in their saliva, feces, and urine. It has also been demonstrated that the etiologic agent can be present in the pharynx and feces of dogs living in the same house with tuberculous patients, even when the animals show no tuberculous lesions. Although few cases of transmission from dog to man have been confirmed, a tuberculous dog (or even an apparently healthy animal living with a tuberculous patient) represents a potential risk and should be destroyed. A dog infected with *M. bovis* can, in turn, be a potential source of reinfection for cattle.

Cats also have a great natural resistance to tuberculosis. *M. bovis* is the most common pathogen in cats, and has been isolated in 90% of the cases. The agent gains entry via the digestive tract when milk or viscera containing tuberculosis bacilli is consumed. Cat-to-cat transmission of *M. bovis* in a scientific institution in Australia has been described (Isaac *et al.*, 1983). In countries where bovine tuberculosis has been brought under control, infection in cats is rare, and the few recorded cases have been caused by *M. tuberculosis* and occasionally MAC.

Destructive lesions are sometimes found; pneumonitis and cutaneous tuberculosis are frequent. In urban areas of Buenos Aires, a cooperative study was conducted by the Pasteur Institute and the Pan American Institute for Food Protection and Zoonoses (INPPAZ). *M. bovis* was isolated from the lesions of 10 of approximately 150 cats studied (I.N. de Kantor. Personal communication). In New Zealand between 1974 and 1986, *M. bovis* was isolated from 57 cats. With the exception of six animals, all came from suburban and rural areas where tuberculosis is also present in wild animals, particularly the opossum (*Trichosurus vulpecula*). Cutaneous lesions were observed in 58% of the cats, with a pyogranulomatous reaction and coagulative necrosis. These lesions had not been described earlier in other geographic areas, where the prevalence of tuberculosis among cats was 2% to 13% before successful control and eradication programs were implemented. Presumably the cats acquired the infection when feeding on tuberculous wild animals (De Lisle *et al.*, 1990). Several cases of reinfection of cattle herds by tuberculous cats have been described.

WILD, CAPTIVE, AND DOMESTIC ANIMALS: Animals living in the wild, far from man and domestic animals, generally do not contract tuberculosis. On the other hand, captive animals in zoos, on pelt farms, in laboratories, and in family homes may be exposed to infection. Monkeys are susceptible to *M. tuberculosis* as well as *M. africanum* and *M. bovis*. Almost 70% of the isolations from these animals are strains of the human bacillus, some are *M. africanum*, and the rest are *M. bovis*. The disease is contracted via the respiratory or digestive route. The infection can be propagated from monkey to monkey and constitutes a grave problem for colonies kept in scientific institutions and zoos. These animals can retransmit the infection to man. It is not unusual to find tuberculous pet monkeys that may have been infected before their acquisition or through contact with a family member. In France, infection due to *M. africanum* has been described in three chimpanzees and a *Cercopithexus* monkey. Three of these animals belonged to a scientific center and one of the chimpanzees belonged to a zoo. Since *M. africanum* has properties intermediate between those of *M. bovis* and *M. tuberculosis*, it is possible that infection by *M. africanum* was not described earlier in nonhuman primates because the species type of strains isolated previously was misidentified. It still has not been determined whether the infection was transmitted to the primates by man or acquired in their natural forest habitat (Thorel, 1980).

Tuberculosis is a problem in cervids, particularly now that deer farming has become popular in several countries. Tuberculosis in deer is caused primarily by *M. bovis*. This presents the possibility of retransmission of the infection to cattle in countries that are practically free of bovine tuberculosis. It is also a potential risk for people who are in contact with these animals. *M. bovis* has been found in free-roaming deer, probably living near cattle operations in Canada, the US (Hawaii), Great Britain, Ireland, and Switzerland. Deer most exposed to the disease are captive animals in zoos or deer on farms.

The first report on infection in farmed deer comes from New Zealand, in a region where the disease exists in cattle and opossum (*Trichosurus vulpecula*). An outbreak of bovine tuberculosis was recorded on farms in England that imported red deer (*Cervus elaphus*) from an eastern European country. Upon necropsy of 106 deer, 26 were found to be infected and 19 had visible lesions. The tuberculin test had 61.3% specificity and 80% sensitivity (Stuart *et al.* 1988). In a case of this type, the test would be used primarily to determine whether or not tuberculosis exists on a farm. An eradication program has been established in New Zealand based on the tuberculin test and slaughter of reactors, but the high percentage of false negatives hampers success.

In South Australia, an outbreak was reported in 1986 in three herds of another deer species (*Dama dama*). Upon necropsy, 47 of 51 animals were found to have bovine tuberculosis (Robinson *et al.*, 1989). In eight US states, the infection was found in 1991 in ten herds of deer. This caused concern because information from Canada indicated the possibility of human infection from this source (Essey *et al.*, 1991).

Outbreaks have been described in farmed fur-bearing animals, such as mink and silver fox; the source of infection was meat or viscera of tuberculous cattle or fowl. Tuberculosis has been found in wild species of ungulates and carnivores in zoos and some nature preserves, and the infection has been confirmed in several animal species in zoos in Latin America and other parts of the world.

Two wild species are reservoirs of and sources of infection by *M. bovis* in cattle. An opossum (*Trichosurus vulpecula*) from Australia—where tuberculous infection has not been found in this species—was introduced into New Zealand, where it contracted bovine tuberculosis. Currently, opossum are attributed a major role in maintaining infection caused by *M. bovis* in cattle in the region of New Zealand where they are found. DNA restriction endonuclease analysis demonstrated that *M. bovis* isolates from cattle and opossum in Upper Hutt (the region where the eradication program encountered difficulties) belong to the same restriction category (Collins *et al.*, 1988).

In southwestern England, reinfection of cattle herds has been attributed to the high rate of *M. bovis* infection found in badgers (*Meles meles*). When the badger population was eliminated from certain areas and prevented from repopulating them, transmission to cattle was halted, thus proving the causal relationship between infection in these species (Wilesmith, 1983).

There is abundant literature on the infection in badgers and cattle. It is estimated that the badger population in Great Britain is approximately 250,000 animals and that infection by *M. bovis* is endemic on the island, regardless of the density of the colonies. A total of 15,000 badgers, most of them killed on roadways, were examined and 3.9% were positive for *M. bovis* (Cheeseman *et al.*, 1989). These researchers and others (Wilesmith *et al.*, 1986) consider the badger an ideal maintenance host or natural reservoir that acts as a source of infection for cattle, although a low level source. In Ireland, it was demonstrated that destroying badger colonies reduced the prevalence of the disease in cattle. The highest incidence of tuberculosis in cattle was found in areas with a high population density of cattle and badgers (McAleer, 1990). Although these researchers admit that badgers may be partially responsible for tuberculosis in cattle, there are other questions that must be investigated and clarified. As badgers scour pastures in search of worms, they excrete *M. bovis* in their feces, urine, and sputum and in pus when they have open abscesses. It is not clear how the cattle become infected, as they suffer primarily from pulmonary tuberculosis, which has a respiratory route of infection, except in the case of calves, many of which become infected by mouth through contaminated milk. Badger colonies with tuberculosis may also coexist with cattle for some time without transmitting the infection to these animals (Grange and Collins, 1987).

In Argentina in 1982 and 1983, 4 million hares (*Lepus europaeus*) were slaughtered under veterinary inspection and 369 animals were confiscated for various causes. *M. bovis* was isolated from only five hares and histopathological examination showed a tuberculous granuloma with significant caseation and little calcification, with the presence of alcohol- and acid-resistant bacilli (de Kantor *et al.*, 1984). Alpacas imported from the Andean highlands to Europe were the cause of small outbreaks of tuberculosis (Veen *et al.*, 1991).

In South Africa, tuberculosis has been diagnosed in many wild species: the Cape buffalo (*Syncerus caffer*), the greater kudu (*Tragelaphus strepsiceros*), and the forest duiker (*Cephalophus grimmia*), among others (Pastoret *et al.*, 1988).

Source of Infection and Mode of Transmission (Figure 20): The main reservoir of *M. bovis* is cattle, which can transmit the infection to many mammalian species, including man. Man contracts the infection primarily by ingesting the agent in raw milk and milk products, and secondarily by inhaling it.

Tuberculosis is transmitted among cattle mainly via aerosols. The digestive tract is an important route of transmission prior to weaning.

A human infected by *M. bovis* who suffers from the pulmonary or urogenital form of tuberculosis can retransmit the infection to cattle. This phenomenon becomes particularly evident during the final stages of bovine tuberculosis eradication.

Tuberculosis in swine, goats, and sheep has as it principal source of infection cattle, fowl, and occasionally man. Swine are infected enterogenously, and retransmission to other swine, other species, and man is thought to be rare. Goats can constitute a source of infection for man and for cattle.

Dogs often contract the infection from humans and, less frequently, from cattle. They may in turn retransmit it to man and cattle. Dogs become infected via the digestive and respiratory tracts. The principal source of infection for cats is cattle and, to a lesser degree, man. The route of entry is mainly oral. At times, cats can be a source of infection for cattle and humans.

Among wild animals in captivity, monkeys are particularly interesting because of their susceptibility to *M. tuberculosis* and *M. bovis*. They contract the infection from man by inhaling the agent. Tuberculous primates constitute a health risk for humans.

Figure 20. Tuberculosis (*Mycobacterium bovis*). Mode of transmission.

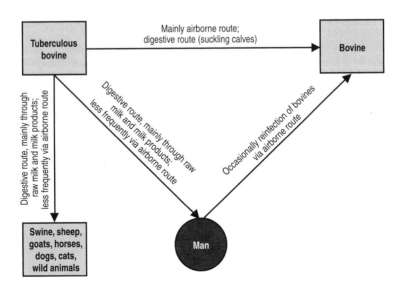

Domestic cattle are the source of infection for wild animals. Once the agent is introduced among wild animals that share pasture with cattle, it can spread among them and represent a risk for domestic animals and for man. This is true of deer and badgers (*Meles meles*) in Great Britain and of opossum (*Trichosurus vulpecula*) in New Zealand.

Role of Animals in the Epidemiology of the Disease: Human-to-human transmission of animal tuberculosis is rare. The infection depends on an animal source.

Diagnosis: Since the human infections caused by *M. tuberculosis* and *M. bovis* are clinically and radiologically indistinguishable, definitive diagnosis can only be achieved by isolating and typing the etiologic agent. In this regard, it should be noted that *M. bovis* grows poorly in media containing glycerin, such as Löwenstein-Jensen culture, which are generally used for culturing *M. tuberculosis*.

For routine diagnosis of bovine tuberculosis, the only approved method for eradication programs is the tuberculin test. The most appropriate tuberculin is the purified protein derivative (PPD), since it is specific and not very costly to produce. It has been made from both human and bovine strains, but research has shown that tuberculin produced with an *M. bovis* strain is more specific. In most countries, only a PPD tuberculin is used in eradication campaigns, and the comparative test (simultaneous application of mammalian and avian tuberculin) is reserved for problem herds in which paraspecific sensitization is suspected. The test is carried out by intradermal inoculation of 0.1 ml of tuberculin into the skin of the caudal fold or the wide part of the neck, depending on standards established in each country. It should be borne in mind that the skin of the neck is much more sensitive than that of the caudal fold. The amount of tuberculin used varies from 2,000 to 10,000 IU in different countries. The test will be more sensitive but less specific when larger doses are used. The test's effectiveness depends not only on the tuberculin and its correct application, but on the response capability of the infected animal. Some herds include anergic animals, which are usually old and have very advanced tuberculosis. Clinical examination and knowledge of the herd's history can help to complete the diagnosis.

The tuberculin test may also be applied to goats, sheep, and swine with satisfactory results. In swine, the preferred inoculation site is the base of the ear, with 2,000 IU of mammalian and avian tuberculin; in goats and sheep, the tuberculin can be applied to the eyelid, the fold of the tail, or the inner thigh.

The tuberculin test is unsatisfactory for horses, dogs, and cats. Some research has suggested that the test using BCG might give better results in dogs. For monkeys, the intrapalpebral test is recommended, as well as radiography in advanced cases.

The tuberculin test has several disadvantages. These include waiting time (reading at 72 hours in cattle) and the need for the veterinarian to visit the herd twice (once to inject the tuberculin and the other to read the test). Similarly, human patients require two medical visits. Old cows with advanced tuberculosis are anergic. This can also happen if there is an intercurrent febrile disease. As an eradication program progresses, the percentage of reactor animals without visible tuberculosis lesions increases at slaughterhouses. These disadvantages have led many researchers to seek serologic tests than can replace or at least complement tuberculin tests.

The enzyme-linked immunosorbent assay (ELISA) using bovine PPD was evaluated in five different groups of cattle, including 53 animals with positive cultures and 101 animals from a tuberculosis-free area. Sensitivity of 73.6% and specificity of 94.1% were obtained (Ritacco *et al.*, 1990). The authors note that ELISA was able to detect IgG against *M. bovis* in the sera of cattle with active tuberculosis, but not in those with a clinically inapparent infection (e.g., at the onset of infection or in the latent state). There was little coincidence between the results from the tuberculin test and results from ELISA. Antibodies were detected in almost three out of four bovines with active tuberculosis. In contrast to what happens with anergic animals, which lose cellular reactivity to the hypersensitivity test with tuberculin, antibodies are more abundant when there is a strong antigenic discharge. Thus, ELISA could be useful as a complement to the intradermal test in detecting anergic tuberculous animals that represent a risk for the rest of the herd (Ritacco *et al.*, 1990). The results obtained in humans infected by *M. tuberculosis* are not unlike those obtained in cattle infected by *M. bovis*. Specificity was 93% in adults and 98% in children; sensitivity was 69% in adults and 51% in children. The conclusion is that enzyme immunoassay can be useful for detecting patients with nonbacilliferous, extrapulmonary, and pediatric tuberculosis (de Kantor *et al.*, 1991).

The enzyme immunoassay can also be used to detect circulating antigens or to diagnose tuberculosis in homogenized animal tissues (Thoen *et al.*, 1981). For a program to eliminate infected badgers, a serological procedure is being sought that could detect individual infected animals and thus prevent indiscriminate slaughter.

In Australia, a simple test has been developed to measure *in vitro* the cell-mediated immune response to bovine PPD tuberculin. The test is based on detecting—using a sandwich enzyme immunoassay—gamma-interferon produced by incubation (for 24 hours) of whole bovine blood in the presence of tuberculin (Rothel *et al.*, 1990). A field study conducted of a large number of cattle compared the analcaudal test with PPD tuberculin and the gamma-interferon assay. Specificity with gamma-interferon was 96% to 98%, while sensitivity was 76.8% to 93.6% (depending on the method of interpretation). If the two diagnostic tests are combined, it is possible to obtain sensitivity of 95.2% (Wood *et al.*, 1991; Wood *et al.*, 1992). The sandwich enzyme immunoassay to detect gamma-interferon in whole bovine blood proved to be more sensitive and specific than the direct enzyme immunoassay for detecting IgG in serum. In a study conducted in Argentina, the gamma-interferon test was positive in 9 of 19 animals that had tuberculous lesions limited to the lymph nodes and no antibodies in the ELISA test. In contrast, cattle with disseminated lesions had a high antibody titer and little or no gamma-interferon production (Ritacco *et al.*, 1991).

Control: Prevention of human infection by *M. bovis* consists of the pasteurization of milk, vaccination with BCG, and above all, control and eradication of bovine tuberculosis.

The only rational approach to reducing and eliminating losses produced by the infection in cattle and preventing human cases caused by *M. bovis* consists of establishing a control and eradication program for bovine tuberculosis. Eradication campaigns are usually carried out by administering tuberculin tests repeatedly, until all infected animals are eliminated from the herd. Application of the tuberculin test and slaughter of reactors has given excellent results in all countries that have undertaken eradication campaigns. At present, many developed countries are free or practically free of bovine tuberculosis. In developing countries, the inability of governments to compensate owners for the destruction of reactors hinders establishment of eradication programs and makes it necessary to find other incentives, such as a surcharge on milk. Campaigns should be begun in regions of low prevalence, where replacing reacting animals is easier, and later extended to areas of higher prevalence. The success of a program depends on the cooperation of the meat inspection agencies so that tuberculosis-free herds are correctly certified, activities are evaluated, and appropriate epidemiologic surveillance is maintained. The cooperation of the health services is also important to prevent persons with tuberculosis from working with animals and either infecting or sensitizing them.

Controlling tuberculosis caused by *M. bovis* in its principal reservoir, cattle, is the best method of preventing transmission to other species, including man.

Several vaccines have been tested for preventing bovine tuberculosis, among them BCG, but none have proved effective. Treatment with anti-tuberculosis drugs, particularly isoniazid, takes many months, is costly, can produce drug-resistant *M. bovis* strains, and the result is uncertain.

Data on the status of bovine tuberculosis in Latin America and the Caribbean, with a summary on other countries, have been compiled and tabulated by de Kantor and Alvarez (1991) and de Kantor and Ritacco (1994).

Bibliography

Argentina, Comisión Nacional de Zoonosis, Subcomisión de Tuberculosis Bovina. *La tuberculosis bovina en la República Argentina.* Buenos Aires: Centro Panamericano de Zoonosis; 1982.

Berggren, S.A.. Field experiment with BCG vaccine in Malawi. *Br Vet J* 137:88–96, 1981. Cited in: Pritchard, D.G. A century of bovine tuberculosis 1888–1988: Conquest and controversy. *J Comp Pathol* 99:357–399, 1988.

Burjanova, B., M. Nagyova. [Tuberculosis due to *Mycobacterium bovis* in the human population in Slovakia 1978–1983]. *Studia Pneumologica Phtiseologica Cechoslavaca* 45:342–346, 1985.

Casal, M., M.J. Linares. Enzymatic profile of *Mycobacterium tuberculosis. Eur J Clin Microbiol* 3:155–156, 1985.

Castets, M., N. Rist, H. Boisvert. Le varieté africaine du bacille tuberculeux. *Medicine de l'Afrique Noire* 16:321, 1969.

Centrángolo, A., L.S. de Marchesini, C. Isola, I.N. de Kantor, M. Di Lonardo. El *Mycobacterium bovis* como causa de tuberculosis humana. Actas, 13r. Congreso Argentino de Tisiología, Mar del Plata, 1973.

Cheeseman, C.L., J.W. Wilesmith, F.A. Stuart. Tuberculosis: The disease and its epidemiology in the badger, a review. *Epidemiol Infect* 103:113–125, 1989.

Collins, D.M., G.W. De Lisle. DNA restriction endonuclease analysis of *Mycobacterium bovis* and other members of the tuberculosis complex. *J Clin Microbiol* 21:562–564, 1985.

Collins, D.M., D.M. Gabric, G.W. De Lisle. Typing of *Mycobacterium bovis* isolates from cattle and other animals in the same locality. *N Z Vet J* 36:45–46, 1988.

Collins, C.H., J.M. Grange. The bovine tubercle bacillus. *J Appl Bacteriol* 55:13–29, 1983.

Collins, C.H., M.D. Yates, J.M. Grange. A study of bovine strains of *Mycobacterium tuberculosis* isolated from humans in South-East England, 1977–1979. *Tubercle* 62:113–116, 1981.

Cordes, D.O., J.A. Bullians, D.E. Lake, M.E. Carter. Observations on tuberculosis caused by *Mycobacterium bovis* in sheep. *N Z Vet J* 29:60–62, 1981.

Davidson, R.M., M.R. Alley, N.S. Beatson. Tuberculosis in a flock of sheep. *N Z Vet J* 29:1–2, 1981.

de Kantor, I.N., E. Alvarez, eds. *Current status of bovine tuberculosis in Latin America and the Caribbean*. Buenos Aires: Pan American Zoonoses Center; 1991. (Special Publication 10).

de Kantor, I.N., L. Barrera, V. Ritacco, I. Miceli. Utilidad del enzimoinmunoensayo en el diagnóstico de la tuberculosis. *Bol Oficina Sanit Panam* 110:461–470, 1991.

de Kantor, I.N., E. de la Vega, A. Bernardelli. Infección por *Mycobacterium bovis* en liebres en la provincia de Buenos Aires, Argentina. *Rev Med Vet* 65:268–279, 1984.

de Kantor, I.N., N. Marchevsky, I.W. Lesslie. Respuesta al PPD en pacientes tuberculosos afectados por *M. tuberculosis* y por *M. bovis*. *Medicina* 36:127–130, 1976.

de Kantor, I.N., J. Pereira, J. Miquet, R. Rovère. Pouvoir pathogène experimental de *Mycobacterium africanum* pour les bovins. *Bull Acad Vet Fr* 52:499–503, 1979.

de Kantor, I.N., V. Ritacco. Bovine tuberculosis in Latin America and the Caribbean: Current status, control and eradication programs. *Vet Microbiol* 40:5–14, 1994.

De Lisle, G.W., D.M. Collins, A.S. Loveday, *et al.* A report of tuberculosis in cats in New Zealand and the examination of strains of *Mycobacterium bovis* by DNA restriction endonuclease analysis. *N Z Vet J* 38:10–13, 1990.

Essey, M.A., A. Fanning, D.A. Saavi, J. Payeur. Bovine tuberculosis in *Cervidae*; human health concerns. *Proc Annu Meet U S Anim Health Assoc* 95:427–436, 1991.

Feldman, W.H. Tuberculosis. *In*: Hull, T.G., ed. *Diseases Transmitted from Animals to Man*. 5th ed. Springfield: Thomas; 1963.

Fernández Salazar, M., V. Gómez Pando, L. Domínguez Paredes. *Mycobacterium bovis* en la patología humana en el Perú. *Bol Inf Col Med Vet* 14:16–18, 1983.

Francis, J. *Tuberculosis in Animals and Man. A Study in Comparative Pathology*. London: Cassel; 1958.

Francis, J., C.L. Choi, A.J. Frost. The diagnosis of tuberculosis in cattle with special reference to bovine PPD tuberculin. *Aust Vet J* 49:246–251, 1973.

García Carrillo, C., B. Szyfres. La tuberculosis animal en las Américas y su transmisión al hombre. Roma: Organización de las Naciones Unidas para la Agricultura y la Alimentación; 1963.

Good, R.C., D.E. Snider, Jr. Isolation of nontuberculous mycobacteria in the United States, 1980. *J Infect Dis* 146:829–833, 1982.

Grange, J.M., C.H. Collins. Bovine tubercle bacilli and disease in animals and man. *Epidemiol Infect* 99:221–234, 1987.

Grange, J.M., M.D. Yates. Incidence and nature of human tuberculosis due to *Mycobacterium africanum* in South-East England: 1977–87. *Epidemiol Infect* 103:127–132, 1989.

Griffith, A.S. Bovine tuberculosis in man. *Tubercle* 18:528–543, 1937. Cited in: Collins, C.H., J.M. Grange. The bovine tubercle bacillus. *J Appl Bacteriol* 55:13–29, 1983.

Hawthorne, V.M., I.M. Lauder. Tuberculosis in man, dog and cat. *Am Rev Resp Dis* 85:858–869, 1962.

Horsburgh, C.R., U.G. Mason III, D.C. Farhi, M.D. Iseman. Disseminated infection with *Mycobacterium avium-intracellulare*. A report of 13 cases and review of the literature. *Medicine* 64:36–48, 1985.

Huitema, H. Development of a comparative test with equal concentrations of avian and bovine PPD tuberculin for cattle. *Tijdschr Diergeneeskd* 98:396–407, 1973.

Huitema, H. The eradication of bovine tuberculosis in cattle in the Netherlands and the significance of man as a source of infection in cattle. *Selected Papers of the Royal Netherlands Tuberculosis Association* 12:62–67, 1969. Cited in: Grange, J.M., C.H. Collins. Bovine tubercle bacilli and disease in animals and man. *Epidemiol Infect* 99:221–234, 1987.

Humble, M.W., A. King, I. Phillips. API ZYM: A simple rapid system for the detection of bacterial enzymes. *J Clin Pathol* 30:275–277, 1977.

Isaac, J., J. Whitehead, J.W. Adams, M.D. Barton, P. Coloe. An outbreak of *Mycobacterium bovis* infection in cats in an animal house. *Aust Vet J* 60:243–245, 1983.

Joint FAO/WHO Expert Committee on Zoonoses. *Joint FAO/WHO Expert Committee on Zoonoses. Third report.* Geneva: WHO; 1967. (Technical Report Series 378).

Karlson, A.G. Tuberculosis. *In*: Dunne, H.W., ed. *Diseases of Swine.* 3rd ed. Ames: Iowa State University Press; 1970.

Kleeberg, H.H. Tuberculosis and other mycobacterioses. *In*: Hubbert, W.T., W.F. McCulloch, P.R. Schnurrenberger, eds. *Diseases Transmitted from Animals to Man.* 6th ed. Springfield: Thomas; 1975.

Konyha, L.D., J.P. Kreier. The significance of tuberculin tests in the horse. *Am Rev Resp Dis* 103:91–99, 1971.

Kubin, M., J. Stastna, M. Havelkova. [Classification of mycobacterial causal agents of tuberculosis and mycobacteriosis in the Czech Republic in 1981–1983]. *Studia Pneumologica Phtisiologica Cechoslovaca* 45:599–603, 1985.

Lesslie, I.W., K.J. Birn, P. Stuart, *et al.* Tuberculosis in the pig and the tuberculin test. *Vet Rec* 83:647–651, 1968.

Liu, S., I. Weitzman, G.G. Johnson. Canine tuberculosis. *J Am Vet Med Assoc* 177:164–167, 1980.

Magnus, K. Epidemiological basis of tuberculosis eradication. 3. Risk of pulmonary tuberculosis after human and bovine infection. *Bull World Health Organ* 35:483–508, 1966.

Magnus, K. Epidemiological basis of tuberculosis eradication. 5. Frequency of pulmonary calcifications after human and bovine infection. *Bull World Health Organ* 36:703–718, 1967.

Matthias, D. Vergleichende Pathologie der Tuberkulose der Tiere. *In*: Meissner, G., A. Schmiedel, eds. *Mykobakterien und Mykobakterielle Krankheiten.* Teil VII. Jena: Fischer; 1970.

McAleer, P.D. The relationship between badger density and the incidence of bovine tuberculosis in County Galway. *Ir Vet J* 43:77–80, 1990.

Myers, J.A., J.H. Steele. *Bovine Tuberculosis Control in Man and Animals.* St. Louis: Green; 1969.

Pan American Health Organization (PAHO). *First International Seminar on Bovine Tuberculosis for the Americas, Santiago, Chile, 21–25 September 1970.* Washington, D.C.: PAHO; 1972. (Scientific Publication 258).

Pastoret, P.P., E.T. Thiry, B. Brochier, *et al.* Maladies de faune sauvage transmissibles aux animaux domestiques. *Rev Sci Tech Off Int Epiz* 7:661–704, 1988.

Patterson, A.B., J.T. Stamp, J.N. Ritchie. Tuberculosis. *In*: Stableforth, A.W., I.A. Galloway, eds. *Infectious Diseases of Animals.* London: Butterworths; 1959.

Pritchard, D.G. A century of bovine tuberculosis 1888–1988: Conquest and controversy. *J Comp Pathol* 99:357–399, 1988.

Ritacco, V., B. López, L. Barrera, *et al.* Further evaluation of an indirect enzyme-linked immunosorbent assay for the diagnosis of bovine tuberculosis. *Zentralbl Veterinarmed [B]* 37:19–27, 1990.

Ritacco, V., B. López, I.N. de Kantor, *et al.* Reciprocal cellular and humoral immune responses in bovine tuberculosis. *Res Vet Sci* 50:365–367, 1991.

Robinson, R.C., P.H. Phillips, G. Stevens, P.A. Storm. An outbreak of *Mycobacterium bovis* in fallow deer (*Dama dama*). *Aust Vet J* 66:195–197, 1989.

Roswurm, J.D., L.D. Konyha. The comparative-cervical tuberculin test as an aid to diagnosing bovine tuberculosis. *Proc Annu Meet U S Anim Health Assoc* 77:368–389, 1973.

Rothel, J.S., S.L. Jones, L.A. Corner, *et al.* A sandwich enzyme immunoassay for bovine interferon-gamma and its use for the detection of tuberculosis in cattle. *Aust Vet J* 67:134–137, 1990.

Ruch, T.C. *Diseases of Laboratory Primates.* Philadelphia: Saunders; 1959.

Schliesser, T. Epidemiologie der Tuberkulose der Tiere. *In*: Meissner, G., A. Schmiedel, eds. *Mykobakterien und Mykobakterielle Krankheiten.* Teil VII. Jena: Fischer; 1970.

Schmiedel, A. Erkrankungen der Menschen durch *Mycobacterium bovis. In*: Meissner, G., A. Schmiedel, eds. *Mykobakterien und Mykobakterielle Krankheiten.* Teil VII. Jena: Fischer, 1970.

Schonfeld, J.K. Human-to-human spread of infection by *M. bovis*. *Tubercle* 63:143–144, 1982.

Shoemaker, S.A., J.H. Fisher, W.D. Jones, C.H. Scoggin. Restriction fragment analysis of chromosomal DNA defines different strains of *Mycobacterium tuberculosis*. *Am Rev Respir Dis* 134:210–213, 1986.

Sjorgen, I., I. Sutherland. Studies of tuberculosis in man in relation to infection in cattle. *Tubercle* 56:127–133, 1974.

Stuart, F.A., P.A. Manser, F.G. McIntosh. Tuberculosis in imported red deer (*Cervus elaphus*). *Vet Rec* 122:508–511, 1988.

Thoen, C.O. Tuberculosis. *In*: Leman, A.D., B.E. Straw, W.L. Mengeling, S. D'Allaire, D.J. Taylor, eds. *Diseases of Swine*. 7th ed. Ames: Iowa State University; 1992.

Thoen, C.O., C. Malstrom, E.M. Himes, K. Mills. Use of enzyme-linked immunosorbent assay for detecting mycobacterial antigens in tissues of *Mycobacterium bovis*-infected cattle. *Am J Vet Res* 42:1814–1815, 1981.

Thorel, M.F. Isolation of *Mycobacterium africanum* from monkeys. *Tubercle* 61:101–104, 1980.

Veen, J., J.V. Kuyvenhoven, E.T.B. Dinkla, *et al.* [Tuberculosis in alpacas; a zoonosis as an imported disease]. *Nederlands Tijdschr Geneesk* 135:1127–1130, 1991.

Vestal, A.L. Procedures for the isolation of *Mycobacteria*. Atlanta: Centers for Disease Control and Prevention; 1969. (Public Health Publication 1995).

Wiessmann, J. Die Rindertuberkulose beim Menschen und ihre epidemiologische Bedentung fur die Veterinarmedizin. *Schweiz Arch Tierhenlkd* 102:467–471, 1960.

Wilesmith, J.W. Epidemiological features of bovine tuberculosis in cattle herds in Great Britain. *J Hyg* 90:159–176, 1983.

Wilesmith, J.W., P.E. Sayers, R. Bode, *et al.* Tuberculosis in East Sussex. II. Aspects of badger ecology and surveillance for tuberculosis in badger populations (1976–1984). *J Hyg* 97:11–26, 1986.

Winkler, W.G., N.B. Gale. Tuberculosis. *In*: Davis, J.W., L.H. Karstad, D.O. Trainer, eds. *Infectious Diseases of Wild Mammals*. Ames: Iowa State University Press; 1970.

Wood, P.R., L.A. Corner, J.S. Rothel, *et al.* Field comparison of the interferon-gamma assay and the intradermal tuberculin tests for the diagnosis of bovine tuberculosis. *Aust Vet J* 68:286–290, 1991.

Wood, P.R., L.A. Corner, J.S. Rothel, *et al.* A field evaluation of serological and cellular diagnostic tests for bovine tuberculosis. *Vet Microbiol* 31:71–79, 1992.

Yates, M.D., J.M. Grange. Incidence and nature of human tuberculosis due to bovine tubercle bacilli in South-East England: 1977–1987. *Epidemiol Infect* 101:225–229, 1988.

Part II

MYCOSES

ADIASPIROMYCOSIS

ICD-10 B48.8

Synonyms: Adiaspirosis, haplomycosis, haplosporangiosis.

Etiology: *Chrysosporium (Emmonsia) parvum* var. *crescens* and *C. parvum* var. *parvum*, saprophytic soil fungi that characteristically form large spherules (adiaspores) in the lungs. In the tissular phase, the fungus does not multiply. *C. crescens* is the most common agent in man and animals. *C. parva* occurs primarily in animals and forms smaller spherules than *C. crescens*. *C. parvum* var. *crescens* and *C. parvum* var. *parvum* differ in size. In the lungs, *C. crescens* measures 200 to 700 microns, whereas *C. parvum* measures 40 microns. In addition, *C. parvum* is mononuclear, even when it reaches its maximum size, while *C. crescens* eventually has hundreds of nuclei.

Geographic Distribution: Worldwide. In the Americas, the infection has been confirmed in Argentina, Brazil, Canada, Guatemala, Honduras, the United States, and Venezuela.

Occurrence in Man: Rare. Eleven human cases have been reported in Asia, Europe, South America, and the United States (Englund and Hochholzer, 1993). According to Moraes *et al.* (1989) there were 23 cases, four of which were extrapulmonary.

Occurrence in Animals: Frequent in small wild mammals. The disease has been confirmed in at least 124 mammalian species or subspecies (Leighton and Wobeser, 1978). Among other mammals, the disease has been diagnosed in skunks (*Mephitis mephitis*) in Argentina, Canada, and the United States.

The Disease in Man and Animals: The only clinically significant form, in man as well as animals, is pulmonary adiaspiromycosis. The few human cases have been diagnosed through biopsy or autopsy specimens. The fungus causes light gray to yellowish lesions in the lungs, without greatly affecting the animal's overall health. The number of spherules (adiaspores) in the lung tissue depends on the number of conidia (spores) inhaled. In the lungs, the fungus increases significantly in size. If few conidia are inhaled, usually only one lung is affected. If the inoculum is large, both lungs are likely to be affected. Adiaspiromycosis usually disappears spontaneously but requires surgical resection if it persists (Englund and Hochholzer, 1993). The etiologic agent may also be found in other organs, though rarely. One case of disseminated adiaspiromycosis was described in an AIDS patient. The most significant clinical characteristic was disseminated osteomyelitis. The fungus, *Chrysosporium parvum* var. *parvum*, was isolated during surgery from the pus of a wrist lesion, as well as from the sputum and bone-marrow aspirate. The mycotic infection was controlled with amphotericin B (Echeverría *et al.*, 1993). A fatal case of adiaspiromycosis was recorded in Brazil in a 35-year-old rural worker who had complained of generalized weakness, dry cough, afternoon fever, and a weight loss of 8 kg during the four weeks prior to hospitalization. Clinical symptoms and radiography were similar to miliary tuberculosis. The fungus was detected in the specimens obtained during autopsy (Peres *et al.*, 1992). Another similar fatal case had occurred previously in Brazil (Moraes *et al.*, 1989).

The disease is generally asymptomatic, but resection of the affected tissue may be necessary if it persists and symptoms appear.

In 7 out of 25 skunks (*Mephitis mephitis*) captured and autopsied in Alberta, Canada, lesions were found that varied from slight and only visible microscopically to severe with grayish-white nodules in the pulmonary parenchyma that spread to the bronchotracheal and mediastinal lymphatic ganglia. Histologically, the lesions were characterized by a centrally located spherule surrounded by granulomatous inflammation (Albassam *et al.*, 1986).

Source of Infection and Mode of Transmission: The great preponderance of pulmonary localizations indicates that the infection is contracted through inhalation. *C. crescens* has been isolated from the soil. Differences in the infection rates for three very similar species of squirrels indicate that the fungus may be present in certain habitats (Leighton and Wobeser, 1978), possibly linked to the root microflora of certain plants. Other authors (cited by Mason and Gauhwin, 1982) suggest that predator-prey interactions affect its distribution: upon ingesting infected animals, carnivores eliminate adiaspores in their feces, where the spores germinate and develop. This was demonstrated in cats, in a mustelid (*Mustela nivalis*), and in birds of prey. Thus, predators could play a role in disseminating the etiologic agent.

Under very windy conditions, both animals and humans may inhale airborne conidia released from the soil.

Role of Animals: The soil is the reservoir for the fungus and the source of infection in humans and other animals. It is believed that some animals may play a role in disseminating the agent.

Diagnosis: Diagnosis may be made by observation of spherules in lung tissue, by stained histological preparations, and by culture and inoculation into laboratory animals. The most effective method for detecting adiaspores in the lungs of animals is tissue digestion with a 2% sodium hydroxide solution (Leighton and Wobeser, 1978). The spherules are stained with acid-Schiff and Gomori methenamine silver nitrate reagents (Englund and Hochholzer, 1993).

Bibliography

Ainsworth, G.C., P.K.C. Austwick. *Fungal Diseases of Animals*. 2nd ed. Farnham Royal, Slough, United Kingdom: Commonwealth Agricultural Bureau; 1973.

Albassam, M.A., R. Bhatnagar, L.E. Lillie, L. Roy. Adiaspiromycosis in striped skunks in Alberta, Canada. *J Wildl Dis* 22:13–18, 1986.

Cueva, J.A., M.D. Little. *Emmonsia crescens* infection (adiaspiromycosis) in man in Honduras. *Am J Trop Med Hyg* 20:282–287, 1971.

Echevarría, E., E.L. Cano, A. Restrepo. Disseminated adiaspiromycosis in a patient with AIDS. *J Med Vet Mycol* 31:91–97, 1993.

England, D.M., L. Hochholzer. Adiaspiromycosis: An unusual fungal infection of the lung. Report of 11 cases. *Am J Surg Pathol* 17:876–886, 1993.

Jellison, W.L. Adiaspiromycosis. *In:* Davis, J.W., L.H. Karstad, D.O. Trainer, eds. *Infectious Diseases of Wild Mammals*. Ames: Iowa State University Press; 1970.

Leighton, F.A., G. Wobeser. The prevalence of adiaspiromycosis in three sympatric species of ground squirrels. *J Wildl Dis* 14:362–365, 1978.

Mason, R.W., M. Gauhwin. Adiaspiromycosis in South Australian hairy-nosed wombats (*Lasiorhinus latifrons*). *J Wildl Dis* 18:3–8, 1982.

Moraes, N.A., M.C. de Almeida, A.N. Raick. Caso fatal de adiaspiromicose pulmonar humana. *Rev Inst Med Trop Sao Paulo* 31:188–194, 1989.

Peres, L.C., F. Figueiredo, M. Peinado, F.A. Soares. Fulminant disseminated pulmonary adiaspiromycosis in humans. *Am J Trop Med Hyg* 46:146–150, 1992.

Salfelder, K. New and uncommon opportunistic fungal infections. *In*: Pan American Health Organization. *Proceedings of the Third International Conference on the Mycoses*. Washington, D.C.: PAHO; 1975. (Scientific Publication 304).

ASPERGILLOSIS

**ICD-10 B44.0 invasive pulmonary aspergillosis;
B44.1 other pulmonary aspergillosis;
B44.7 disseminated aspergillosis; B44.8 other forms of aspergillosis**

Synonyms: Pneumonomycosis, bronchomycosis (in animals).

Etiology: *Aspergillus fumigatu*s and occasionally other species of the genus *Aspergillus*, such as *A. flavus*, *A. nidulans*, *A. niger*, and *A. terreus*. These saprophytic fungi are common components of the soil microflora; they play an important role in the decomposition of organic matter.

Aspergillus flavus and *A. parasiticus* are known for their production of aflatoxins in oleaginous grains and seeds such as corn, rice, peanuts, and cottonseeds stored under damp conditions. Aflatoxin B_1 is hepatotoxic and carcinogenic for humans and animals. These fungi do not produce the aflatoxin in animal tissue. Thus, this chapter covers only infection by *Aspergillus* spp.

Geographic Distribution: The fungus is ubiquitous and distributed worldwide. The disease has no particular distribution.

Occurrence in Man: Aspergillosis occurs sporadically and is uncommon. Its incidence, as is that of other opportunistic mycoses[1] (candidiasis, zygomycosis), is increasing due to the growing use of antibiotics, antimetabolites, and corticosteroids. It occurs frequently in advanced cases of cancer. Small nosocomial outbreaks have also been reported (see section on the disease in man).

In Mexico, aspergillosis lesions were found in 1.2% of more than 2,000 random autopsies performed in a general hospital (González-Mendoza, 1970).

Occurrence in Animals: Sporadic cases have been described in many species of domestic and wild mammals and birds. The disease in fowl and cattle has economic

---

[1] Mycoses that attack debilitated persons or those treated over a long period with antibiotics, antimetabolites, or corticosteroids.

implications. The incidence is low in adult domestic fowl, but outbreaks in chicks and young turkeys can cause considerable losses on some farms.

The Disease in Man: Aspergillosis establishes itself in patients debilitated by chronic diseases (such as diabetes, cancer, tuberculosis, deep mycoses) and diseases of the immune system, as well as in persons treated with antibiotics, antimetabolites, and corticosteroids for prolonged periods. Persons occupationally exposed for long periods to materials contaminated by fungus spores (grain, hay, cotton, wool, and others) run a greater risk.

A study group on aspergillosis in AIDS patients conducted a retrospective review of 33 patients with invasive aspergillosis in different medical facilities in France. Of this group of 33 patients, 91% were recorded from 1989 to 1991, suggesting that invasive aspergillosis is an emerging complication of AIDS. *Aspergillus* spp. cultures were obtained from bronchopulmonary lavage of 28 patients, and no other pathogenic agents were found. Of 15 patients who underwent biopsy or autopsy, 14 were histologically positive. The clinical and radiological symptoms were comparable to aspergillosis in non-AIDS patients with neutropenia, though the AIDS patients had a higher incidence of neurological complications (Lortholary *et al.*, 1993).

There are two differentiated clinical forms of the disease: localized and invasive. Aspergillosis is essentially a respiratory system infection acquired through inhalation of *Aspergillus* spp. conidia. Patients with pronounced granulocytopenia may contract an acute and rapidly progressing pneumonia. The symptoms are high fever, pulmonary consolidation, and cavitation. Normal children who inhale a large number of conidia may develop fever, dyspnea, and miliary infiltration (Bennett, 1990). Allergic bronchopulmonary aspergillosis (ABPA) occurs in patients with preexisting asthma who present eosinophilia and intermittent bronchial obstruction (Bennett, 1990). Eosinophilia, precipitant antibodies, and high serum IgE concentration are found in these patients; the intradermal [skin prick] test produces an immediate reaction to *Aspergillus* antigens, with papules and reddening. Despite recurring exacerbations, some patients do not experience any permanent loss of pulmonary function. Other patients, however, suffer corticoid-dependent asthma or permanent obstructive disease (Bennett, 1990). ABPA patients may expectorate bronchial plugs in which hyphae of the fungus can be detected microscopically. Even during remission, 33% of patients evidenced circulating immune complexes, primarily involving IgG (Bhatnagar *et al.*, 1993).

Allergic bronchopulmonary aspergillosis is more common than was thought in the past. The disease may begin during childhood and continue without being clinically recognized for many years or decades, until the patient begins to suffer from fibrotic pulmonary disease. In this regard, it must be noted that aspergillosis infection may be asymptomatic and suspected only due to a significant increase in serum IgE. Often the diagnosis comes too late for chemotherapy treatment to be effective. When corticoids are discontinued, dyspnea and wheezing occur, requiring a return to medication with prednisolone (Greenberger, 1986). A later study concluded that inhaled beclomethasone dipropionate may be more effective in treating ABPA than traditional prednisolone by mouth (Imbeault and Cormier, 1993).

Another form of the disease is the fungus ball or aspergilloma, which occurs when the fungus colonizes respiratory cavities caused by other preexisting diseases (bronchitis, bronchiectasis, tuberculosis). This form is relatively benign, but it occasionally produces hemoptysis.

Other clinical forms are otomycosis (often caused by *A. niger*) and invasion of the paranasal sinuses by the fungus. Though rare, the cutaneous form of the disease may appear in immunodeficient patients.

The invasive form is usually very serious. The fungi penetrate the blood vessels and can spread throughout the body. Cases of pulmonary aspergillosis have also been described in patients who are not immunodeficient. There is general insistence that the invasive form of the disease occurs only in patients with neutropenia. Neutrophil polymorphonuclear leukocytes are very important in the defense against aspergillosis or in those who have serious defects in cell-mediated immunity (Karam and Griffin, 1986). Karam and Griffin describe three cases over five years in a university hospital and cite 32 cases found in the literature. Of the 32 cases cited, 14 had no underlying disease.

Surgical intervention in the case of pulmonary or pleuropulmonary aspergillosis may be indicated to treat pleural empyemas and bronchopleural fistulae. In these cases, myoplasty, thoracomyoplasty, and omentoplasty are the procedures most recommended (Wex *et al.*, 1993). Surgical removal is also justified in the case of invasive aspergillosis in the brain and paranasal sinuses, as well as in noninvasive colonization of the paranasal sinuses (Bennett, 1990). When colonization is invasive, it is advisable to discontinue or reduce the use of immunosuppressants and to start treatment with intravenous amphotericin B or itraconazole.

Several small outbreaks have occurred during the renovation, expansion, or remodeling of hospitals and the construction of highways near hospitals. During these projects, large numbers of conidia are made airborne, and may become concentrated due to ventilation systems with defective filters. Between July 1981 and July 1988, 11 immunodeficient patients in a military hospital contracted disseminated aspergillosis and died as a result. The hospital's project involved the renovation of the intensive care unit and several other rooms. The infection spread no further after several simultaneous measures were taken, such as installing floor-to-ceiling partitions in the construction area, negative pressure in the same area, antifungal decontamination using copper 8-hydroxyquinoline, and high-efficiency particulate air (HEPA) filters in air conditioning units and in rooms with immunodeficient patients (Opal *et al.*, 1986). However, a certain percentage of patients with lymphoma who received bone marrow transplants and were located in single-occupancy rooms with positive air pressure and high efficiency air filters did acquire aspergillosis. Of 417 lymphoma patients studied, 22 (5.2%) contracted invasive aspergillosis. These 22 patients were treated with amphotericin B, 17 of them prior to being diagnosed with aspergillosis; seven survived. All of the patients with disseminated aspergillosis died (Iwen *et al.*, 1993).

The Disease in Animals: Although aspergillosis occurs sporadically in many animal species, where it primarily causes respiratory system disorders, the following discussion only deals with the disease in cattle, horses, dogs, and fowl.

CATTLE: It is estimated that 75% of mycotic abortions are due to *Aspergillus*, particularly *A. fumigatus*, and 10% to 15% to fungi of the order *Mucorales*. As brucellosis, campylobacteriosis, and trichomoniasis are brought under control, the relative role of fungi as a cause of abortions increases. Mycotic abortion is seen mainly in stabled animals; thus, it occurs during the winter in countries with cold or temperate climates. Generally, only one or two females in a herd abort.

The pathogenesis of the disease is not well known. It is thought that the fungus first localizes in the lungs or the digestive system, where it multiplies before invading the placenta via the bloodstream and causing placentitis. Most abortions occur during the third trimester of pregnancy. The cotyledons swell and turn a brownish gray color. In serious cases, the placenta becomes wrinkled and leathery. The fungus may invade the fetus as well, causing dermatitis and bronchopneumonia. Retention of the placenta is common. Other forms of the infection are the pulmonary forms, also due primarily to *A. fumigatus*, and skin aspergillomas, caused by *A. terreus* (Schmitt, 1981).

HORSES: Invasive pulmonary aspergillosis is relatively rare in horses. As in cattle, the disease is generally associated with abortion. There is also an association between enterocolitis (*Salmonella, Ehrlichia ristici*) and invasive pulmonary aspergillosis (Hattel *et al.*, 1991).

DOGS: Aspergillosis in dogs is generally confined to the nasal cavity or paranasal sinuses. *A. fumigatus* is the most common fungus. Disseminated aspergillosis is rare and has been found in dry, warm regions. In Australia, 12 cases due to *A. terreus* were recorded during 1980–1984. Eleven of the 12 dogs were German Shepherds. The disease was characterized by granulomas in several organs, particularly in the kidneys, spleen, and bones. Lumbar diskospondylitis and focal osteomyelitis were common, generally in the epiphysis of the long bones (Day *et al.*, 1986). Six cases of disseminated aspergillosis were recorded in the United States with characteristics similar to those in Australia (Dallman *et al.*, 1992).

FOWL: Outbreaks of acute aspergillosis occur in chicks and young turkeys, sometimes causing considerable losses. The symptoms include fever, loss of appetite, labored breathing, diarrhea, and emaciation. In chronic aspergillosis, which occurs sporadically in adult birds, the clinical picture is varied and depends on the localization. The affected birds may survive for a long time in a state of general debilitation. Yellowish granulomas of 1 to 3 mm (or larger, if the process is chronic) appear in the lungs. Plaques develop in the air sacks and may gradually cover the serosa; the same lesions or a mucoid exodate are found in the bronchial tubes and the trachea. Granulomatous lesions are also found frequently in different organs, as either nodules or plaques. The principal etiologic agents are *A. fumigatus* and *A. flavus*. Many species of domesticated and wild birds are susceptible to the disease. Captive penguins frequently are victims (Chute and Richard, 1991).

Clinical forms other than the pulmonary form occur in birds. These are dermatitis, osteomycosis, ophthalmitis, and encephalitis. Osteomycosis and encephalitis are probably spread through the bloodstream (Chute and Richard, 1991).

Source of Infection and Mode of Transmission: The reservoir is the soil. The infecting element is the conidia (exospores) of the fungus, which are transmitted to man and animals through the air. The causal agent is ubiquitous and can survive in the most varied environmental conditions. Despite this, the disease does not occur frequently in man, indicating natural resistance to the infection. This resistance may be undone by the use of immunosuppressant medications or factors that impair the immune system (see the section on the disease in man for other details on predisposing factors and diseases). In domestic mammals and birds, as well as in people who work with them, an important source of infection is fodder and bedding contaminated by the fungus, which releases conidia upon maturing. Apparently, exposure must be prolonged or massive for the infection to become established. Airborne conidia are found in incubators, hatcheries, incubation rooms, and air ducts; these may be the source of infection for chicks or young turkeys (Chute and Richard, 1991).

Role of Animals in Epidemiology: The source of infection is always the environment. The infection is not transmitted from one individual to another (man or animal).

Diagnosis: Due to the ubiquitous nature of the agent, isolation by culture is not a reliable test, since the agent may exist as a contaminant in the environment (laboratory or hospital) or as a saprophyte in the upper respiratory tract. A conclusive test may be obtained by simultaneously conducting a histological examination using biopsy material and confirming the presence of the fungus in the preparations. The agent may also be isolated by culturing aseptically obtained specimens from lesions not exposed to the environment. The species can only be identified by means of a culture. The immunodiffusion test has yielded very good results, as have counter-immunoelectrophoresis and enzyme-linked immunosorbent assay (ELISA). Serological tests are useful for diagnosing aspergillomas and in allergic bronchopulmonary aspergillosis, but not in invasive aspergillosis (Bennett, 1990). High levels of *A. fumigatus*-specific IgE and IgG are detected in the sera of ABPA patients, while IgG alone is detected in aspergillomas (Kurup, 1986). In fowl, it is enough to confirm the presence of the fungus through direct observation or by culturing materials from lesions of sacrificed birds.

Control: Due to the ubiquitous nature of the fungus, it is impossible to establish practical control measures. Prolonged treatment with antibiotics or corticosteroids should be limited to cases in which such therapy is essential. It is advisable to take special precautionary measures to avoid nosocomial outbreaks and to protect immunodeficient patients when construction work is done inside or near hospitals. Patients with lymphoma who receive bone marrow transplants should receive prophylactic treatment with amphotericin B (Iwen *et al.*, 1993). Moldy bedding or fodder should not be handled or given to domestic mammals and birds. Hygienic conditions in incubators and incubation rooms are important in preventing avian aspergillosis.

Bibliography

Ainsworth, G.C., P.K.C. Austwick. *Fungal Diseases of Animals*. 2nd ed. Farnham Royal, Slough, United Kingdom: Commonwealth Agricultural Bureau; 1973.

Ajello, L., L.K. Georg, W. Kaplan, L. Kaufman. *Laboratory Manual for Medical Mycology*. Washington, D.C.: U.S. Government Printing Office; 1963. (Public Health Service Publication 994).

Bennett, J.E. *Aspergillus* species. *In*: Mandell, G.L., R.G. Douglas, Jr., J.E. Bennett, eds. Vol 2: *Principles and Practice of Infectious Disease*. 3rd ed. New York: Churchill Livingstone, Inc.; 1990.

Bhatnagar, P.K., B. Banerjee, P.V. Sarma. Serological findings in patients with allergic bronchopulmonary aspergillosis during remission. *J Infect* 27:33–37, 1993.

Chute, H.L., J.L. Richard. Fungal infections. *In*: Calnek, B.W., H.J. Barnes, C.W. Beard, W.M. Reid, H.W. Yoder, Jr., eds. *Diseases of Poultry*. 9th ed. Ames: Iowa State University Press; 1991.

Dallman, M.J., T.L. Dew, L. Tobias, R. Doss. Disseminated aspergillosis in a dog with diskospondylitis and neurologic deficits. *J Am Vet Med Assoc* 200:511–513, 1992.

Day, M.J., W.J. Penhale, C.E. Eger, *et al*. Disseminated aspergillosis in dogs. *Aust Vet J* 63:55–59, 1986.

González-Mendoza, A. Opportunistic mycoses. *In*: Pan American Health Organization. *Proceedings: International Symposium on Mycoses*. Washington, D.C.: PAHO; 1970. (Scientific Publication 205).

Gordon, M.A. Current status of serology for diagnosis and prognostic evaluation of opportunistic fungus infections. *In*: Pan American Health Organization. *Proceedings of the Third International Conference on the Mycoses*. Washington, D.C.: PAHO; 1975. (Scientific Publication 304).

Greenberger, P.A. Aspergillosis: Clinical aspects. *Zbl Bakt Hyg A* 261:487–495, 1986.

Hattel, A.L., T.R. Drake, B.J. Anderholm, E.S. McAllister. Pulmonary aspergillosis associated with acute enteritis in a horse. *J Am Vet Med Assoc* 199:589–590, 1991.

Imbeault, B., Y. Cormier. Usefulness of inhaled high-dose corticosteroids in allergic bronchopulmonary aspergillosis. *Chest* 103:1614–1617, 1993.

Iwen, P.C., E.C. Reed, J.O. Armitage, *et al*. Nosocomial invasive aspergillosis in lymphoma patients treated with bone marrow or peripheral stem cell transplants. *Infect Control Hosp Epidemiol* 14:131–139, 1993.

Karam, G.H., F.M. Griffin, Jr. Invasive pulmonary aspergillosis in nonimmunocompromised, nonneutropenic hosts. *Rev Infect Dis* 8:357–363, 1986.

Kurup, V.P. Enzyme-linked immunosorbent assay in the detection of specific antibodies against *Aspergillus* in patient sera. *Zbl Bakt Hyg A* 261:509–516, 1986.

Lortholary, O., M.C. Meyohas, B. Dupont, *et al*. Invasive aspergillosis in patients with acquired immunodeficiency syndrome: Report of 33 cases. French Cooperative Study Group on Aspergillosis in AIDS. *Am J Med* 95:177–187, 1993.

Mishra, S.K., S. Falkenberg, N. Masihi. Efficacy of enzyme-linked immunosorbent assay in serodiagnosis of aspergillosis. *J Clin Microbiol* 17:708–710, 1983.

Opal, S.M., A.A. Asp, P.B. Cannady, Jr., *et al*. Efficacy of infection control measures during a nosocomial outbreak of disseminated aspergillosis associated with hospital construction. *J Infect Dis* 153:634–637, 1986.

Schmitt, J.A. Mycotic diseases. *In*: Ristic M., I. McIntyre, eds. *Diseases of Cattle in the Tropics*. The Hague: Martinus Nijhoff; 1981.

Utz, J.P. The systemic mycoses. *In*: Wyngaarden, J.B., L.H. Smith, Jr., eds. *Cecil Textbook of Medicine*. 16th ed. Philadelphia: Saunders; 1982.

Wex, P., E. Utta, W. Drozdz. Surgical treatment of pulmonary and pleuropulmonary *Aspergillus* disease. *Thorac Cardiovasc Surg* 41:64–70, 1993.

Winter, A.J. Mycotic abortion. *In*: Faulkner, L.C., ed. *Abortion Diseases of Livestock*. Springfield: Thomas; 1968.

BLASTOMYCOSIS

ICD-10 B40.0 acute pulmonary blastomycosis; B40.1 chronic pulmonary blastomycosis; B40.3 cutaneous blastomycosis; B40.7 disseminated blastomycosis; B40.8 other forms of blastomycosis

Synonyms: North American blastomycosis, Chicago disease, Gilchrist's disease.

Etiology: *Blastomyces dermatitidis*, a dimorphic fungus existing in mycelial form in cultures and as a budding yeast in the tissues of infected mammals. The fungus also exists as yeast in enriched culture media at 37°C. The mycelial form in culture media at 25°C is cottony white, turning to brown over time.

Sandy, acidic soil close to rivers or other freshwater reservoirs is the microecosystem most favorable to *B. dermatitidis*. It remains in an infective sporulated state in this biotope, as its spores (conidia) can detach and become airborne. High ambient humidity seems to favor the release of spores.

B. dermatitidis is subdivided into two serotypes (1 and 2) based on the presence of an exoantigen, called A and recognized by a specific precipitin. Strains examined from India, Israel, and the United States, and one strain examined from Africa all contained A antigen (serotype 1). Eleven of 12 African strains examined were type 2. The African strains are deficient in A antigen, but contain K antigen (Kaufman *et al.*, 1983).

Geographic Distribution: The disease has been observed in eastern Canada, India, Israel, South Africa, Tanzania, Tunisia, Uganda, the United States, and the former Zaire. Autochthonous cases have also occurred in some Central and South American countries (Klein *et al.*, 1986). In the United States, endemic areas are located along the Mississippi, Missouri, and Ohio rivers, and in parts of New York State. In Canada, they are located along the St. Lawrence River and near the Great Lakes.

Occurrence in Man: Predominantly sporadic. Most of the cases have been recorded in the United States, with the highest prevalence in the Mississippi and Ohio river basins. From 1885 to 1968, there were 1,573 cases in that country (Menges as cited by Selby, 1975). Klein *et al.* (1986) summarized from the literature the incidence in different endemic U.S. states: from 0.1 to 0.7 cases per 100,000 inhabitants per year in Arkansas from 1960 to 1965; 0.61, 0.44, and 0.43 cases per 100,000 inhabitants per year in Mississippi, Kentucky, and Arkansas, respectively, from 1960 to 1967; and 0.48 cases per 100,000 inhabitants per year in Wisconsin from 1873 to 1982. Hyperendemic areas in these states have an incidence of 4 cases per 100,000 per year. These data do not include slight cases of the disease that do not generally receive medical attention.

In Louisiana (USA), an attempt was made to identify all cases that occur in the state and to study one district in detail (Washington Parish) that is considered endemic. The average annual incidence for the entire state during 1976–1985 was 0.23 cases per 100,000 inhabitants, while the incidence for Washington Parish was 6.8 cases per 100,000. In 30 cases studied in this district, the patients' ages ranged from 3 weeks to 81 years. Five people died, and one of these was probably infected *in utero* (Lowry *et al.*, 1989).

In Canada, about 120 cases of blastomycosis were recorded up until 1979. Most of the cases occurred in Quebec, followed by Ontario and the maritime provinces. More recently, 38 cases were reported in Ontario, as was a new focus to the north and east of Lake Superior that accounted for 20 of the patients (Bakerspigel *et al.*, 1986).

The disease also occurs in the form of outbreaks. Klein *et al.* (1986) reported seven of them, mainly in the northern part of the mid-western United States. The largest outbreak affected 48 people in Wisconsin who traveled to a beaver pond and also visited their dens and dams. Only one outbreak occurred in an urban area (near Chicago), and in nine months affected five people living close to a highway under construction. Another outbreak in a wooded, marshy area of Virginia simultaneously affected four raccoon hunters and their four hunting dogs (Armstrong *et al.*, 1987). The disease occurs more frequently among males and the highest rate of infection is found in men over 20 years of age. Most cases occur in winter (Klein *et al.*, 1986).

Occurrence in Animals: Sporadic. Canids are the most affected, and the greatest concentration of cases is seen in Arkansas (USA). A study was conducted on the accumulated data of 20 university veterinary hospitals in terms of the risk factors for blastomycosis in dogs. From 1980 to 1990, 971 cases were recorded. The prevalence of blastomycosis in dogs was 205 per 100,000 hospital admissions. The highest incidence of the disease occurred in autumn. The principal victims were hunting dogs weighing between 23 and 45 kg and aged 2 to 4 years. The endemic areas were the same as for man. Hunting dogs generally cover large distances and can enter endemic areas with ecological niches of the fungus (Rudmann *et al.*, 1992). Cases have also been described in cats, a horse, a captive sea lion (*Eumetopias jubata*), an African lion (*Panthera leo*) in a zoo, a dolphin, and a ferret. Cats follow dogs in terms of numbers of cases, but the total number of cats affected is small. In a university hospital in Tennessee (USA), 5 out of 5,477 cats treated presented blastomycosis (Breider *et al.*, 1988).

The Disease in Man: The incubation period is not well known, but is estimated to be from 21 to 106 days (an average of 43 days) (Klein *et al.*, 1986). Blastomycosis may develop insidiously and silently, or acutely with symptoms of a febrile disease, arthralgia, myalgia, and pleuritic pain. It may start with a dry cough that becomes productive with hemoptysis, chest pain, and weight loss. Fever, cough, dyspnea, and diffuse pulmonary infiltration indicated by chest x-ray were seen in a description of acute respiratory distress syndrome in 10 adult patients. Six of the patients had no underlying disease associated with a change in immunity and two had no recent exposure to environmental reservoirs of *B. dermatitidis*. Microscopic examination of tracheal secretions showed budding yeasts. Five of the 10 patients died, despite intravenous treatment with amphotericin B (Meyer *et al.*, 1993). However, in most cases, the disease is asymptomatic at the outset and is diagnosed in a chronic state. The principal clinical form is pulmonary blastomycosis. It is a systemic disease with a wide variety of pulmonary and extrapulmonary manifestations. The pulmonary form has the symptoms of chronic pneumonia. The lesions are similar to those produced by other granulomatous diseases (Chapman, 1990).

The extrapulmonary forms are attributed to dissemination from the lungs. The cutaneous form is the form most commonly seen in patients. Some patients do not present simultaneous pulmonary involvement. The disease is evidenced by verruciform lesions on exposed parts of the body or by an irregularly shaped scabby ulcer with raised borders. A single patient may present both types of cutaneous lesions (Chapman, 1990). Other forms consist of subcutaneous nodules and particularly lesions in the joints, long bones, vertebrae, and ribs. The lesions are osteolytic and well defined, with abscesses forming in the soft tissue. A large number of patients may have prostate and epididymis lesions (Chapman, 1990).

Of 15 AIDS patients in six endemic and four nonendemic areas, seven suffered from a localized pulmonary blastomycosis and eight from disseminated or extrapulmonary blastomycosis. Localization in the CNS was frequent (40% of cases). Six of the patients died in the first 21 days after admission to the medical facility with a clinical picture of blastomycosis, two of them with fulminant pneumonia (Pappas *et al.*, 1992). The authors conclude that blastomycosis is a late and often fatal complication that occurs in a small number of AIDS patients.

The preferred medication for disseminated cases is intravenous amphotericin B; ketoconazole is preferred for patients with more limited lesions, as it does not have the amphotericin B side effects.

The Disease in Animals: The highest incidence is seen in dogs around two years of age. Symptoms consist of weight loss, chronic cough, dyspnea, cutaneous abscesses, fever, anorexia, and, with some frequency, blindness. The lesions localize in the lungs, lymph nodes, eyes, skin, and joints and bones. Of the 47 clinical cases described, 72% occurred in large males. Lesions were present in the respiratory tract in 85% of the cases (Legendre *et al.*, 1981). The number of cases in dogs is increasing in the United States; between January 1980 and July 1982, 200 cases of canine blastomycosis were recorded in Wisconsin alone. Cases also have been reported east of the Mississippi River (Archer *et al.*, 1987). The preferred treatment is the same as for man—intravenous amphotericin B. A large percentage of sick dogs are euthanized due to the high cost of treatment and the possible side effect of nephrotoxicity (Holt, 1980).

Source of Infection and Mode of Transmission: The reservoir is environmental. Epidemiologic studies conducted in recent years reveal that the optimum microecosystem is sandy, acidic soil along waterways, and probably around artificial reservoirs as well (see the section on etiology). When environmental conditions change, the agent isolated once often cannot be isolated again. Exposed men and dogs are those who come into contact with the foci in endemic areas (see the section on geographic distribution), for work or recreation, particularly hunting. Transmission to man and animals is via the airborne route; fungal conidia are the infecting element.

Role of Animals in the Epidemiology of the Disease: None. It is a disease common to man and animals. There are no known cases of transmission from one individual to another (man or animal).

Diagnosis: Diagnosis is based on direct microscopic examination of sputum and material from lesions, on isolation of the agent in culture media, and on histological preparations. *B. dermatitidis* grows well in Sabouraud's culture medium or another suitable culture medium. It is most distinctive in its budding yeast form, and thus the inoculated medium should be incubated at 37°C (the mycelial form of the fungus is obtained at ambient temperature). *B. dermatitidis* in its yeast form (in tissues or cultures at 37°C) is characterized by a single bud attached to the parent cell by a wide base from which it detaches upon reaching a size similar to that of the parent cell. In contrast, *Paracoccidioides brasiliensis*, the agent of paracoccioidomycosis ("South American blastomycosis"), has multiple buds in the yeast-forming phase. A commercial DNA probe can be used to confirm the identity of the *B. dermatitidis* culture (Scalarone *et al.*, 1992).

Serological tests used are complement fixation and gel immunodiffusion; the latter yields the best results. Sensitivity is much greater in disseminated than in localized blastomycosis. An antigen-capture ELISA test proved to be more specific than the conventional enzymatic immunoassays: of eight serum samples obtained from patients in an early stage of the disease, seven tested positive with this method, whereas three tested positive with gel immunodiffusion and three with complement fixation. There were no cross reactions with sera from patients with histoplasmosis or coccidioidomycosis (Lo and Notenboom, 1990), though it should be borne in mind that cross reactions with *Histoplasma* and *Coccidioides* may occur. At present, the intradermal test is considered to have no diagnostic value. In dogs, serological tests have not yielded reliable results.

Control: There are no adequate control measures.

Bibliography

Ajello, L. Comparative ecology of respiratory mycotic disease agents. *Bact Rev* 31: 6–24, 1967.

Archer, J.R., D.O. Trainer, R.F. Schell. Epidemiologic study of canine blastomycosis in Wisconsin. *J Am Vet Med Assoc* 190:1292–1295, 1987.

Armstrong, C.W., S.R. Jenkins, L. Kaufman, *et al.* Common-source outbreak of blastomycosis in hunters and their dogs. *J Infect Dis* 155:568–570, 1987.

Bakerspigel, A., J.S. Kane, D. Schaus. Isolation of *Blastomyces dermatitidis* from an earthen floor in southwestern Ontario, Canada. *J Clin Microbiol* 24:890–891, 1986.

Benenson, A.S., ed. *Control of Communicable Diseases in Man.* 15th ed. An official report of the American Public Health Association. Washington, D.C.: American Public Health Association; 1990.

Breider, M.A., T.L. Walker, A.M. Legendre, R.T. VanEl. Blastomycosis in cats: Five cases (1979–1986). *J Am Vet Med Assoc* 193:570–572, 1988.

Chapman, S.W. *Blastomyces dermatitidis. In:* Mandell, G.L., R.G. Douglas, Jr., J.E. Bennett, eds. *Principles and Practice of Infectious Diseases.* 3rd ed. New York: Churchill Livingstone, Inc.; 1990.

Drutz, D.J. The mycoses. *In:* Wyngaarden, J.B., L.H. Smith, Jr., eds. *Cecil Textbook of Medicine.* 16th ed. Philadelphia: Saunders; 1982.

Holt, R.J. Progress in antimycotic chemotherapy, 1945–1980. *Infection* 8:5284–5287, 1980.

Kaplan, W. Epidemiology of the principal systemic mycoses of man and lower animals and the ecology of their agents. *J Am Vet Med Assoc* 163:1043–1047, 1973.

Kaufman, L. Current status of immunology for diagnosis and prognostic evaluation of blastomycosis, coccidioidomycosis, and paracoccidioidomycosis. *In:* Pan American Health Organization. *Proceedings of the Third International Conference on the Mycoses.* Washington, D.C.: PAHO; 1975. (Scientific Publication 304).

Kaufman, L., P.G. Standard, R.J. Weeks, A.A. Padhye. Detection of two *Blastomyces dermatitidis* serotypes by exoantigen analysis. *J Clin Microbiol* 18:110–114, 1983.

Klein, B.S., J.M. Vergeront, J.P. Davis. Epidemiologic aspects of blastomycosis, the enigmatic systemic mycosis. *Semin Respir Infect* 1:29–39, 1986.

Legendre, A.M., M. Walker, N. Buyukmihci, R. Stevens. Canine blastomycoses: A review of 47 clinical cases. *J Am Vet Med Assoc* 178:1163–1168, 1981.

Lo, C.Y., R.H. Notenboom. A new enzyme immunoassay specific for blastomycosis. *Am Rev Resp Dis* 141:84–88, 1990.

Lowry, P.W., K.Y. Kelso, L.M. McFarland. Blastomycosis in Washington Parish, Louisiana, 1976–1985. *Am J Epidemiol* 130:151–159, 1989.

Menges, R.W. Blastomycosis in animals. *Vet Med* 55:45–54, 1960. Cited in: Selby, L.A. Blastomycosis. *In*: Hubbert, W.T., W.F. McCulloch, P.R. Schnurrenberger, eds. *Diseases Transmitted from Animals to Man*. 6th ed. Springfield: Thomas; 1975.

Meyer, K.C., E.J. McManus, D.G. Maki. Overwhelming pulmonary blastomycosis associated with the adult respiratory distress syndrome. *N Engl J Med* 329:1231–1236, 1993.

Pappas, P.G., J.C. Pottage, W.G. Powderly, *et al.* Blastomycosis in patients with acquired immunodeficiency syndrome. *Ann Intern Med* 116:847–853, 1992.

Rudmann, D.G., B.R. Coolman, C.M. Pérez, L.T. Glickman. Evaluation of risk factors for blastomycosis in dogs: 857 cases (1980–1990). *J Am Vet Med Assoc* 201:1754–1759, 1992.

Scalarone, G.M., A.M. Legendre, K.A. Clark, K. Pusatev. Evaluation of a commercial DNA probe assay for the identification of clinical isolates of *Blastomyces dermatitidis* from dogs. *J Med Vet Mycol* 30:43–49, 1992.

Selby, L.A. Blastomycosis. *In*: Hubbert, W.T., W.F. McCulloch, P.R. Schnurrenberger, eds. *Diseases Transmitted from Animals to Man*. 6th ed. Springfield: Thomas; 1975.

CANDIDIASIS

ICD-10 B37.0 candidal stomatitis; B37.1 pulmonary candidiasis; B37.2 candidiasis of skin and nail; B37.3 candidiasis of vulva and vagina; B37.4 candidiasis of other urogenital sites; B37.5 candidal meningitis; B37.6 candidal endocarditis; B37.7 candidal septicaemia

Synonyms: Moniliasis, candidosis, thrush, candidomycosis.

Etiology: *Candida albicans (Monilia albicans, Oidium albicans)* is the most common species in man and animals. Other less frequent species are *Candida tropicalis, C. parapsilosis, C. krusei, C. guillermondi, C. pseudotropicalis,* and *C. lusitaniae.*

C. albicans in young cultures measures approximately 3 x 5 microns. It is gram-positive and reproduces by budding. In Sabouraud's medium it forms creamy white, convex colonies. Old cultures have septate hyphae and sometimes chlamydospores (enlarged spherical cells with thick walls). *C. albicans* forms part of the normal flora in the human and animal digestive system, mucosa and, to a lesser extent, the skin. It is also found in the soil, in plants, and in fruits. In its normal habitat, *Candida* takes the form of a budding yeast. In infected tissue, it can produce hyphae or pseudohyphae (filaments consisting of elongated budding cells that did not detach from the parent cell). Odds and Abbott (1980, 1983) developed a biotyping method for *Candida albicans*, later modified by Childress *et al.* (1989). This method consists of evaluating the growth of the strain in nine agar plates with various biochemical compositions in order to differentiate the strains for epidemiological purposes.

Geographic Distribution: Worldwide. There are no delimited endemic zones.

Occurrence in Man: It is the most frequent opportunistic mycosis. Its incidence has increased in recent years due to the increase in prolonged treatments with antibiotics and corticosteroids. Candidiasis is a sporadic disease; epidemics have occurred in nurseries, particularly among premature babies in intensive care units; some epidemics are due to the use of contaminated medicinal solutions or parenteral feeding fluids. It is estimated that the disease is responsible for nearly one-quarter of mycotic deaths. In a general hospital in Mexico, candidiasis lesions were found in 5.4% of random autopsies conducted (González-Mendoza, 1970).

Occurrence in Animals: The disease has been confirmed in numerous mammalian and avian species. Moniliasis in chicks and poults is common and sometimes has economic implications. Outbreaks have been described in various parts of the world.

The Disease in Man: *Candida* is found as a commensal in the digestive tract and vagina of a high percentage of healthy individuals. Diaper rash and cheilitis (lip sores) are often caused by *Candida*. In adults, candidiasis is always associated with debilitating diseases or conditions, such as diabetes (which particularly favors superficial candidiasis), AIDS, tuberculosis, syphilis, cancer, obesity, and others. The agent often is responsible for intertrigo of large skin folds, balanitis, and onychia with paronychia (especially in women whose work frequently requires them to immerse their hands in water).

The most frequent form of the mucosal infection presents clinically as a mycotic stomatitis (thrush) characterized by lightly adhering white plaques on the tongue and other parts of the mouth that can leave a bloody surface when removed. Some have observed that this clinical form increased in asthmatic children treated with inhaled steroids. The infection often heals spontaneously (Edwards, 1990).

The high incidence of thrush in cancer or AIDS patients should lead a physician treating a patient with thrush to test for these diseases (Syrjanen *et al.*, 1988).

Another form of mucosal infection is esophageal candidiasis, which may or may not be an extension of oral thrush. It is particularly frequent in patients receiving treatment for malignant processes of the hematopoietic or lymphatic system. The most common symptoms of esophagitis are pain upon swallowing and substernal pain (Edwards, 1990).

Gastrointestinal candidiasis follows the esophageal form in frequency among cancer patients. The small intestine is the third most frequent site of infection. Ulcers are the most common lesions in the stomach and intestine.

Mucosal candidiasis recently has been surpassing *Trichomonas* as a cause of vulvovaginitis. This form is commonly accompanied by vaginal discharge of varying intensity and pruritus vulvae.

Although candidiasis is usually limited to mucocutaneous forms, systemic infection can occur through hematogenous transmission, particularly in very weak patients who are treated with antibiotics over a long period. These cases often develop as a result of lesions caused by medical explorations using catheters, insertion of these instruments in the urethra, or surgical interventions. Though localization may occur in any organ, it is most frequent in the eyes, kidneys, lung, spleen, and the CNS, as well as around a cardiac value prosthesis or in the bones.

The antimycotic recommended for mucosal and skin candidiasis is nystatin; clotrimazole is also effective. Amphotericin B or fluconazole are used to treat other sites.

A cooperative study in 18 medical centers in Europe evaluated the efficacy, harmlessness, and tolerance of oral fluconazole (50 mg/day in a single dose) and of polyenes (oral amphotericin B at 2 g/day or nystatin at 4 million units/day in four or more doses) in preventing mycotic infection. The study included 536 patients hospitalized with a malignant disease who were about to receive chemotherapy, radiotherapy, or bone marrow transplants, including patients who already had neutropenia or who were expected to develop it. Treatment was administered for approximately 30 days. Oral fluconazole proved to be more effective than the oral polyenes in preventing buccopharyngeal infection and was equally effective in preventing infections in other parts of the body in patients with neutropenia. Side effects were recorded in 5.6% of 269 patients in the group treated with fluconazole and 5.2% of 267 patients treated with polyenes. These reactions led to a discontinuation of treatment in seven patients in each group (Philpott-Howard *et al.*, 1993).

The Disease in Animals: Candidiasis in chicks, poults, and other fowl is usually sporadic. Epidemic outbreaks sometimes occur, particularly in poults, with mortality ranging from 8% to 20%. Avian candidiasis is an infection of the upper respiratory system. In young birds it sometimes has an acute course, with nervous symptoms. However, the disease is generally asymptomatic and diagnosis occurs postmortem. The most frequent lesion is found in the crop and consists of plaques that resemble curdled milk and adhere lightly to the mucosa. In adult birds, candidiasis has a chronic course and causes thickening of the crop wall, on which a yellowish necrotic material accumulates. In Israel, a strange epidemic of a venereal disease in geese that affected many farms was described. The disease began with reddening and tumefaction of the mucosa of the penis or cloaca; the lesion later became gangrenous and a portion of the penis was lost. Examinations indicated a mixed flora of bacteria and *C. albicans*. Experimental inoculation of the bacterial flora did not affect the birds; in contrast, it was possible to reproduce the disease with *C. albicans* isolated from the lesions.

Oral candidiasis occurs sporadically in calves, colts, lambs, swine, dogs, cats, laboratory mice and guinea pigs, as well as in zoo animals. *Candida* spp. can, on rare occasions, lead to mastitis and abortions in cattle. A systemic disease due to *C. albicans*, with lesions in various organs, was reported in calves that underwent prolonged treatment with antibiotics. Skin lesions and thrush have been described in cats.

Source of Infection and Mode of Transmission: *C. albicans* occurs as a component of the normal flora in the digestive system of a high percentage of healthy individuals and animals. The yeast is also found in nature.

In young fowl, *C. albicans* is probably a primary etiologic agent, while in man candidiasis is almost always associated with other diseases. Prolonged treatment with antibiotics, cytotoxic agents, and corticosteroids is a predisposing factor. The use and abuse of antibiotics over an extended period is an important factor in the proliferation of and later infection by *Candida* and other fungi, in that they alter the natural flora of the mucosal surfaces.

Most infections have an endogenous source. The infection can be spread through contact with oral secretions, skin, vagina, and feces of sick individuals or carriers. A mother with vaginal candidiasis can infect her child during childbirth. Balanitis may in some cases be due to sexual relations with women suffering from vaginitis caused by *C. albicans*. In nurseries, particularly in units for premature infants, the infection may have an environmental source (see the section on occurrence in man). An exogenous infection probably occurred due to indirect contact between patients in a hospital bone marrow transplant unit and an intensive care unit (Vázquez *et al.*, 1993).

Role of Animals in the Epidemiology of the Disease: It is a disease common to man and animals. There are no known cases of transmission from animal to animal, but human-to-human transmission has occurred, as in the case of mothers who infect their children during childbirth.

Diagnosis: Given the ubiquitous nature of the yeast, laboratory diagnosis must be conducted with great care. Direct examination of lesions in the nails, skin (in potassium hydroxide) or the mucous membranes (in lactophenol-cotton blue), or microscopic observation of gram-stained films, is diagnostically significant if the microorganism is found in great numbers. The examination should be carried out with fresh specimens. The presence in lesions of the budding yeast form together with forms with hyphae or pseudohyphae has diagnostic value. Isolation of the agent from blood, pleural or peritoneal fluid, cerebrospinal fluid, or biopsy material obtained aseptically from closed localized foci permits diagnosis of disseminated candidiasis. However, it should be kept in mind that fungemia may be transient and is not always indicative of systemic infection. Hemocultures can detect candidemia in 35% to 44% of patients with disseminated candidiasis. *C. albicans* grows well in a medium of blood agar and Sabouraud agar at 25°C and 37°C. It can be identified by demonstrating the presence of chlamydospores upon seeding in depth a plate of corn meal agar and observing it at 24 and 48 hours. Since another characteristic of this species is the production of germinating tubes, identification can be performed by adding a small amount of culture to a small amount of serum and incubating the mixture at 37°C for two to four hours (Carter and Chengappa, 1991). The other species of *Candida* can be identified by their biochemical properties of carbohydrate fermentation and assimilation. A labeled anti-*C. albicans* globulin for immunofluorescence testing of smears of pathologic or cultured materials is available.

The most widely used serologic test to diagnose systemic candidiasis is immunodiffusion or double diffusion in ouchterlony agar gel, which cumulative experience has shown to be highly sensitive and specific. The immunoelectrophoresis test correlates well with the immunodiffusion test and results are obtained in only two hours. Nonetheless, serologic diagnosis of systemic candidiasis presents serious difficulties and an increase in patients' titers should be confirmed. Immunosuppressed patients have a poor humoral response, and thus an attempt has been made to use techniques that detect antigenemia rather than circulating antibodies. To date the results have not been very encouraging. Sensitivity is low (Lemieux *et al.*, 1990; Bougnoux *et al.*, 1990). Tube agglutination, indirect immunofluorescence, and indirect hemagglutination are also useful tests if the antibody level detected is above that prevalent in the normal population. The predominant or sole antibodies in healthy individuals are IgM. In contrast, with systemic candidiasis there is an initial rapid increase of IgM and then IgG, with subsequent reduction of IgM and persistence of IgG.

Control: Neonatal candidiasis can be prevented by treating the mother's vaginal candidiasis with nystatin during the third trimester. This antimycotic antibiotic can also be used in patients undergoing prolonged treatment with broad-spectrum antibiotics. Plastic catheters should be avoided. Generalized thrush in weakened patients can be halted by treating the oral lesions. To prevent epidemics in nurseries, patients with oral thrush should be isolated and strict hygiene measures established. As a preventive measure, nutritional deficiencies should be corrected, given that candidiasis occurs with greater frequency in patients with vitamin deficiencies or inadequate diets (Ajello and Kaplan, 1980).

Recommended control measures in case of a moniliasis outbreak among fowl include destroying all sick birds and administering copper sulphate (1:2,000) in the drinking water and nystatin (110 mg/kg) in the feed.

To date there is no vaccine.

Bibliography

Ainsworth, G.C., P.K.C. Austwick. *Fungal Diseases of Animals.* 2nd ed. Farnham Royal, Slough, United Kingdom: Commonwealth Agricultural Bureau; 1973.

Ajello, L., W. Kaplan. Systemic mycoses. *In*: Stoenner, H., W. Kaplan, M. Torten, eds. Section A, Vol 2: *CRC Handbook Series in Zoonoses.* Boca Raton: CRC Press; 1980.

Anderson, K.L. Pathogenic yeasts. *In*: Hubbert, W.T., W.F. McCulloch, P.R. Schnurrenberger, eds. *Diseases Transmitted from Animals to Man.* 6th ed. Springfield: Thomas; 1975.

Beemer, A.M., E.S. Kuttin, Z. Katz. Epidemic venereal disease due to *Candida albicans* in geese in Israel. *Avian Dis* 17:639–649, 1973.

Benenson, A.S., ed. *Control of Communicable Diseases in Man.* 15th ed. An official report of the American Public Health Association. Washington, D.C.: American Public Health Association; 1990.

Bougnoux, M.E., C. Hill, D. Moissenet, *et al.* Comparison of antibody, antigen, and metabolite assays for hospitalized patients with disseminated or peripheral candidiasis. *J Clin Microbiol* 28:905–909, 1990.

Carter, G.R. *Diagnostic Procedures in Veterinary Microbiology.* 2nd ed. Springfield: Thomas; 1973.

Carter, G.R., M.N. Chengappa. *Essentials of Veterinary Bacteriology and Mycology.* 4th ed. Philadelphia: Lea & Febiger; 1991.

Childress, C.M., J.A. Holder, A.N. Neely. Modifications of a *Candida albicans* biotyping system. *J Clin Microbiol* 27:1392–1394, 1989.

Edwards, J.E., Jr. *Candida* species. *In*: Mandell, G.L., R.G. Douglas, Jr., J.E. Bennett, eds. *Principles and Practice of Infectious Diseases.* 3rd ed. New York: Churchill Livingstone, Inc.; 1990.

González-Mendoza, A. Opportunistic mycoses. *In*: Pan American Health Organization. *Proceedings: International Symposium on Mycoses.* Washington, D.C.: PAHO; 1970. (Scientific Publication 205).

Gordon, M.A. Current status of serology for diagnosis and prognostic evaluation of opportunistic fungus infections. *In*: Pan American Health Organization. *Proceedings of the Third International Conference on the Mycoses.* Washington, D.C.: PAHO; 1975. (Scientific Publication 304).

Lemieux, C., G. St.-Germain, J. Vincelette, *et al.* Collaborative evaluation of antigen detection by a commercial latex agglutination test and enzyme immunoassay in the diagnosis of invasive candidiasis. *J Clin Microbiol* 28:249–253, 1990.

Negroni, P. *Micosis cutáneas y viscerales.* 5.ª ed. Buenos Aires: López; 1972.

Odds, F.C., A.B. Abbott. A simple system for the presumptive identification of *Candida albicans* and differentiation of strains within the species. *Sabouraudia* 18:301–317, 1980.

Odds, F.C., A.B. Abbott. Modification and extension of tests for differentiation of *Candida* species and strains. *Sabouraudia* 21:79–81, 1983.

Philpott-Howard, J.N., J.J. Wade, G.J. Mufti, *et al.* Randomized comparison of oral flucanozole versus oral polyenes for the prevention of fungal infection in patients at risk of neutropenia. Multicentre Study Group. *J Antimicrob Chemother* 31:973–984, 1993.

Soltys, M.A. *Bacteria and Fungi Pathogenic to Man and Animals.* London: Baillière-Tindall; 1963.

Syrjanen, S., S.L. Valle, J. Antonen, *et al.* Oral candidal infection as a sign of HIV infection in homosexual men. *Oral Surg Oral Med Oral Pathol* 65:36–40, 1988.

Vázquez, J.A., V. Sánchez, C. Dmuchowski, *et al.* Nosocomial acquisition of *Candida albicans*: An epidemiologic study. *J Infect Dis* 168:195–201, 1993.

COCCIDIOIDOMYCOSIS

ICD-10 B38.0 acute pulmonary coccidioidomycosis; B38.1 chronic pulmonary coccidioidomycosis; B38.3 cutaneous coccidioidomycosis; B38.7 disseminated coccidioidomycosis; B38.8 other forms of coccidioidomycosis

Synonyms: Posada's disease, San Joaquin Valley fever, desert fever.

Etiology: *Coccidioides immitis,* a diphasic fungus that exists in the mycelial phase when it is a soil saprophyte, and in the spherule phase in organic tissues and fluids. The life cycle of *C. immitis* is unique among pathogenic fungi. The fungus occurs in one phase in the natural environment, i.e., the soil of semiarid regions, and in another when it is parasitic in the mammalian host. In the soil, *C. immitis* develops as a mycelium (a mass of filamentous hyphae that make up the fungus). The cycle begins with the arthroconidium, or arthrospore (spore formed in the hyphae), which in a suitable medium germinates and forms a branching, septate mycelium. When the mycelium fragments, it releases into the air arthroconidia 2 to 5 microns in size. The parasitic phase begins with the inhalation of arthroconidia by man and animals. Arthroconidia grow to form thick-walled spherules 10 to 80 microns in diameter. The cytoplasm of the spherules divides to produce hundreds of endospores which, when released, disperse into the surrounding tissue and give rise to new spherules. The parasitic cycle lasts from four to six days (Drutz and Huppert, 1983) and can revert to the saprophytic or mycelial phase if the endospores reach the soil upon the death of the infected animal or through bodily excretions. The endospores give rise to hyphae and renew the cycle (Stevens, 1990). However, the mycelial cycle does not depend on this reversion as the hyphae contain large amounts of arthroconidia that are dispersed by the wind and colonize new sites in the soil.

Geographic Distribution: Limited to the Americas. The fungus is found in arid and semiarid areas of the United States Southwest, northwestern Mexico, Argentina,

Colombia, Guatemala, Honduras, Paraguay, Venezuela, and probably Bolivia. The endemic area in Latin America is estimated to cover 1.5 million km^2, more than 1 million km^2 of which are in Mexico (Borelli, 1970).

Occurrence in Man: In some endemic areas the rate of infection seems to be very high and it is estimated that in some of these areas in the United States nearly 100% of the population could contract the infection within a few years (Fiese, cited by Ajello, 1970). There are an estimated 25,000 to 100,000 cases in the US each year. Approximately 20% of the cases involve people who live outside endemic areas and become infected while visiting them (Drutz and Huppert, 1983). Some cases have also been described in Europe (the former Czechoslovakia, Great Britain, and Denmark). The rate of reactors to the skin test in different endemic areas varies from 5% to more than 50% of the population. There is a significant increase in cases in the United States. In 1991, 1,208 new cases were recorded in California as compared to 450 cases per year on average in the previous five years. Of these cases, 80% came from Kern County, a known endemic area. Sixty-three percent of the cases were reported from October through December. The outbreak in California could have been associated with prolonged drought, followed by occasional heavy rains. Another important factor could be migration to California of people not previously exposed to the fungus. In the United States, endemic areas are found in Arizona, California, Nevada, New Mexico, Texas, and Utah (CDC, 1993). The data on South America are more fragmentary, but the rate of infection appears to be lower in this region.

Occurrence in Animals: Natural infection has been found in many species of mammals. Infection is very frequent in cattle and dogs in endemic areas. Veterinary inspection has discovered coccidioidomycosis lesions in 5% to 15% of the cattle slaughtered in abattoirs in central Arizona (USA). Several million cattle are thought to be infected in the endemic areas of the southwestern United States. Infection has also been demonstrated in sheep, horses, swine, and wild rodents.

Several studies were carried out on animals in the endemic region of Mexico. In the state of Sinaloa, sera from 100 hogs and 200 cattle were examined by immunoelectrophoresis and reactions were found in 12% and 13%, respectively (Velasco Castrejón and Campos Nieto, 1979). In the state of Sonora, when the intradermal test using coccidioidin was conducted on 459 cattle, 6.75% tested positive. Another study performed histological examinations of granulomatous lesions discovered in 3,032 slaughtered cattle and found that the lesions in 77 (44%) of 175 animals confiscated for suspected tuberculosis were actually caused by *C. immitis*, indicating a rate of infection of 2.5% in all the animals (Cervantes *et al.*, 1978).

The Disease in Man: The incubation period lasts from one to four weeks. An estimated 60% of infections occur asymptomatically and are only recognizable with the intradermal test. The remaining 40% present as a respiratory disease with acute symptoms similar to those of influenza and that generally pass without sequelae. About 5% of primary infections develop either an erythema multiforme or an erythema nodosum arthralgia. What is more common, however, is a light erythroderma or maculopapular eruption. Chest pain can be strong and pleuritic. The radiological picture is varied, but hilar adenopathy with alveolar infiltrates and infiltrates that change area are indicative of coccidioidal pneumonia (Ampel *et al.*, 1989). When the primary respiratory disease does have sequelae, these consist of fibrotic or cavernous lesions in the lungs. Pneumonia may persist in some patients for six to eight weeks, accompanied by fever, chest pain, cough, or postration (persistent coccidioidal pneumonia). Mortality in these cases is high in immunocompromised patients. Another disease form is the chronic form, which can be confused with tuberculosis (Drutz, 1982).

Extrapulmonary dissemination generally occurs following the primary disease in approximately 0.5% of infections (CDC, 1993). Thoracic radiography may or may not show abnormalities. The most common localization is in the cutaneous and subcutaneous tissues. Cutaneous lesions generally consist of verruciform granulomas (usually on the face), erythromatous plaques, and nodules. Sometimes there are subcutaneous abscesses. Osteomyelitis occurs in 10% to 50% of disseminated cases and may affect one or more bones. Meningitis cases are frequent (33% to 50% of patients) and generally fatal within two years. Eosinophilic pleocytosis is frequent in coccidioidal meningitis and has diagnostic value (Ragland et al., 1993). Other manifestations are thyroiditis, tenosynovitis, and prostatis (Drutz, 1982). Clinical coccidioidomycosis is more frequent among migrant workers and soldiers transferred to endemic zones. In endemic areas of C. immitis the symptomatic form of the disease is frequent in individuals infected by the human immunodeficiency virus. Immunodeficiency is an important risk factor for developing the disease (Ampel et al., 1993).

Treatment is difficult and often unpredictable. Fungicides that were effective in some cases were not in other similar cases. It is estimated that less than 5% of those infected need treatment. Those who are suffering from a progressive illness, patients with severe primary pulmonary disease, and those who have disseminated infection should be treated. Treatment should also be considered for patients with a compromised immune system. Amphotericin B and ketoconazole are the medications most frequently used (Ampel et al., 1989). The administration of 400 mg of fluconazole daily for up to four years to 47 patients with coccidioidal meningitis produced a favorable result in 37 patients (Galgiani et al., 1993).

The Disease in Animals: The infection is asymptomatic in cattle. Lesions are generally limited to the bronchial and mediastinal lymph nodes. On rare occasions, small granulomatous lesions are found in the lungs and the submaxillary and retropharyngeal lymph nodes. Macroscopic lesions resemble those seen in cases of tuberculosis.

Ziemer et al. (1992) conducted a retrospective study of 15 cases of coccidioidomycosis in horses recorded from 1975 to 1984 in a university hospital in California, with diagnosis confirmed by culture or histopathology. The most common symptom in 53% of the horses was chronic weight loss, which ranged from 45.5 kg to 91 kg in three horses. One of the horses lost 24% of its body weight in three months. Thirty-three percent of the horses had a persistent cough. Sixty percent of the animals had respiratory abnormalities detected through auscultation. Other symptoms were depression and superficial abscesses.

Various cases have been described in sheep, with lesions similar to those in cattle.

In the same university hospital in California, 19 cases of coccidioidomycosis were recorded in llamas (10 from Arizona and 9 from California). Eighteen of the animals had disseminated mycosis, with pyogranulomas in the lungs, thoracic ganglia, liver, and kidneys. The llama seems to be highly susceptible to infection by *C. immitis*. It is not known whether there are unapparent or slight infections in this species (Fowler *et al.*, 1992).

After man, the dog is the species most affected. In addition to the lungs, granulomatous lesions are found in nearly all organs. The disseminated form of the disease is frequent in dogs and the disease advances progressively until death (Timoney *et al.*, 1988).

Source of Infection and Mode of Transmission: *C. immitis* is a soil saprophyte in arid and semiarid regions. Its distribution in endemic zones is not uniform. The infection is transmitted to man and animals through inhalation of wind-borne arthrospores of the fungus; it occurs more frequently after dust storms. The infection can be contracted in the laboratory by inhaling the spores from fungus cultures.

Exposure to soil with a high concentration of the agent increases the risk of a symptomatic and severe disease. This was probably the case with two archeology students on a dig in southern California (Larsen *et al.*, 1985; Ampel *et al.*, 1989).

Those most exposed to contracting the infection are individuals without a history of the infection who visit or migrate to endemic areas.

Coccidioidomycosis is currently increasing in the United States due to significant growth in population and tourism in endemic areas.

In recent decades, due to the great increase in the use of immunosuppressant drugs for transplants, oncology, and rheumatology, as well as to AIDS, the severe form of the disease is seen more frequently (Ampel *et al.*, 1989).

Role of Animals: The soil is the common source of infection for man and animals. The fungus is not transmitted from one individual to another, because man and other infected animals do not produce arthroconidia, the infecting agent. An exceptional case due to aerosolization of endospores occurred during the autopsy of a horse with disseminated coccidioidomycosis. The veterinarian who performed the autopsy contracted the infection by inhaling the endospores (Kohn *et al.*, 1992).

Diagnosis: Diagnosis is based on confirmation of the fungus's presence by means of: (1) direct microscopic examination that reveals spherules with endospores in sputum, pus, pleural fluid, or gastric juices (treated with a 10% solution of potassium hydroxide); (2) culture of clinical material; and (3) histopathology. Cultures should not be prepared in Petri dishes but in closed tubes so as to avoid infection of the handler and laboratory personnel. Appropriate biosafety equipment should also be used.

The skin test using coccidioidin or spherulin (considered to be more sensitive) is very valuable in epidemiologic studies. It is administered in the same way as tuberculin. The test should be read at 24 and 48 hours. A reaction of 5 mm or more is considered positive. This test is very useful for delimiting endemic areas. In infections by *C. immitis* there may be cross-reactions with other fungal antigens, especially histoplasmin. In clinical diagnosis, the intradermal test with a positive result is only significant if the patient had no reaction at the beginning of the illness. In a study comparing the tests with coccidioidin (prepared from the mycelial phase fungus) and spherulin (parasitic phase fungus) in patients with coccidioidomycosis, one preparation could not be shown superior to the other for diagnosis. Forty-three percent of the patients reacted positively to both preparations, another 43% reacted negatively to both, and 14% has contradictory results. The lack of reaction in a high percentage of patients is perhaps due to defects in immune function, particularly in the case of advanced disease (Gifford and Catanzaro, 1981). Serologic tests in use are complement fixation (CF), precipitation, immunodiffusion, and latex agglutination. The combination of immunobiological tests provides useful information for both diagnosis and prognosis. In the first two weeks of the disease, IgM antibodies predominate, as can be demonstrated by the tube precipitation, latex agglutination, and immunodiffusion tests. IgG antibodies appear somewhat later and may be detected through CF or immunodiffusion. A persistent high CF titer with loss of reactivity to the skin test indicates dissemination of the infection. In 75% to 95% of meningitis cases, antibodies can be detected with the CF test (Drutz, 1982). Radioimmunoassay is useful for diagnosis and prognosis of the pulmonary disease. As patients improve, the test titer decreases (Catanzaro and Flataner, 1983). The CF test also indicates the efficacy of the treatment.

Control: It is recommended that persons from nonendemic areas not work in endemic areas, since they lack immunity against coccidioidomycosis. In the United States, dust control measures (paving roads, seeding lawns, sprinkling dust with oil) have been used successfully to protect military personnel.

People at risk of contracting disseminated coccidioidomycosis (pregnant women, immunocompromised patients) should be advised to avoid endemic areas. Trials of a vaccine made from formalin-inactivated spherules are being conducted in California and Arizona (USA). Animal tests have shown that the vaccine does not prevent the infection, but does arrest its progress and prevent dissemination of the disease (Drutz and Huppert, 1983). A test conducted from 1980 to 1985 with 1,436 vaccinated subjects and 1,431 subjects given a placebo showed a slight but statistically insignificant reduction in the incidence of coccidioidomycosis in the vaccinated group as compared to the group receiving the placebo. There was no difference between the two groups in the severity of the disease (Pappagianis, 1993). Treatment with antifungal drugs may be useful to prevent dissemination in high-risk patients with primary coccidioidomycosis.

Bibliography

Ajello, L. Comparative ecology of respiratory mycotic disease agents. *Bact Rev* 31: 6–24, 1967.

Ajello, L. The medical mycological iceberg. *In*: Pan American Health Organization. *Proceedings: International Symposium on Mycoses*. Washington, D.C.: PAHO; 1970. (Scientific Publication 205).

Ajello, L., L.K. Georg, W. Kaplan, L. Kaufman. *Laboratory Manual for Medical Mycology*. Washington, D.C.: U.S. Government Printing Office; 1963. (Public Health Service Publication 994).

Ampel, N.M., C.L. Dols, J.N. Galgiani. Coccidioidomycosis during human immunodeficiency virus infection: Results of prospective study in a coccidioidal endemic area. *Am J Med* 94:235–240, 1993.

Ampel, N.M., M.A. Wieden, J.N. Galgiani. Coccidioidomycosis: Clinical update. *Rev Infect Dis* 11:897–911, 1989.

Benenson, A.S., ed. *Control of Communicable Diseases in Man*. 15th ed. An official report of the American Public Health Association. Washington, D.C.: American Public Health Association; 1990.

Borelli, D. Prevalence of systemic mycoses in Latin America. *In*: Pan American Health Organization. *Proceedings: International Symposium on Mycoses*. Washington, D.C.: PAHO; 1970. (Scientific Publication 205).

Catanzaro, A., F. Flataner. Detection of serum antibodies in coccidioidomycosis by solid-phase radioimmunoassay. *J Infect Dis* 147:32–39, 1983.

Cervantes, R.A., A.J. Solózano, C.B.J. Pijoan. Presencia de coccidioidomicosis en bovinos del Estado de Sonora. *Rev Latinoam Microbiol* 20:247–249, 1978.

Davis, J.W. Coccidioidomycosis. In: Davis, J.W., L.H. Karstad, D.O. Trainer, eds. *Infectious Diseases of Wild Mammals*. Ames: Iowa State University Press; 1970.

Drutz, D.J. The mycoses. *In*: Wyngaarden, J.B., L.H. Smith, Jr., eds. *Cecil Textbook of Medicine*. 16th ed. Philadelphia: Saunders; 1982.

Drutz, D.J., M. Huppert. Coccidioidomycosis: Factors affecting the host-parasite interaction. *J Infect Dis* 147:372–390, 1983.

Fiese, M.J. *Coccidioidomycosis*. Springfield: Thomas; 1958. Cited in: Ajello, L. The medical mycological iceberg. *In*: Pan American Health Organization. *Proceedings: International Symposium on Mycoses*. Washington, D.C.: PAHO; 1970. (Scientific Publication 205).

Fowler, M.E., D. Pappagianis, I. Ingram. Coccidioidomycosis in llamas in the United States: 19 cases (1981–1989). *J Am Vet Med Assoc* 201:1609–1614, 1992.

Galgiani, J.N., A. Catanzaro, G.A. Cloud, *et al*. Fluconazole therapy for coccidioidal meningitis. The NIAID-Mycoses Study Group. *Ann Intern Med* 119:28–35, 1993.

Gifford, J., A. Catanzaro. A comparison of coccidioidin and spherulin skin testing in the diagnosis of coccidioidomycosis. *Am Rev Resp Dis* 124:440–444, 1981.

Kohn, G.J., S.R. Linne, C.M. Smith, P.D. Hoeprich. Acquisition of coccidioidomycosis at necropsy by inhalation of coccidioidal endospores. *Diagn Microbiol Infect Dis* 15:527–530, 1992.

Larsen, R.A., J.A. Jacobson, A.H. Morris, B.A. Benowitz. Acute respiratory failure caused by primary pulmonary coccidioidomycosis. Two case reports and a review of the literature. *Am Rev Resp Dis* 131:797–799, 1985.

Maddy, K.T. Coccidioidomycosis. *Adv Vet Sci* 6:251–286, 1960.

Negroni, K.T. *Micosis cutáneas y viscerales*. 5.ª ed. Buenos Aires: López; 1972.

Pappagianis, D. Evaluation of protective efficacy of the killed *Coccidioides immitis* spherule vaccine in humans. The Valley Fever Vaccine Study Group. *Am Rev Resp Dis* 148:656–660, 1993.

Ragland, A.S., E. Arsura, Y. Ismail, R. Johnson. Eosinophilic pleocytosis in coccidioidal meningitis: Frequency and significance. *Am J Med* 95:254–257, 1993.

Stevens, D.A. *Coccidioides immitis*. *In*: Mandell, G.L., R.G. Douglas, Jr., J.E. Bennett, eds. *Principles and Practice of Infectious Diseases*. 3rd ed. New York: Churchill Livingstone, Inc.; 1990.

Timoney, J.F., J.H. Gillespie, F.W. Scott, J.E. Barlough. *Hagan and Bruner's Microbiology and Infectious Diseases of Domestic Animals*. 8th ed. Ithaca: Comstock; 1988.

United States of America, Department of Health and Human Services, Centers for Disease Control and Prevention (CDC). Coccidioidomycosis—United States, 1991–1992. *MMWR Morb Mortal Wkly Rep* 42:21–24, 1993.

Velasco Castrejón, O., E. Campos Nieto. Estudio serológico de la coccidioidomicosis bovina y porcina del Estado de Sinaloa (México). *Rev Latinoam Microbiol* 21:99, 1979.

Ziemer, E.L., D. Pappagianis, J.E. Madigan, *et al*. Coccidioidomycosis in horses: 15 cases (1975–1984). *J Am Vet Med Assoc* 201:910–916, 1992.

CRYPTOCOCCOSIS

ICD-10 B45.0 pulmonary cryptococcosis; B45.1 cerebral cryptococcosis; B45.2 cutaneous cryptococcosis; B45.3 osseous cryptococcosis; B45.7 disseminated cryptococcosis; B45.8 other forms of cryptococcosis

Synonyms: Torulosis, European blastomycosis, Busse-Buschke's disease.

Etiology: *Cryptococcus neoformans (Saccharomyces neoformans, Torulopsis neoformans, Torula histolytica)*, a saprophytic yeast growing in certain soils. The agent has a spheroid or ovoid shape, is encapsulated, ranges from 4 to 7 microns in diameter, and is gram-positive. It reproduces by means of buds attached by a delicate base to the parent cell. Research in recent years has demonstrated that *C. neoformans* has a sexual form and is a basidiomycete.

Of epidemiological interest is *C. neoforman*'s subdivision into four serotypes (A, B, C, and D) on the basis of capsular polysaccharide antigens. In turn, the serotypes are categorized in two varieties: *C. neoformans* var. *neoformans* (serotypes A and D) and *C. neoformans* var. *gattii* (serotypes B and C). In addition to biochemical, serological, and genetic differences, serotypes A and D are different in their perfect (sexual) state from serotypes B and C. Although a few A and D strains can be conjugated with B and C, their survival is short-lived (Diamond, 1990).

Geographic Distribution: Worldwide. In the Americas the disease has been confirmed in Argentina, Brazil, Canada, Colombia, Mexico, the United States, and Venezuela. Serotype A is prevalent throughout the world. Serotype D is common in some European countries (Denmark, Italy, and Switzerland), but rare in the United States. In contrast, serotypes B and C are more localized and are recognized as disease agents, particularly in southern California, southeastern Oklahoma, and some other areas of the United States, as well as in Asia (Kaplan *et al.*, 1981; Fromtling *et al.*, 1982). In some regions of Australia, a high percentage of isolated strains have the characteristics of the *gattii* strain, as in the case of the indigenous population in the Northern Territory. In one study, 25 of 26 isolates (24 of them from meningitis patients) corresponded to *gattii*. In another study, 21 of 22 strains (95.5%) were also of the *gattii* variety. In South Australia, which has a primarily urban population, 65.2% of 23 strains were classified as *gattii* (Ellis, 1987). Other sites with a high prevalence of *gattii* var. are Brazil (10 of 31 strains) and southern California (30 of 73) (Kwon-Chung and Bennett, 1984). In Argentina, 101 of 105 isolates from 1981–1990 were classified as *C. neoformans* var. *neoformans* and 4 as var. *gattii* (serotype B). These data are similar to those found in the United States (Bava and Negroni, 1992).

Occurrence in Man: Cases are sporadic, with a higher incidence in men than in women. From 1965 to 1997, 1,264 cases of cryptococcosis were documented in the United States. Of 848 cases confirmed between 1973 and 1997, 608 patients had meningitis and 240 had extrameningeal localizations. These data indicate a great increase as compared to earlier periods (Kaufman and Blumer, 1978). There were 85 cases in Malaysia between 1974 and 1980, predominantly among ethnic Chinese (Pathmanathan and Soo-Hoo, 1982). In the United States and Europe, cryptococcosis occurs primarily in patients with immune system defects (especially AIDS) or who are undergoing immunosuppressant treatment. The prevalence of the disease has grown worldwide as the number of AIDS patients has increased. In Argentina, the annual number of cases ranged from four to eight until 1987, began to increase in 1988, and reached 35 cases in 1990. The age group most affected was 20- to 39-year-olds. More men were affected than women, particularly when the underlying disease was AIDS (Bava and Negroni, 1992). It is estimated that the male-female ratio was 3:1. The percentage of AIDS patients who contracted cryptococcosis in Argentina increased from 12.5% in 1990 to 25.9% in 1991. This percentage is similar to the incidence of cryptococcosis in AIDS patients in central Africa and southeast Asia (20% to 35%), but greater than that in Europe and the United States (6% to 10%). In greater Buenos Aires, cryptococcosis is second among the tracer diseases of AIDS, after esophageal candidiasis (Bava *et al.*, 1992). In Malaysia, on the other hand, only 14% of the patients studied had AIDS.

Epidemiologic studies based on the intradermal test indicate that many individuals exposed to the agent show no symptoms of the disease.

Occurrence in Animals: Rare, sporadic cases. Some epizootic outbreaks of mastitis and cryptococcal pneumonia have been described in cattle. The disease has been described in goats, horses, and cats.

The Disease in Man: The large majority of cases are meningitis or meningoencephalitis. This form is preceded by a pulmonary infection, which is often asymptomatic or, if symptomatic, may resolve spontaneously. In most cases of localization in the CNS, pulmonary invasion is not evident (Diamond, 1990). The initial pulmonary infection can resolve spontaneously, give rise to a granulomatous mass ("cryptococcoma"), or disseminate via the bloodstream. The pulmonary form manifests with fever, cough, chest pain, and hemoptysis. Radiography shows single or multiple nodules or large cryptococcomas. The course is usually chronic. When dissemination from the original pulmonary focus occurs, the infection localizes primarily in the meninges, spreading to the brain. The most obvious symptoms of the meningeal form of the disease are headache and visual disturbances. Other symptoms may include confusion, personality changes, agitation, and lethargy. Cryptococcal meningoencephalitis can follow a course lasting for weeks or months and is almost always fatal if not properly treated. The characteristic lesion in the brain is comprised of groups of fungal cysts without inflammation. This lesion can also be found in other sites (Diamond, 1990). Asymptomatic meningitis sometimes occurs when there are other locations and the disease is discovered through lumbar puncture and culture of the cerebrospinal fluid (Liss and Rimland, 1981). The lesion can affect the skin, the mucosa, and the bones, as well as various other organs. Cutaneous infection is characterized by the formation of papules and abscesses and subsequent ulceration.

Man is resistant to *C. neoformans*. There are cryptococcosis patients who show no obvious predisposing factors. However, the fungus is to a large extent an opportunistic pathogenic agent. The number of cases increased significantly with the HIV epidemic. In the United States, cryptococcosis is the fourth potential leading case of death in AIDS patients, after *Pneumocystis carinii*, cytomegaloviruses, and mycobacteria. A retrospective study of AIDS patients was conducted in a hospital in Porto Alegre, Brazil to determine the diseases that could affect the CNS. Between 1985 and 1990, 138 autopsies were performed and all the brains were examined macro- and microscopically. According to the results, 29 (21%) suffered from cerebral toxoplasmosis; 17 (12%), from cryptococcosis; 2 (1%), from tuberculosis; and 1 (0.7%), from candidiasis. In addition, there were cadavers with vascular lesions and gliosis; 5% had encephalopathy due to HIV (Wainstein *et al.*, 1992).

Cryptococcosis often appears in patients weakened by other diseases (reticuloen-dothelial system disorders, particularly Hodgkin's disease) and by corticosteroid treatment. The incubation period is unknown. Pulmonary lesions may precede cerebral lesions by months or years. It is estimated that some 100 deaths per year in the United States are due to cryptococcosis.

Intravenous amphotericin B in doses of 0.4–0.6 mg/kg per day for six weeks can be effective in many cases. Recently, the preferred therapy is a combination of intravenous amphotericin in reduced doses and oral flucytosine. This combination is not indicated for AIDS patients due to the early development of signs of flucytosine poisoning. Fluconazole is useful for preventing relapses after administering amphotericin B (Diamond, 1990; Benenson, 1990).

The Disease in Animals: The disease has been recognized in cattle, horses, sheep, goats, dogs, cats, nonhuman primates, and several species of wild animals (in zoos), but not in birds. Various cases have been described in sheep and goats with pulmonary disease and mastitis. Of four cases described in goats in Western Australia, the pulmonary form predominated in two animals; one had accumulated fluid in the pleural and peritoneal cavities, atelectatic lungs, and dark red plaque in the trachea from which *C. neoformans* was isolated; the fourth animal had an alopecic lesion on the head from which a yellow exudate seeped, which showed *Cryptococcus* spp. upon microscopic examination (Chapman *et al.*, 1990). The disseminated form of the disease is the form most commonly diagnosed in dogs and cats. Of 21 cases in dogs with a clinical history, 13 manifested the meningeal form, 4 the nasal form, and 1 osteoarticular involvement; the remaining animals had lesions in other organs. Six cases described in Australia all had the meningeal form (Sutton, 1981). The primary diagnosis in cats has been a disorder of the central nervous system, with granulomas in the eyes and nasal passages, as well as the cutaneous form. Of 29 cats with cryptococcosis, 24 (83%) had the nasal form and 15 had the cutaneous and subcutaneous form. One cat with a significant involvement of the nasal cavity developed meningoencephalitis and optical neuritis. Antibodies to feline immunodeficiency virus were detected in eight cats. These animals suffered from advanced or disseminated cryptococcosis. *C. neoformans* var. *neoformans* was isolated from 21 cats and *C. neoformans* var. *gattii* was isolated from 6 cats. Treatment with oral fluconazole yielded very good results. All the cats were cured except for one that died four days after treatment began (Malik *et al.*, 1992). Nasal and pulmonary tumors with a myxomatous consistency have been observed in various animal species. Several outbreaks of mastitis have been confirmed in cows, with visible abnormalities in the udder and changes in the milk. A few cases of meningoencephalitic and pulmonary cryptococcosis, cases affecting the frontal sinuses and para-orbital area, and abortions have been described in horses.

Source of Infection and Mode of Transmission: Serotypes A and D (*C. neoformans* var. *neoformans*) are ubiquitous and have been isolated from various environmental sources, such as soil, certain plants, bird feces, raw milk, and fruit juices. The causal agent is found frequently in pigeon roosts and in soil contaminated by pigeon feces. The creatinine in pigeon fecal matter serves as a source of nitrogen for *C. neo-*

formans, favoring its development and prolonging its survival in the soil. Pigeons do not become ill with cryptococcosis.

The environmental source of *C. neoformans* var. *gattii* was unknown until a few years ago. A study conducted in Australia succeeded in isolating var. *gattii* from 35 samples of bark and plant remains accumulated under the foliage of a species of eucalyptus, *Eucalyptus camaldulensis*. Attempts to isolate samples from other eucalyptus species were unsuccessful. *E. camaldulensis* has been exported to various countries in the Americas, Africa, and Asia. The air sample taken from beneath the foliage demonstrated that the presence of the agent in the air coincided with the eucalyptus' blooming season in late spring. These findings would explain the high incidence of *C. neoformans* var. *gattii* among the aborigines in Australia's Northern Territory, where these trees are abundant and the indigenous population lives in close contact with them (Ellis and Pfeiffer, 1990). Man and animals become infected by inhaling dust containing the causal agent. *C. neoformans,* which has no capsule in nature, becomes encapsulated in the lungs, allowing it to resist phagocytosis. Although all researchers agree that the infection is contracted through inhalation, there is still debate regarding the infecting element. Some believe it is the yeast form of the agent while others believe it is the basidiospores of the agent's sexual phase. It has also been pointed out that the yeast form would be too large (4 to 7 microns) to enter the alveoli, while basidiospores measure only about 2 microns (Cohen, 1982).

Role of Animals in the Epidemiology of the Disease: There are no known cases of transmission of the disease from animal to animal, from animal to man, or from man to man, except in the case of a corneal transplant (Beyt and Waldman, 1978).

Diagnosis: Diagnosis can be made through microscopic observation of encapsulated *C. neoformans* in tissues and body fluids, and can be confirmed by culture. The use of culture media to differentiate serotypes A and D from serotypes B and C now facilitates serotyping (Salkind and Hurd, 1982; Kwon-Chung *et al.*, 1982). The direct immunofluorescence test can be used for the same purpose for cultures and for some histological preparations (Kaplan *et al.*, 1981).

As the etiologic agent multiplies in the human host, the capsular polysaccharide of *C. neoformans* neutralizes antibodies. Excess antibodies can be detected in blood and urine, as well as in cerebrospinal fluid in cases in which the central nervous system is affected. Cases that come to receive medical attention are frequently far advanced. Consequently, better results are obtained if the medical examination is directed toward detecting the specific antigen rather than the antibodies. The plate latex agglutination test with particles sensitized by anticryptococcal globulin is used to detect the cryptococcal antigen. The enzyme-linked immunosorbent assay (ELISA) test is also available to detect the capuslar polysaccharide antigen of the etiologic agent. This test is much more sensitive than latex agglutination and permits earlier diagnosis (Scott *et al.*, 1980). In patients with meningoencephalitis, a sample of the cerebrospinal fluid is used for direct microscopic examination and a cell count, another examination with India ink to detect encapsulated fungus cells, and culture in Sabouroud's dextrose agar with incubation at 30°C to 37°C to isolate the fungus. The antigen is sought in serum and cerebrospinal fluid.

In England, 828 HIV-positive patients with fever were examined (in the United Kingdom, 85% of cases occur in immunodeficient individuals, while in the United States, 50% of patients apparently have a normal immune system). Sixty-nine of the

828 patients had meningitis. The cryptococcal antigen detection test was performed using the latex technique for the capsulated polysaccharide antigen. The test was positive in 16 of 17 patients with meningitis and with positive cultures (Nelson *et al.*, 1990).

A study conducted on 20 cats with cryptococcosis and 184 uninfected animals used the latex agglutination test. The latex particles were sensitized with rabbit antibodies to *C. neoformans* to detect the antigen in the cats' serum. The test was positive in 19 of the 20 cats with cryptococcosis and in none of the controls (Medlean *et al.*, 1990). According to some authors, the test has prognostic value in humans, in that a progressive disease is accompanied by a rise in titer, whereas there is generally a decline in the agglutinating titer when there is clinical improvement.

Control: There are no specific measures for preventing the disease. It is important to control underlying diseases and to reduce prolonged treatment with corticosteroids as much as possible.

Controlling the pigeon population might prevent some cases. Human exposure to accumulations of pigeon excrement should be avoided, particularly on windowsills, in roosts, perches, and nests. Removal of pigeon excrement should be preceded by chemical decontamination or by wetting down with water or oil to prevent aerosolization (Benenson, 1990).

Bibliography

Ainsworth, G.C., P.K.C. Austwick. *Fungal Diseases of Animals.* 2nd ed. Farnham Royal, Slough, United Kingdom: Commonwealth Agricultural Bureau; 1973.

Bava, A.J., R. Negroni. Características epidemiológicas de 106 casos de criptococosis diagnosticados en la República Argentina entre 1981–1990. *Rev Inst Med Trop Sao Paulo* 34:335–340, 1992.

Bava, A.J., R. Negroni, A.M. Robles, *et al.* Características epidemiológicas de 71 casos de criptococosis diagnósticos en diferentes centros asistenciales de la ciudad de Buenos Aires y sus alrededores durante 1991. *Infect Microbiol Clin* 4:85–89, 1992.

Benenson, A.S., ed. *Control of Communicable Diseases in Man.* 15th ed. An official report of the American Public Health Association. Washington, D.C.: American Public Health Association; 1990.

Beyt, B.E., Jr., S.R. Waltman. Cryptococcal endophthalmitis after corneal transplantation. *N Engl J Med* 298:825–826, 1978.

Chapman, H.M., W.F. Robinson, J.R. Bolton, J.P. Robertson. *Cryptococcus neoformans* infection in goats. *Aust Vet J* 67:263–265, 1990.

Cohen, J. The pathogenesis of cryptococcosis. *J Infect* 5:109–116, 1982.

Diamond, R.D. *Cryptococcus neoformans. In*: Mandell, G.L., R.G. Douglas, Jr., J.E. Bennett, eds. *Principles and Practice of Infectious Diseases.* 3rd ed. New York: Churchill Livingstone, Inc.; 1990.

Drutz, D.J. The mycoses. *In*: Wyngarden, J.B., L.H. Smith, Jr., eds. *Cecil Textbook of Medicine.* 16th ed. Philadelphia: Saunders; 1982.

Ellis, D.H. *Cryptococcus neoformans* var. *gattii* in Australia. *J Clin Microbiol* 25: 430–431, 1987.

Ellis, D.H., T.J. Pfeiffer. Natural habitat of *Cryptococcus neoformans* var. *gattii. J Clin Microbiol* 28:1642–1644, 1990.

Fromtling, R.A., S. Shadomy, H.J. Shadomy, W.E. Dismukes. Serotypes B/C *Cryptococcus neoformans* isolated from patients in nonendemic areas. *J Clin Microbiol* 16:408–410, 1982.

Gordon, M.A. Current status of serology for diagnosis and prognostic evaluation of opportunistic fungus infections. *In*: Pan American Health Organization. *Proceedings of the Third International Conference on the Mycoses*. Washington, D.C.: PAHO; 1975. (Scientific Publication 304).

Kaplan, W., S.L. Bragg, S. Crane, D.G. Ahearn. Serotyping *Cryptococcus neoformans* by immunofluorescence. *J Clin Microbiol* 14:313–317, 1981.

Kaufman, L., S. Blumer. Cryptococcosis: The awakening giant. *In*: Pan American Health Organization. *Proceedings of the Fourth International Conference on Mycoses: The Black and White Yeasts*. Washington, D.C.: PAHO; 1978. (Scientific Publication 356).

Kwon-Chung, K.J., J.E. Bennett. Epidemiologic differences between the two varieties of *Cryptococcus neoformans*. *Am J Epidemiol* 120:123–130, 1984.

Kwon-Chung, K.J., I. Polacheck, J.E. Bennett. Improved diagnostic medium for separation of *Cryptococcus neoformans* var. *neoformans* (serotypes A and D) and *Cryptococcus neoformans* var. *gattii* (serotypes B and C). *J Clin Microbiol* 15:535–537, 1982.

Liss, H.P., D. Rimland. Asymptomatic cryptococcal meningitis. *Am Rev Resp Dis* 124:88–89, 1981.

Malik, R., D.I. Wigney, D.B. Muir, *et al.* Cryptococcosis in cats: Clinical and mycological assessment of 29 cases and evaluation of treatment using orally administered flucanozole. *J Med Vet Mycol* 30:133–144, 1992.

Medlean, L., M.A. Marks, J. Brown, W.L. Borges. Clinical evaluation of a cryptococcal antigen latex agglutination test for diagnosis of cryptococcosis in cats. *J Am Vet Med Assoc* 196:1470–1473, 1990.

Muchmore, H.G., F.G. Felton, S.B. Salvin, E.R. Rhoades. Ecology and epidemiology of cryptococcosis. *In*: Pan American Health Organization. *Proceedings: International Symposium on Mycoses*. Washington, D.C.: PAHO; 1970. (Scientific Publication 205).

Negroni, P. *Micosis cutáneas y viscerales*. 5.ª ed. Buenos Aires: López; 1972.

Nelson, M.R., M. Bower, D. Smith, *et al.* The value of serum cryptococcal antigen in the diagnosis of cryptococcal infection in patients infected with the human immunodeficiency virus. *J Infect* 21:175–181, 1990.

Pathmanathan, R., T.S. Soo-Hoo. Cryptococcosis in the University Hospital Kuala Lumpur and review of published cases. *Trans Roy Soc Trop Med Hyg* 76:21–24, 1982.

Salkind, I.F., N.J. Hurd. New medium for differentiation of *Cryptococcus neoformans* serotype pairs. *J Clin Microbiol* 15:169–171, 1982.

Scott, E.N., H.G. Muchmore, F.G. Felton. Comparison of enzyme immunoassay and latex agglutination methods for detection of *Cryptococcus neoformans* antigen. *Am J Clin Pathol* 73:790–794, 1980.

Sutton, R.H. Cryptococcosis in dogs: A report on 6 cases. *Aust Vet J* 57:558–564, 1981.

Wainstein, M.V., L. Ferreira, L. Wolfenbuttel, *et al.* Achados neuropatológicos na síndrome da imunodeficiência adquirida (SIDA): revisão de 138 casos. *Rev Soc Brasil Med Trop* 25:95–99, 1992.

DERMATOPHYTOSIS

ICD-10 B35

Synonyms: Tinea, dermatomycosis, ringworm.

Etiology: Several species of *Microsporum* and *Trichophyton* and the species *Epidermophyton floccosum*. Ecologically and epidemiologically, three groups of species are distinguished according to the reservoir: anthropophilic, zoophilic, and geophilic. This discussion will consider only zoophilic species transmissible to man.

Dermatophytes were formerly considered imperfect fungi, *Fungi imperfecti* or *Deuteromycotyna*. However, several species have been shown to reproduce sexually. The most important zoophilic species are *Microsporum canis* (whose perfect state received the name *Nannizzia otae*), *Trichophyton mentagrophytes (Arthroderma benhamiae)*, and *T. verrucosum*. Species of more limited interest are *M. equinum, T. equinum, M. gallinae, M. nanum, M. persicolor*, and *T. simii*. The species *T. mentagrophytes* is subdivided into two varieties: *T. mentagrophytes* var. *erinacei* and var. *quinckeanum*.

The infecting element is the arthrospore (an asexual spore formed in the hyphae and released when these break down) of the parasitic phases. Conidia that form in organic material substrates (where the fungus may form sexual and asexual spores) may also be infective.

A notable characteristic is that the hyphae and spores are highly resistant in desquamated epithelium, where they may remain viable for several months or even years if they don't dry up.

Geographic Distribution: Among the zoophilic species, *M. canis, T. verrucosum, T. equinum*, and *T. mentagrophytes* are distributed worldwide. *T. mentagrophytes* var. *erinacei* has limited distribution (France, Great Britain, Italy, and New Zealand) and *T. simii* is limited to Asia. The geographic distribution of these fungi depends on the dispersion of the host animals. The host hedgehog of *T. mentagrophytes* var. *erinacei* exists only in Europe and in New Zealand, where it was introduced from Europe. The abundance or rarity of a dermatophyte species depends largely on the rural or urban habitat and the relationship between man and animals. *M. canis* is a fungus that occurs primarily in urban areas where its natural hosts, the dog and cat, are abundant and in close contact with humans. In contrast, *T. verrucosum* is found in rural areas, particularly among stabled cattle, i.e., generally in areas with cold or temperate climates.

Occurrence in Man: Dermatophytic infections are common, but their exact prevalence is unknown. The disease is not notifiable and, moreover, many people with minor infections do not see a doctor. Most of the data come from dermatologists, mycology laboratories, and epidemiologic investigations. Economically advanced countries have experienced a marked reduction in some species of anthropophilic dermatophytes. This is true of *M. audouinii*, which causes epidemic outbreaks of tinea capitis. In such countries, zoophilic dermatophytes are now much more significant. A study conducted in England on 23 families to evaluate the prevalence of the infection among family members who were in contact with clinically or sub-clinically infected young cats found that 46 (50%) out of 92 individuals contracted the infection due to

M. canis. The percentage of adults infected was 44.2% and that of children and young people was 80% (12 out of 15) (Pepin and Oxenham, 1986). A retrospective study of 1,717 Ministry of Agriculture veterinarians in the United Kingdom found that dermatophytosis was the most common zoonosis, with a prevalence of 24% (Constable and Herington, cited by Pepin and Oxenham, 1986). In northeast Madrid (Spain), the annual incidence of dermatophytosis was found to be 84 cases per 10,000 inhabitants, and the most frequent agents in 135 patients were *Epidermophyton floccosum*, an anthropophilic dermatophyte (35.5%), *Microsporum canis* (26.6%), and *Trichophyton mentagrophytes* (20.7%) (Cuadros *et al.*, 1990). A retrospective study conducted in Argentina on 1,225 samples of superficial mycoses (95% adult patients and 5% children) indicated that 60% were dermatophytes. The most common agent was *T. rubrum* (66.6%), followed by *T. mentagrophytes* (20%), *M. canis* (8%), and others (Canteros *et al.*, 1993). In Peru, it is likely that zoophilic species are responsible for 21% of human dermatomycoses (Gómez Pando and Matos Díaz, 1982). A study conducted in India found that *T. verrucosum* and *T. mentagrophytes* var. *mentagrophytes* were responsible for 56 (38.6%) of 145 human isolates and for 50 (53.8%) of the 93 human cases in the rural area (Chatterjee *et al.*, 1980).

Many human cases originated in Hungary, in a nursery of 5,500 rabbits. Over the course of six months, all the rabbits were infected by *T. mentagrophytes* var. *mentagrophytes* (var. *granulosum*) and 38 human cases appeared among workers and their families (Szili and Kohalmi, 1983).

Occurrence in Animals: In recent years, epidemiologic studies have demonstrated that dermatophytic infection in animals is very common. Tinea occurs more frequently among stabled animals than those kept in open pastures throughout the year.

Infection by *M. canis* is very common in cats and dogs and is often asymptomatic. In Lima (Peru) and its environs, *M. canis* was found in 12 (15%) of 79 cats without apparent lesions examined and *T. mentagrophytes* in 8 (10%). *M. canis* was isolated from 17 (3.9%) of 432 samples from dogs, and *T. mentagrophytes* from 22 (5%) (Gómez Pando and Matos Díaz, 1982). In the United Kingdom, in 1,368 dermatophytes isolated between 1956 and 1991, *Microsporum canis* was diagnosed in 92% of infected cats and in 65% of dogs (Sparkes *et al.*, 1993). Long-haired cats and dogs under one year of age were most affected (Sparkes *et al.*, 1993).

The cat is the most common host and reservoir of *M. canis.* Some studies have found infection in between 6.5% and 88% or more of the cats examined. These studies were conducted in areas where the cats were in contact with other cats. A completely different picture was obtained in a study conducted at the University of Wisconsin (USA). Fifteen genera of fungi, 13 of which were considered saprophytes, were isolated from the skin of 172 cats that lived alone with their owners. *T. rubrum*, considered an anthropophilic dermatophyte, was isolated from 14 cats; *T. gypseum* and *M. vanbreuseghemii*, both geophilic, were isolated from 1 cat each; but *M. canis* was isolated from none. *T. rubrum* is a common agent in human dermatophytosis, but the role that cats might play in its transmission to man is unknown (Moriello and De Boer, 1991).

The Disease in Man: Dermatophytosis, or tinea, is a superficial infection of the keratinized parts of the body (skin, hair, and nails). As a general rule, zoophilic and geophilic dermatophytes produce more acute inflammatory lesions than the anthropophilic species, which are parasites better adapted to man. The *Microsporum* species cause most cases of tinea capitis and tinea corporis, but are rarely responsible for infection of the nails (onychomycosis) or skin folds (intertrigo). However, the *Trichophyton* species can affect the skin in any part of the body.

There are two varieties of *T. mentagrophytes*: an anthropophilic variety (var. *interdigitale*) that is relatively nonvirulent in humans and localizes in the feet (athlete's foot), and a zoophilic variety (morphologically granular) that causes a very inflammatory dermatophytosis on different areas of the human body. The zoophilic variety is usually found in rodents, cats, dogs, and other animals. Transmission to man is probably caused by contamination of his habitat by hair from infected animals. Several epidemic outbreaks of inflammatory dermatophytoses on different parts of the body among the U.S. troops in Vietnam were caused by *T. mentagrophytes* var. *mentagrophytes* (var. *granulosum*). About one-fourth of the rats trapped in the vicinity of military camps were infected with strains of the same variety of fungus. Among the inhabitants of the region, the disease was seen only in children, suggesting that adults were probably immunized by infections contracted during childhood.

Currently, *M. canis* is one of the principal etiologic agents of tinea and, in many countries, has displaced the anthropophilic species *M. audouinii* as the cause of tinea capitis. In South America, *M. canis* is the most common of the microspora.

The incubation period of the disease is one to two weeks. Tinea of the scalp is most frequent among those aged 4 to 11 years and its incidence is higher among males. The disease begins with a small papule, the hair becomes brittle, and the infection spreads peripherally, leaving scaly, bald patches. Suppurative lesions (kerions) are frequent when the fungus is of animal origin. Tinea caused by *M. canis* heals spontaneously during puberty.

Suppurative tinea barbae, which affects rural populations, is caused by *T. mentagrophytes* of animal origin. However, in the United States dry tinea barbae is caused by *T. mentagrophytes* of human origin and by *T. rubrum* (Silva-Hunter *et al.*, 1981).

Tinea corporis is characterized by flat lesions that tend to be annular. The borders are reddish and may be raised, with microvesicles or scales.

Tinea corporis in children is usually an extension of tinea capitis to the face and is caused by *M. canis* or *M. audouinii*. Active lesions may also appear on the wrists and neck of mothers or young adults who have contact with the infected child. Tinea corporis in adults, occurring primarily on the limbs and torso, is chronic in nature and usually is caused by the anthropophilic dermatophyte *T. rubrum* (Silva-Hunter *et al.*, 1981).

Tinea pedis (athlete's foot), the incidence of which is increasing worldwide, is caused by anthropophilic species of *Trychophyton* and, to a lesser extent, by *Epidermophyton floccosum* (also anthropophilic).

In AIDS patients, mycosis caused by *T. mentagrophytes* and *M. canis* can be cutaneous and disseminated (Lowinger-Seoane *et al.*, 1992). AIDS patients may suffer from extensive dermatophytosis caused by a fungus as rare in humans as *M. gallinae*, a zoophilic dermatophyte; there are only seven known cases, all of them localized (del Palacio *et al.*, 1992).

The recommended treatment is topical application of antimycotics. The azoles (miconazole, clotrimazole, econazole, bifonazole, oxiconazole, tioconazaole, and others) are used most frequently. These antimycotics produce good results in all forms of dermal tinea caused by zoophilic dermatophytes.

Topical treatment should continue for two to four weeks. Naftifine is another powerful antimycotic (Hay, 1990).

The Disease in Animals: The most important species considered reservoirs of dermatophytes transmissible to humans are cats, dogs, cattle, horses, and rodents.

CATS AND DOGS: The most important etiologic agent in these animals is *M. canis*. This dermatophyte species is very well adapted to cats and approximately 90% of infected animals manifest no apparent lesions. When lesions do occur, they appear primarily on the face and paws.

Lesions are frequent and apparent in dogs and may appear on any part of the body in the form of tinea circinata (ringworm).

Dogs and cats may also be infected by other dermatophytes, particularly *T. mentagrophytes*.

CATTLE: The principal etiologic agent of tinea in cattle is *T. verrucosum* (*T. faviforme, T. ochraceum, T. album,* and *T. discoides*). The disease is more common in countries where animals are kept in stables during winter, and its incidence is higher in calves than in adults. Lesions may be as small as 1 cm in diameter or may cover extensive areas; they are most frequently located on the face and neck, but lesions are also found with some frequency on other parts of the body, such as the flanks and legs. The lesion is initially characterized by grayish white, dry areas with a few brittle hairs. The lesion then thickens and resembles a light brown scab. The scab falls off, leaving an alopecic area. The condition clears up spontaneously within two to four months.

HORSES: Dermatophytosis in horses is caused by *T. equinum* and *M. equinum*; the latter is rare in the Americas. Lesions are usually found in areas where the harness causes friction. They are dry, bald, covered with scales, and the skin is thickened. Colts are the most susceptible. Infections caused by *Trichophyton equinum* are usually more severe, with pruritus and exudative lesions causing the hair to stick together in clumps. When they drop off, they leave alopecic areas. Infections due to *M. equinum* cause less serious lesions with small scaly areas with brittle hairs.

RODENTS AND LAGOMORPHS: Tinea favus of mice, caused by *T. mentagrophytes* var. *quinckeanum*, is widely distributed throughout the world and is transmissible to domestic animals and man. The lesion is white and scabby and localized on the head and trunk. *T. mentagrophytes* (var. *mentagrophytes*) is another dermatophyte common to rodents. Laboratory mice and guinea pigs are mostly infected by *T. mentagrophytes*, and may not have apparent lesions; the agent's presence is often detected when humans contract the infection. It is also transmissible to dogs.

Dermatophytosis in rabbits is also caused by *T. mentagrophytes* and usually occurs in animals that have recently been weaned. Scabby areas of alopecia are seen clinically around the eyes and nose. Secondary lesions appear on the feet. This disease is self-limiting.

SHEEP AND GOATS: Tinea is rare in these species. The lesions localize on the head and face. The most frequent agent is *T. verrucosum*. The lesions are limited to areas of the head covered by hair; they are circular, balding, and have thick scabs. Two outbreaks of dermatophytosis caused by *M. canis* were described in Australia. In the first outbreak, transmission was attributed to cats and to the use of contaminated shearing implements. In the second, with 20% of 90 sheep infected, it was not possible to determine how the infection had been introduced, but its spread throughout the establishment was undoubtedly due to shearing implements and close contact among the animals immediately after being sheared (Jackson *et al.*, 1991).

SWINE: The most common agent of swine tinea is *M. nanum*. Infection has been confirmed in Australia, Canada, Cuba, Kenya, Mexico, New Guinea, New Zealand, and the United States. This dermatophyte was isolated in only a few human cases. The lesion is characterized by a wrinkled area covered by a thin, brown scab that detaches easily. *M. nanum* lives as a soil saprophyte in areas where swine are raised and is classified as geophilic.

FOWL: Tinea favus in hens occurs sporadically throughout the world and is rarely transmitted to man. Its agent is *T. gallinae*.

Source of Infection and Mode of Transmission: The natural reservoirs of zoophilic dermatophytes are animals. Transmission to man occurs through contact with an infected animal (either sick or a carrier) or indirectly through spores contained in the hair and dermal scales shed by the animal. Dermatophytes remain viable in shed epithelium for several months or even years. The same animal can infect several people within a family, but a zoophilic dermatophyte does not usually spread from person to person and, unlike the anthropophilic dermatophytes, does not cause epidemic tinea. Cases of human-to-human transmission of *M. canis* have been observed, but the agent loses its infectiveness for man after a few intermediaries (Padhye, 1980). A nosocomial infection was described in a nursery for newborns. Although tinea of the scalp is common among children, it is rarely found in newborns. The common source of the infection turned out to be a nurse who had an indolent infection due to *M. canis* (Snider *et al.*, 1993). *T. verrucosum*, whose principal reservoir is cattle, is found in infections in rural populations. A study conducted in Switzerland found that 14% of those working with infected cattle contracted dermatophytosis caused by *T. verrucosum* (Haub, as reported to Gudding *et al.*, 1991). This mycosis also has economic consequences, in that skins from the infected animal depreciate in value. It is a reportable disease in Norway. In contrast, *M. canis* is transmitted by cats and dogs to urban and rural populations. The cat is considered the principal source of infection for humans due to the custom of picking up and petting a cat, as well as to its high rate of infection. Cats can also host the anthropophilic dermatophyte, *T. rubrum*, in their hair, but it has not been demonstrated that they can transmit it to man. Infection due to *T. mentagrophytes* var. *mentagrophytes* (var. *granulosum*) and *T. mentagrophytes* var. *quinckeanum* is indirectly transmitted from rodents to man via residues of shed epithelium in the environment. Cats and dogs can also become infected by these dermatophytes in the same way or by direct contact when they hunt rodents and can, in turn, transmit the infection to man.

Animal-to-animal transmission occurs in the same ways. Crowding and reduced organic resistance influence the incidence of infection.

Role of Animals in the Epidemiology of the Disease: Animals are the reservoir of zoophilic dermatophytes and the source of infection for man. As in other zoonoses, human-to-human transmission is rare. Transmission of anthropophilic dermatophytes from humans to animals is also rare.

The dermatophyte *M. gypseum* is the causal agent of sporadic cases of tinea in humans and animals; its reservoir is the soil (geophilic).

Diagnosis: Clinical diagnosis can be confirmed by the following methods: a) microscopic observation of hair and scales from lesions; this method can provide a diagnosis at the genus level, since the spores surround the hair shaft in an irregular mosaic when infection is due to *Microsporum* and are arranged in chains when infection is due to *Trichophyton*; b) the use of Wood's light (filtered ultraviolet light), under which hair infected by many species of *Microsporum* exhibits a bright blue-green fluorescence; c) isolation in culture media, the only method that permits identification of the species.

Control: Prevention of human dermatophytoses caused by zoophilic species should be based on controlling the infection in animals, although this is difficult to accomplish. Avoiding contact with animals that are obviously sick can prevent a certain percentage of human cases. These animals should be isolated and treated with topical antimycotics or griseofulvin administered orally. Remains of hair and scales should be burned and rooms, stables, and all utensils should be disinfected. Apparently healthy cats can be examined with Wood's light. Controlling the rodent population is a useful measure.

In cold climates where animals are stabled over long periods of time, dermatophytoses can be a problem in cattle and horses. Man and animals respond to infection with a humoral and cellular immunity, as has been demonstrated by experiments as well as by the observation that animals once infected are protected against reinfection. Two vaccines were developed in the former Soviet Union: one for cattle, made from an attenuated strain of *T. verrucosum*, and another for horses, made from *T. equinum*. Both vaccines yielded satisfactory results in preventing dermatophytoses. The vaccine was used in Norway in 200,000 cattle with very good results (Aamodt *et al.*, 1982). An eradication program was established in Gausdal, Norway; vaccination was required for all cattle for a period of six years, followed by voluntary vaccination thereafter. The prevalence of infected herds was 70% and eradication was achieved in 1987. A live attenuated vaccine was used (two doses with an interval of 14 days) along with disinfection of stables, isolation of infected animals, and other hygiene methods (Gudding *et al.*, 1991).

Bibliography

Aamodt, O., B. Naess, O. Sandvik. Vaccination of Norwegian cattle against ringworm. *Zbl Vet Med B* 29:451–456, 1982.

Ainsworth, G.C., P.K.C. Austwick. *Fungal Diseases of Animals*. 2nd ed. Farnham Royal, Slough, United Kingdom: Commonwealth Agricultural Bureau; 1973.

Allen, A.M., D. Taplin. Epidemiology of cutaneous mycoses in the tropics and subtropics: Newer concepts. *In*: Pan American Health Organization. *Proceedings of the Third International Conference on the Mycoses*. Washington, D.C.: PAHO; 1975. (Scientific Publication 304).

Benenson, A.S., ed. *Control of Communicable Diseases in Man*. 15th ed. An official report of the American Public Health Association. Washington, D.C.: American Public Health Association; 1990.

Canteros, C.E., G.O. Davel, W. Vivot, S. D'Amico. Incidencia de los distintos agentes etiológicos de micosis superficiales. *Rev Argent Microbiol* 25:129–135, 1993.

Chatterjee, A., D. Chattopadhyay, D. Bhattacharya, A.K. Dutta, D.N. Sen Gupta. Some epidemiological aspects of zoophilic dermatophytosis. *Int J Zoonoses* 7:19–33, 1980.

Chmel, L. Epidemiological aspects of zoophilic dermatophytes. *In*: Chmel, L., ed. *Recent Advances in Human and Animal Mycology*. Bratislava: Slovak Academy of Sciences; 1967.

Cuadros, J.A., J. García, J.I. Alos, R. González-Palacios. Dermatofitosis en un medio urbano: un estudio prospectivo de 135 casos. *Enferm Infecc Microbiol Clin* 8:429–433, 1990.

del Palacio, A., M. Pereiro-Miguens, C. Gimeno, *et al*. Widespread dermatophytosis due to *Microsporum* (*Trichophyton*) *gallinae* in a patient with AIDS: A case report from pain. *Clin Exp Dermatol* 17:449–453, 1992.

Emmons, C.W. Mycoses of animals. *Adv Vet Sci* 2:47–63, 1955.

English, M.P. The epidemiology of animal ringworm in man. *Br J Dermatol* 86(Suppl)8:78–87, 1972.

Gentles, J.C. Ringworm. *In*: Graham-Jones, O., ed. *Some Diseases of Animals Communicable to Man in Britain*. Oxford: Pergamon Press; 1968.

Georg, L.K. *Animal Ringworm in Public Health, Diagnosis and Nature*. Atlanta, Georgia: U.S. Centers for Disease Control and Prevention; 1960. (Public Health Service Publication 727).

Gómez Pando, V., J. Matos Díaz. Dermatofitos: aspectos epidemiológicos. *Bol Inf Col Med Vet Peru* 17:16–19, 1982.

Gudding, R., B. Naess, O. Aamodt. Immunisation against ringworm in cattle. *Vet Rec* 128:84–85, 1991.

Hay, R.J. Dermatophytosis and other superficial mycoses. *In*: Mandell, G.L., R.G. Douglas, Jr., J.E. Bennett, eds. *Principles and Practice of Infectious Diseases*. 3rd ed. New York: Churchill Livingstone Inc.; 1990.

Jackson, R.B., B.F. Peel, C. Donaldson-Wood. Endemic *Microsporum canis* infection in a sheep flock. *Aust Vet J* 68:122, 1991.

Lowinger-Seoane, M., J.M. Torres-Rodríguez, N. Madrenys-Brunet, *et al*. Extensive dermatophytosis caused by *Trichophyton mentagrophytes* and *Microsporum canis* in a patient with AIDS. *Mycopathologia* 120:143–146, 1992.

Moriello, K.A., D.J. De Boer. Fungal flora of the coat of pet cats. *Am J Vet Res* 52:602–606, 1991.

Negroni, P. *Micosis cutáneas y viscerales*. 5.ª ed. Buenos Aires: López; 1972.

Padhye, A.A. Cutaneous mycoses. *In*: Stoenner, J., W. Kaplan, M. Torten, eds. Section A, Vol 2: *CRC Handbook Series in Zoonoses*. Boca Raton: CRC Press; 1980.

Pepin, G.C., P.K.C. Austwick. Skin diseases of domestic animals. II. Skin disease, mycological origin. *Vet Rec* 82:208–214, 1968.

Pepin, G.A., M. Oxenham. Zoonotic dermatophytosis (ringworm) [letter]. *Vet Rec* 118:110–111, 1986.

Raubitscheck, F. Fungal diseases. *In*: Van der Hoeden, J., ed. *Zoonoses*. Amsterdam: Elsevier; 1964.

Rebell, G., D. Taplin. *Dermatophytes: Their Recognition and Identification*. Miami: University of Miami Press; 1970.

Sarkisov, A.K. New methods of control of dermatomycoses common to animals and man. *In*: Lysenko, A., ed. Vol 2: *Zoonoses Control*. Moscow: Centre of International Projects; 1982.

Silva-Hunter, M., I. Weitzman, S.A. Rosenthal. Cutaneous mycoses (dermatomycoses). *In*: Balows, A., W.J. Hausler, Jr., eds. *Diagnostic Procedures for Bacterial, Mycotic and Parasitic Infections*. 6th ed. Washington, D.C.: American Public Health Association; 1981.

Smith, J.M.B. Superficial and cutaneous mycoses. *In*: Hubbert, W.T., W.F. McCulloch, P.R. Schnurrenberger, eds. *Diseases Transmitted from Animals to Man*. 6th ed. Springfield: Thomas; 1975.

Snider, R., S. Landers, M.L. Levy. The ringworm riddle: An outbreak of *Microsporum canis* in the nursery. *Pediatr Infect Dis J* 12:145–148, 1993.

Sparkes, A.H., T.J. Gruffyd-Jones, S.E. Shaw, *et al*. Epidemiological and diagnostic features of canine and feline dermatophytosis in the United Kingdom from 1956 to 1991. *Vet Rec* 133:57–61, 1993.

Szili, M., I. Kohalmi. Endemic *Trichophyton mentagrophytes* infection of rabbit origin. *Mykosen* 24:412–420, 1981. *Abst Rev Med Vet* 64:65, 1983.

HISTOPLASMOSIS

ICD-10 B39.0 acute pulmonary histoplasmosis capsulati; B39.1 chronic pulmonary histoplasmosis capsulati; B39.3 disseminated histoplasmosis capsulati; B39.5 Histoplasma duboisii

Synonyms: Reticuloendothelial cytomycosis, cavern disease, Darling's disease.

Etiology: *Histoplasma capsulatum*, a dimorphic fungus that has a yeast form in the parasitic phase and develops a filamentous mycelium in the saprophytic phase, producing macroconidia and microconidia. The yeast form may also be grown in the laboratory by culturing the fungus in an enriched medium at 37°C. The perfect (or sexual) state of the fungus is also known and has been given the name *Emmonsiela capsulata*.

There are two known varieties of the agent: *H. capsulatum* var. *capsulatum* and *H. capsulatum* var. *duboisii*. They are indistinguishable in the mycelial phase but in infected tissue the yeast-form cells of var. *duboisii* are much larger (7–15 microns) than those of var. *capsulatum* (2–5 microns). The tissue reactions they produce are also different. In regions in which the two varieties of the fungus coexist, the use of monoclonal antibodies in the ELISA or Western blot tests has been suggested for differentiating them in the yeast phase (Hamilton *et al.*, 1990).

Geographic Distribution: Distribution of var. *capsulatum* is worldwide and more abundant in the Americas than other continents. Autochthonous human cases are rare in Europe and Asia. The var. *duboisii* is known only in Africa between 20° S and 20° N (there are known cases in Madagascar) (Coulanges, 1989), where the other variety is known to exist as well. Distribution of the fungus in the soil is not uniform, as some regions are more contaminated than others and microfoci exist where the agent is highly concentrated. The assumption is that endemic areas would be determined by the number of microfoci. As for the *duboisii* variety, efforts to determine its habitat in the environment have been unsuccessful.

Occurrence in Man: Judging from the results of the histoplasmin intradermal test, the rate of infection is very high in endemic areas. It has been estimated that in the United States, where the infection is concentrated in the Missouri, Ohio, and Mississippi river basins, 30 million inhabitants have been infected by *Histoplasma* and some half million people become infected each year (Selby, 1975). The disease appears sporadically or in epidemic outbreaks. Isolated cases frequently elude diagnosis. There was an outbreak in 1980 with 138 cases of acute pulmonary disease among workers in a lime quarry in northern Michigan, an area not considered endemic (Waldman et al., 1983). Another outbreak occurred in 1978–1979 at the Indianapolis campus of Indiana University, affecting 435 people. Again in 1980–1981, an outbreak in an area close to the same university affected 51 people (Schlech et al., 1983). Histoplasmosis is considered the most common systemic mycotic infection in the United States (Loyd et al., 1990). There are also endemic regions in Latin America. Although prevalence varies from region to region, it has been claimed that the entire population of Latin America lives within or near areas where the infection can be contracted (Borelli, 1970). In Mexico, epidemic outbreaks or isolated cases of the disease have been recorded in all but two states. There was a study of 11 outbreaks affecting 75 people in 1979, with mortality at 5.3%, and 12 outbreaks affecting 68 people in 1980. Most of the cases occurred in people who for occupational, educational, or recreational reasons had visited caves, abandoned mines, and tunnels in which bat droppings had accumulated. More than 2,000 large mines have had to be abandoned because of the presence of *H. capsulatum* due to large bat colonies (OPS, 1981). There are also endemic areas in Guatemala, Peru, and Venezuela (Ajello and Kaplan, 1980). In Cuba, three outbreaks, one of which affected 521 people, occurred between 1962 and 1963. In 1978 there was an outbreak among students who visited a cave in the province of Havana; more recently, in a cave in the city of Morón, seven of eight spelunkers contracted the disease (González Menocal et al., 1990).

Although the infection is common, the clinical disease is much less so. Radiography revealed pulmonary calcifications in a high percentage (about 25%) of people reacting to histoplasmin. Approximately 90% of those who have a positive reaction to the histoplasmin hypersensitivity skin test are clinically normal.

In Africa, there are some 200 known cases of histoplasmosis due to the *duboisii* variety (Coulanges, 1989).

Occurrence in Animals: Many species of domestic and wild mammals are susceptible to the infection. Surveys using the histoplasmin test have shown that infection is frequent in cattle, sheep, and horses in endemic areas. Dogs are the animal species in which the infection appears most frequently with clinical symptoms. Of 14,000 dogs admitted to the University of Ohio clinic (USA) over the course of four years, histoplasmosis was diagnosed in 62 (0.44%) (Cole et al., 1953).

The Disease in Man: When conidia are inhaled, they can lodge in the bronchioles and alveoli. After a few days, they germinate and produce yeasts that are phagocytized by macrophages where they proliferate. The macrophages move toward the mediastinal lymph nodes and the spleen. When immunity develops, the macrophages acquire the ability to destroy the phagocytized yeasts, and the infiltrates in the nodes and other infection sites disappear (Loyd et al., 1990). Most infections occur asymptomatically. The development of the disease depends on the number of conidia inhaled and on the individual's cellular immunity. The incubation period lasts from 5 to 18 days. There are essentially three clinical forms of the disease: acute pulmonary, chronic cavitary pulmonary, and disseminated. The acute pulmonary form is the most frequent and resembles influenza with febrile symptoms that may last from one day to several weeks. A high percentage of patients also experience cough and chest pain. In most patients, chest radiographs show no changes, but in other cases small infiltrates and an increase in the hilar and mediastinal nodes can be seen. Erythema nodosum or multiforme, diffuse eruption, and arthralgia may be present. This form of the disease often goes unnoticed. In mild cases, recovery occurs without treatment, with or without pulmonary calcification. The chronic form of the disease occurs most frequently in people over the age of 40, with a high prevalence among males, and almost always with a preexisting pulmonary disease (particularly emphysema). Its clinical form resembles pulmonary tuberculosis, with cavitation. The course may vary from months to years and cure may be spontaneous. The disseminated form of the disease is the most serious and is seen primarily in the very young or elderly, where it can take an acute or chronic course. The acute course occurs primarily among nursing babies (immature immunity) and small children and is characterized by different degrees of hepatosplenomegaly, fever, and prostration. It is often confused with miliary tuberculosis and is highly fatal if the patient is not treated. Leukopenia, thrombocytopenia, and anemia are frequent. The agent can be isolated from blood and bone marrow. Between 1934 and 1988, the medical literature recorded only 73 pediatric cases of disseminated histoplasmosis (Miranda Novales et al., 1993). The symptomatology in the chronic disseminated form depends on the localization of the fungus (pneumonia, hepatitis, endocarditis, etc.). There is frequently ulceration of the mucosa and hepatosplenomegaly in these cases. It usually occurs in adults, who may survive for many years, but it can be fatal if the patient is not treated.

Disseminated histoplasmosis occurs in immunodeficient patients, including patients with AIDS. It is sometimes the first manifestation of the syndrome and in some endemic areas it is the most common infection in AIDS (Johnson et al., 1988). The forms of the disease and their symptoms are very varied. The most frequent clinical symptoms in 27 patients (23 men and 4 women) were fever, weight loss, anemia, cutaneous lesions, micronodules in the lungs, hepatosplenomegaly, and adenomegaly (Negroni et al., 1992). Some cases follow a fulminant course with respiratory insufficiency; other cases involve encephalopathy (AIDS dementia), gastrointestinal histoplasmosis with intestinal perforation, and cutaneous histoplasmosis with papules on the limbs, face, and torso.

Fifty radiographs of AIDS patients suffering from disseminated histoplasmosis indicated no changes in 27 patients and different abnormalities (nodular opacities and irregular or linear opacities) in 23 patients. Radiographic results in these patients were varied and nonspecific (Conces et al., 1993).

In the United States, an annual average of only 68 deaths due to histoplasmosis was recorded for 1952–1963, despite the high prevalence of the disease in endemic areas. This confirms that the disease is usually benign.

In African histoplasmosis caused by var. duboisii, lesions occur most frequently on the skin, in subcutaneous tissue, and bones. Skin granulomas appear as nodules or ulcerous or eczematous lesions. Abscesses can be observed in subcutaneous tissue. Isolated or multiple lesions are found in osseous histoplasmosis, sometimes asymptomatically (Manson-Bahr and Apted, 1982). When the disease is progressive and severe, giant cell granulomas may form in many internal organs.

Treatment of acute pulmonary histoplasmosis is justified only in severe and prolonged cases. Short-term treatment with intravenous amphotericin B for three or four weeks is generally sufficient. Patients with disseminated histoplasmosis should usually be treated for a longer period with intravenous amphotericin B or oral ketoconazole (Loyd et al., 1990).

Twenty-seven AIDS patients with disseminated histoplasmosis were given oral itraconazole (200 mg per day to 24 patients and 400 mg per day to 3 patients) for six months. Patients who were considered cured continued to take 100 mg per day. A total of 23 patients responded well to the treatment, three showed questionable results, and one had a negative result (Negroni *et al.*, 1992). Forty-two patients with AIDS and disseminated histoplasmosis who successfully completed treatment with amphotericin B for 4 to 12 weeks (15 mg/kg of body weight) were given itraconazole (200 mg twice a day) to prevent relapses, with satisfactory results (Wheat *et al.*, 1993).

The Disease in Animals: Dogs manifest clinical symptoms most often but, as in man, most infections are asymptomatic. The primary respiratory form of the disease almost always heals by encapsulation and calcification. In disseminated cases, the dogs lose weight and have persistent diarrhea, anorexia, and chronic cough; hepatosplenomegaly and lymphadenopathy may also be observed.

Cats follow dogs in terms of frequency of clinical histoplasmosis. The symptoms of feline disseminated histoplasmosis are anemia, weight loss, lethargy, fever, and anorexia. In chest radiographs, the lungs of 7 of 12 cats indicated anomalies. Kittens one year of age or younger were most affected (Clinkenbeard *et al.*, 1987).

H. capsulatum has also been isolated from the intestinal contents and various organs of bats. High rates of reactors have been found in different domesticated species (cattle, horses, sheep) in endemic areas and the agent has been isolated from the lymph nodes of dogs and cats as well as from a wild rodent (*Proechimys guyanensis*) and a sloth in Brazil. Birds are not susceptible to histoplasmosis, perhaps because their high body temperature does not allow the fungus to develop.

Source of Infection and Mode of Transmission: The reservoir of the agent is the soil, where it lives as a saprophyte. Its distribution in the soil is not uniform and depends on various factors such as humidity, temperature, and others yet to be determined. Microfoci that have led to sporadic cases and epidemic outbreaks have usually been associated with soils in which excreta from certain species of bird or bats have accumulated over some time. These excreta apparently allow the fungus to compete with other microorganisms in the soil, ensuring its survival. In contrast to birds, which are not infected by *H. capsulatum* and whose role in the epidemiology is limited to the enabling function of their excreta, certain bat species, particularly species that live in colonies, do become infected and eliminate the fungus in their droppings, thus contributing to its dissemination. Humans frequently become infected when they visit caves, tunnels, and abandoned mines and other places where there are large populations of bats and much accumulated guano. Most infections in Mexico were due to exposure to bat droppings; cases occurred among explorers, tourists, spelunkers, geologists, biologists, and others entering such places for work or study.

Man and animals acquire the infection from the same source (the soil) through inhalation. Microconidia of the fungus are the infecting element. The infection usually starts when natural foci are disturbed by activities that scatter the etiologic agent in the air, such as bulldozing, cleaning or demolishing rural structures (especially henhouses), and visits to caves inhabited by bats.

Histoplasmosis occurs predominantly in rural areas, but outbreaks have also occurred among urban dwellers, particularly construction workers. This was the case in outbreaks on the Indianapolis campus of Indiana University, where building demolition and excavation led to many human cases (see the section on occurrence in man).

In dogs, the disease appears more frequently in working and sporting breeds.

Role of Animals in the Epidemiology of the Disease: Both man and animals are accidental hosts of the etiologic agent and do not play a role in maintaining or transmitting the infection. Only certain bat species are thought to play an active role in disseminating the infection, in addition to contributing to its development by means of their droppings. However, further study is needed to assess the role of bats in spreading the agent from one roost to another, and to determine the susceptibility of certain species to histoplasmosis (Hoff and Bigler, 1981).

Diagnosis: Laboratory diagnosis can be performed through microscopic examination of stained smears; immunofluorescence using clinical specimens such as sputum, ulcer exudate, and other materials; isolation in culture media; inoculation of mice; and examination of histopathologic sections (bone marrow, lung, liver, and spleen). In the acute pulmonary form, radiological findings of pulmonary infiltrates and hilar adenopathy, combined with data indicating that the patient comes from an endemic area and has symptoms compatible with histoplasmosis, are enough to establish a presumptive diagnosis.

Disseminated histoplasmosis is diagnosed by culturing the blood, bone marrow, urine, or other extrapulmonary tissues, or through biopsy and histopathology. Severe acute, but not chronic, histoplasmosis can be diagnosed using a peripheral blood smear with Wright or Giemsa stain. Biopsy material from the liver or material from oropharyngeal ulcers stained with silver methenamine yields good results (Loyd *et al.*, 1990).

The histoplasmin test is administered like the tuberculin test and read at 24 and 48 hours. Sensitivity is established one to two months after infection and lasts for many years. Although this test is extremely value for epidemiological research, its usefulness is limited in clinical diagnosis. It is advisable to administer the test together with the coccidioidin and blastomycin tests because of cross-reactions. A negative test in a patient can indicate that the infection is recent or that the disease has a different etiology.

Serological tests (complement fixation, immunodiffusion, radioimmunoassay, enzyme immunoassay, precipitation, latex agglutination) are useful for diagnosis but not very sensitive or specific. Tests for blastomycosis and coccidioidomycosis should be performed at the same time. It should be kept in mind that a histoplasmin test can produce antibodies; thus, it is recommended that the blood sample be taken when the allergy test is conducted. It is expected that a test that detects *H. capsulatum* antigen in serum and urine will give more specific results (Wheat *et al.*, 1986).

Control: The principal protection measure consists of reducing people's exposure to dust by spraying with a 3%–5% formalin solution on the ground when cleaning henhouses or other potentially contaminated sites. The use of protective masks has been recommended. Control of natural foci is difficult. During one outbreak, it was possible to eradicate the fungus from its natural foci by spraying the soil with formol.

Bibliography

Ajello, L. Comparative ecology of respiratory mycotic disease agents. *Bact Rev* 31:6–24, 1967.

Ajello, L., W. Kaplan. Systemic mycoses. In: Stoenner, H., W. Kaplan, M. Torten, eds. Section A, Vol 2: *CRC Handbook Series in Zoonoses*. Boca Raton: CRC Press; 1980.

Benenson, A.S., ed. *Control of Communicable Diseases in Man.* 15th ed. An official report of the American Public Health Association. Washington, D.C.: American Public Health Association; 1990.

Borelli, D. Prevalence of systemic mycoses in Latin America. In: Pan American Health Organization. *Proceedings: International Symposium on Mycoses.* Washington, D.C.: PAHO; 1970. (Scientific Publication 205).

Clinkenbeard, K.D., R.L. Cowell, R.D. Tyler. Disseminated histoplasmosis in cats: 12 cases (1981–1986). *J Am Vet Med Assoc* 190:1445–1448, 1987.

Cole, C.R., R.L. Farrell, D.M. Chamberlain, *et al.* Histoplasmosis in animals. *J Am Vet Med Assoc* 122:471–473, 1953.

Conces, D.J., S.M. Stockberger, R.D. Tarver, I.J. Wheat. Disseminated histoplasmosis in AIDS: Findings on chest radiographs. *Am J Roentgenol* 160:15–19, 1993.

Coulanges, P. L'histoplasmose a grandes formes *(H. duboisii)* a Madagascar (A propos de 3 cas). *Arch Inst Pasteur Madagascar* 56:169–174, 1989.

González Menocal, I., M. Suárez Menéndez, L. Pérez González, J. Díaz Rodríguez. Estudio clínico-epidemiológico de un brote de histoplasmosis pulmonar en el Municipio de Morón. *Rev Cubana Hig Epidemiol* 28:179–183, 1990.

Hamilton, A.J., M.A. Bartholomew, L. Fenelon, *et al.* Preparation of monoclonal antibodies that differentiate between *Histoplasma capsulatum* variant *capsulatum* and *H. capsulatum* variant *duboisii*. *Trans Roy Soc Trop Med Hyg* 84:425–428, 1990.

Hoff, G.L., W.J. Bigler. The role of bats in the propagation and spread of histoplasmosis: A review. *J Wild Dis* 17:191–196, 1981.

Johnson, P.C., N. Khardori, A.F. Naijar, *et al.* Progressive disseminated histoplasmosis in patients with acquired immunodeficiency syndrome. *Am J Med* 85:152–158, 1988.

Kaplan, W. Epidemiology of the principal systemic mycoses of man and lower animals and the ecology of their etiologic agents. *J Am Vet Med Assoc* 163:1043–1047, 1973.

Loyd, J.E., R.M. Des Prez, R.A. Goodwin, Jr. *Histoplasma capsulatum. In* Mandell, G.L., R.G. Douglas, Jr., J.E. Bennett, eds. *Principles and Practice of Infectious Diseases.* 3rd ed. New York: Churchill Livingstone Inc.; 1990.

Manson-Bahr, P.E.C., F.I.C. Apted. *Manson's Tropical Diseases.* 18th ed. London: Baillière-Tindall; 1982.

Menges, R.W., R.T. Habermann, L.A. Selby, H.R. Ellis, R.F. Behlow, C.D. Smith. A review and recent findings of histoplasmosis in animals. *Vet Med* 58:334–338, 1963.

Miranda Novales, M.G., F. Solórzano Santos, H. Díaz Ponce, *et al.* Histoplasmosis diseminada en pediatría. *Bol Med Hosp Infant Mex* 50:272–275, 1993.

Negroni, P. *Histoplasmosis: Diagnosis and Treatment.* Springfield: Thomas; 1965.

Negroni, P. *Micosis cutáneas y viscerales.* 5.ª ed. Buenos Aires: López; 1972.

Negroni, R., A. Taborda, A.M. Robles, A. Archevala. Itraconazole in the treatment of histoplasmosis associated with AIDS. *Mycoses* 35:281–287, 1992.

Organización Panamericana de la Salud (OPS). Histoplasmosis en México, 1979–1980. *Bol Epidemiol* 2:12–13, 1981.

Sanger, V.L. Histoplasmosis. In: Davis, J.W., L.H. Karstad, D.O. Trainer, eds. *Infectious Diseases of Wild Mammals.* Ames: Iowa State University Press; 1970.

Schlech, W.F., L.J. Wheat, J.L. Ho, M.L.V. French, R.J. Weeks, R.B. Kohler, *et al.* Recurrent urban histoplasmosis, Indianapolis, Indiana. 1980–1981. *Am J Epidemiol* 118:301–302, 1983.

Selby, L.A. Histoplasmosis. In: Hubbert, W.T., W.F. McCulloch, P.R. Schnurrenberger, eds. *Diseases Transmitted from Animals to Man.* 6th ed. Springfield: Thomas; 1975.

Sweany, H.C., ed. *Histoplasmosis.* Springfield, Illinois: Thomas; 1960.

Waldman, R.J., A.C. England, R. Tauxe, T. Kline, R.J. Weeks, L.A. Ajello, *et al.* A winter outbreak of acute histoplasmosis in northern Michigan. *Am J Epidemiol* 117:68–75, 1983.

Wheat, J., R. Hafner, M. Wulfsohn, *et al.* Prevention of relapse of histoplasmosis with itraconazole in patients with acquired inmunodeficiency syndrome. The National Institute of Allergy and Infectious Diseases. Clinical Trials and Mycoses Study Group Collaborators. *Ann Intern Med* 118:610–616, 1993.

Wheat, L.J., R.B. Kohler, R.P. Tewari. Diagnosis of disseminated histoplasmosis by detection of *Histoplasma capsulatum* antigen in serum and urine specimens. *N Engl J Med* 314:83–88, 1986.

MYCETOMA

ICD-10 B47.0 eumycetoma; B47.1 actinomycetoma

Synonyms: Maduromycosis, Madura foot, maduromycotic mycetoma, eumycotic mycetoma, actinomycetoma.

Etiology: Mycetomas may be caused by many species of fungi (eumycetoma) or by bacterial agents (actinomycetoma). The principal agents of eumycetoma are *Madurella mycetomatis, M. grisea, Leptosphaeria senegalensis* (all of which produce black granules), *Pseudallescheria (Petriellidium, Allescheria) boydii,* various species of *Acremonium* (white or yellow granules), *Exophiala jeanselmei,* and other species of fungi. Actinomycetomas are caused by *Nocardia brasiliensis, N. asteroides,* and *N. otitidiscaviarum, Streptomyces somaliensis, Actinomadura madurae,* and *A. pelletieri.* The principal agents of animal mycetomas are *P. boydii, Curvularia geniculata, Cochliolobus spicifer, Acremonium* spp., and *Madurella grisea.*

Both the fungi and the actinomycetes are soil saprophytes that accidentally enter the host's tissues, where they form granules (colonies). Eumycetoma granules contain thick hyphae whereas actinomycetoma granules contain fine filaments.

Geographic Distribution: The agents of maduromycosis are distributed worldwide but occur primarily in the tropics. In tropical areas of Africa and India, infection is most frequently caused by *Madurella mycetomatis* and *Streptomyces somaliensis.* In Mexico, Central America, and South America, mycetomas are caused primarily by *Nocardia brasiliensis* and *Actinomadura madurae*; in Canada and the United States, they are caused primarily by *Pseudallescheria boydii*; and in Japan they are due to *Nocardia asteroides* (Mahgoub, 1990).

Occurrence in Man: Infrequent. It is more common in tropical and subtropical zones, particularly where people go barefoot.

Most cases occur in Africa. In Sudan, 1,231 patients required hospitalization in a two-and-a-half-year period. In many African countries, such as Cameroon, Chad, Kenya, Mauritania, Niger, Senegal, Somalia, and Sudan, mycetoma is considered the most frequent deep mycosis (Develoux *et al.*, 1988). The responsible agents in Africa vary by geographic area. In India, mycetoma is endemic in many areas. In the Americas, it occurs most frequently in Mexico and Central America (due primarily to *Nocardia brasiliensis*) (Manson-Bahr and Apted, 1982). In São Paulo (Brazil) there were 154 cases between 1944 and 1978; 73.4% of these were actinomycetomas and 26.6% were eumycetomas. In Niger, men are infected more frequently than women (4:1). The disease occurs in rural areas.

Occurrence in Animals: Rare.

The Disease in Man: Mycetoma is a slow-developing, chronic infection that usually localizes on the foot, the lower leg, sometimes the hand, and rarely on some other part of the body. The incubation period is several months from the time of inoculation. The lesion may begin as a papule, nodule, or abscess. The mycetoma spreads to deep tissue and the foot (or hand) swells to two or three times its normal size. Numerous small abscesses form, as well as fistulous tracks in the subcutaneous tissue that branch out to the tendons and may reach the bones. Pus discharged to the surface contains characteristic granules (microcolonies) that may be white or another color depending on the causal agent. The skin does not lose sensitivity nor does the patient generally feel any pain. Actinomycetomas almost always respond to treatment with antibacterial antibiotics (streptomycin, co-trimoxazole), but eumycetomas are quite resistant (ketoconazole, myconazole) and often lead to amputation. Oral dapsone is preferred for cases of *Actinomadura madurae*. The same treatment is recommended for patients affected by *Streptomyces somaliensis* but should be changed to trimethoprim/sulfamethoxazole tablets if no improvement is seen after one month. The latter treatment is also used for infections caused by *Nocardia* spp. (Mahgoub, 1990).

The Disease in Animals: Almost all confirmed cases have occurred in the United States. In animals (dogs, cats, horses), eumycetomas are localized in the feet, lymph nodes, abdominal cavity, and other areas of the body. The most common agents of eumycetoma in animals are *Curvularia geniculata* and *Pseudallescheria boydii*. Mycetomas are frequently preceded by traumas. Intraabdominal infections have been described in dogs in association with ovariohysterectomies or a surgical incision that had opened up, with surgery occurring two years prior to the appearance of clinical symptoms. Lesions seen in animals are similar to those in humans. They generally start with a small subcutaneous nodule that grows gradually for months or years. They may become deeper and destroy underlying tissues (McEntee, 1987).

Cases of keratomycosis and other ophthalmic conditions due to *Pseudallescheria boydii* have been described in humans as well as horses and dogs (Friedman *et al.*, 1989).

Source of Infection and Mode of Transmission: The etiologic agents of this disease are saprophytes in soil and vegetation. The fungus is introduced into subcutaneous tissue of humans and animals through wounds. Contaminated thorns or splinters may be the immediate source of the infection. In animals, there are cases of post-operative wounds being infected by *P. boydii*.

Role of Animals in the Epidemiology of the Disease: None.

Diagnosis: Microscopic examination of pus or material from curettage or biopsy can distinguish eumycetoma granules from actinomycetoma (nocardiosis) granules. The agent is identified through isolation in culture media such as Lowenstein-Jensen medium for actinomycetoma granules and blood agar for eumycetoma granules. Sabouraud's agar is used for subculturing with antimicrobial antibiotics. It is recommended that biopsy material, rather than material from the fistulae, be used to obtain the granules aseptically (Mahgoub, 1990). It is advisable to determine the agent's sensitivity to different medications in order to ensure correct treatment.

In a study conducted in Sudan, specific diagnosis was achieved for 78% of the specimens by using histologic methods, and for 82% of the cases by immunodiffusion (Mahgoub, 1975). The choice of strains for serological testing is very important.

Control: Humans can avoid becoming infected by wearing shoes.

Bibliography

Benenson, A.S., ed. *Control of Communicable Diseases in Man*. 15th ed. An official report of the American Public Health Association. Washington, D.C.: American Public Health Association; 1990.

Brodey, R.S., H.F. Schryver, M.J. Deubler, W. Kaplan, L. Ajello. Mycetoma in a dog. *J Am Vet Med Assoc* 151:442–451, 1967.

Conant, N.F. Medical mycology. *In*: Dubos, R.J., J.G. Hirsch, eds. *Bacterial and Clinical Mycology*. 2nd ed. Philadelphia: Saunders; 1963.

Conant, N.F. Medical mycology. *In*: Dubos, R.J., J.G. Hirsch, eds. *Bacterial and Mycotic Infections of Man*. 4th ed. Philadelphia: Lippincott; 1965.

Develoux, M., J. Audoin, J. Tregner, *et al.* Mycetoma in the Republic of Niger: Clinical features and epidemiology. *Am J Med Trop Hyg* 38:386–390, 1988.

Friedman, D., J.V. Schoster, J.P. Pickett, *et al. Pseudallescheria boydii* keratomycosis in a horse. *J Am Vet Med Assoc* 195:616–618, 1989.

Jang, S.S., J.A. Popp. Eumycotic mycetoma in a dog caused by *Allescheria boydii. J Am Vet Med Assoc* 157:1071–1076, 1970.

Mahgoub, E.S. Serologic diagnosis of mycetoma. *In*: Pan American Health Organization. *Proceedings of the Third International Conference on the Mycoses*. Washington, D.C.: PAHO; 1975. (Scientific Publication 304).

Mahgoub, E.S. Agents of mycetoma. *In*: Mandell, G.L., R.G. Douglas, Jr., J.E. Bennett, eds. *Principles and Practice of Infectious Diseases*. 3rd ed. New York: Churchill Livingstone Inc.; 1990.

Manson-Bahr, P.E.C., F.I.C. Apted. *Manson's Tropical Diseases*. 18th ed. London: Baillière-Tindall; 1982.

McEntee, M. Eumycotic mycetoma: Review and report of a cutaneous lesion caused by *Pseudallescheria boydii* in a horse. *J Am Vet Med Assoc* 191:1459–1461, 1987.

Segretain, G., F. Mariar. Mycetoma. *In*: Warren, K.S., A.A.F. Mahmoud, eds. *Tropical and Geographical Medicine*. New York: McGraw-Hill; 1984.

PROTOTHECOSIS

Synonyms: Algal infections.

Etiology: In recent years, mycologists have called attention to infections in humans and animals caused by microorganisms of the genus *Prototheca*, the nature and taxonomy of which have not yet been clearly defined. Most authors believe they are unicellular algae, but others describe them as algae-like fungi.

The cells of *Prototheca* spp. are round or oval and measure between 2 and 16 microns in diameter. The species of interest are *P. wickerhamii* and *P. zopfii*. These microorganisms reproduce asexually. Hyaline cells, called sporangia when mature, produce from 2 to 20 endospores in their interior that increase in volume and repeat the reproductive cycle when they reach maturity.

Geographic Distribution: The agents are distributed worldwide.

Occurrence in Man: Slightly more than 30 cases of protothecosis have been described, 60% of them in men. With the exception of one case due to *P. zopfii*, the causal agent in all other cases in which the species was identified was *P. wickerhamii*. Recently, an infection caused by green algae was described (Jones, 1983).

Occurrence in Animals: Protothecosis occurs in many animal species, but above all in cattle and dogs. Numerous isolations have been recorded (McDonald *et al.*, 1984). Most infections are due to *P. zopfii*. Occurrence is sporadic. Nevertheless, 23 infected animals were found in one dairy herd of 90 cows.

Mastitis caused by *P. zopfii* in cattle is more frequent than was formerly thought. In the United States, there were 400 reported cases in 1982 in New York State alone (Mayberry, 1984, cited in Pore *et al.*, 1987). In Australia, mastitis due to *P. zopfii* was diagnosed in 17 of the 120 cows in a herd (Hodges *et al.*, 1985). There were 10 cases in a herd of 192 cows in Denmark and 5 cases in a herd of 130 cows in Great Britain (Pore *et al.*, 1987).

The Disease in Man: The incubation period is unknown. Protothecosis manifests itself in two principal clinical forms (Kaplan, 1978). One is progressive ulcerative or verrucous lesions of the cutaneous and subcutaneous tissue on exposed skin. The other is chronic olecranon bursitis, with pain and swelling. In one case of dissemination, intraperitoneal and facial nodules were observed.

Treatment consists of surgical excision of the lesion. Antibacterial medications are ineffective. Of the antimycotics, amphotericin B has produced satisfactory results.

The Disease in Animals: The predominant form of protothecosis in cattle is mastitis, which at times may affect all four quarters of the udder. Temperature and appetite may remain normal. Inflammation of the udder is mild in comparison with bacterial mastitis, but it is invasive and chronic. The etiological agent causes pyogranulomas in the mammary gland and the regional lymph nodes (Pore *et al.*, 1987). Milk production in the affected quarter diminishes, and small clots may be found in the milk. The disease was reproduced experimentally using a small number of *P. zopfii* (McDonald *et al.*, 1984).

Protothecosis in dogs is usually a systemic disease, with dissemination of the infection to many internal organs. The severity of the disease varies according to the organs affected. Weakness and weight loss were observed in all cases of dissemination (Kaplan, 1978).

Approximately one-half of the cases in dogs are caused by *P. wickerhamii* and the other half by *P. zopfii* (Dillberger *et al.*, 1988). Other animal species in which protothecosis has been diagnosed are Atlantic salmon and cats. In salmon, *P. salmonis* causes a disseminated and fatal disease (Gentles and Bond, 1977). The clinical manifestation of protothecosis in cats more closely resembles the cutaneous disease in humans and does not tend to disseminate as it does in dogs. The infection in cats is caused by *P. wickerhamii* (Dillberger *et al.*, 1988).

Source of Infection and Mode of Transmission: *Prototheca* spp. and green algae are saprophytes found in nature, primarily in stagnant or slow-moving waters. Humans acquire the infection, possibly through skin lesions, when they come into contact with contaminated water or other habitats of these agents. The profusion of these agents in the environment, as well as the few cases described in humans, indicate that they are not very virulent and that lowered host resistance is required for them to act as pathogens. In fact, five of nine patients with cutaneous or subcutaneous protothecosis had a preexisting or intercurrent disease. Similarly, seven of eight patients with the olecranon bursitis form had previously sustained a trauma to the elbow (Kaplan, 1978). Cattle contract mastitis caused by *P. zopfii* in the environment itself; the portal is probably the teat. *P. zopfii* is abundant in dairies, in cow feces as well as in drinking troughs, feed, and mud. A study conducted on various dairy cows, some with mastitis caused by *Prototheca* and others without any history of the disease, isolated the agent (94% *P. zopfii* and 6% *P. wickerhamii*) in 48 (25.3%) of 190 samples (Anderson and Walker, 1988). Little is known of the predisposing conditions in dogs, which almost always manifest systemic protothecosis.

In cattle, the retropharyngeal and mandibular lymph nodes affected by green algae indicate that the infection is possibly contracted by ingestion of contaminated water. The few cases described in cattle and sheep suggest that these species are not very susceptible to green algal infection.

Diagnosis: Special stains such as Gomori, Gridley, and PAS (periodic acid-Schiff) applied to histological sections from affected tissues permit detection of *Prototheca* in all developmental stages. To determine the species, cultures or the immunofluorescence test with species-specific reagents must be used. The immunofluorescence technique can be used for cultures as well as for histological sections stained with hematoxylin-eosin, but not for those stained with the methods mentioned above.

Control: Treatment of underlying conditions or diseases in humans.

Bibliography

Anderson, K.L., R.L. Walker. Sources of *Prototheca* spp. in a dairy herd environment. *J Am Vet Med Assoc* 193:553–556, 1988.

Dillberger, J.E., B. Homer, D. Daubert, N.H. Altman. Protothecosis in two cats. *J Am Vet Med Assoc* 192:1557–1559, 1988.

Gentles, J.C., P.M. Bond. Protothecosis of Atlantic salmon. *Sabouraudia* 15: 133–139, 1977.

Hodges, R.T., J.T.S. Holland, F.J.A. Neilson, N.M. Wallace. *Prototheca zopfii* mastitis in a herd of dairy cows. *N Z Vet J* 33:108–111, 1985.

Jones, J.W., H.W. McFadden, F.W. Chandler, W. Kaplan, D.H. Conner. Green algal infection in a human. *Am J Clin Pathol* 80:102–107, 1983.

Kaplan, W. Protothecosis and infections caused by morphologically similar green algae. *In:* Pan American Health Organization. *Proceedings of the Fourth International Conference on Mycoses: The Black and White Yeasts.* Washington, D.C.: PAHO; 1978. (Scientific Publication 356).

Kaplan, W., F.W. Chandler, C. Choudary, P.K. Ramachandran. Disseminated unicellular green algal infection in two sheep in India. *Am J Trop Med Hyg* 32:405–411, 1983.

Mayberry, D. Colorless alga can pollute water, cause mastitis. *Agri Res* March: 4–5, 1984. Cited in: Pore, R.S., *et al.* Occurrence of *Prototheca zopfii*, a mastitis pathogen, in milk. *Vet Microbiol* 15:315–323, 1987.

McDonald, J.S., J.L. Richard, N.F. Cheville. Natural and experimental bovine intramammary infection with *Prototheca zopfii. Am J Vet Res* 45:592–595, 1984.

Pore, R.S., T.A. Shahan, M.D. Pore, R. Blauwiekel. Occurrence of *Prototheca zopfii*, a mastitis pathogen, in milk. *Vet Microbiol* 15:315–323, 1987.

Rogers, R.J., M.D. Connole, J. Norton, A. Thomas, P.W. Ladds, J. Dickson. Lymphadenitis of cattle due to infection with green algae. *J Comp Pathol* 90:1–9, 1980.

RHINOSPORIDIOSIS

ICD-10 B48.1

Etiology: *Rhinosporidium seeberi*, a fungus that in tissue forms sporangia containing a large number of sporangiospores. Its environmental habitat is unknown and its taxonomy uncertain.

Geographic Distribution: The disease has been confirmed in the Americas, Asia (endemic zones in India and Sri Lanka), Africa, Europe, Australia, and New Zealand.

Occurrence in Man and Animals: The disease is rare throughout the world. Up to 1970, data from Latin America show 108 cases in humans. Most occurred in Paraguay (56), Brazil (13), and Venezuela (13) (Mayorga, 1970). According to more recent data, more than 50 cases have occurred in Venezuela, mainly in the states of Barinas and Portuguesa. In addition to the Latin American countries already cited, the disease has been confirmed in Argentina and Cuba. In the United States, some 30 cases have been recorded, primarily in the south. Five cases have been reported in Trinidad (Raju and Jamalabadi, 1983), four of them affecting the conjunctiva. Most of the cases in Africa were recorded in Uganda. A retrospective study (1948–1986) of 91,000 biopsies was conducted at the Central Hospital of Maputo, Mozambique; rhinosporidiosis was diagnosed in 33 (0.036%) (Moreira Díaz *et al.*, 1989). Some 1,000 cases have occurred in India and Sri Lanka, and 72 occurred in Iran over a 30-year period.

The disease is seen mostly in children and young people, predominantly in males (Mahapatra, 1984).

Rhinosporidiosis in animals occurs in cattle, horses, dogs, cats, and geese. More than 90% of the cases occur in males (Carter and Chengappa, 1991). The disease occurs sporadically, as it does in humans. An unusual case occurred in a province in northern Argentina where an outbreak was described in a herd of cattle that was kept in a flooded field for two years. Twenty-four percent of the animals examined had polyps (Luciani and Toledo, 1989).

The Disease in Man and Animals: Rhinosporidiosis is characterized by pedunculated or sessile polyps on the mucous membranes, particularly of the nose and eyes. The polyps are soft, lobular, and reddish with small white spots (the sporangia). These excrescences are not painful but they do bleed easily. In humans, these granulomatous formations can also be found in the pharynx, larynx, ear, vagina, penis, rectum, and on the skin. Cases of dissemination to internal organs are rare.

The clinical picture in animals consists of a chronic polypoid inflammation that may cause respiratory difficulty and sneezing if the disease lodges in the nasal mucosa and if the lesion is sufficiently large. Another common symptom is epistaxis.

Treatment for humans and animals consists of surgical excision of the polyp. Recurrence is rare. Successful treatment with dapsone has been described in three patients (Job *et al.*, 1993).

Source of Infection and Mode of Transmission: The natural habitat of the agent is unknown. It is suspected that the infection enters the body with soil particles through lesions of the mucous membranes. Those affected almost always live in rural areas, thus the assumption that the agent lives in the soil. In India and Sri Lanka, where most cases have been recorded, the source of infection has been associated with stagnant waters, but it has not yet been possible to demonstrate the presence of the fungus in such waters or in aquatic animals. The route of infection and the mode of transmission are also unknown.

Role of Animals in the Epidemiology of the Disease: Rhinosporidiosis is a disease common to humans and animals, contracted from an as yet unknown environmental source. It is not transmitted from one individual to another.

Diagnosis: Since the fungus cannot be cultured, diagnosis depends on the clinical appearance of the lesions and demonstration of the agent's presence in tissues. Best results are obtained by using stained histological preparations.

Control: No practical control measures are available.

Bibliography

Ajello, L., L.K. Georg, W. Kaplan, L. Kaufman. *Laboratory Manual for Medical Mycology*. Washington, D.C.: U.S. Government Printing Office; 1963. (Public Health Service Publication 994).

Carter, G.R., M.M. Chengappa. *Essentials of Veterinary Bacteriology and Mycology*. 4th ed. Philadelphia: Lea & Febiger; 1991.

Job, A., S. VanKateswaran, M. Mathan, *et al.* Medical therapy of rhinosporidiosis with dapsone. *J Laryngol Otol* 107:809–812, 1993.

Luciani, C.A. H.O. Toledo. *Rhinosporidium seeberi* en bovinos criollos (*Bos taurus*). *Vet Arg* 6(57):451–455, 1989.

Mahapatra, L.N. Rhinosporidiosis. *In*: Warren, K.S., A.A.F. Mahmoud, eds. *Tropical and Geographical Medicine*. New York: McGraw-Hill; 1984.

Mayorga, R. Prevalence of subcutaneous mycoses in Latin America. *In*: Pan American Health Organization. *Proceedings: International Symposium on Mycoses*. Washington, D.C.: PAHO; 1970. (Scientific Publication 205).

Moreira Díaz, E.E., B. Milán Batista, C.E. Mayor González, H. Yokoyama. Rinosporidiosis: estudio de 33 casos diagnosticados por biopsias en el Hospital Central de Maputo, desde 1944 hasta 1986. *Rev Cubana Med Trop* 41:461–472, 1989.

Negroni, P. *Micosis cutáneas y viscerales*. 5.ª ed. Buenos Aires: López; 1972.

Raju, G.C., M.H. Jamalabadi. Rhinosporidiosis in Trinidad. *Trop Geogr Med* 35: 257–258, 1983.

Sauerteig, E.M. Rhinosporidiosis in Barinas, Venezuela. *In*: Pan American Health Organization. *Proceedings of the Fifth International Conference on the Mycoses: Superficial, Cutaneous, and Subcutaneous Infections*. Washington, D.C.: PAHO; 1980. (Scientific Publication 396).

Utz, J.P. The mycoses. *In*: Beeson, P.B., W. McDermott, J.B. Wyngaarden, eds. *Cecil Textbook of Medicine*. 15th ed. Philadelphia: Saunders; 1979.

SPOROTRICHOSIS

ICD-10 B42.0 pulmonary sporotrichosis; B42.1 lymphocutaneous sporotrichosis; B42.7 disseminated sporotrichosis; B42.8 other forms of sporotrichosis

Etiology: *Sporothrix schenckii* (*Sporotrichum schenckii, Sporotrichum beurmanni*), a saprophytic fungus that lives in soil, plants, wood, and decaying vegetation. *S. schenckii* is a dimorphic fungus that occurs in a mycelial form in nature and a yeast form in infected animal tissues or on enriched culture media (such as blood agar) at 37°C. The latter form generally produces multiple buds and occasionally a single bud.

Geographic Distribution: Worldwide; more common in tropical regions.

Occurrence in Man: Sporadic; its frequency varies from region to region. The disease has been confirmed in all Latin American countries except Bolivia, Chile, and Nicaragua. It is more frequent in Asia, Brazil, the Central American countries, Mexico, South Africa, and Zimbabwe than in other countries. Although it is a relatively rare disease, an epidemic affecting 3,000 workers was recorded in South African gold mines. One group of cases also occurred in the United States among forestry workers who contracted the disease while planting pine trees, and another group of cases occurred among students who came in contact with contaminated bricks (Mitchell, 1983). The largest outbreak in the United States, encompassing 15 states, occurred in the spring of 1988 and affected 84 people. The outbreak was due to *S. schenckii* in sphagnum moss that was used to pack young plants for shipment

(Coles *et al.*, 1992). In the area around Ayerza Lagoon in Guatemala, 53 cases were seen between 1971 and 1975 (Mayorga *et al.*, 1979). Results of skin hypersensitivity tests using *S. schenckii* and *Ceratocystis stenoceras* (a closely related species) antigens indicated that asymptomatic infection is probably frequent among people who work with plants. The study done in the Ayerza Lagoon region (Mayorga *et al.*, 1979) found that cutaneous hypersensitivity was at least 10 times higher among local inhabitants than among residents of Guatemala City.

The disease is much more frequent in males than in females.

Occurrence in Animals: Occasional. Horses are the most frequently affected. Cases have been recorded in dogs, cats, rodents, cattle, swine, camels, birds, and wild animals.

The Disease in Man: The incubation period can range from three weeks to three months. The most common clinical form is the cutaneous form; it begins with a nodule or pustule at the point where broken skin allowed inoculation. The primary lesion is usually located on exposed extremities. The infection may remain confined to the entry site or may eventually spread and produce subcutaneous nodules along the enlarged lymph nodes. The nodules may ulcerate, and a gray or yellowish pus appears. The patient's general state of health is usually not affected. There are also vegetative and verrucous dermal and epidermal forms.

Disseminated forms, which are rare, may give rise to localizations in different organs, especially the bones and joints (80% of extracutaneous forms) as well as the mouth, nose, kidneys, and subcutaneous tissue over large areas of the body. Of more than 3,000 miners who contracted cutaneous sporotrichosis, only five developed systemic infections and none developed the pulmonary form (Lurie, 1962). Some researchers have concluded that dissemination occurs via the bloodstream or the lymphatic system from the inoculation site on the skin, while others believe that a primary focus in the lungs is involved.

Pulmonary sporotrichosis, a rare form of the disease, results from inhalation of the fungus. Its course may be acute, but in general it is chronic and can be confused with tuberculosis. The number of cases described is probably less than 90, and most patients lived in states bordering the Mississippi and Missouri rivers in the United States. Many of them had underlying diseases, such as alcoholism and tuberculosis. The most common symptoms are cough (69%), expectoration (59%), dyspnea, pleuritic pain, and hemoptysis. Patients frequently complain of weight loss, fatigue, and a slight rise in body temperature. The most frequent lesion in the lungs occurs in the upper lobe, and radiography shows cavitation, surrounded by parenchymatous densities (Pluss and Opal, 1986).

Oral potassium iodide may be used to treat the cutaneous form. Extracutaneous cases have been treated successfully with ketoconazole and itraconazole, or with the new oral triazole, saperconazole. Treatment with this last antimycotic requires a dose of 100 to 200 mg per day for a period of three-and-a-half months (Franco *et al.*, 1992).

Because of their occupation, farmers, gardeners, and floriculturists are the persons most exposed to the infection.

The Disease in Animals: The disease in horses and mules is similar to that in humans; it must be differentiated from epizootic lymphangitis caused by

Histoplasma farciminosum (Cryptococcus farciminosum). The skin covering the spherical nodules becomes moist, the hair falls out, and a scab forms. The ulcers heal slowly and leave alopecic scars. The affected extremity swells due to lymphatic stasis. No cases of dissemination have been described in horses.

The disease in dogs may manifest as the cutaneo-lymphatic form, but it frequently affects the bones, liver, and lungs.

The disease in cats is of particular interest because it has often served as the source of infection for humans. One of these epizootic episodes occurred in Malaysia, where four veterinary students became infected when caring for cats with sporotrichosis on their forelegs and faces. Five cats with lesions inflicted during fights in the clinic of the Veterinary School were treated with antibacterial medications for two weeks, but the wounds did not heal. During this period, various ulcerative nodules appeared on the eyes, behind the ears, and in the nose. *S. schenckii* was isolated from these lesions. The four students who treated the cats contracted sporotrichosis, as did the owner of one of the cats (Zamri-Saad *et al.*, 1990). Three members of a family caught the infection from their cat and became ill with cutaneous sporotrichosis, which disappeared completely after two weeks of treatment with ketoconazole (Haqvi *et al.*, 1993). Other cases of zoonotic transmission occurred in Brazil (Larsson *et al.,* 1989) and the United States (Dunstan *et al.,* 1986). Reed *et al.* (1993) described the case of a veterinarian who contracted the infection from a cat; the authors also reviewed the relevant literature.

Source of Infection and Mode of Transmission: The reservoirs of the fungus are soil and plants. Humans and animals almost always become infected through a cutaneous lesion. The infection can be contracted from handling moss, wood splinters, firewood, or dead vegetation on which the fungus has developed. The source of infection in a gold mine epidemic in the Transvaal (South Africa) was timber on which *S. schenckii* was growing. Nevertheless, the source of infection is not always easily recognized. Out of the 53 cases of sporotrichosis that occurred in the Ayerza Lagoon area of Guatemala, 24 (45.3%) patients attributed the wound and subsequent ulceration to handling fish, 6 (11.3%) attributed it to wood splinters, and 20 (37.7%) could not remember any trauma. An attempt to isolate *S. schenckii* from 58 environmental samples yielded negative results (Mayorga *et al.*, 1979).

Inhalation provides another entry route for the fungus and is responsible for the small number of pulmonary sporotrichosis cases that have been recorded.

Feline sporotrichosis is known for its ability to transmit the infection to humans. Of 19 people who contracted the disease from a cat in the United States, none had experienced any traumatic lesion at the site of infection. Transmission occurred through direct contact with the ulcerous lesions on the cats' skin, which contained a large amount of fungus. The principal victims of zoonotic sporotrichosis are veterinarians. Of the 19 zoonotic cases, 12 involved veterinarians or their assistants (Dunstan *et al.*, 1986). Outside the United States, transmission was attributed to cat scratches or bites.

Cats (usually male) may carry decaying vegetation containing the fungus between their nails and may transmit the infection to other cats when they fight.

Role of Animals in the Epidemiology of the Disease: Sporotrichosis is a disease common to man and animals. Feline sporotrichosis is zoonotic.

Diagnosis: Diagnosis can be confirmed by culture and identification of the fungus. A specific and rapid method is direct immunofluorescence applied to biopsy samples from affected tissues or smears from sputum and bronchial lavages. Serological tests (latex agglutination, immunodiffusion, indirect immunofluorescence) are useful for patients with extracutaneous sporotrichosis. The disadvantage of serological tests is that antibodies may take some time to develop or may disappear after a while even though the disease persists (Pluss and Opal, 1986).

Control: It is recommended that wood in industries where cases occur be treated with fungicides. Moss must be wetted only immediately prior to packing plants so as to keep the fungus from developing.

Veterinarians and their assistants should use gloves to handle and treat cats with cutaneous legions suspected of being sporotrichosis.

Bibliography

Ainsworth, G.C., P.K.C. Austwick. *Fungal Diseases of Animals.* 2nd ed. Farnham Royal, Slough, United Kingdom: Commonwealth Agricultural Bureau; 1973.

Benenson, A.S., ed. *Control of Communicable Diseases in Man.* 15th ed. An official report of the American Public Health Association. Washington, D.C.: American Public Health Association; 1990.

Bruner, D.W., J.H. Gillespie. *Hagan's Infectious Diseases of Domestic Animals.* 6th ed. Ithaca, New York: Comstock; 1973.

Coles, F.B., A. Schuchat, J.R. Hibbs, *et al.* A multistate outbreak of sporotrichosis associated with sphagnum moss. *Am J Epidemiol* 136:475–487, 1992.

Dunstan, R.W., K.A. Reimann, R.F. Langham. Feline sporotrichosis. Zoonosis update. *J Am Vet Med Assoc* 189:880–883, 1986.

Franco, L., I. Gómez, A. Restrepo. Saperconazole in the treatment of systemic and subcutaneous mycoses. *Int J Dermatol* 31:725–729, 1992.

Haqvi, S.H., P. Becherer, S. Gudipati. Ketoconazole treatment of a family with zoonotic sporotrichosis. *Scand J Infect Dis* 25:543–545, 1993.

Larsson, C.E., M.A. Goncalves, V.C. Araujo, *et al.* Esporotricosis felina: aspectos clínicos e zoonóticos. *Rev Inst Med Trop Sao Paulo* 31:351–358, 1989.

Lima, L.B., A.C. Pereira, Jr. Esprotricose-Inquerito epidemiológico. Importancia como doença profissional. *An Bras Dermatol* 56:243–248, 1981.

Lurie, H.I. Five unusual cases of sporotrichosis from South Africa showing lesions in muscles, bones, and viscera. *Br J Surg* 50:585–591, 1962.

Mackinnon, J.E. Ecology and epidemiology of sporotrichosis. *In:* Pan American Health Organization. *Proceedings: International Symposium on Mycoses.* Washington, D.C.: PAHO; 1970. (Scientific Publication 205).

Mayorga, R., A. Cáceres, C. Toriello, G. Gutiérrez, O. Álvarez, M.E. Ramírez, *et al.* Investigación de una zona endémica de esporotricosis en la región de la laguna de Ayarza, Guatemala. *Bol Oficina Sanit Panam* 87:20–34, 1979.

Mitchell, T.G. Micosis subcutáneas. *In:* Joklik, W.K., H.P. Willet, D.B. Amos, eds. *Zinsser Microbiología.* 17.ª ed. Buenos Aires: Editorial Médica Panamericana; 1983.

Negroni, B. *Micosis cutáneas y viscerales.* 5.ª ed. Buenos Aires; López; 1972.

Pluss, J.L., S.M. Opal. Pulmonary sporotrichosis: Review of treatment and outcome. *Medicine* 65:143–153, 1986.

Reed, K.D., F.M. Moore, G.E. Geiger, M.E. Stemper. Zoonotic transmission of sporotrichosis: Case report and review. *Clin Infect Dis* 16:384–387, 1993.

Richard, J.L. Sporotrichosis. In: Hubbert, W.T., W.F. McCulloch, P.R. Schnurrenberger, eds. *Diseases Transmitted from Animals to Man*. 6th ed. Springfield: Thomas; 1975.

Zamri-Saad, M., T.S. Salmiyah, S. Jasni, *et al*. Feline sporotrichosis: An increasingly important zoonotic disease in Malaysia. *Vet Rec* 127:480, 1990.

ZYGOMYCOSIS

ICD-10 B46.0 pulmonary mucormycosis; B46.1 rhinocerebral mucormycosis; B46.2 gastrointestinal mucormycosis; B46.3 cutaneous mucormycosis; B46.4 disseminated mucormycosis; B46.8 other zygomycoses

Synonyms: Mucormycosis, entomophthoromycosis.

Etiology: Zygomycosis denotes a group of diseases caused by several genera and species of fungi belonging to the class *Zygomycetes*, orders *Entomophthorales* and *Mucorales*. Consequently, the etiologic agents are numerous; the principal ones are mentioned below in connection with the different diseases they cause, which can be subdivided into entomophthoromycoses and mucormycoses (CIOMS, 1982).

All the zygomycetes develop as hyphae and appear in the environment as well as in tissue as filamentous fungi. Sabouraud's agar is an excellent culture medium for these fungi, in which they develop at ambient temperature. The sporangiophores (specialized hyphae that support sporangia) contain many asexual spores (Carter and Chengappa, 1991).

Geographic Distribution: Worldwide. Mucormycosis has no defined geographic distribution. Entomophthoromycosis predominates in the tropics, particularly in Africa and Asia.

Occurrence in Man: It occurs sporadically, particularly in patients weakened by other diseases. However, in the 1970s there was an epidemic of cutaneous zygomycosis in the United States caused by contamination of elastic bandages with the fungus. The clinical manifestation was cellulitis, caused by direct inoculation of the fungus through the bandages. The infection was invasive in some patients and affected muscles and internal organs (Sugar, 1990). At present, the incidence of zygomycosis is increasing because of the longer survival of diabetics and the growing number of immunosuppressed patients. Despite its broad diffusion in nature and the likelihood that humans will come into contact with spores, this is not a very frequent mycosis.

It is possible that the incidence of mucormycoses is higher in the developed countries, given the higher survival rate of diabetics and the number of immunosuppressed patients. In a hospital in Washington, D.C., 730 cases of mucormycoses were recorded between 1966 and 1988. Of 170 cases of entomophthoromycosis caused by *Basidiobolus haptosporus* described up to 1975, 112 occurred in Africa. To these cases should be added 75 cases in Uganda that became known later (Kelly *et al.*, 1980). This disease also occurs in Southeast Asia and Latin America. Entomophthoromycosis due to the genus *Conidiobolus* also occurs in the tropics and is more common among men (CIOMS, 1982).

Occurrence in Animals: It occurs sporadically in many animal species, such as domestic and wild mammals (including marine mammals), birds, reptiles, amphibians, and fish. There was a significant epizootic outbreak in New South Wales and Queensland, Australia, affecting 52 sheep farms; 700 sheep died in three months. The causal agent was *Conidiobolus incongruens* of the order Entomophthorales (Carrigan *et al.*, 1992).

The Disease in Man: The agents of mucormycoses are potential pathogens that are classified as opportunistic, since they invade the tissues of patients debilitated by other diseases or treated for a long time with antibiotics or corticosteroids. About 40% of the cases have been associated with diabetes mellitus. In contrast, in Africa and Asia entomophthoromycoses occur in individuals without histories of preexisting illness (Bittencourt *et al.*, 1982).

The mucormycoses are caused by fungi of the genera *Absidia, Mucor, Rhizopus, Cunninghamella, Rhizomucor*, and several others. The infection begins in the nasal mucosa and paranasal sinuses, where the fungi may multiply rapidly and spread to the eye sockets, meninges, and brain. The clinical forms caused by these fungi are rhinocerebral, pulmonary, gastrointestinal, disseminated, cutaneous, and subcutaneous mucormycoses. The rhinocerebral form appears mainly in diabetes mellitus patients with acidosis and in leukemia patients with prolonged neutropenia. Patients have fever, facial pain, and headache. As rhinocerebral mucormycosis progresses, there may be loss of vision, ptosis, and pupillary dilatation. This form of the disease is highly fatal. Patients with a malignant blood disease and those receiving immunosuppressants primarily suffer from pulmonary or disseminated mucormycoses and, less frequently, from the rhinocerebral form. The gastrointestinal form has occurred in a few cases in malnourished children and in adult patients with advanced malnutrition; it is generally diagnosed postmortem. The cutaneous and subcutaneous form may be due to deep burns, injections, and application of contaminated bandages. Mucormycosis is characterized by vascular occlusion with fungal hyphae, thrombosis, and necrosis.

Localized mucormycosis may disseminate (disseminated mucormycosis) to various organs and systems. The underlying diseases are generally leukemia, solid neoplasias, chronic renal deficiency (dialysis treatment with deferoxamine seems to predispose the patient to mucormycosis, particularly to *Rhisopus* spp.), hepatic cirrhosis, organ transplants (particularly bone marrow transplants), and diabetes. The largest group of disseminated mucormycoses involves cancer patients (51% of 185 cases analyzed) (Ingram *et al.*, 1989).

Treatment consists of controlling the underlying disease, controlling hyperglycemia and acidosis in diabetics, and reducing immunosuppressant use in other cases. Surgical intervention and systemic administration of amphotericin B yielded favorable results in pulmonary and rhinocerebral mucormycosis when diagnosis occurred early. In primary cutaneous mucormycosis, débridement and topical treatment with amphotericin B are indicated. Generally, the earlier the infection is detected, the smaller the amount of dead tissue that will have to be removed and the greater the chances for avoiding major tissue damage (Sugar, 1990).

Treatment of entomophthoromycosis consists primarily of surgical excision of the subcutaneous nodules (*Basidiobolus*) or corrective surgery (*Conidiobolus*) of the nose and other parts of the face. It is advisable at the same time to treat the patient with ketoconazole or some other oral antimycotic azole derivative (Yangco et al., 1984).

Entomophthoromycoses due to *Basidiobolus haptosporus* are characterized by the formation of granulomas with eosinophilic infiltration in subcutaneous tissues. Generally, the region affected is the buttock or thigh, with hard tumefaction of the subcutaneous tissue and a clear delimitation from the healthy tissue. The disease is usually benign, but can sometimes be invasive and cause death (Greenham, 1979; Kelly et al., 1980).

Entomophthoromycoses due to *Conidiobolus coronatus* and *C. incongruens* generally originate in the lower nasal conchae and invade the subcutaneous facial tissues and paranasal sinuses. Lesions in the pericardium, mediastinum, and the lungs have also been described (CIOMS, 1982).

The Disease in Animals: Zygomycosis in animals is usually found during necropsy or postmortem inspection in abattoirs. Few cases are confirmed by isolation and identification of the causal agent. Lesions are granulomatous or ulcerative. Zygomycosis in cattle, sheep, and goats usually appears as ulcers of the abomasum. A 10-year study of gastrointestinal mycoses in cattle was conducted in Japan. Of 692 cattle autopsied, 45 had systemic mycosis, 38 of them in the gastrointestinal tract. The large majority (94.7%) of stomach infections were due to mucormycoses and the lesions consisted of focal hemorrhagic necroses. Many of the cattle were affected by predisposing factors for ruminal acidosis, such as ruminal atony (Chihaya et al., 1992). In cattle, lesions can also be found in nasal cavities and bronchial, mesenteric, and mediastinal nodes (Carter and Chengappa, 1991). In some countries, these fungi are an important cause of mycotic abortions. In Great Britain, they account for 32% of abortions caused by fungi, and in New Zealand for 75%.

In horses, zygomycosis takes the form of a chronic, localized disease that causes the formation of cutaneous granulomas on the extremities. A clinical study of 266 cases of zygomycosis conducted in tropical Australia found that 18% involved *Basidiobolus haptosporus* and 5.3% involved *Conidiobolus coronatus*.

In the disease caused by *B. haptosporus* (*B. ranarum*), lesions are found primarily on the trunk and face. In contrast, lesions due to *C. coronatus* are located in the nasal region (Miller and Campbell, 1982). Pulmonary infection, disease of the guttural pouch, systemic infection, and some mycotic abortions have also been described in horses.

Zygomycosis in piglets produces a gastric ulceration and appears in adult animals as a disseminated infection. Gastroenteritis with diarrhea, dehydration, and some deaths attributed to zygomycosis have been described in suckling pigs (Reed et al., 1987). Disseminated zygomycosis appears as granulomas in the submaxillary, cervical, and mesenteric nodes, and in the abdominopelvic organs. Three herd animals weighing between 50 and 80 kg were found with very swollen submandibular nodes; systemic dissemination was confirmed postmortem in three of them (Sanford et al., 1985).

An epidemic occurred in 52 sheep farms in Australia, leading to the death of 700 sheep within a period of three months. The affected animals had marked, asymmetrical swelling of the face, extending from the nostrils to the eyes. They were depressed, without appetite, and had marked dyspnea and frequent bloody discharge from the nose. The animals would die between 7 and 10 days later. Necropsy confirmed severe necrogranulomatous rhinitis that went as deep as the palate. Lesions were also confirmed in the lymph nodes and thorax. *Conidiobolus incongruens* was isolated from the nasal lesions, parotid gland, submandibular glands, and the lungs. The most important histopathological change was a severe granulomatous inflammation that contained small eosinophilic foci of coagulative necrosis. There were fungal hyphae in the center of these foci.

To explain an outbreak of this magnitude, the authors assume that the infection was influenced by environmental factors. After a rainy winter, grass grew plentifully; it was cut, and the cuttings began to decompose. Additional rain, heat, humidity, and the presence of decomposing plants created conditions favorable to proliferation of the etiologic agent (Carrigan *et al.*, 1992).

In dogs and cats, the disease usually affects the gastrointestinal tract and mortality is very high. Lesions of the stomach or small intestine are accompanied by vomiting, and lesions in the colon are accompanied by diarrhea and tenesmus (Ader, 1979).

Source of Infection and Mode of Transmission: Zygomycetes are ubiquitous saprophytes that produce a large number of spores; they are common inhabitants of decomposing organic material and food, and are found in the gastrointestinal tract of reptiles and amphibians. Humans contract the infection through inhalation, inoculation, and contamination of the skin by spores, and sometimes through ingestion. The common route of entry is the nose, by inhalation of spores. Debilitating diseases, such as diabetes mellitus, and prolonged treatment with immunosuppressants and antibiotics, are important causal factors of mucormycosis. *Mucoraceae* spores probably do not germinate in individuals with intact immune systems, judging from experimental tests in laboratory animals. However, some cases have been described in apparently normal people with no known underlying disease. Subcutaneous entomophthoromycosis due to *Basidiobolus* develops as a result of direct inoculation by thorns, and the disease caused by *Conidiobolus* spp. is contracted through inhalation.

Entomophthoromycosis generally occurs in healthy individuals with no preexisting disease.

In domestic animals, the digestive route of infection seems to be more important than inhalation.

Role of Animals in the Epidemiology of the Disease: Humans and animals contract the infection from a common source in the environment. The infection is not transmitted from one individual to another (man or animal).

Diagnosis: Diagnosis is based on confirmation of the agent's presence in scrapings or biopsies of lesions by means of direct microscopic examination or by culture. Zygomycetes in tissue can be identified by their large nonseptate hyphae. The species of fungus can only be determined by culture and spore identification (Ader, 1979). An indirect ELISA test with a homogenate of *Rhizopus arrhizus* and *Rhizomucor pusillus* can be useful for diagnosing mucormycosis. This test was able to detect 33 of 43 cases of mucormycosis. The sensitivity of the test is 81% and the specificity is 94%. It cannot determine the genus or the species of the causal agent (Kaufman *et al.*, 1989).

Control: Human zygomycosis can be prevented in many cases by proper treatment of metabolic disorders, especially diabetes mellitus. Prolonged treatment with antibiotics and corticosteroids should be limited to those cases in which it is absolutely necessary. Animals should not be allowed to consume moldy fodder.

Bibliography

Ader, P.L. Phycomycosis in fifteen dogs and two cats. *J Am Vet Med Assoc* 174: 1216–1223, 1979.

Ainsworth, G.C., P.K.C. Austwick. *Fungal Diseases of Animals*. 2nd ed. Farnham Royal, Slough, United Kingdom: Commonwealth Agricultural Bureau; 1973.

Ajello, L., L.K. Georg, W. Kaplan, L. Kaufman. *Laboratory Manual for Medical Mycology*. Washington, D.C.: U.S. Government Printing Office; 1963. (Public Health Service Publication 994).

Bittencourt, A.L., G. Serra, M. Sadigursky, M.G.S. Araujo, M.C.S. Campos, L.C.M. Sampaio. Subcutaneous zygomycosis caused by *Basidiobolus hapthoporus*: Presentation of a case mimicking Burkitt's lymphoma. *Am J Trop Med Hyg* 31:370–373, 1982.

Carter, G.R. *Diagnostic Procedures in Veterinary Microbiology*. 2nd ed. Springfield: Thomas; 1973.

Carter, G.R., M.M. Chengappa. *Essentials of Veterinary Bacteriology and Mycology*. 4th ed. Philadelphia: Lea & Febiger; 1991.

Carrigan, M.J., A.C. Small, G.H. Perry. Ovine nasal zygomycosis caused by *Conidiobolus incongruus*. *Aust Vet J* 69:237–240, 1992.

Chihaya, Y., K. Matsukawa, K. Ohshima, *et al*. A pathological study of bovine alimentary mycosis. *J Comp Pathol* 197:195–206, 1992.

Council for International Organizations of Medical Sciences (CIOMS). Vol 2: Infectious Diseases; Part 2: Mycoses. In: *International Nomenclature of Diseases*. Geneva: CIOMS; 1982.

González-Mendoza, A. Opportunistic mycoses. *In:* Pan American Health Organization. *Proceedings: International Symposium on Mycoses*. Washington, D.C.: PAHO; 1970. (Scientific Publication 205).

Greenham, R. Subcutaneous phycomycosis: Not always benign. *Lancet* 1:97;98, 1979.

Ingram, C.W., J. Sennesh, J.N. Cooper, J.R. Perfect. Disseminated zygomycosis: Report of four cases and review. *Rev Infect Dis* 11:741–754, 1989.

Kaufman, L., L.F. Turner, D.W. McLaughlin. Indirect enzyme-linked immunosorbent assay for zygomycosis. *J Clin Microbiol* 27:1979–1982, 1989.

Kelly, S., N. Gill, M.S.R. Hutt. Subcutaneous phycomycosis in Sierra Leone. *Trans Roy Soc Trop Med Hyg* 74:396–397, 1980.

Miller, R.I., R.S.F. Campbell. Clinical observations on equine phycomycosis. *Aust Vet J* 58:221–226, 1982.

Reed, W.M., C. Hanika, N.A.Q. Mehdi, C. Shackelford. Gastrointestinal zygomycosis in suckling pigs. *J Am Vet Med Assoc* 191:549–550, 1987.

Richard, J.L. Phycomycoses. *In:* Hubbert, W.T., W.F. McCulloch, P.R. Schnurrenberger, eds. *Diseases Transmitted from Animals to Man*. 6th ed. Springfield: Thomas; 1975.

Sanford, S.E., G.K.A. Josephson, E.H. Waters. Submandibulary and disseminated zygomycosis (mucormycosis) in feeder pigs. *J Am Vet Med Assoc* 186:171–174, 1985.

Soltys, M.A. *Bacteria and Fungi Pathogenic to Man and Animals*. London: Baillière-Tindall; 1963.

Sugar, A.M. Agents of mucormycosis and related species. *In:* Mandell, G.L., R.G. Douglas, Jr., J.E. Bennett, eds. *Principles and Practice of Infectious Diseases*. 3rd ed. New York: Churchill Livingstone Inc.; 1990.

Yangco, B.G., J.I. Okafor, D. TeStrake. *In vitro* susceptibilities of human and wild-type isolates of *Basidiobolus* and *Conidiobolus* species. *Antimicrob Agents Chemother* 25: 413–416, 1984.

INDEX

A

Abortion
  brucellosis, 43, 44-49, 55, 61, 62
  campylobacteriosis, 69, 72, 73-75, 76
  colibacillosis, 94, 95
  contagious (*see* Brucellosis)
  epizootic
    sheep (*see* Diseases caused by
      Campylobacter fetus)
    vibrionic (*see* Diseases caused by
      Campylobacter fetus)
    (*see also* Brucellosis)
  infectious (*see* Brucellosis)
  leptospirosis, 159, 160, 161
  listeriosis, 170-173, 175, 176
  nocardiosis, 196
  salmonellosis, 238
  streptococcosis, 260
  tetanus, 266, 268, 269
  tularemia, 278
  yersiniosis
    enterocolitic, 126
    pseudotuberculous, 220
Absidia, 357
Acremonium, 345
Actinobacillus, 142, 199
Actinomadura
  madurae, 345, 346
  pelletieri, 345
Actinomyces, 3, 5
  bovis, 3-5
  israelii, 3-5
  meyeri, 3
  naeslundi, 3
  odontolytical, 3
  suis, 4
  viscosus, 3, 4
Actinomycetales, 103, 195, 229
Actinomycetoma (*see* Mycetoma)
Actinomycosis, 3-6
Actinostreptotrichosis, (*see*
  Actinomycosis)
Adiaspiromycosis, 303-305
Adiaspirosis (*see* Adiaspiromycosis)
Aedes aegypti, 188
Aeromonas, 6-8, 10-12
  caviae, 6, 8
  hydrophila, 6-12
  jandae, 6

  salmonicida, 6, 7
  schuberti, 6
  sobria, 6-9, 11, 12
  trota, 6, 9
  veronii, 6
Aeromoniasis, 6-14
Afipia felis, 78, 80
Allantiasis (*see* Botulism)
Allescheria boydii (*see*
  Pseudallescheria boydii)
Alligators, animal erysipelas, 14
Alpacas
  brucellosis, 49
  listeriosis, 171
  tuberculosis, zoonotic, 292
Amblyomma americanum, 279
Amphibians
  aeromoniasis, 8, 9, 10, 12
  salmonellosis, 236
  zygomycosis, 357, 359
Animals, domestic
  aeromoniasis, 11
  anthrax, 21, 25
  aspergillosis, 305, 306, 308
  botulism, 33, 35
  brucellosis, 41, 49, 50
  campylobacteriosis, 68, 69-70
  coccidioidomycosis, 321
  cryptococcosis, 327, 328
  dermatophilosis, 104, 105
  dermatophytosis, 335
  diseases caused by nontuberculous
    mycobacteria, 109
  food poisoning
    clostridial, 82
    staphylococcal, 252, 254
  histoplasmosis, 340, 342
  leptospirosis, 158, 162-165
  listeriosis, 171, 172-173
  Lyme disease, 180, 181
  melioidosis, 185, 186
  mycetoma, 346
  nocardiosis, 195
  pasteurellosis, 199, 203
  protothecosis, 348-349
  rhinosporidiosis, 351
  rhodococcosis, 229
  salmonellosis, 236, 237, 239, 241
  tetanus, 268
  tuberculosis, zoonotic, 291, 294

S

NOTES

NOTES

NOTES

NOTES

NOTES

NOTES